Osteoarthritis of the knee

T0205671

Springer

Paris
Berlin
Heidelberg
New York
Hong Kong
London
Milan
Tokyo

Michel Bonnin
Pierre Chambat

Osteoarthritis of the knee

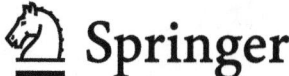 Springer

Michel Bonnin
Centre orthopédique Santy
24, avenue Paul Santy
69008 Lyon - France

Pierre Chambat
Centre orthopédique Santy
24, avenue Paul Santy
69008 Lyon - France

ISBN-13 : 978-2-287-74174-6 Springer Paris Berlin Heidelberg New York

© Springer-Verlag France, Paris, 2008
Imprimé en France

Springer-Verlag France est membre du groupe Springer Science + Business Media

Apart from any fair dealing for the purposes of the research or private study, or criticism or review, as permitted under the Copyright, Designs and Patents Act 1998, this publication may only be reproduced, stored or transmitted, in any forrn or by any means, with the prior permission in writing of the publishers, or in the case of reprographic reproduction in accordance with the terms of licenses issued by the copyright. Enquiry concerning reproduction outside those terms should be sent to the publishers.
The use of registered names, trademarks, etc., in this publication does not imply, even in the absence of a specific statement that such names are exempt from the relevant laws and regulations and therefore free for general use.

Maquette de couverture : Nadia Ouddane

DANGER

LE PHOTOCOPILLAGE
TUE LE LIVRE

Titles already published in *Approche pratique en orthopédie – traumatologie – Series*

Editors: Christian Fontaine, Alain Vannineuse

– *Fractures de l'extrémité proximale du fémur*
A. Vannineuse, Ch. Fontaine, Springer-Verlag France, 2000

– *La gonarthrose*
M. Bonnin, P. Chambat, Springer-Verlag France, 2003, 2005

– *Pathologie ligamentaire du genou*
Ph. Landreau, P. Christel, Ph. Djian, Springer-Verlag France, 2003

– *Fractures du genou*
Ch. Fontaine, A. Vannineuse, Springer-Verlag France, 2005

– *Biomécanique de l'épaule – De la théorie à la clinique*
P. Blaimont, A. Taheri, Springer-Verlag France, 2006

– *Approche pratique de la couverture des pertes de substance cutanée de la main et des doigts*
D. Le Nen, W. Hu, J. Laulan, Springer-Verlag France, 2007

Authors

Aglietti P.
First Orthopaedic Clinic
of the University of Florence,
Largo P. Pallagi 1, 50139 Firenze - Italy

Aït Si Selmi T.
Centre Livet, 8, rue de Margnolles
69300 Caluire - France

Almquist K.F.
University Hospital De Pintelaan 185
Orthopedie P5,
Gent B-9000 - Belgium

Amendola A.
Fowler Kennedy Sport Medicine
Clinic, University of Western Ontario,
London, Ontario - Canada

Argenson J.N.
CHR Sainte-Marguerite,
Service d'orthopédie,
270, boulevard Sainte-Marguerite,
13274 Marseille Cedex 09 - France

Aubaniac J.M.
CHR Sainte-Marguerite,
Service d'orthopédie,
270, boulevard Sainte-Marguerite,
13274 Marseille Cedex 09 - France

Baldini A.
First Orthopaedic Clinic
of the University of Florence,
Largo P. Pallagi 1, 50139 Firenze - Italy

Beaufils P.
Hôpital Mignot, 177, route de Versailles,
78150 Le Chesnay - France

Bellemans J.
University Hospital Pallenberg,
Weligerveld 1, 3212 Pallenberg - Belgium

Besse J.L.
Centre hospitalier Lyon-Sud,
Service de chirurgie orthopédique,
Chemin du Grand Revoyet,
69495 Pierre Bénite Cedex - France

Biot V.
Centre de rééducation Iris,
271, rue des Sources, BP 22,
69280 Marcy L'Étoile - France

Bizot P.
Clinique Arago, 95, boulevard Arago,
75014 Paris - France

Boldt J.G.
Schulthess Klinik, Lengghalde 2,
CH-8008 Zurich - Switzerland

Bonnin M.
Centre orthopédique Santy,
24, avenue Paul Santy,
69008 Lyon - France

Breton P.
Centre hospitalier Lyon-Sud,
69495 Pierre Bénite - France

Brilhault J.
CHU De Tours,
37044 Tours Cedex 01 - France

Burdin P.
CHU Trousseau,
37044 Tours Cedex 1 - France

Carrillon Y.
Clinique Saint-Jean, 30, rue Bataille
69008 Lyon - France

Cerullo G.
Clinica Valle Giulia,
via G. de Notaris 2B,
00197 Roma - Italy

Chambat P.
Centre orthopédique Santy,
24, avenue Paul Santy,
69008 Lyon - France

Cipolla M.
Clinica Valle Giulia,
via G. de Notaris 2B,
00197 Roma - Italy

Clatworthy M.
Aukland Bone and Joint Surgery,
Ascot Hospital, Level 1,
90 Greenlane Raod East,
Private bag 28912, Remuera,
Auckland - New Zealand

Dejour D.
Clinique de la Sauvegarde,
avenue Ben Gourion 69009 Lyon - France

Deroche P.
Centre orthopédique,
71640 Dracy-le-Fort - France

Deschamps G.
Centre orthopédique,
71640 Dracy-le-Fort - France

DiGioia A.M. III
Institute for Computer-Assisted
Orthopaedic Surgery,
The Western Pennsylvania Hospital,
4815 Liberty Avenue, Mellon Pavillion,
Suite 242, Pittsburgh,
PA 15224 - United States

Ferreira A.
Clinique du Parc,
86, boulevard des Belges,
69006 Lyon - France

Fu F.H.
Department of Orthopaedic Surgery,
Kaufmann Building, Suite 1010,
3471 Fifth Avenue,
Pittsburgh PA 15213 - United States

Gacon G.
Clinique du Parc,
86, boulevard des Belges,
69006 Lyon - France

Gallet D.
Centre orthopédique Santy,
24, avenue Paul Santy,
69008 Lyon - France

Gianni E.
Clinica Valle Giulia,
via G. de Notaris 2B,
00197 Roma - Italy

Giffin J.R.
Department of Orthopaedic Surgery,
Kaufmann Building, Suite 1010,
3471 Fifth Avenue,
Pittsburgh PA 15213 - United States

Girard J.
Hôpital Roger Salengro,
Service traumatologie-orthopédie,
59037 Lille - France

Giroud A.
Centre de rééducation Iris,
271, rue des Sources, BP 22,
69280 Marcy L'Étoile - France

Godenèche A.
Centre orthopédique Santy,
24, avenue Paul Santy,
69008 Lyon - France

Gougeon F.
Hôpital Roger Salengro,
Service traumatologie-orthopédie,
59037 Lille - France

Graveleau N.
Espace Médical Vauban,
2a., avenue de Ségur 75007 Paris - France

Guyen O.
Hôpital Édouard Herriot, Pavillon T,
Place d'Arsonval, 69003 Lyon - France

Huten D.
Hôpital Pontchaillou,
2, rue Henri Le Guilloux,
35033 Rennes Cedex 9- France

Jacquemard C.
Le Val Rosay,
centre de réadaptation fonctionnelle,
133, route de Saint-Cyr,
69370 Saint-Didier-au-Mont-d'Or -France

Landreau P.
Espace médical Vauban,
2, avenue de Ségur, 75007 Paris - France

Lautman S.
Centre hospitalier universitaire de Tours,
2, boulevard Tonnellé,
37000 Tours - France

Lerat J.L.
Centre hospitalier Lyon-Sud,
Service de chirurgie orthopédique,
Chemin du Grand Revoyet,
69495 Pierre Bénite Cedex - France

Malo M.
Department of Orthopaedic Surgery,
Hôpital du Sacré-cœur,
5400, boulevard Gouin Ouest,
Montréal, Québec- Canada

Margheritini F.
Department of Orthopaedic Surgery,
Kaufmann Building, Suite 1010,
3471 Fifth Avenue,
Pittsburgh PA 15213 - United States

Mathelin J.
Centre de rééducation Iris,
271, rue des Sources, BP 22,
69280 Marcy L'Étoile - France

Ménétrey J.
Clinique et polyclinique d'orthopédie
et de chirurgie de l'appareil moteur,
Hôpitaux universitaires de Genève,
24, rue Micheli-di-Crest,
CH-1211 Genève - Switzerland

Migaud H.
Hôpital Roger Salengro,
Service traumatologie-orthopédie,
59037 Lille - France

Moyen B.
Centre hospitalier Lyon-Sud,
Service de chirurgie orthopédique,
Chemin du Grand Revoyet,
69495 Pierre Bénite Cedex - France

Munzinger U.
Schulthess Klinik, Lengghalde 2,
CH-8008 Zurich - Switzerland

Musahl V.
Department of Orthopaedic Surgery,
Kaufmann Building, Suite 1010,
3471 Fifth Avenue,
Pittsburgh PA 15213 - United States

Neyret P.
Centre Livet, 8, rue de Margnolles
69300 Caluire - France

Nissen M.J.
Hôpital Édouard Herriot, Pavillon F,
Place d'Arsonval,
69003 Lyon - France

Noël E.
Centre orthopédique Santy,
24, avenue Paul Santy,
69008 Lyon - France

Nordin J.Y.
Hôpital Bicêtre,
78, rue du général Leclerc,
94270 Le Kremlin Bicêtre - France

Parker D.A.
Fowler Kennedy Sport Medicine Clinic,
University of Western Ontario, London,
Ontario - Canada

Picard F.
Golden Jubilee National Hospital,
Beardmore Street,
Clydebank G81 4HX,
Glasgow United Kingdom

Puddu G.
Clinica Valle Giulia,
via G. de Notaris 2B,
00197 Roma - Italy

Rivat P.
Clinique Pasteur,
294, avenue du Général De Gaulle,
07500 Guilherand-Granges - France

Roberto J.
Centre de rééducation Iris,
271, rue des Sources, BP 22,
69280 Marcy L'Étoile - France

Saragaglia D.
Service d'orthopédie et traumatologie
du sport, Hôpital Sud CHU,
38042 Grenoble Cedex 09 - France

Stern R.
Clinique et polyclinique d'orthopédie
et de chirurgie de l'appareil moteur,
Hôpitaux universitaires de Genève,
24, rue Micheli-di-Crest,
CH-1211 Genève - Switzerland

Tavernier T.
Clinique de la Sauvegarde,
avenue Ben Gourion 69009 Lyon - France

Tirveilliot F.
Centre hospitalier, 4, rue Roger-Aini,
14100 Lisieux - France

Trivett A.J.
Fowler Kennedy Sport Medicine Clinic,
University of Western Ontario, London,
Ontario - Canada

Vasconcelos W.
Clinique de la Sauvegarde,
avenue Ben Gourion
69009 Lyon - France

Verdonk R.
University Hospital De Pintelaan 185
Orthopedie P5, Gent B-9000 - Belgium

Vince K.G.
50, Monterey Boulevard,
Hermosa Beach,
CA 90254 - United States

Vinel H.
CHR Sainte-Marguerite,
Service d'orthopédie,
270, boulevard Sainte-Marguerite,
13274 Marseille Cedex 09 - France

Vittorio F.
Clinica Valle Giulia,
via G. de Notaris 2B,
00197 Roma - Italy

Westphal M.
Centre de rééducation Iris,
271, rue des Sources, BP 22,
69280 Marcy L'Étoile - France

Table of Contents

Specialized Aspects

GENERALITY

Imaging knee osteoarthritis

Y. Carrillon

Introduction

Knee osteoarthritis (OA) is a disease caused by biomechanical stresses affecting the articular cartilage and subchondral bone of the knee. This disease will cause pain and functional impotence. OA may involve either medial tibiofemoral compartment, lateral tibiofemoral compartment or patellofemoral compartment according to the localization of cartilage deterioration. It is necessary to keep in mind that the diagnosis of knee OA is made at first at clinical examination. Pain, morning stiffness and swelling of the knee in a patient older than 50 must be considered as consequences of OA. However, imaging modalities also play an important role in knee OA, since they may confirm the diagnosis of OA, determine the involved compartments, and evaluate the stage of the disease. Imaging may also confirm the responsibility for OA in the onset of symptoms and give also information about the evolution of the disease during treatment. Several types of imaging techniques are useful to evaluate knee OA: conventional radiography, MRI and arthro CT-scanner. CT-scanner does not bring any additional information to Conventional Radiography and ultra-sonography is not well suited for this purpose.

Conventional radiography

Conventional radiography is still today the technique of reference for evaluating knee OA. It is the only imaging technique which was scientifically evaluated in OA. However, conventional radiography gives an indirect appreciation of the articular cartilage status, since the cartilage is not apparent on X-ray.

Technical aspects

Conventional radiography must be performed according to strict criteria of quality and reproducibility. Three different views may be helpful to evaluate knee OA: frontal view, lateral view and tangential view of the patellofemoral compartment.

Frontal view of the knee

Frontal view (AP or PA view) must be performed in standing position in order to precisely demonstrate joint space narrowing (JSN), reflecting cartilage thickness. In non standing position, this view does not reflect precisely cartilage thickness (fig. 1). Weight-bearing position could be performed in either bipodal, or monopodal standing position. To our knowledge, no study has shown the superiority of one of these positions compared to the other. Monopodal standing position seems more logical, reflecting the functional position of the knee during walk.

The frontal view is performed generally upright, the knee locked in hyperextension. It appeared that this type of view could underestimate JSN since the preferential topography of cartilage damage is the posterior part of the femoral condyle. For this reason, several authors have proposed to perform frontal views in semi-flexed position, allowing a contact between the posterior part of the condyles with the shinbone (fig. 2). Railhac (1) was the first to describe this view, followed laterly by Buckland-Wright (2) who used macro-radiography and gave for the first time the name of "semi-flexed view".

The frontal view must be performed in a precise and reproducible way. That poses the problem of the alignment of the X-ray beam. This alignment conditions JSN and the reproducibility of the views. Lateral tibiofemoral compartment does not pose a problem since lateral condyle and shinbone are together convex in shape and therefore do not create superimposition on the film. On the other hand, the medial shinbone is concave, presenting a shape resembling to a cup with a bottom and two edges, one anterior and one posterior. The ideal inclination and alignment for the directing X-ray beam must be performed in order to overlap the two edges, letting appear only two lines: for the bottom and for the overlapped anterior and posterior edges (fig. 3). For this reason, radiographic examination of the knee, in an ideal way, must be carried out under radioscopic control, paying attention to align properly the medial compartment.

In certain cases, frontal view can be performed upright, on a large film, in order to evaluate the frontal axis of the knees and lower limbs. This kind of view may be helpful to plan surgery.

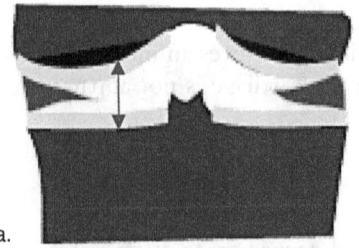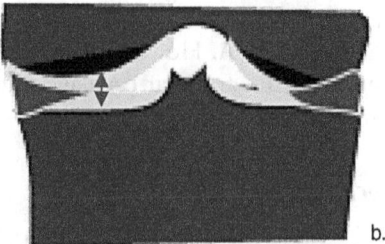

a.   b.

Fig. 1. – JSN variation between AP views performed without (**a.**) and with support (**b.**). Without support, cartilaginous surfaces are not in contact making it impossible to potentiate JSN. It will be noted that the meniscus is an element which can disturb the evaluation of JSN.

Lateral view of the knee

Lateral view is not regarded as useful for analysing knee OA. It however allows a relatively reliable analysis of joint space. Contours of the condyles and tibial plateau surfaces are easy to identify. The lateral view allows also a reliable and reproducible analysis of the patellofemoral joint objectifying not only marginal osteophytes and joint space narrowing but also the associated lesions such as the disorders of patellar engagement 3).

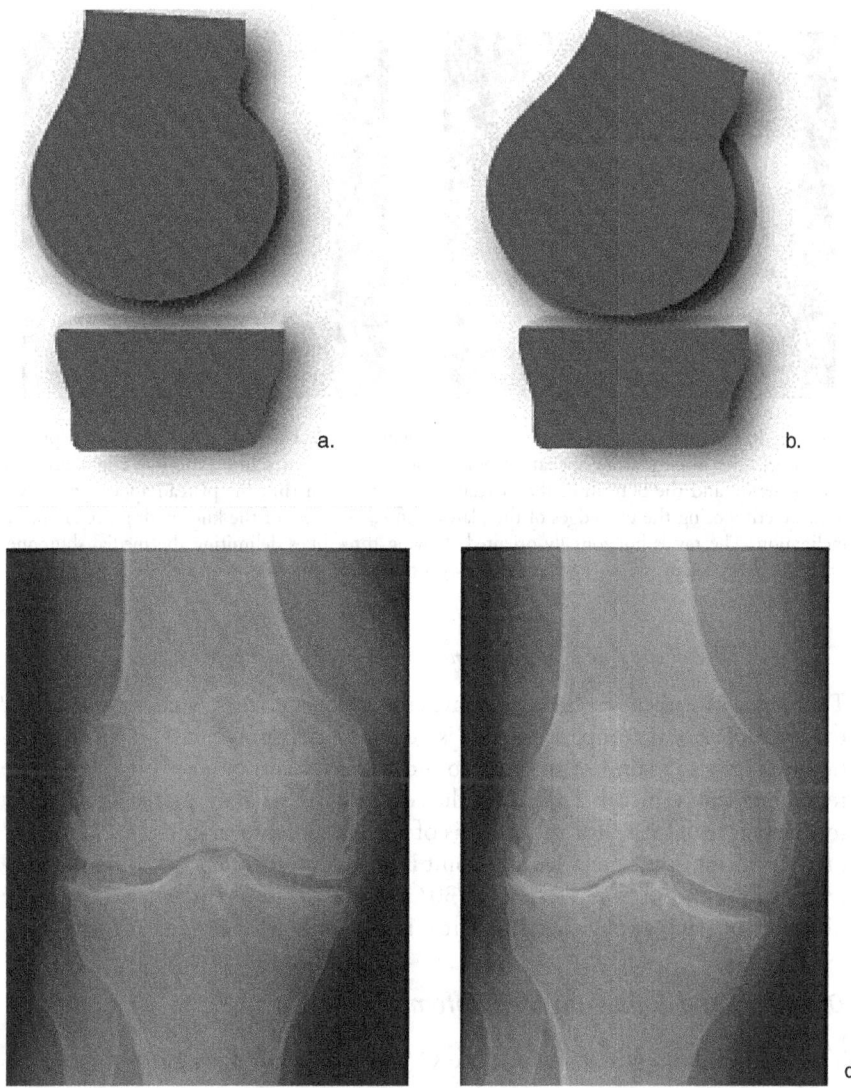

Fig. 2. – Usefulness of semi-flexed view. The cartilage loss is preferentially located on the posterior aspect of the femoral condyle. If the frontal view is performed with no knee flexion (**a., c.**), JSN is not well evaluated. If the frontal view is performed in semi-flexed position (**b., d.**), JSN is more prominent.

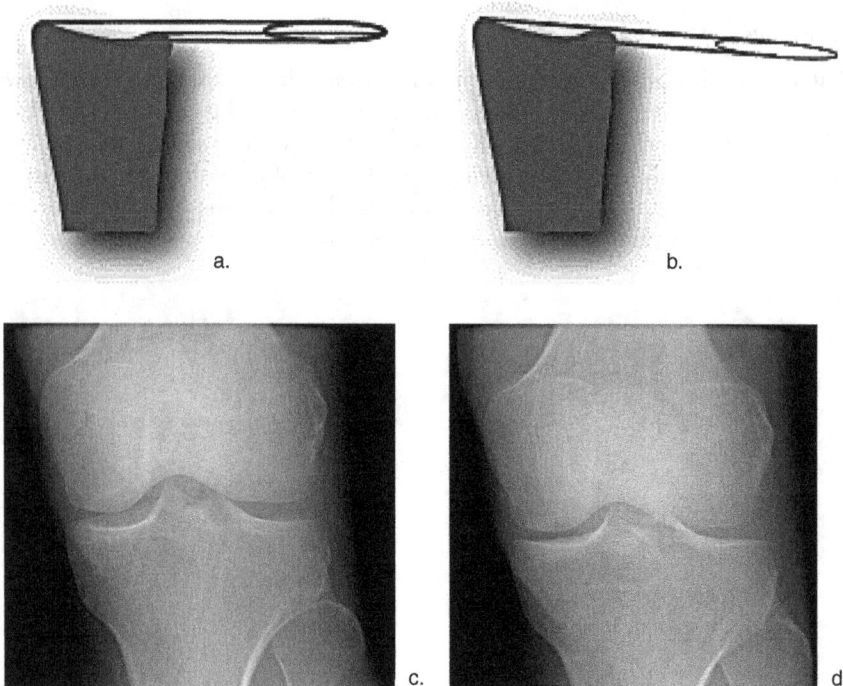

Fig. 3. – In **a.** and **b.**, diagram representing the medial tibial plateau and the X-ray beam projection. In **a.**, the tibial plateau appears as three distinct lines, representing the two edges, anterior and posterior, and the bottom of the plateau; with inclination (**b.**), the plateau appears with two lines superimposing the two edges of the plateau. In **c.**, AP view of the knee with no X-ray beam inclination. The ray is horizontally oriented showing three lines delimiting the medial shinbone, in **d.** the X-ray beam is tilted to be tangent with the medial plateau, two lines are apparent.

Tangential view of the patellofemoral joint

This view, as indicated, does not have any interest for the analysis except for the patellofemoral compartment. It is generally performed in laid down position, less often in support in order to increase JSN and patellar offsetting. The technique can sometimes be difficult, certain authors may prefer lateral view to this tangential view for the analysis of the patellofemoral joint (3). With 45° of knee flexion, the patellofemoral joint is well demonstrated, allowing the analysis of JSN and osteophytes. With 30° of knee flexion, it is possible to study disorders of patellar engagement, but joint space is less better seen.

Diagnosis and follow-up of tibiofemoral OA

The main radiological signs of knee OA on conventional radiography are:

– JSN corresponding to the loss of cartilage;
– osteophytes which represent marginal bone reaction proportional to the loss of cartilage. Their etiology is still discussed but some says they can be due to OA synovitis;

– subchondral bone reactions, geodes or condensation, which are the consequences of the overlying cartilaginous damages.

JSN analysed on a radiography performed in weight-bearing position is the only sign which corresponds exactly to the loss of cartilaginous substance. This sign presents the disadvantage to be not very sensitive, giving the diagnosis of pre-osteoarthritis difficult. This sign is on the other hand very specific.

Osteophyte is the most specific radiographic sign of knee OA. It can however occur tardily reducing its sensitivity probably more than JSN. The majority of classifications of the knee OA are interested either in JSN, or in osteophytes, or in both. The classification of Menkes is based mainly on JSN (4):

– Stage 1: JSN less than 50% of the articular surface;
– Stage 2: JSN from 50 to 90%;
– Stage 3: complete JSN;
– Stage 4: moderated JSN (2-3mm in depth);
– Stage 5: marked (4-6mm);
– Stage 6: severe;
– + 1 if osteophytes marked.

Ahlbäck (5) had earlier described a classification taking account of JSN and subchondral bone reactions which were considered as appearing latterly:

– Stage 1: JSN (width < 3mm);
– Stage 2: complete JSN;
– Stage 3: moderate subchondral bone condensation (0-5mm);
– Stage 4: significant bone condensation (attrition) (5-10mm);
– Stage 5: major bone condensation (> 10mm).

Kellgreen (6) and Lawrence were interested more particularly in osteophytes:
– Stage 1: minor osteophytes;
– Stage 2: osteophytes without JSN;
– Stage 3: moderate JSN;
– Stage 4: JSN with subchondral bone condensation.

Two more recent classifications deserve a detailed attention. Piperno (7) tries to individualize JSN and osteophytes. In counterpart, this classification doesn't make it possible to classify the patients in a completely progressive and uniform way.

– JSN:
• 0: no JSN;
• 1: doubtful JSN;
• 2: unquestionable JSN;
• 3: JSN> 2/3 at the opposite side;
• 4: complete JSN;
• 5: JSN and bone erosion.

– Osteophytes:
• 0: no osteophyte;
• 1: doubt on an osteophyte;

- 2: osteophyte of the shinbone;
- 3: broad osteophyte of the shinbone.

The Osteoarthritis Association Research Society (OARS) has developed a classification based on an atlas where it is thus possible to compare and to classify the stereotypes in an evolutionary way (8). This atlas takes into account: JSN (fig. 4), osteophytes, subchondral bone sclerosis, erosion, and desaxation.

This superabundance of classification shows that the evaluation of OA still poses problems with conventional radiography. In routine, it seems that marginal osteophyte is the most specific and most reproducible sign (9, 10). Desaxation of the knee may be found on patients with knee OA. Erosion of

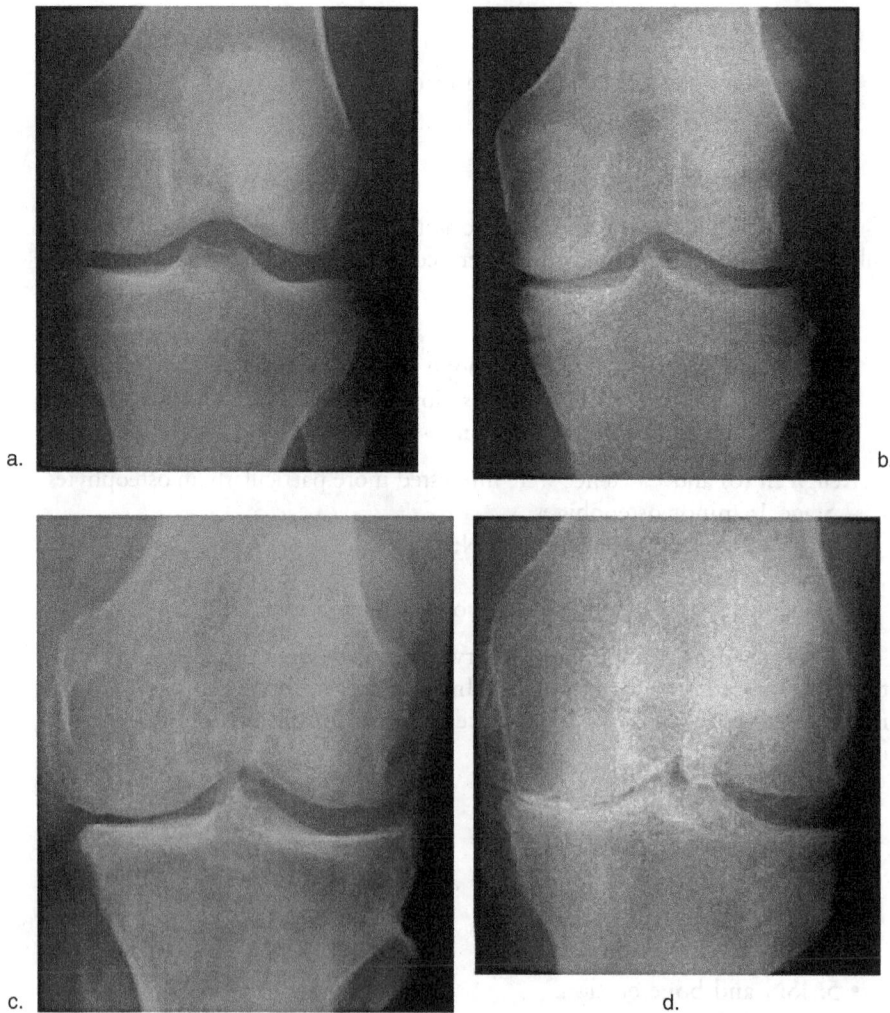

a.   b.

c.   d.

Fig. 4. – Radiographic aspects of medial tibiofemoral OA according to the OARS. In **a.**, normal aspect; in **b.**, moderate JSN; in **c.**, JSN more marked with moderate osteophyte; in **d.**, complete JSN with marked osteophytes.

tibial plateau, wear of femoral condyles will cause degenerative ligamentar lesions and thus knee desaxation which, generally, will further increase the anomalies of axis of the lower limbs (varus or valgus). The surgeons adopt for the majority a classification which takes account of these desaxations:

- Stage 1: moderate JSN;
- Stage 2: complete JSN;
- Stage 3: JSN with "depression" of the adjacent shinbone;
- Stage 4: JSN with lateral desaxation testifying degenerative tear of the Anterior Cruciate Ligament.

A particular case: patellofemoral OA

Patellofemoral OA may be primitive (patellar instability, traumatic after-effects...) or secondary (medial tibiofemoral OA...). Loss of cartilage can be electively localized on lateral, medial patellar articular surfaces. To our know-ledge, there is no specific classification, but classifications used in tibiofemoral OA can also be used for this joint.

Recent techniques

Arthro CT-scanner and MRI allow a direct visualization of the articular cartilage. The real place of these techniques between conventional radiography and arthroscopy still remains to be evaluated. However, these techniques may be useful in a certain number of cases to support the diagnosis of OA. They also make differential diagnosis (meniscal tear, arthritis...).

Arthro CT-scanner (fig. 5)

Arthro CT-scanner comes to substitute or supplement conventional arthrography. The most usually used technique is the simple iodised articular injection. This injection allows a good visualization of intra-articular structures and especially

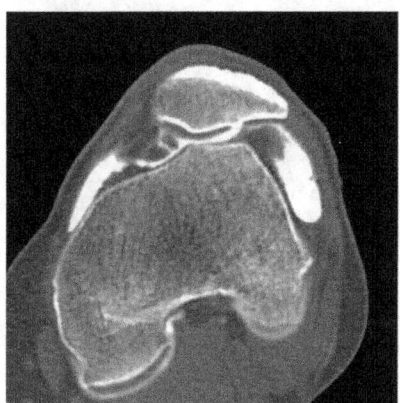
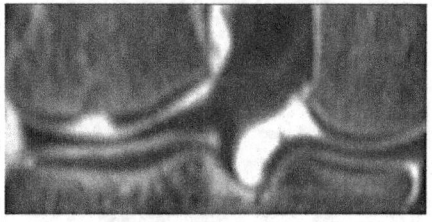

b.

Fig. 5. – Arthro CT-scanner. In **a.**, axial slice demonstrating a stage 4 lesion on the lateral patellar facet of the patella. In **b.**, a frontal reformation shows a stage 4 lesion of the medial condyle.

a.

cartilage. CT-scanner performed using spiral technique makes it possible to obtain very fine slices (< 1mm) and survey of all the knee area in a very short time (< 30sec). The acquisition performed in the transverse axial plan (horizontal) may be secondarily reformated in all desired planes. These reformations, taking into account the narrowness of the slices and the overlapping obtained, can be of a quality as good as a direct acquisition. It is thus possible to obtain slices in frontal, sagittal or axial transverse plane. Even if there does not exist much articles in the literature describing the performances of arthro CT-scanner in knee OA, it is obvious that this technique is an excellent tool to assess cartilaginous losses.

Magnetic Resonance Imaging (fig. 6 and 7)

Magnetic Resonance Imaging (MRI) is the most recent imaging technique and appears to be particularly suited for the study of cartilage. It is able to perform very thin images with an optimal contrast giving good demonstration of cartilaginous losses and also information on the quality of the cartilage itself. MRI must be carried out in a suitable way to obtain a satisfactory analysis of articular cartilage. The choice of the type of sequence (T1, T2, or proton density weighted images) is crucial. Image weighting is the result of the presetting of a whole of parameters such as flip angle, time of echo, time of repetition... These adjustments will condition image contrast and allow a good discrimination between cartilage and articular liquid. T2 or proton density weighted sequences with fat-suppression technique allow best discrimination (11, 12, 13). With these sequences, cartilage will appear in intermediate signal (gray), water in hypersignal (white) and subchondral bone in hyposignal (black). Slice thickness is also a paramount element for image quality. One can consider that a thickness of

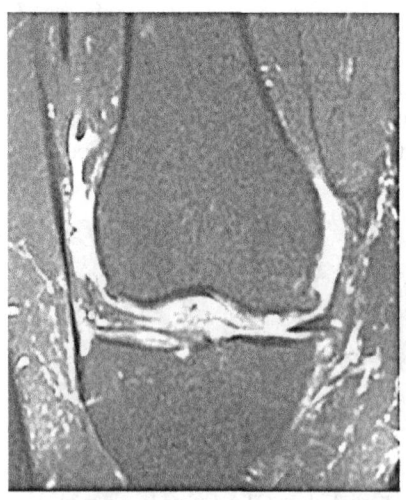 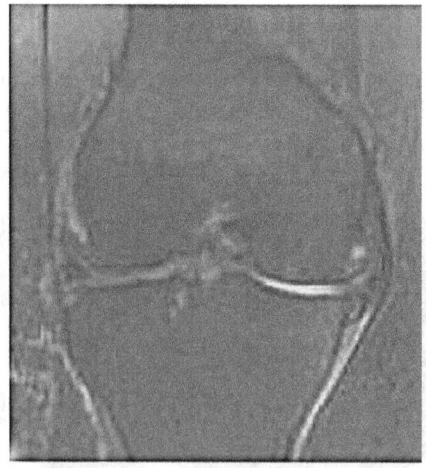

a.   b.

Fig. 6. – Two different examples tibiofemoral OA demonstrated on density of protons weighted MR images. In **a.**, there is an irregular, central lesion of stage 3. In **b.**, OA is total, condylar cartilage has disappeared and is replaced by liquid. There is an osteophyte with an associated marginal oedema.

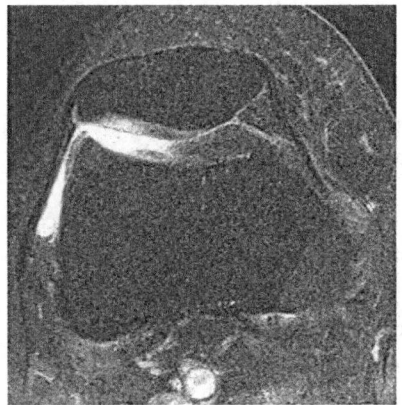 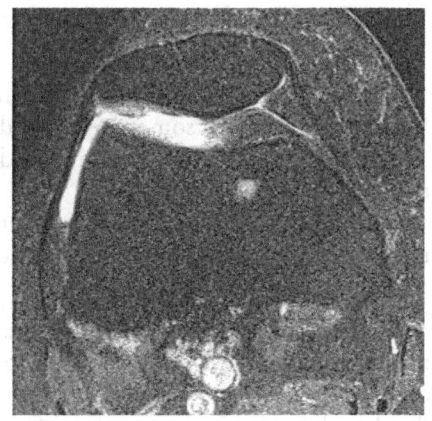

a.   b.

Fig. 7. – MR T2-weighted with fat-saturation technique axial transverse slices. In **a.**, the image shows an intermediate hypersignal corresponding to chondromalacia without loss of substance of the lateral patellar articular surface. In **b.**, the image demonstrates loss of cartilaginous substance corresponding to stage 2 (SFA).

less than 2mm allows a good analysis of the cartilage. The signal/noise ratio is the last element which influences the image quality. This factor also depends on MR parameters used. It also depends on the intrinsic quality of the machine, the antennas used as well as time spent to obtain images. The question of knowing whether MRI performed on high field (1,5T) is preferable to MRI performed with low field (0,15-0,3T) to analyze the cartilage does not seem crucial being given the numbers of intricate factors which manage the quality of the image. In our opinion, a suitable examination of the articular cartilage of the knee must include at least sequences in three different planes: axial transverse, sagittal and frontal in either T2 or proton density weighted images with fat-saturation technique. MRI may give also a quantitative evaluation of cartilage. By using special 3D sequences, it is possible to measure the total amount of knee cartilage (14, 15, 16, 17). Nevertheless, this evaluation does not make sense today, as there is still no calculated references in normal subject. It is logical to imagine that there could be a great variation in the general population. MRI would be also able to analyze the intrinsic quality of cartilage, thus making it possible to make the diagnosis of chondromalacia before the loss of substance (18, 19). Chondromalacia, non visualized on conventional radiography or arthro CT-scanner, can be detected on MRI (fig. 6). Once again, T2 or proton density weighted images with fat-saturation technique may demonstrate chondromalacia.

MR classifications of cartilage lesions

Many classifications have been proposed to evaluate cartilaginous knee lesions on MRI. However, the use of an arthroscopic classification may be particularly interesting for analyzing cartilage on MRI or arthro CT-scanner. SFA classification is then particularly interesting. This classification evaluates the lesions qualitatively but also quantitatively (20, 21, 22).

The SFA classification is defined by:

– Stage 0: normal cartilage;
– Stage 1: closed chondromalacia with discrete lesions of the under-surface layer of the cartilage sometimes only detectable to palpation;
– Stage 2: superficial opened chondropathy concerning less than 50% of cartilage depth;
– Stage 3: major opened chondropathy concerning more than 50% of cartilage depth but without naked subchondral bone;
– Stage 4: naked subchondral bone.

This classification is reproducible but does not give information on neither the aspect, neither the topography, nor the total surface of cartilage loss. In order to evaluate more precisely cartilage losses in terms of surface, the SFA developed a score and a new staging.

Score SFA is the resultant of: Stage 1 × 0,14 + Stage 2 × 0,34 + Stage 3 × 0,65 + Stade 4. SFA stages correspond to:

– SFA Stage 0
  • 100% Stage 0
– SFA Stage 1
  • 0% Stage 4
  • 80-100% Stage 0
– SFA Stage 2
  • 0% Stage 4
  • < 80% Stage 0
  • < 15% Stage 3
– SFA Stage 3
  • Either: 0% Stage 4
  • < 80% Stage 0
  • > 15% Stage 3
  • Or: > 1%
  Stage 4
  • < 65% Stage 0
– SFA Stage 4
  • > 1% Stage 4
  • < 65% Stage 0

These classifications are not easy to use in routine practice. They can however be used for the follow-up of patients during treatment.

Pain and osteoarthritis

It is sometimes difficult to make sure that OA is the real cause of a painful knee. MRI, for certain authors, would be an ideal examination technique to affirm the origin of pain.

Articular fluid collection, marginal or subchondral oedema are major elements that may suggest the responsibility of the OA in the onset of symptoms (23).

Conclusion

Conventional radiography remains the imaging technique of reference in knee OA. This technique assesses the diagnosis of knee OA and is validated for the follow-up of the disease during treatment. However, in certain cases, this technique is not sufficient. Arthro CT-scanner and MRI are excellent techniques for analyzing knee OA. MRI seems even more interesting since this technique may not only make the diagnosis of knee OA, but also assumes its responsibility in the symptoms onset. However, these techniques need to be more largely validated in order to assess their real role in knee OA.

References

1. Railhac JJ, Fournie A, Gay R *et al.* (1981) Étude radiologique du genou en incidence antéro-postérieure avec légère flexion en appui. Intérêt pour détecter l'arthrose fémoro-tibiale. J Radiol 62(3): 157-66
2. Buckland-Wright C (1995) Protocols for precise radio-anatomical positioning of the tibio-femoral and patellofemoral compartments of the knee. Osteoarthritis Cartilage 3 Suppl A: 71-80
3. Chaisson CE, Gale DR, Gale E *et al.* (2000) Detecting radiographic knee osteoarthritis: what combination of views is optimal? Rheumatology (Oxford) 39(11): 1218-21
4. Menkes CJ (1991) Radiographic criteria for Classification of osteoarthrosis. J Rheumatol Supp 27(28): 13-15
5. Ahlbäck S. (1968) Osteoarthrosis of the knee: a radiographic investigation. Acta Radiol Stockholm Suppl 227: 7-72
6. Kellgreen JH, Lawrence JS (1957) Radiological assessment of ostoearthrosis. Ann Rheum Dis 16: 494-501
7. Vignon E, Conrozier T, Piperno M *et al.* (1999) Radiographic assessment of hip and knee osteoarthritis. Recommendations: recommended guidelines. Osteoarthritis Cartilage 7(4): 434-6
8. Altman RD, Hochberg M, Murphy WA Jr *et al.* (1995) Atlas of individual radiographic features in osteoarthritis. Osteoarthritis Cartilage 3 Suppl A: 3-70
9. Fife RS, Brandt KD, Braunstein EM *et al.* (1991) Relationship between arthroscopic evidence of cartilage damage and radiographic evidence of joint space narrowing in early osteoarthritis of the knee. Arthritis Rheum 34(4): 377-82
10. Lysholm J, Hamberg P, Gillquist J (1987) The correlation between osteoarthrosis as seen on radiographs and on arthroscopy. Arthroscopy 3(3): 161-5
11. Bredella MA, Tirman PF, Peterfy CG *et al.* (1999) Accuracy of T2-weighted fast spin-echo MR imaging with fat saturation in detecting cartilage defects in the knee: comparison with arthroscopy in 130 patients. AJR Am J Roentgenol 172(4): 1073-80
12. Broderick LS, Turner DA, Renfrew DL *et al.* (1994) Severity of articular cartilage abnormality in patients with osteoarthritis: evaluation with fast spin-echo MR vs arthroscopy. AJR Am J Roentgenol 162(1): 99-103
13. Trattnig S, Huber M, Breitenseher MJ *et al.* (1998) Imaging articular cartilage defects with 3D fat-suppressed echo planar imaging: comparison with conventional 3D fat-suppressed gradient echo sequence and correlation with histology. J Comput Assist Tomogr 22(1): 8-14
14. Drape JL, Pessis E, Auleley GR *et al.* (1998) Quantitative MR imaging evaluation of chondropathy in osteoarthritic knees. Radiology 208(1): 49-55
15. Dye SF, Merchant AC (1999) Magnetic resonance imaging of articular cartilage in the knee. An evaluation with use of fast-spin-echo imaging. J Bone Joint Surg Am 81(9): 1349-50
16. Eckstein F, Westhoff J, Sittek H *et al.* (1998) *In vivo* reproducibility of three-dimensional cartilage volume and thickness measurements with MR imaging. AJR Am J Roentgenol. 170(3): 593-7

17. Piplani MA, Disler DG, McCauley TR *et al.* (1996) Articular cartilage volume in the knee: semi-automated determination from three-dimensional reformations of MR images. Radiology198(3): 855-9
18. Goodwin DW, Zhu H, Dunn JF (2000) *In vitro* MR imaging of hyaline cartilage: correlation with scanning electron microscopy. AJR Am J Roentgenol 174(2): 405-9
19. Mosher TJ, Dardzinski BJ, Smith MB (2000) Human articular cartilage: influence of aging and early symptomatic degeneration on the spatial variation of T2 – preliminary findings at 3 T. Radiology 214(1): 259-66
20. Dougados M, Ayral X, Listrat V *et al.* (1994) The SFA system for assessing articular cartilage lesions at arthroscopy of the knee. Arthroscopy 10(1): 69-77
21. Ayral X (1996) Diagnostic and quantitative arthroscopy: quantitative arthroscopy. Baillieres Clin Rheumatol 10(3): 477-94. Review
22. Ayral X, Dougados M, Listrat V *et al.* (1996) Arthroscopic evaluation of chondropathy in osteoarthritis of the knee. J Rheumatol 23(4): 698-706
23. Felson DT, Chaisson CE, Hill CL *et al.* (2001) The association of bone marrow lesions with pain in knee osteoarthritis. Ann Intern Med 134(7):5 41-9

Patellofemoral osteoarthritis

D. Dejour, W. Vasconcelos, T. Tavernier

Introduction

Patellofemoral osteoarthritis (OA) is a common feature of three-compartment knee joint OA. More rarely, the patellofemoral compartment is affected in isolation.

The subject has been investigated by a number of authors (11, 35, 36). McAlindon et al. (35, 36) studied 2,101 individuals over the age of 55 years, and found a greater prevalence in females: of the women in the study population, 24% had patellofemoral OA; of the men, only 11% were affected. Falconnet (20) thought the prevalence to be 15%, while Ahlbäck and Mattson (2) found a rate of 35% of isolated patellofemoral OA in their study.

The aetiological factors involved in patellofemoral OA are less easy to determine than those responsible for tibiofemoral OA. The best known are rheumatological conditions, such as chondrocalcinosis, and trauma (patellar fractures). Equally, patients with a history of patellar dislocation or patellar surgery may develop patellofemoral OA. Where none of these predisposing factors is found, the condition is described as primary OA.

Establishing the causative factor(s) is important, since – similar to the situation in tibiofemoral OA – a knowledge of the aetiology may lead to therapeutic, preventive, or palliative strategies being devised.

In the literature on patellofemoral OA, the emphasis tends to be upon the biomechanics of the joint, and upon possible treatment modalities; this chapter highlights also the epidemiology and the various features of the condition.

History, signs, and symptoms

Patellofemoral OA tends to be well tolerated for a long time. The early manifestations will depend on the aetiology of the condition. A detailed history is essential in establishing the cause. The patient should be carefully questioned about any dislocations, trauma involving fractures, and previous surgery.

History-taking is important, since it allows the type of OA to be ascertained. The clinical signs do not allow this discrimination, since they are the same regardless of the aetiology of the condition.

Patellofemoral OA tends to be well tolerated for a long time; in particular, walking on level ground is not painful. Pain occurs mainly as the loaded knee

is being flexed during the ascent or descent of stairs. When sitting for prolonged periods of time, the patient has to get up from time to time to relieve
the patellofemoral pain. There will also be so-called reflex instability, from
quadriceps inhibition as a result of painful stimuli. This instability is different from that seen in mechanical instability (dislocation), which tends to
disappear as the degenerative process gets under way. Reflex instability occurs
while walking, and is not triggered by knee movements performed in sports.
Often, there will be a sense of something catching, or of the knee locking.
Some of the manifestations are more specific to the different aetiologies; these
features are discussed in the relevant sections of this chapter. In population
of 367 patients with isolated OA we found similar alteration in terms of IKS
score to femoro-tibial arthritis (1).

Radiology

Once the history has been obtained, the patient is worked up with radiology.
This is another key element in establishing the cause of the condition and in
deciding on the most suitable treatment modality.

In the first instance, standard radiographs (30° axial view, AP view, and
lateral view in single-leg stance and 20° of flexion) should be obtained. In
patients over the age of 50 years, and in those with a history of orthopaedic
surgery (meniscectomy etc.), a Rosenberg view (weight-bearing PA view in
45° of flexion) should be added.

Two criteria are essential for an analysis of the patellofemoral joint (14, 40):

– the posterior femoral condyles must be superimposed on the lateral view
(fig. 1);

– true 30° axial view must be obtained, using Knutsson's technique (26).

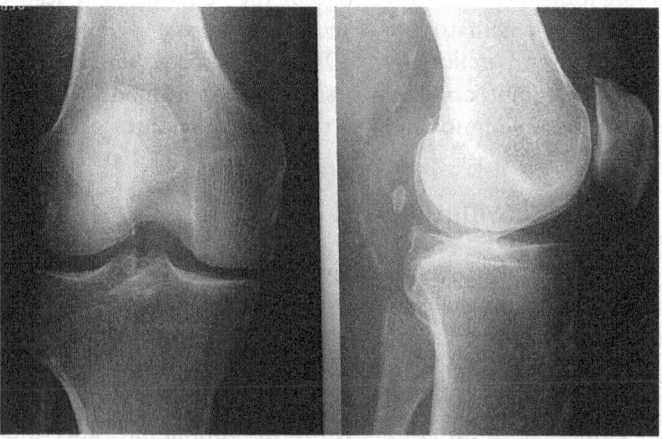

Fig. 1. – The AP radiograph shows the tibiofemoral compartments to be healthy (note superimposition of the posterior condyles). The lateral radiograph shows discreet narrowing of the
joint space. Figure 2 provides more detailed information.

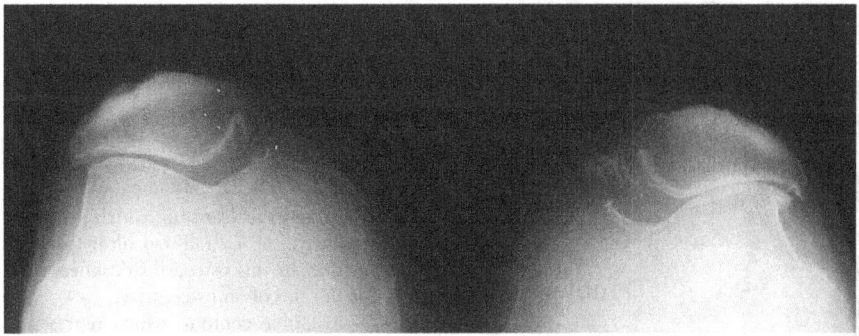

Fig. 2. – 30° axial view: The lateral slope of the trochlea accounts for two thirds of the trochlea. There is bony contact, and secondary subluxation following the loss of cartilage. Note enthesophytes in the lateral retinaculum, and trochlear osteophytes.

This is a craniopodal view taken with the patient lying supine, with the quadriceps relaxed. On a good 30° axial view, the lateral slope of the trochlea will occupy about two thirds of the total trochlear width (fig. 2). Isolated patellar arthritis is defined using Iwanno's classification on the axial view at 30° flexion, this classification has four stages (25).

Features to be analyzed

Dysplasia of the trochlea

A dysplastic trochlea is the main cause of patellar instability (14, 17, 19). It manifests itself in a gradual infilling of the trochlea, leading to the disappearance of the groove, which becomes flat or even convex. On the true lateral radiograph, dysplasia is defined by the crossing of the line representing the deepest part of the trochlear groove with the anterior border of the two condyles (14). At this crossing point, the trochlea is completely flat. This crossing sign was found in 96% of patients with objective evidence of patellar instability, in 12% of patients with anterior knee pain, but was seen in only 3% of the healthy controls (14). Initially, three stages of trochlear dysplasia were described. A recent study of 177 cases of proven patellar instability involved a comparison of conventional radiographs and CT scans. This allowed the analysis to be refined, and led to the definition of a four-grade system (16, 40).

On the true lateral view, two new radiological signs have been described (fig. 3):

– the *supratrochlear spur*, which is formed by a bone spicule proximal to the trochlea. This feature is seen where the entire trochlea projects beyond the anterior cortex of the femur. In OA, this will be the site of an osteophyte;

– the *double contour* is produced, on the lateral radiograph, by the projection of the medial facet of the trochlea. It is abnormal if it finishes below the crossing described above.

Once OA has set in, the crossing sign becomes difficult to discern; however, the supratrochlear spur and the double contour will still be seen.

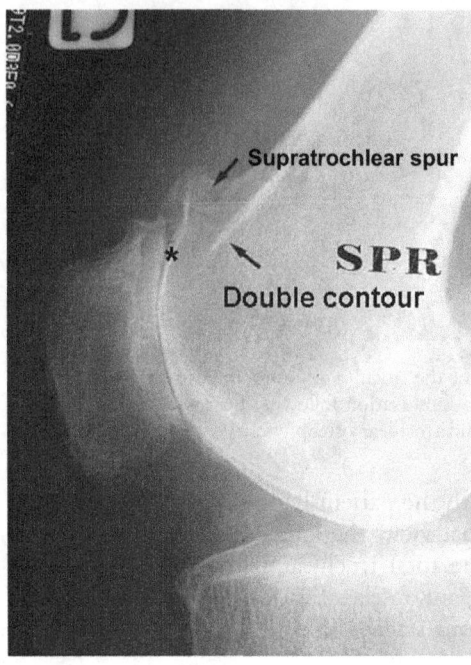

Supratrochlear spur

SPR

Double contour

*

Fig. 3. – The lateral radiograph shows:
– a supratrochlear spur, which provides evidence of overall trochlear prominence. In this osteoarthritic knee, this is the site of an osteophyte;
– a double contour, which represents the projection of the hypoplastic medial facet of the trochlea.

Note the crossing sign (*), which is specific to trochlear dysplasia, and narrowing of the patellofemoral joint space.

Other authors have used different radiographic criteria. Thus, Malghem and Maldague (31) looked at the depth of the trochlea at a point 1cm below the upper limit of the trochlear groove. This depth corresponds to the mean of the distances from the deepest part of the groove to the anterior borders of the medial and lateral condyles. The mean depth was found to be 6 ± 1.5mm. The authors stated that a proximal trochlear depth of less than 5mm was evidence of dysplasia.

The trochlear angle, measured on a 30° axial view, has been proposed as yet another yardstick of trochlear dysplasia. Bernageau and Goutallier (4) found a mean trochlear angle of 144 ± 6.75°. According to other authors, a trochlea with an angle of > 150° on the 30° axial view should be considered as dysplastic.

The trochlea dysplasia is the highest predisposing factor; the incidence is 78% in the isolated arthritis population (1), 55% are a dysplasia with a supratrochlear spur type B and D. The proeminence of the trochlea leads to an antimaquet effet and increases the patellofemoral forces in flexion. The second predisposing factor is the patella dysplasia with an incidence of 42% of patella wiberg II.

Patellar height

The height of the patella is the sole factor which, by itself, could cause objective patellar instability. Normally, the patella enters the trochlea during the first few degrees of flexion, and is thus stabilized and guided by the bony groove. If the patella is too high in relation to the trochlea, it will not engage until flexion has advanced further, and will be at risk for dislocation.

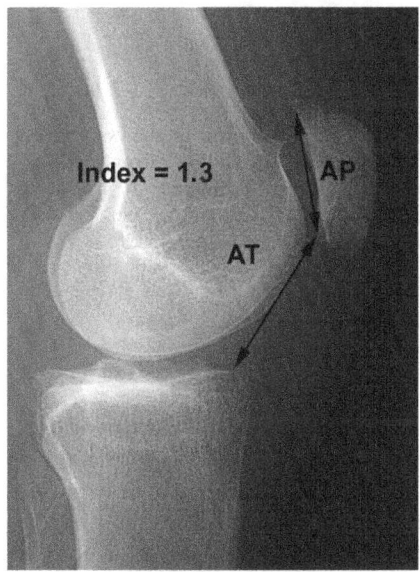

Fig. 4. – Caton-Deschamps method of establishing the patellar index. The index is the ratio of AT to AP. A patella with an index > 1.2 is considered to be high-riding.

The Caton-Deschamps patellar index (9) is a reliable yardstick (fig. 4). A normal index is equal to 1; a patella with an index > 1.2 is a high-riding patella (patella alta). An index > 1.2 has been found in 30% of patients with proven patellar instability, whilst not being encountered at all in healthy controls (14). Patellar height may also be specified in terms of the Blackburne-Peel index (5) and the Insall-Salvati index (24), details of which may be found in the literature cited.

Loss of joint space

The patellofemoral joint space is studied on the 30° axial view, which, in OA, will show narrowing of the joint space and, in severe cases, bone-to-bone contact between the trochlea and the patella. The axial view also shows which side of the compartment is affected (usually, the lateral side is involved). Information is also provided on the size of osteophytes, and on whether the patella is well centred or subluxed.

Iwano *et al.* (25) have produced a simple staging system of lateral patellofemoral OA:

- stage 1: mild OA; joint space at least 3mm;
- stage 2: moderate OA; joint space less than 3mm, but no bony contact;
- stage 3: severe OA; bony contact less than one-quarter of the joint surface;
- stage 4: very severe OA, joint surfaces entirely touch each other.

Further investigations

CT arthrography (fig. 5)

There are two reasons why this is the most important of the further investigations to be considered.

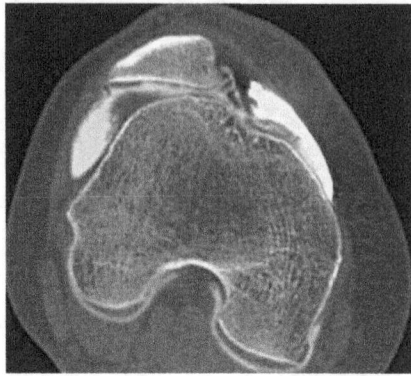

Fig. 5. – The CT arthrogram shows the extent of cartilage damage, and the factors predisposing to instability. In this case, the trochlea is dysplastic and convex, and the patellar cartilage has completely disappeared.

– In incipient OA in a patient with patellar instability, CT arthrography will show the extent of the cartilage damage, and will indicate whether surgical recentring of the patella, as practised for unstable patella, may be expected to restore a satisfactory pattern. The scans should show whether such factors as the distance between the tibial tubercle and the bottom of the trochlear groove (22), and patellar tilt, can be corrected.

– Where there is medial patellofemoral impingement, as a result of excessive medialization, CT arthrography will show cartilage lesions on the medial facet, and the extent of medialization as compared with the pattern in the contralateral knee, which is used as the reference (fig. 6).

Magnetic resonance (MR) imaging is not indicated in the work-up of patients with OA or a pre-osteoarthritic condition of the patellofemoral joint.

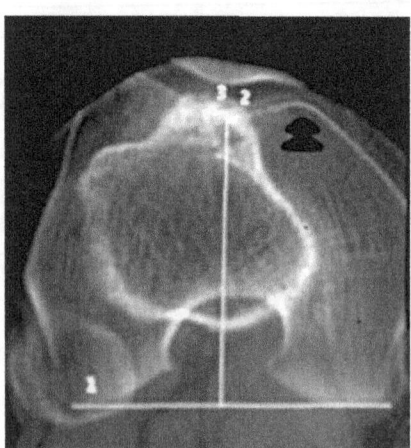

Fig. 6. – The distance from the tibial tubercle to the deepest part of the trochlea is measured on superimposed CT scans. Here, the TT–TG is 0mm (as a result of excessive medialization).

Differential diagnosis: patella infera (15)

Clinically, patella infera manifests itself by anterior knee pain, which may be perceived as a burning sensation. The knee will feel extremely tight. The pain is constant, and made worse by effort. The patients will invariably have had several previous surgeries, with a difficult and painful postoperative course.

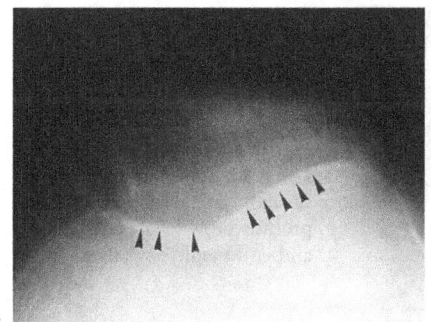
a.

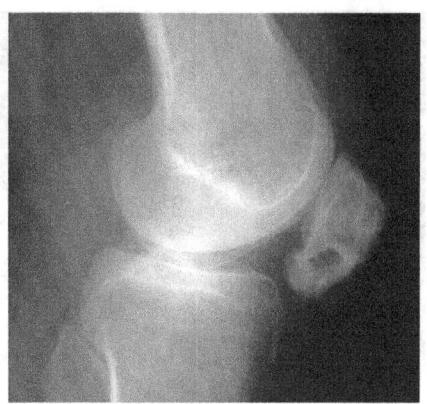
b.

Fig. 7. – Patella infera.
a. The axial view of a knee with patella infera shows complete loss of joint space, since the trochlea is superimposed on the patella, which is wedged in the intercondylar fossa ("sunset" pattern).
b. The lateral radiograph allows the diagnosis of patella infera to be made: the Caton-Deschamps patellar index is < 0.6. The CT scan and the two radiographs must be considered together.

The diagnosis may be made from the radiographs. The lateral film shows a Caton-Deschamps patellar index ≤ 0.6. On a correctly produced 30° axial view, the patella will have an unmistakable pattern: It appears wedged in the intercondylar notch, producing a superimposition of the trochlear groove and the patella mimicking complete loss of patellofemoral joint space (fig. 7). Compared with the 30° "sunrise" view on the healthy side, the affected knee will show a "sunset" pattern. The three views (AP, lateral, axial) must be studied together, to extract all the relevant information.

The different forms of patellofemoral OA, and their features

Primary OA

Epidemiology and clinical manifestations

49% of the isolatead patellofemoral arthritis. This form of patellofemoral OA occurs late in life, around the age of 70; it is often bilateral. The prevalence is greater in women (35, 36). It tends to be very well tolerated for a long time, with patients able to walk virtually normally on level ground, whereas uneven ground, and above all stairs and steep slopes, become progressively more difficult to negotiate. The patients complain of a sense of instability; this is due to reflex quadriceps inhibition as a result of painful stimuli. Catching and locking sensations as the knee goes through its range of movement are due to patellar osteophytes catching on the lateral facet of the trochlea, and to the bony spurs on the trochlea.

Radiological features

Both knees are affected. The 30° axial view shows loss of joint space, with bony contact between the lateral patellar facet and the trochlea. The patella

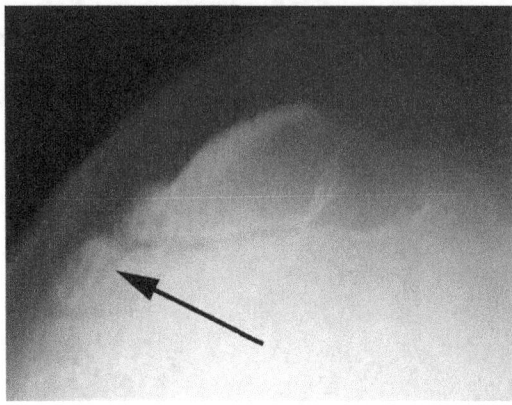

Fig. 8. – Primary patellofemoral OA, with total loss of articular cartilage, lateral subluxation, and profuse growth of osteophytes and enthesophytes (arrow).

is subluxed. This subluxation is due to cartilage wear, rather than to malalignment of the extensor system. The lateral retinaculum contains enthesophytes, and there are osteophytes on the lateral border of the patella and on the trochlea (fig. 8). The lateral film shows osteophytes on the proximal part of the trochlea, as well as subchondral sclerosis of the patellofemoral joint, and joint space narrowing. (The lateral film does not, however, provide the most pertinent information on which a diagnosis of patellofemoral OA could be based.)

Patellofemoral chondrocalcinosis

Epidemiology and clinical manifestations

8% of the isolatead patellofemoral arthritis. The cause of this condition is unknown. The pathological pattern involves the deposition of microcrystals in various parts of the joint; the most common material deposited is calcium pyrophosphate dihydrate (CPPD). Chondrocalcinosis is a metabolic joint disease which may affect any joint in the body. Its forms range from the comparatively benign to the severely destructive.

The knee is among the most commonly affected joints. In the patellofemoral joint, chondrocalcinosis occurs in a form that mimics OA, and, above all, in a destructive form.

The clinical picture is marked by spontaneous serosanguinous effusions of increasing frequency and severity. Otherwise, the signs and symptoms are those of primary OA.

Radiological features

Both knees are affected. The patella is thinned out overall, with the lateral facet worst affected. The trochlea is worn or even destroyed, resulting in patellar subluxation (fig. 9). The joint surfaces are jagged and irregular, a feature that distinguishes chondrocalcinosis from primary OA. If earlier radiographs are available, they may be scrutinized for calcium deposits, which will show up either as a thin linear deposit along all or part of the joint line, or, in some cases, as discrete densities in the patellar cartilage. Patellofemoral

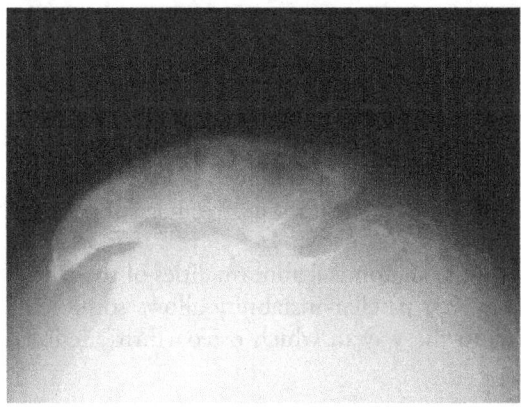

Fig. 9. – Typical pattern in chondrocalcinosis: The joint surfaces are jagged and irregular.

involvement may occur in the absence of tibiofemoral or meniscal disease; however, for treatment purposes, chondrocalcinosis must be looked upon as a disorder affecting the entire joint as well as other joints in the body.

Post-traumatic OA

Epidemiology and clinical manifestations

9% of the isolatead patellofemoral arthritis. The mean age is 54 years old. Patellar fractures account for 0.5% to 1.7% of all fractures involving the knee joint (7).

These fractures typically produce patellofemoral OA in the long term (38).

The factors that may give rise to OA are linked to the accident pattern, and to the fracture mechanism. A direct blow to the patella, with crushing of the cartilage and the production of a comminuted fracture, is notorious as a source of OA (8, 10); equally, suboptimal treatment of the injury, with poor reduction, gaps > 2mm, and/or residual joint incongruity > 1mm, is likely to result in OA (8,10).

Two further factors tend to put the patient at increased risk of OA developing in the long term: manipulation under anaesthesia to mobilize a stiff knee, which leads to diffuse cartilage damage, and infections.

Radiological features

The radiographic appearance is very variable. Usually, the pattern is one of global patelolofemoral OA. One of the most common features is patella magna (an enlarged patella overhanging the trochlea on both the medial and the lateral sides).

OA and patellar instability

Epidemiology and clinical manifestations

33% of the isolatead patellofemoral arthritis. This is perhaps the most important of the aetiologies of OA, since it is the only one in which preventive treatment may be considered. The mean age is 55 years old, a little bit younger than the primary arthritis.

The percentage of OA patients with a history of proven patellar instability varies with the series. Different authors have quoted between 8% and 53% (3, 13, 27). Few study results are available concerning patellar dislocation as an aetiological factor predisposing to OA (12, 30). However, all the studies of patellofemoral arthroplasty (3, 13, 27) have included a percentage of patients with a history of patellar dislocation.

A study of the biomechanics and the anatomical abnormalities of the patellofemoral joint in patients with proven patellar instability allows some tentative conclusions to be drawn as to the way in which osteoarthritic lesions have come about.

Dislocation (fig. 10)

As the patella dislocates, the patellar cartilage is damaged; sometimes, there are small articular fractures. Mirror-image lesions will be found on the lateral aspect of the trochlea, or even on the lateral condyle.

Extensor mechanism malalignment (fig. 11)

This malalignment has been extensively discussed in the English-language literature, where the underlying defect has been defined in terms of an excessive Q angle. To our way of thinking, malalignment is due to an increase in the distance between the tibial tubercle and the deepest part of the trochlear groove (TT-TG) (23), which increases the dislocating force acting on the patella. Excessively high and asymmetrical pressure peaks occur on the lateral facet of the trochlea and on the lateral facet of the patella.

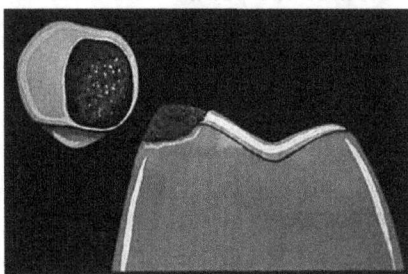

Fig. 10. – Dislocation involves patellar and trochlear cartilage trauma; a chondral or osteochondral fragment may be chipped off. These cartilage lesions may lead to OA.

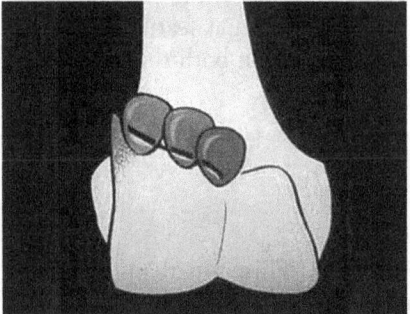

Fig. 11. – Extensor mechanism malalignment, with an increase in the TT-TG, will increase the dislocating forces and the pressure in the lateral patellofemoral compartment. These changes may give rise to OA.

Lack of congruency between the patella and the trochlea

Trochlear dysplasia (14, 17, 21) and, to a lesser extent, patellar dysplasia (41) will lead to a lack of congruency between the two mating surfaces. Pressure will be asymmetrically distributed, and the patellofemoral joint will become unstable. Under these circumstances, two factors may produce OA.

– *Overall trochlear* prominence, in severe (grade B or D) dysplasia, will cause impingement of the patella on the trochlea every time the knee is flexed, and increase the patellofemoral contact stresses as the angle of flexion increases (fig. 12). Mirror-image grade 3 and 4 cartilage lesions will be seen, typically extending the entire length of the patella (fig. 13). These lesions are the harbingers of OA.

– The *asymmetry of the trochlear facets* seen in grade C and grade D trochlear dysplasia will lead to permanent tilting of the patella, which, in turn, will worsen the asymmetrical pressure distribution in the patellofemoral joint (17).

It follows that whenever a young patient presents with patellofemoral OA, a careful search should be made for any episodes of dislocation in the patient's history, and radiographs should be scrutinized with meticulous care to detect any anatomical abnormalities that may cause patellar instability.

A detailed history should be taken to obtain further information on any patellar dislocation in the past. The sort of incident to elicit would be a frankly traumatic event, during which the patient felt his or her patella dislocate and then reduce. At least in the early stages, such incidents will invariably be followed by massive effusion (haemarthrosis). As the events become more frequent, dislocation tends to be followed by hydarthrosis caused by the cartilage lesions.

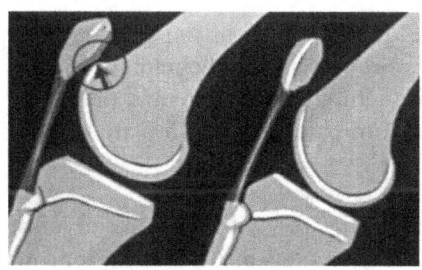

Fig. 12. – Trochlear prominence in high-grade trochlear dysplasia leads to impingement between the proximal trochlea and the central portion of the patella. This will damage a strip of cartilage across the patella.

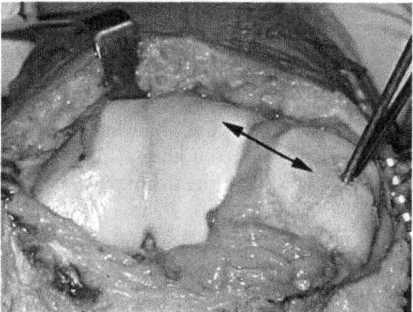

Fig. 13. – Patellar instability seen at surgery. There are mirror-image lesions on the trochlea and the patella. These lesions, going down to subchondral bone, are pre-osteoarthritic.

Osteoarthritic lesions are seen only in cases of severe trochlear dysplasia. This form of OA occurs in subjects under the age of 50 years.

As the conditon of the joint progressively worsens, it becomes increasingly difficult to analyze the causative factors of instability on the radiographs.

Medial patellofemoral OA following medialization for anterior knee pain (18)

Epidemiology and clinical manifestations

This form of patellofemoral OA involves the medial compartment, a pattern that is extremely rare in primary OA. The patients concerned will have had anterior knee pain in the past, with the condition affecting one or both knees, and attributed to a patellar syndrome. There will be no history of trauma with effusion, and no report of any sensation of the patella dislocating. Typically, these patients will have been managed, some ten years previously, with tibial tubercle anteriorization plus medialization combined with a lateral release. After an initial period of relief from anterior knee pain, the former clinical manifestations will have gradually reappeared, together with recurrent effusions. Eventually, the pain will have become constant and disabling.

Radiographic features

The clinical history plus the radiographic pattern allow the diagnosis to be made.

On the preoperative radiographs, there will be no evidence of trochlear dysplasia or patella alta. If, at the time of the index surgery, a CT had been made, it would not have shown an increased TT-TG, nor excessive tilting of the patella.

If no radiological records are available from the time of the index procedure, the fellow knee should be studied. The contralateral radiograph will show a perfectly healthy patella. This pattern is useful for the differential diagnosis of the condition, since the factors that lead to patellar instability are known to be often bilateral.

The radiographs of the affected knee are very typical.

The axial view shows medial impingement (fig. 14), with some loss of joint space. This view must be truly axial in 30°, or even in 60°, of flexion, in

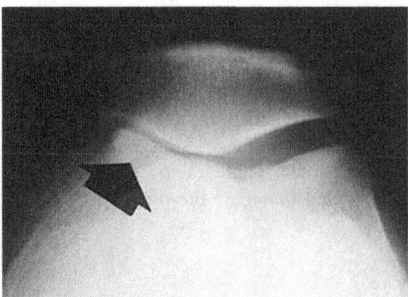

Fig. 14. – The 30° axial view shows iatrogenic medial patellofemoral OA following excessive medialization for anterior knee pain. The trochlear angle is > 145°; the trochlea is not dysplastic.

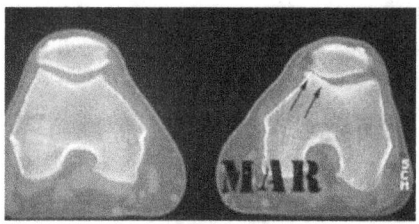

Fig. 15. – The CT scan shows medial loss of patellofemoral joint space, and a negative tilt of the patella. A comparison with the healthy fellow knee shows the extent to which the involved knee has been affected by prior surgery.

order to bring out the loss of joint space. The radiological work-up should also include two CT cuts of the patella, to establish the TT-TG, which will be found to be short (between 0 and 5mm), and may be negative (fig. 6). The value found is then compared with that on the healthy side, which is typically between 15mm and 20mm. The CT scan will also provide the best evidence of medial patellofemoral impingement, and of the virtual absence of patellar tilt (fig. 15). If CT arthrography is available, the medial loss of cartilage space may be quantified, as may the amount of cartilage remaining at the bottom of the trochlear groove, on the lateral facet of the trochlea, and on the lateral facet of the patella.

The height of the patella should be carefully measured. Excessive medialization may be associated with a low-riding patella, which could be corrected at surgery for the lateralization of the tibial tubercle.

Treatment modalities as a function of the aetiology of the condition (excluding prosthetic patellofemoral joint replacement)

The treatment modalities described below apply to patients aged under 60 years suffering from incipient patellofemoral OA.

The first line of treatment is non-surgical. The medical side of regimen consists in the use of anti-inflammatories, to reduce effusion and synovitis. This is complemented by physical therapy and rehabilitation, which involve two major approaches:

– *"running-in" of the joint* – this is done through bicycling, to polish the remaining cartilage and to smooth any uneven surfaces;

– *extensor and hamstring stretching exercises* – these are designed to diminish patellofemoral pressure during flexion.

The programme is controlled by a physiotherapist. However, in order to work, it must be performed by the patient himself or herself several times a week, without the physiotherapist being present. The patient is reassessed at three months. Only if this non-surgical approach fails will surgery be considered.

Lateral release and vertical lateral patellectomy (fig. 16)

This procedure is designed to reduce the pressure in the lateral patellofemoral compartment. It also aims to abolish the impingement of the lateral patellar

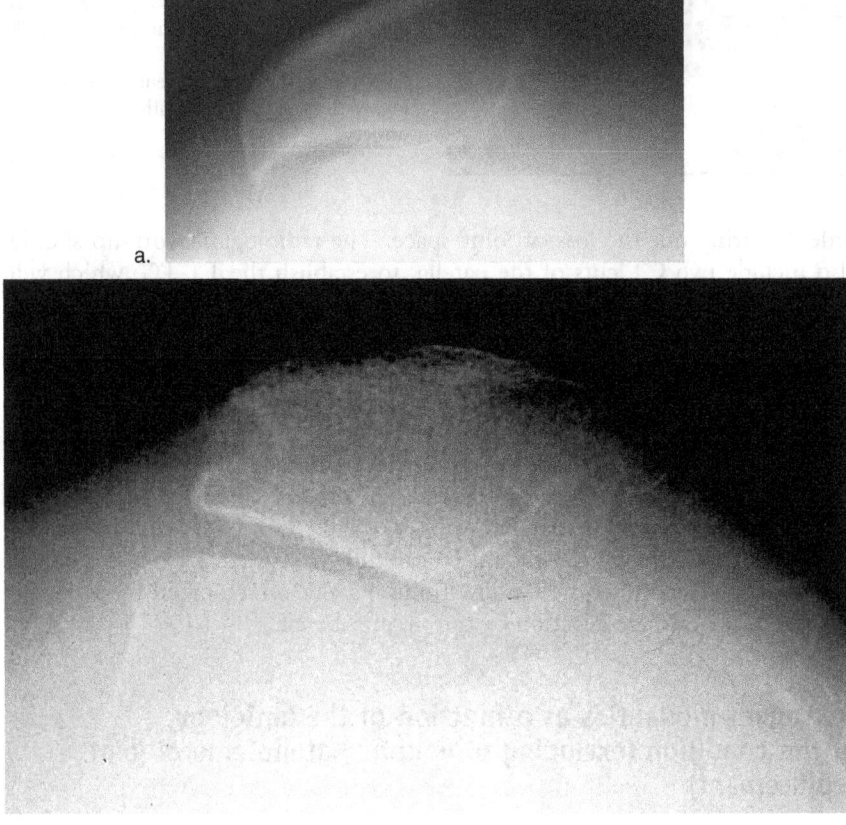

Fig. 16. – Lateral release and vertical lateral patellectomy.
a. 30° axial view before surgery. The patella is laterally subluxed; there is total loss of lateral joint space, and a lateral enthesophyte.
b. 30° axial view after vertical lateral patellectomy and lateral release. Restoration of correct patellar tracking has opened up the patellofemoral joint space. Patellectomy has to be generous (removing a fragment ca. 1.5cm wide).

enthesophytes and the osteophytes on the lateral facet of the trochlea, which causes the catching, locking, reflex instability, and recurrent episodes of hydarthrosis. A procedure confined to a simple lateral release cannot be expected to effect a lasting cure, and must be combined with a vertical lateral patellectomy. Resection must be wide enough (1.5cm) to remove more than just the bony spurs. The superolateral osteophytes on the trochlea may be trimmed at the same time.

Tibial tubercle medialization and/or advancement

This is the most extensively described procedure (32, 33) for the palliative treatment of patellofemoral OA. It may be done in isolation, or combined with a Maquet procedure involving a graft (22). An isolated Maquet tibial tubercle elevation is probably no longer indicated: Whilst the procedure is biomechanically sound (6, 33), the outcomes in patients with patellofemoral pain have not been universally satisfactory (37). The patient is left with difficulty kneeling, because of the prominence of the tibial tubercle; the bulge on the front of the tibia is also unsightly. Medialization tends to produce 70% of good and excellent results (22). The studies published in the literature do not state whether the patients had any coexisting risk factors for instability, and do not break down the treatments by aetiological groups.

CT arthrography or CT can guide the decision on whether to operate, and on the most appropriate procedure to be adopted.

Where there is an excessive TT-TG, a very dysplastic trochlea, and, above all, a tilted patella associated with chronic subluxation, the surgeon may opt for realignment through medialization, if need be combined with trochlear remodelling (trochleoplasty) (17, 19, 34). These procedures should be combined with a vertical lateral patellectomy and a lateral release. The course of action should be considered very carefully, since there is a danger of making things worse rather than better for the patient. The severity of the patient's disability must be carefully assessed.

Distal transfer of the patella is no longer an appropriate treatment of OA, since it increases the patellofemoral contact stresses, and since the risk of patellar dislocation diminishes as the OA advances.

Peripheral patellar remodelling (29)

This procedure is designed specifically for cases of post-traumatic OA with patella magna.

It consists in wide medial and lateral release plus a reduction in the overall bony bulk of the patella. Particular care should be taken to ensure that the quadriceps and patellar tendon attachments are left intact, so as not to weaken the extensor mechanism (fig. 17).

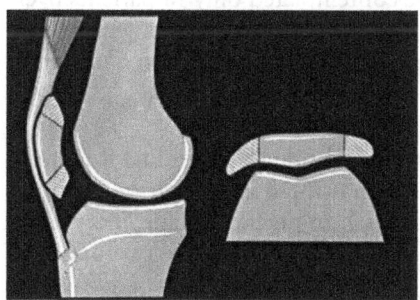

Fig. 17. – Peripheral patellar remodelling is indicated in knees with patella magna. First, a medial and a lateral release are performed; next, the patella is trimmed superiorly, inferiorly, medially, and laterally. Particular care should be taken to leave the quadriceps and patellar tendon attachments intact, so as not to weaken the extensor mechanism. The lateral retinaculum is left unsutured.

Tibial tubercle lateralization

This procedure is indicated only in cases of medial patellofemoral OA following excessive medialization. CT arthrography should be performed to confirm that there is cartilage remaining at the bottom of the trochlear groove and on the lateral trochlear facet. The lateral retinaculum is not released; the medial retinaculum is lengthened. Lateralization should be generous (on average ca. 15mm). In cases of patella infera, lateralization may be combined with a proximal transfer of the tibial tubercle.

The radiological result should not be expected to be perfect: in 26% of the cases, the axial view will still show undercorrection, with a certain amount of medial impingement. However, the clinical outcome has been found to be satisfactory in 81% of the cases (18).

PatelloFemoral Joint Arthroplasty (1)

In case of PFJ replacement we have to deal with the anatomy, the extensor mechanism alignment and the patellofemoral dysplasia. Two types of PFJ prosthesis are available.

The first is a "resurfacing prosthesis" with no bony trochlear cut, the positioning of this implant has to follow the anatomy and the landmark is the trochlear groove.

The second type of implant is the "anatomic prosthesis" which corresponds to a TKA trochlea and the medio-lateral positioning is free and done after the trochlea cut as it is done in a TKA.

The analysis of 211 PFJAs showed that the best results were with the resurfacing prosthesis combined to a distal realignment (93% at 11 years) and with an anatomic prosthesis with a trochlea lateralisation (proximal realignment) (95% at 7 years). The survival curves were 76% with the resurfacing prosthesis with no distal realignment. This shows that the PFJ dysplasia has to be corrected in the use of a PFJA. In this series the failure by instability were always in PFJA without any realignment.

Total knee replacement

Total knee r eplacement (TKR) should be contemplated only in patients over the age of 60, with a low-demand sedentary life style. In patients with patellofemoral primary OA, certain technical points will need to be borne in mind.

Thickness of the patella

The patella is often thin, especially on the lateral side. The residual thickness of the patella after resection must be such that there is no risk of fracture. The fracture's risk increased in patella wiberg III. In practical terms, this means a thickness of at least 13mm. If the patella is too thin, there are two options:

– the surgeon may perform peripheral patellar remodelling, and refrain from inserting a patellar prosthesis;
– the more ambitious alternative (to be considered where the inadequate thickness is confined to the lateral one-third of the patella) consists in placing a cancellous graft between the polyethylene prosthesis and the patella, at the cementing stage.

Extensor mechanism realignment

Patients with a history of patellar surgery (medialization, advancement, distal transfer, etc.) may well have been left with malalignment of the extensor mechanism; in particular, there may be excessive medialization. The preoperative CT scans will allow the TT-TG to be measured, and to compare the value obtained with that in the fellow knee (providing that the contralateral knee has not previously been operated on).

It may be necessary to perform tibial tubercle osteotomy to restore a normal TT-TG (39). In this context, knee prostheses with a mobile bearing may be useful, since they allow minor differences to be corrected without the need for transferring the tibial tubercle.

In all knees undergoing TKR, a lateral release must be performed (28, 39); where required, this release should be associated with a vertical lateral patellectomy.

Laskin and Davis (28) compared the results of arthroplasty in patellofemoral OA and in tricompartmental OA, and found patients who had undergone TKR for patellofemoral OA to have better ROM recovery and better Knee Scores and Function Scores. Parvizi *et al.* (39) stressed the quality of the clinical results, and considered TKR to be a treatment of choice in advanced patellofemoral OA.

Conclusion

Patellofemoral OA is a condition with very specific treatment principles. Research is still required to establish the relationship between patellar instability and the development of OA in the long term, since this aetiology may be amenable to preventive treatment. Attention should be paid to the iatrogenic medial patellofemoral OA which may occur following medialization for anterior knee pain rather than for patellar instability. Careful scrutiny of the current and, where available, any previous radiographs to detect factors predisposing to instability is of great importance in establishing the aetiology of the condition. CT and CT arthrography may help to establish the most appropriate form of treatment.

Advanced patellofemoral OA is best managed with TKR.

References

1. Dejour D, Allain J (2004) Histoire naturelle de l'arthrose fémoro-patellaire isolée. Rev Chir Orthop 90 1S69-1S129 suppl. au n°5
2. Ahlbäck S, Mattsson S (1978) Patella alta and gonarthrosis. Acta Radiol Diagn 19: 578-84
3. Argenson JN, Guillaume JM, Aubaniac JM (1995) Is there a place for patellofemoral arthroplasty? Clin Orthop 321: 162-7
4. Bernageau J, Goutallier D (1984) Examen radiologique de l'articulation fémoro-patellaire. In: Actualités rhumatologiques, Expansion Scientifique Française, Paris, p. 105
5. Blackburne JS, Peel TE (1977) A new method of measuring patellar height. J Bone Joint Surg Br 59: 241-2

6. Blaimont P, Van Elegem P, Alamech M *et al.* (1985) Contribution à l'étude des contraintes patellaires : hypothèse pathogénique de l'arthrose fémoro-patellaire. Rev Chir Orthop 71, Suppl. II: 99-101

7. Bonnel F, Hafdi CH (1985) Résultats précoces du traitement des fractures de la rotule. In: L'appareil extenseur du genou, Masson, Paris, p. 143

8. Carpenter JE, Kasman R, Matthews LS (1993) Fractures of the patella. Bone Joint Surg Am 75: 1550-61

9. Caton J, Deschamps G, Chambat P *et al.* (1982) Les rotules basses : à propos de 128 observations. Rev Chir Orthop 68: 317-25

10. Chrisman OD, Ladenbauer-Bellis IM, Panjabi M *et al.* (1981) The relationship of mechanical trauma and the early biochemical reactions of osteoarthritic cartilage. Clin Orthop 161: 275-84

11. Cooper C, McAlindon T, Snow S *et al.* (1994) Mechanical and constitutional risk factors for symptomatic knee osteoarthritis: differences between medial tibiofemoral and patellofemoral disease. J Rheumatol 21: 307-13

12. Crosby EB, Insall J (1976) Recurrent dislocation of the patella. Relation of treatment to osteoarthritis. J Bone Joint Surg Am 58: 9-13

13. De Cloedt P, Legaye J, Lokietek W (1999) Femoro-patellar prosthesis. A retrospective study of 45 consecutive cases with a follow-up of 3-12 years. Acta Orthop Belg 65: 170-5

14. Dejour H, Walch G, Neyret P *et al.* (1990) La dysplasie de la trochlée fémorale. Rev Chir Orthop 76: 45-54

15. Dejour D, Levigne C, Dejour H (1995) La rotule basse post-opératoire. Traitement par allongement du tendon rotulien. Rev Chir Orthop 81: 286-95

16. Dejour D, David MD, Lecoultre B (2007) Osteotomies in Patello-Femoral Instabilities. Sports Medicine & Arthroscopy Review 15 (1): 39-46

17. Dejour D, Nove-Josserand L, Walch G (1998) Patellofemoral Disorders – Classification and an Approach to Operative Treatment for Instability. In: Chang KM (ed) Controversies in Orthopedic Sports Medicine, Williams & Wilkins, Baltimore, p. 235

18. Dejour D, Panisset JC, Dejour H (1999) Résultats de 32 lateralisations de tubérosité tibiale antérieure après hypermédialisation. Rev Chir Orthop 85, Suppl. III: 93

19. Dejour D, Locatelli E (2001) Patellar instability in adults. Surgical techniques. In: Orthopaedics and Traumatology. Éditions Scientifiques et Médicales Elsevier, Paris, 55-520-A-10, 6

20. Falconnet M (1985) Étude et devenir des gonarthroses. Rhumatologie 37: 41-5

21. Fitoussi F, Akoure S, Chouteau Y *et al.* (1994) Profondeur de la trochlée et arthrose fémoropatellaire. Rev Chir Orthop 80: 520-4

22. Fulkerson JP (1983) Anteromedialization of the tibial tuberosity for patellofemoral malalignment. Clin Orthop 177: 176-81

23. Goutailler D, Bernageau J, Lecudonnec B (1978) Mesure de l'écart tubérosité tibiale antérieure-gorge de la trochlée (TA-GT). Technique. Résultats. Intérêt. Rev Chir Orthop 64: 423-8

24. Insall J, Salvati E (1971) Patella position in the normal knee joint. Radiology 101: 101-4

25. Iwano T, Kurosawa H, Tokuyama H *et al.* (1990) Roentgenographic and clinical findings of patellofemoral osteoarthrosis. With special reference to its relationship to femorotibial osteoarthrosis and etiologic factors. Clin Orthop 252: 190-7

26. Knutsson F (1941) Über die Röntgenologie des Femoropatellargelenks sowie eine gute Projektion für das Kniegelenk. Acta Radiol 22: 371-6

27. Krajca-Radcliffe JB, Coker TP (1996) Patello-femoral arthroplasty. A 2- to 18-year follow-up study. Clin Orthop 330: 143-51

28. Laskin RS, Davis J (1999) Total knee replacement in patients with patellofemoral arthritis. American Academy of Orthopaedic Surgeons, Anaheim, CA, 4-8 February

29. Lerat JL, Moyen B (1992) La patelloplastie périphérique ou remodelage périphérique de la rotule. 67th Annual Meeting of SOFCOT, Paris, 11 November

30. Mäenpää H, Lehto MU (1997) Patellofemoral osteoarthritis after patellar dislocation. Clin Orthop 339: 156-62

31. Malghem J, Maldague B (1989) Depth insufficiency of the proximal trochlear groove on lateral radiographs of the knee: relation to patellar dislocation. Radiology 170: 507-10
32. Maquet P (1976) Advancement of the tibial tuberosity. Clin Orthop 115: 225-30
33. Maquet P (1984) Biomechanics of the knee. 2nd ed. Springer, Berlin, Heidelberg New York
34. Masse Y (1978) La trochléoplastie : restauration de la gouttière trochléenne dans les sub-luxations et luxations de la rotule. Rev Chir Orthop 64: 3-17
35. McAlindon T, Zhang Y, Hannan M et al. (1996) Are risk factors for patellofemoral and tibiofemoral knee osteoarthritis different? J Rheumatol 23: 332-7
36. McAlindon TE, Snow S, Cooper C et al. (1992) Radiographic patterns of osteoarthritis of the knee joint in the community: the importance of the patellofemoral joint. Ann Rheum Dis 51: 844-9
37. Morshuis WJ, Pavlov PW, De Rooy KP (1990) Anteromedialisation of the tibial tubero-sity in the treatment of patellofemoral pain and malalignment. Clin Orthop 255: 242-50
38. Neyret P, Selmi TAS, Chatain F et al. (1999) De la fracture de rotule à l'arthrose fémoro-patellaire In: Pathologie fémoro-patellaire. Expansion Scientifique Publication, Paris, p. 103
39. Parvizi J, Pagnano MW, Stuart MJ et al. (2001) Total knee arthroplasty in patients with isolated patellofemoral arthritis. American Academy of Orthopaedic Surgeons, San Francisco, CA, 28 February-4 March
40. Tavernier T, Dejour D (2001) Imagerie du genou : quel examen choisir ? In: Encyclopédie Médico-Chirurgicale. Éditions Scientifiques et Médicales Elsevier, Paris, 30-433-A-20, 18
41. Wiberg G (1941) Roentgen graphic and anatomic studies on the femoropatellar joint. Acta Orthop Scand 12: 319-410

ACL and arthritis

M. Clatworthy

Introduction

The treatment of the young ACL deficient patients with an osteoarthritic knee has been a great dilemma for orthopaedic surgeons. The treatment options in the past have been limited and the literature gave us little direction. Patients were granted analgesics, anti-inflammatories, physical therapy and were braced until they were old enough for total knee replacement. However in the last eight years surprisingly good results have been reported in these patients with anterior cruciate reconstruction, high tibial osteotomies, meniscal allografts and combined procedures.

In this review we will assess the natural history of osteoarthritis in the anterior cruciate deficient knee and examine the factors which may influence its progression. These include meniscal damage, osteochondral lesions, malalignment, concomitant ligamentous pathology, biological factors and surgery. We critique the recent literature. The role of anterior cruciate reconstruction, high tibial osteotomy in the coronal and sagittal plane, meniscal allografts and combined procedures are reviewed. Finally we will present our approach.

Natural history

The incidence and progression of osteoarthritis following an anterior cruciate disruption is not clearly determined. It is likely that it is dependant not solely on the ligament tear but also the sequelae of this injury; meniscal tears, osteochondral lesions and cytokine release following the injury. Limb alignment also plays a significant role.

Radiographic degenerative changes following an ACL injury have been reported in 20%-88% of cases (5, 43, 56, 60, 66, 69, 75, 80, 84). Increased anterior translation of the tibia places abnormal load on the medial meniscus leading to a high incidence of medial meniscal damage. The combination of an ACL deficient knee and posterior medial meniscal dysfunction results in posteromedial osteoarthritis (fig. 1). The posterior slope of the tibia increases and a cupped posterior osteophyte (cupola) may develop with time (fig. 2). This prevents further anterior translation, reducing instability.

Most studies show a correlation with a meniscectomy. MacDaniel and Dameron (61) in an average 10 years follow-up of untreated ACL's exhibited

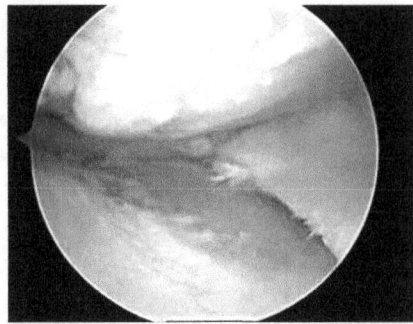

Fig. 1. – Arthroscopic photo of posteromedial arthritis.

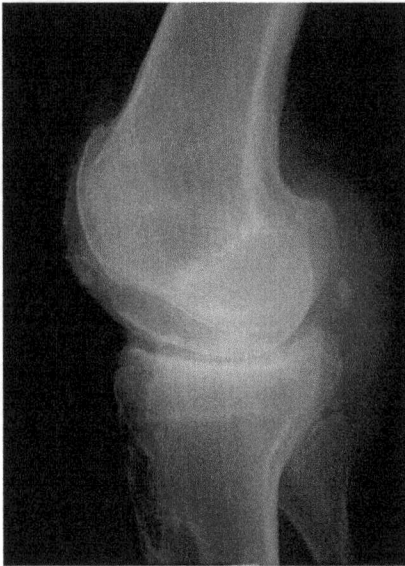

Fig. 2. – Lateral radiographs 12 years following a conservatively treated ACL knee. Note the increased in posterior slope and posterior osteophyte.

radiographic osteoarthritis in 33% of cases. They revealed a definite relationship between osteoarthritis and a varus deformity, medial meniscectomy and medial joint space narrowing. Sherman (80) reported that patients with chronic ACL deficient knees and a meniscectomy showed more progressive degenerative changes by radiographic criteria. However at 10 years all knees were doing poorly regardless of meniscal status. Allen (3) in a follow-up of 210 knees 10-22 years after meniscectomy reported a higher incidence of osteoarthritis after lateral meniscectomy or with abnormal alignment. Lynch (56) in his evaluation of stable ACL reconstructions reported that only 3% of knees with both menisci intact had greater than two Fairbank changes in comparison with 88% in the knees that had a partial or total meniscectomy. In contrast Sommerlath (85) found no correlation with osteoarthritic changes and meniscal integrity however the incidence of radiographic changes was universally high: 50%-60% at 6-8 years.

Indelicato (35) has demonstrated an increased incidence of articular surface disease in the chronically lax ACL (54%) compared with the acute knee (23%) however we are unaware of any published study that has correlated the extent of chondral damage with osteoarthritic progression.

By reconstructing the anterior cruciate ligament we seek stability and consequently protection of the menisci and articular cartilage. We endeavour to alter the natural history of osteoarthritic progression. Four recent studies (23, 40, 42, 76) have compared the incidence and progression of osteoarthritis in patients with an isolated ACL injury treated acutely with a chronic group that have had meniscal and osteochondral pathology. All demonstrate better outcome and decreased osteoarthritis if surgery is performed early and if the menisci and articular cartilage are intact at the time of surgery.

Factors affecting the progression of osteoarthritis

Meniscal lesions

Fairbank (25) was the first to associate the loss of the meniscus with an accelerated development of osteoarthritis. Meniscectomy has been shown not only to alter the load bearing characteristics of the knee joint but also influence stability. This is of major importance in the cruciate deficient knee.

The meniscus serves many roles. These include transmission of weight bearing load (2, 6, 10, 12, 30, 45, 72, 83), shock absorption thus protecting the articular cartilage (72, 88), joint stability by contouring the tibial plateau to match the femoral condyles (16) and distribution of synovial fluid and nutrients.

In the anterior cruciate deficient knee the posterior horn of the medial meniscus is the primary stabilizer to anterior translation (82). This places the posterior horn under high loads with translation and explains the high incidence of secondary meniscal tears in chronic ACL insufficiency. Rupture of the posterior horn leads to even greater anterior translation (22, 49, 57) resulting in increased instability. Osteoarthritis is likely to ensue.

Clinical studies support this biomechanical rationale (22, 29, 37). A long term follow-up (29) (minimum 15 years, range 15-52 years) of 328 patients with an ACL deficient knee from four centers found that best correlation with the degree of osteoarthritis was the time to meniscectomy. Stabilization decreased the progression of arthritis but to a lesser degree than meniscal retention. They concluded that preservation of as much meniscus tissue as possible is the best warranty for slowing down degenerative arthritis after cruciate ligament injury. De Jour (22) found that in patients who underwent an ACL reconstruction two years post injury medial meniscal tears occurred in 30% and lateral meniscal tears in 7%. This increased to 60% for the medial meniscus and 15% for the lateral meniscus 10 years from injury. Two studies have evaluated the incidence of a secondary meniscal lesion following an isolated ACL injury without initial meniscal damage. Shelton *et al.* (79) followed 44 conservatively treated ACL deficient patients prospectively who elected to return to sports with a brace. They had a normal meniscus on MRI post injury. In the 29 patients requiring reconstruction 23 menisci were torn in 17 patients. Finsterbush (28) reviewed 98 patients who had an isolated ACL rupture at diagnostic arthroscopy. A re-look arthroscopy was performed in 34 patients who had been treated conservatively at a mean of 4.2 years. A meniscal lesion was seen in 71% of these patients.

Osteochondral lesions

At the time of an ACL rupture there is anterior subluxation of the tibia on the femur with an associated valgus force. This results in a compressive load and shear force on the articular cartilage. Characteristic osteochondral lesions occur on the posterolateral aspect of the tibia and the anterolateral aspect of the lateral femoral condyle in approximately 80% of patients with an acute ACL injury (31, 44, 58, 61, 74, 85). On T1 weighted images a decreased signal is observed, while T2 weighted images reveal an increased signal. Although the MRI findings are dramatic, the radiographic and arthroscopic appearances are often normal and thus the terms "occult osteochondral lesion" or "bone bruise" have been popularized.

The long term sequelae of these bone bruises has yet to be determined. A clinical and MR imaging evaluation of occult osteochondral lesions in 23 reconstructed patients has recently been reported 6 years following the initial injury (24). All patients had T1 weighted low signal intensity changes in the subchondral bone on the lateral tibial plateau and the lateral femoral condyle

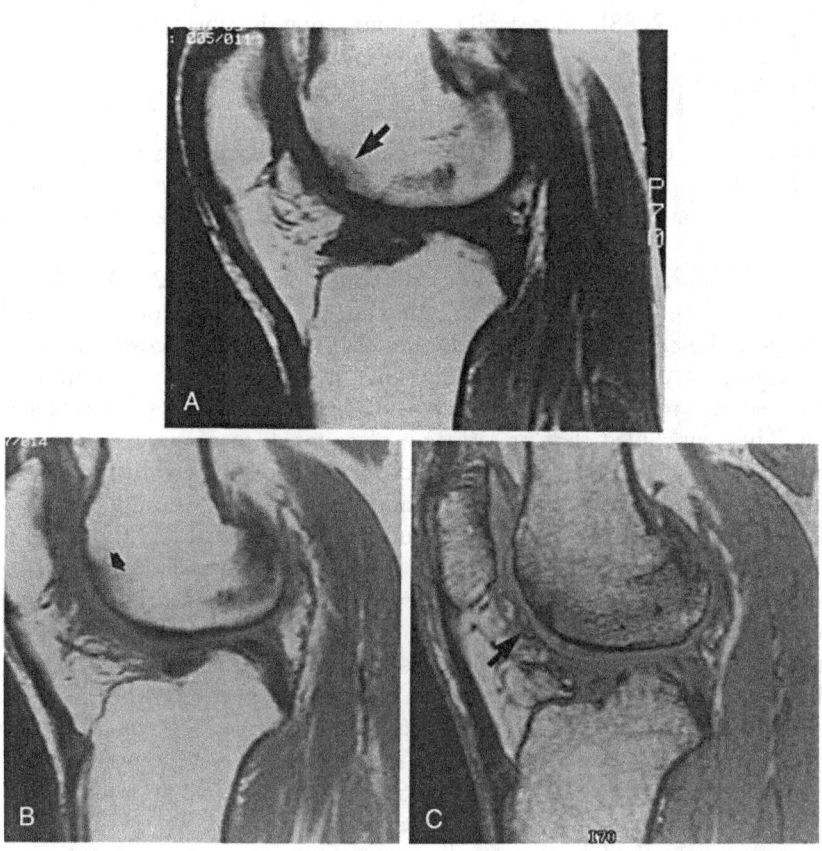

Fig. 3.
A: Sagittal T1 at the time of injury. Note decreased signal in subchondral bone in the lateral femoral condyle (arrow).
B: Sagittal T1 6.5 years after injury. Note persistent decreased signal in the area (arrow).
C: Sagittal three dimensional volume GRASS 6.5 years after injury. Note focal articular thinning (intermediate signal at arrow, superficial to dark line of cortical bone) overlying area of subchondral bone injury.

on index MRI. The follow-up MRI revealed that the subchondral changes initially present on the lateral femoral condyle reverted to normal marrow signal in only 8 of 23 patients. Chondral thinning was identified in two patients in the index MRI compared with 13 at 6 years (fig. 3A-3C). In all cases the area of cartilage thinning was adjacent to the initial subchondral lesions. There was greater resolution in the lateral tibial plateau. Only 8 patients had persistent subchondral marrow changes however no chondral thinning was seen. In this small group of patients no significant clinical differences could be found between patients with normal and abnormal MRI findings.

Concomitant ligamentous pathology

Two studies demonstrate an increased incidence of arthritis with a concomitant PCL rupture. Kullmer *et al.* (46) in their review of 77 patients treated with a synthetic ACL reconstruction evaluated the risk factors for osteoarthritis. The greatest risk factor was an additional PCL rupture. The second and only other significant risk factor was a meniscal injury.

For conservatively treated patients Jacobsen (39) reported that severe osteoarthritis developed in all patients with a combined cruciate injury 5 years post injury.

To our knowledge there are no studies that evaluate the contribution of a posterolateral corner injury to the development of osteoarthritis in the anterior cruciate deficient knee however these injuries result in a varus tilt on unilateral weight bearing. This significantly increases the varus stresses and thus is likely to be highly arthrogenic (22).

Two papers show no arthritic progression with an associated collateral ligament injury (27, 46).

Alignment

An alteration in the coronal alignment of the knee will place the mechanical axis eccentrically leading to an increased load through this compartment and subsequent osteoarthritis. The most common and arthrogenic cause of malalignment is a meniscectomy. An ACL rupture itself is accompanied by displacement of the centre of rotation towards the medial compartment (51). This increase in stress is explained by medial hyper-rotation of the tibia or femoral lateral rotation, both of which lead to increased medial forces. Another cause of the more common varus knee associated with ACL deficiency is posterolateral instability. This leads to lateral de-coaptation i.e. loss of contact between the femur and tibia during stance. If progressive it can lead to a varus thrust with further loading of the medial compartment during weight bearing. The significance of congenital genu varum in the development of osteoarthritis is controversial. De Jour (22) states that in the absence of a meniscoligamentous lesion the patient with constitutional genu varum of 6° does not have an increased risk.

The relationship between tibial slope and anterior tibial translation on monopodal weight bearing has been demonstrated in an analysis of 281 cases of unilateral rupture of the ACL (8) (fig. 4). There is a significant linear relationship between tibial slope and anterior translation for both the normal and injured knee. Thus as the slope increased so did the translation. The regression curve demonstrates that for every 10° increase in the backward inclination of the tibial plateau anterior tibial translation is increased 6mm. At present no relationship has been established between increased tibial slope and arthritic progression.

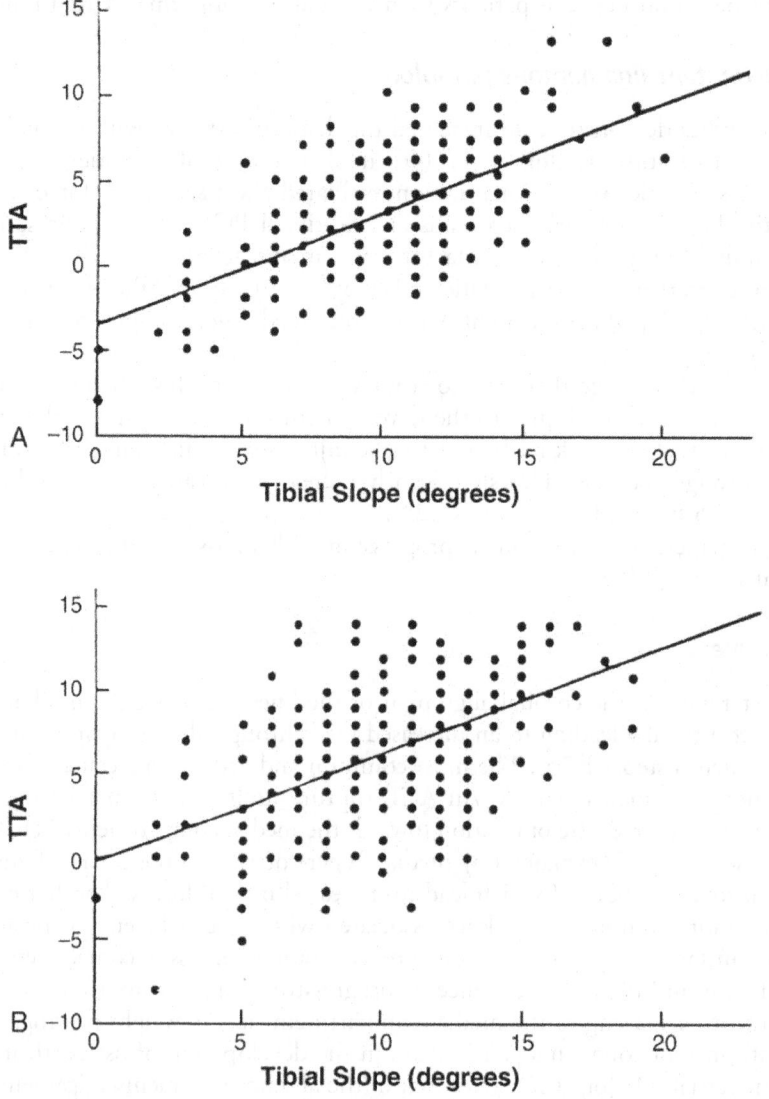

Fig. 4. – Relationship between tibial slope and anterior tibial translation on monopodal weight bearing. **A:** Normal knee, **B:** ACL tear. (From Bonnin M: La subluxation tibiale antérieure en appui monopodal dans les ruptures du ligament croisé antérieur. Étude clinique et bio-mécanique. Thèse Med Lyon, 1990.)

Surgery

Until recently there has been great controversy as to whether a reconstruction delays or hastens osteoarthritis. There are no randomised prospective trials to evaluate this dilemma. Studies performed in the 1980's (19, 26, 41, 81) suggest that surgery may speed the development of osteoarthritis. However problems exist with these studies. Most pre-date modern arthroscopic techniques with anatomical placement of the graft and accelerated postoperative rehabilitation. The extremely important variables of meniscal lesions, osteochondral injuries and chronicity of the injury have not been controlled. The most commonly quoted study was that of Daniels (19). In a prospective outcome study he found that the reconstructed patients had a higher level of arthrosis documented by radiographs and bone scan. Although this paper exceeds others, it still has major flaws. The study was not controlled. Younger and more active patients underwent early reconstruction. Patients who had ongoing instability and wanted to remain active had a delayed reconstruction. The more stable and less active were treated conservatively. Thus similar groups were not compared. The study was also performed during a period of evolution in ACL reconstruction techniques. At least 6 different types of ACL reconstruction were performed on 93 patients.

In the last two years five studies have correlated timing of surgery and chondral and meniscal damage at the time of surgery with outcome and arthritic progression. All demonstrate better results with early surgery in patients with no articular cartilage or meniscal damage. Osteoarthritis is negligible in these patients 5-15 years post surgery.

Shelbourne et al. (76) evaluated 928 patients 5 to 15 years after surgery. A normal or nearly normal IKDC rating was found in 87% of patients who had both menisci intact, 70% with partial or total lateral meniscectomies, 63% with partial or total medial meniscectomies, and 60% with both menisci removed.

Jomha, Pinczewski et al. (42) evaluated 72 patients at 7 years. They demonstrated increased osteoarthritic changes in chronic patients even if their menisci were intact as well as a significant deterioration in outcome with torn menisci at the time of surgery. Acute anterior cruciate ligament reconstruction with meniscal preservation was shown to have the lowest incidence of degenerative change. They conclude that their study support early reconstruction of anterior cruciate ligament deficient knees before episodes of giving way occur in individuals intent on continuing activities that involve sidestepping and pivoting. In a later study Pinczewski et al. (20) evaluated a group of 90 patients who had normal menisci at the time of surgery five years post surgery. Patient rating was 90% normal or nearly normal, 98% had a Grade 0 pivot shift and 97% had no degenerative changes seen radiographically. Their study support the view that reconstruction of the ACL is a reliable technique allowing full rehabilitation of the previously injured knee. In the presence of normal menisci there is a low incidence of osteoarthritic change despite continued participation in sporting activity.

Jarvela et al. (40) assessed 91 patients 5-9 years after a patella-tendon bone graft. Patients with early reconstruction had fewer degenerative changes and were more satisfied with the result. They also returned to their pre-injury level of sports activity more often than those patients in the late reconstruction group.

Erickson *et al.* (23) evaluated 164 patients with a median follow-up of 31 months. Patients with associated meniscal injuries had lower IKDC, visual analogue and Lysholm scores than those without such injuries. Patients in whom reconstruction had been carried out less than five months after the injury had better final IKDC scores than the more chronic cases. They conclude that associated meniscal pathology significantly affects the final outcome and early reconstruction seems to be beneficial.

Biological factors

Recent analysis of cytokine levels (14, 15), breakdown products of cartilage (53) and markers of cartilage matrix metabolism (14, 54, 55) in the synovial fluid of cruciate deficient knee suggests that biological as well as biomechanical factors may contribute to osteoarthritis.

Many different cytokines have been implicated in the pathogenesis of osteoarthritis (71). Commonly cited cytokines include interleukin-1 (IL-1), IL-6, IL-8, basic fibroblastic growth factor (bFGF), tumor necrosis factor-α (TNF-α) and granulocyte macrophage colony stimulating factor (GM-CSF). Interleukin-1 receptor antagonist protein (IRAP) and transforming growth factor-β (TGF-β) are two cytokines that have been found to neutralize some of the cartilage catabolic effects of these aforementioned cytokines.

Cameron *et al.* (14) measured the levels of seven cytokine modulators of cartilage metabolism and keratan sulfate, a product of articular cartilage catabolism, in synovial fluid after anterior cruciate ligament rupture. 96 patients were evaluated. 10 knees had an uninjured knee joint, 60 had an acute ACL, 18 a subacute injury and 8 a chronic injury. Normal synovial fluids contained high levels of the IRAP but low concentrations of other cytokines. Immediately after ligament rupture there were large increases in IL-6 and IL-8, TNFα and keratan sulfate. IL-1 levels remained low throughout the course. As the injury became subacute and then chronic, IL-6, TNFα and keratan sulfate levels fell but remained considerably elevated 3 months after injury. Concentrations of IRAP fell dramatically. GM-CSF concentrations were normal acutely and subacutely but 3 months post injury they were elevated ten-fold.

They concluded that their data revealed a persistent and evolving disturbance in cytokine and keratan sulfate profiles within the anterior cruciate ligament deficient knee, suggesting an important biochemical dimension to the development of osteoarthritis.

Other biological risk factors for arthritis are gene variations and mutations. It is evident that there is a differing genetic expression for type II collagen (87, 89). Thus certain patients are predisposed to premature chondral degeneration.

Treatment review

The treatment of osteoarthritis and ACL deficiency is complex and controversial. The patients are often young and active with extensive degenerative changes. Their disease is progressive and there is no cure, rather temporizing options.

Historically these patients have been advised to follow a conservative course. The mainstay of treatment has been analgesics, anti-inflammatories, physical therapy, bracing and modification of activities. These patients persevere with pain and loss of function until they are old enough for total knee replacement. However in the last seven years there have been a number of studies which report encouraging results with osteotomy, isolated ACL reconstructions and combined procedures. More recently combined meniscal transplant and ACL reconstruction is showing encouraging results.

Conservative measures

Conservative modalities include analgesics, anti-inflammatories, chondroprotective agents such as glucosamine and chondrotin sulphate, synovial fluid replacements such as Synvisc, physical therapy and bracing. Bracing can be an excellent modality for these patients as it prevents instability at low loads (7, 52) and can relieve arthritic pain. Recent studies (50, 59) have shown that pain, function, and biomechanical axis can be altered by a brace designed to unload the medial compartment of the knee.

ACL reconstruction

The role of an ACL reconstruction in the osteoarthritic knee is controversial. Some authors have suggested that osteoarthritis is a contraindication to ACL reconstruction (4, 32, 47). Concerns include increased pain, joint contact forces and constraint leading to an increase in the progression of osteoarthritis. Others contend that reconstruction is worthwhile to improve stability, function and proprioception and helps reduce pain with the hope of halting arthritic advancement.

Four recent papers have addressed the success of ACL reconstruction in patients with arthrosis.

Shelbourne (78) reported on 33 patients who had chronic ACL reconstructions at a mean 44.8 months post injury. Inclusion criteria were meniscectomies prior to reconstruction, grade 3 to 4 chondral changes in at least one compartment at arthroscopy and at least mild degeneration on X-ray. Alignment was not determined. Patients who complained of pain and instability tested a brace preoperatively to confirm a decrease in pain from the increased stability achieved with the brace. Patients reported a decrease in pain and increased subjective function measured by a modification of the Cincinnati knee score. They improved from 55 preoperatively to 81 postoperatively. There was a significant increase in stability measured with the KT-1000 from 8.3mm preoperatively to 2.7mm postoperatively. There was no difference in range of motion and strength. The progression of osteoarthritic change was not analyzed.

In a later report Shelbourne (77) expanded this group to 58 patients. 30 of these had a follow up of greater than 5 years (mean 7.2 years). Patients reported similar improvement in pain relief, stability and knee scores. He was able to further show that patients with medial compartment arthrosis reported a better subjective total score (mean 87) than patients with lateral compartment (mean 73) or bicompartmental (mean 79) arthrosis, but there was not a statistically significant difference. There was no correlation between pain, stability, or total scores and time from surgery however patients greater than 5 years post surgery reported a lower activity level. Alignment was not determined however he states that many patients had unicompartmental osteoarthritis, thus were candidates for an osteotomy. No correlation was performed to assess alignment and operative result, however he predicts that this procedure may delay the need for osteotomy.

Noyes (62) evaluated 53 patients who underwent autogenous patella tendon graft ACL reconstruction at a mean of 27 months post surgery. The inclusion criteria were extensive fissuring and fragmentation involving greater than 50% of the articular cartilage (62%) or exposure of subchondral bone (38%). The lesions had to be at least 15mm in diameter. Alignment had to be in the normal range as determined by weight bearing radiographs. He showed that pain was reduced in 70%, giving way was eradicated in 89% and recreational activities were resumed in 79%. The patients' opinion of overall knee condition improved dramatically. Only 71% rated their knee as very good or normal postoperatively compared with 22% preoperatively. Again no assessment was made of arthritic progression. He concludes that the contraindication to ACL reconstruction is subchondral bone exposure on opposing articular surfaces and knees where secondary osseous changes confer stability.

Noyes (63) also reported on a similar group of patients who had an allograft patella tendon reconstruction. He evaluated 40 patients at a mean follow up of 37 months. The inclusion criteria were the same as in the autograft study. Significant improvements were found for pain, giving way, functional limitations with daily and sports activities and the overall knee rating. 55% had returned to mostly light athletics avoiding high impact sports based on advice and were asymptomatic. A follow-up arthroscopy was performed in 60% at a mean of 15 months. None of the articular cartilage lesions noted at the reconstruction had progressed, however in 15% of cases lesions were found in other areas.

Interestingly the allograft group exhibited considerably higher arthrometer side to side differences than the autografts. The mean difference in the allograft group was 4.3mm compared with 0.8mm in the autograft group.

In summary good results are obtained in patients with at least moderate arthritic changes with an ACL reconstruction. Pain, instability and activity level are increased in all four papers however both authors emphasize that the patients must modify their activity level to avoid contact, pivoting and repetitive high loading sports. A brace is a useful adjunct in helping the clinician determine whether the patient's symptoms are coming primarily from the instability or the osteoarthritis.

Osteotomy: coronal and sagittal

Many reports in the literature have addressed the role of a high tibial osteotomy in the older population for predominantly unicompartmental osteoarthritis (1, 17, 18, 33, 36, 38). To our knowledge no published paper has specifically addressed the role of osteotomy alone in the patient with cruciate deficiency and varus osteoarthritis.

Fowler *et al.* have recently reviewed this scenario (44). The inclusion criteria for the study were patients with chronic ACL insufficiency, varus alignment, grade 2 or greater medial compartment degeneration, a varus thrust and symptoms of pain and instability. 8 patients meet the criteria, 7 were reviewed. Patients demonstrated a significant improvement in pain, instability and overall function. Only 2 patients had ongoing instability requiring stabilization 2.5 years following the osteotomy.

Two studies have assessed high tibial osteotomies in young patients. Both studies include patients with cruciate deficient however they did not review these patients as a separate entity. Holden *et al.* (34) reviewed 51 knees at a mean of ten years. The average age of the patients was 41 (range 23-50). 14 of these patients were cruciate deficient. They state "deficiency of the anterior cruciate ligament at the time of injury did not prevent a good result". However instability was not a major complaint in these patients. When all patients were evaluated, 66% were able to participate in recreational activities such as bicycling, swimming, weight lifting, golf and tennis. Only 10% could run. The most important factor in determining a good result was the preoperative level of the patient. The higher the preoperative HSS knee score, the better the result. There was no correlation with the severity of the preoperative arthritis radiographically. They thus conclude that osteotomy provides the best long term results when it is done early.

There is only one report (68) that analyzed results according to level of sports activity or occupation. Odenbring *et al.* reported on 27 patients younger than 50 who underwent HTO for medial osteoarthritis. The mean follow-up was 11 years (range 7-18). They found that 32% performed high activity sports or heavy work and only 13% had no pain with running, while 50% had unlimited painless walking. 4 out of 5 patients with an associated ACL had a high activity level and no patient demonstrated arthritic progression.

Noyes introduced the concept of the double varus knee (varus malalignment and lateral ligamentous laxity) and triple varus knee (double varus with varus recurvatum due to arcuate ligament complex deficiency (67). Gait laboratory analysis of these ACL deficient knees shows high adduction moments. It is postulated that these knees are at increased risk for arthritic progression due to increased medial loads particularly as a partial or total meniscectomy is frequent in these patients. Noyes thus advocates early realignment.

Bonnin (8) developed the technique of altering the tibial slope in the sagittal plane to alter tibial translation. Reducing the tibial slope will increase stability in the anterior cruciate knee while increasing the slope will increase the stability in the posterior cruciate deficient knee. To date no paper has been published analyzing the results of an anterior closing wedge high tibial osteotomy for anterior cruciate insufficiency. However De Jour (21) noted in his paper on ACL reconstruction with tibial osteotomy that postoperative tibial translation correlated with the change in tibial slope. The greater the slope, the greater the translation. A lateral closing wedge tends to decrease tibial slope as surgeons tend to resect less posterior bone resulting in increased slope. If the surgeon favours an anterior opening wedge technique, care must be taken to place the plate posteriorly. This technique is aided by using a sloped puddu plate.

In summary the osteotomy is effective in relieving pain and improves stability in many patients.

Combined ACL reconstruction and osteotomy

The combined procedure is indicated in patients who complain of comparable instability and pain with a malaligned knee. Five papers in the last eight years have evaluated the efficacy of this procedure.

The largest series is from De Jour (21). He reports on 50 knees with chronic ACL deficiency combined with acquired varus alignment at a mean follow up of 3.6 years. The mean age at surgery was 29 (range 18-42). The osteotomy was performed first. Patients predominantly had a lateral closing wedge osteotomy (74%). Those who had tibia varus as a component of the malalignment underwent a medial opening wedge osteotomy (26%). Care was taken to evaluate the tibial slope. An autogenous central third patella tendon graft usually augmented when a Lemaire extra-articular procedure (56%) was performed for the ACL reconstruction. He reported low morbidity and significantly improved clinical symptoms, clinical stability and functional stability. Patient satisfaction was high (91%). The number of patients playing contact and pivotal sport dropped from 37% preoperatively to 14% at assessment however the number playing leisure sports increased from 45% to 60%. At review there was no radiological progression of osteoarthrosis which is an improvement over the previously reported series where varus malalignment was not corrected at the time of ACL reconstruction (11). He conclude that the combined procedure is indicated in symptomatic sportsmen with a chronic rupture of the ACL who have developed varus malalignment from medial compartment disease or lateral opening from posterolateral instability.

Noyes (65) reviewed 41 patients with varus malalignment and chronic anterior cruciate deficiency at an average of 58 months post surgery. The patients were young, mean 32 years (range 16-47). All had significant degenerative changes in the medial compartment. Fissuring and fragmentation were present in 56% while subchondral bone was evident in 44%. Not all patients had an ACL reconstruction. The indication for reconstruction was frequent instability during light recreational activity. An extra-articular Losee type procedure was performed in 14 patients, an intra-articular allograft bone patella bone reconstruction in 16 patients and an HTO alone in 11 patients. A lateral closing wedge osteotomy was performed. If the procedure was combined, the HTO was completed first. In their evaluation they combined all three groups. Statistically significant improvements were found in the mean overall rating scores for pain, swelling, and giving way. Preoperatively, 73% had pain with activities of daily living or with any sports activity; 27% could perform only light sports activities without pain. At follow-up, 78% had no pain with activities of daily living or light sports. 10 of 15 patients with advanced medial tibiofemoral arthrosis (subchondral bone exposure) had a significant improvement in symptoms. Patients who had the allograft reconstruction had significantly lower anterior-posterior displacements at follow-up than those who had the extra-articular procedure. They did not evaluate arthritic progression. In a latter series Noyes *et al.* (64) treated 41 young patients who had anterior cruciate ligament deficiency, lower limb varus angulation, and varying amounts of posterolateral ligament deficiency. 73% of the patients had lost the medial meniscus and 63% had marked articular cartilage damage in the medial compartment. All patients were treated with high tibial osteotomy and, in the 34 anterior cruciate ligament, reconstruction was performed at a mean of 8 months later. Posterolateral reconstructions were also required in 18 knees. A 100% follow-up was obtained at a mean of 4.5 years after osteotomy. At follow-up, a reduction in pain was found in 71%; elimination of giving way in 85%, and resumption of light recreational activities without symptoms in 66%. The patient rating of the knee condition was normal or very good in 37% and good in 34%. The mean Cincinnati Knee Rating Score significantly improved from 63 to 82 points. The mean adduction moment, 35% higher than controls preoperatively, significantly decreased to below normal values postoperatively. Correction of varus alignment was maintained in 33 knees (80%). They recommend osteotomy in addition to ligament reconstructive procedures in these knees with complex injury patterns

Lattermann and Jakob (48) reported on 27 patients with medial compartment osteoarthritis and chronic anterior cruciate instability. Patients were divided into three treatment groups: HTO alone (11 patients), HTO and ACL staged (8 patients) and combined ACL and HTO (8 patients). Patients were treated according to a treatment algorithm (table 1). An opening wedge osteotomy was performed on 10 patients while a closing wedge was performed in 17 patients. The ACL reconstruction was done arthroscopically using a bone patella bone autograft. In the combined procedure the osteotomy was performed first. No statistical analysis was performed due to the low numbers in each group. In the HTO group 91% of patients felt significant pain relief and some even returned to recreational sports. The instability improved in this group. Whether this was due to an alteration in knee kinematics or arthritic progression they were unable to determine.

In the staged group an HTO was performed and if this did not restore sufficient stability an ACL reconstruction was performed 9-12 months later. 8 of 9 HTO patients required the delayed stabilization. Only 38% felt signi-

Table I. – Latterman & Jakob Treatment Algorithm.

Group	Age	Pain	Instability	Arthroscopy	Treatment
1	> 40	+++	+	Subchondral bone	HTO alone
2	25-40	+ or ++	+ or ++	Severe fissuring and fragmentation	Staged
3	< 20-35	+	+++	Fissuring	Combined

ficant pain relief however the remaining patients despite ongoing pain were able to perform pain-free, light daily activities. There was no instability in 6 patients, with partial giving way in 2.

In the combined group all patients had undergone a partial medial meniscectomy and all but one had a failed ACL reconstruction. Significant pain relief was achieved in 50% with the remainder having pain with moderate activity. Instability symptoms were reduced in 63%.

They report a high complication rate in all three groups. 10 major complications are reported. Again their results show that surgery in these patients does not allow them to return to their previous sport. Only 2 of 16 patients achieved this if they underwent an ACL and reconstruction. They conclude that a simultaneous ACL reconstruction and HTO can be a valuable procedure if patient selection is thorough. A shorter rehabilitation period is balanced by an increased complication rate. They note that a two stage procedure is equally effective in the long run.

The longest follow-up is reported by Boss *et al.* (9). They evaluated 27 patients with a closing wedge osteotomy and ACL reconstruction. They divided the patients into three groups: 2-5 years, 5-10 years and > 10 years postop. The results are comparable with those of the other studies. 89% practiced their preoperative job, over 50% had a higher level of sports activities than preoperatively, and more than 25% regained their pretraumatic sports capacity. Two-thirds had no giving way and less than 3mm translation difference in comparison to the contralateral knee. There was no difference in the subjective or clinical results between the three groups suggesting there is no significant deterioration with time however the numbers are small in each group.

All of these papers report good relief of pain and instability with only a moderate return to pre-injury activities. All of the patients had a chronic ACL with extensive degenerative changes and multiple surgeries. In this setting the combined operation appears to be a good salvage procedure. It is important to inform the patients that their chances of a return to their pre-injury athletic level is slim. All authors advocate early intervention for the varus, anterior cruciate deficient knee. We await with anticipation evaluation of the prophylactic rather than salvage procedure reported in the above papers.

An extension tibial osteotomy (anterior closing wedge) combined with an ACL reconstruction has been described by De Jour (22). Their indications are patients with prearthrosis, anterior tibial translation greater than 10mm and excessive tibial slope > 13°. They describe their technique only. We await their results with interest.

Meniscal transplantation

Meniscal transplants are becoming increasingly promoted for patients with a previous subtotal meniscectomy and instability. The surgical technique is becoming better defined and three recent studies have shown encouraging results.

The study with the longest follow-up evaluates 18 patients who had cryopreserved meniscal allograft transplantation for compartmental pain after total meniscectomy 2 to 8 years (mean 5.4 years) after the operation (73). The SF-

36 scores revealed a decrease in pain with a significant improvement in function, although function remained limited. There was no significant decrease in joint space on 45° PA weight bearing radiographs through the duration of the study. 8 of 22 allograft menisci (36%) tore during the study period, necessitating 6 partial and 2 total meniscectomies. Two patients subsequently underwent reimplantation. Histologic examination of the removed tissue revealed reduced cellularity as compared with normal or torn native menisci. Four specimens also underwent detailed cytokine evaluation and demonstrated reduced cytokine expression compared with controls. These cells also demonstrate potentially reduced function, as measured by decreased growth factor production. This decreased biologic activity may be a factor that contributes to the high frequency of retears noted in this and prior studies.

Cameron (13) reported on 67 meniscal allografts with a mean follow-up of 31 months. The menisci were gamma irradiated and bone plugs were not utilised.

5 of these underwent a concomitant ACL reconstruction with 80% obtaining a good to excellent result. 7 patients had a combined ACL reconstruction and osteotomy. A satisfactory result was obtained in 85.7%. The most significant gains were in pain and swelling while all patients with a favourable result report that post surgery activities were much less painful and several were able to resume vigorous activities.

Fu and Harner (90) evaluated 22 patients with 25 fresh frozen non irradiated transplants with a follow-up of 1 to 4 years. Bone plugs were used for the medial meniscus and a bone bridge for the lateral meniscus. 9 had an accompanying ACL reconstruction. The best results were obtained in this group (mean Lysholm 92.44) while good results were obtained in the 3 patients who had a transplant and revision ACL (mean Lysholm 88.33). No allograft failed.

Van Arkel and de Boer (86) in a prospective study evaluated the clinical results of 23 patients with a cryopreserved meniscal transplant at a follow-up of 2 to 5 years. The early results were satisfactory in 20 patients. 3 transplants failed. 6 patients had an associated ACL rupture. No mention is made of a concomitant reconstruction. Post-transplantation arthroscopy showed that most meniscal transplants had healed to the knee capsule. Histological examination showed revascularization of the transplant and evidence of viable meniscal chondrocytes. The failures were thought to be caused by malalignment, resulting in impaired revascularization.

Despite early encouraging results we still await longer term studies to determine the role of this procedure in halting progressive degenerative changes.

My approach

Patient evaluation

This consists of a thorough history, physical examination and radiographic evaluation. Patients complain of two predominant symptoms: pain and instability. The key is determining which is the primary symptom and what is the severity of this complaint. This is often not straightforward. It is important to determine the type of instability. When instability occurs with activities of daily living rather than during rapid deceleration or a change in direction, it is likely that the ACL deficiency is not the crux of the problem rather the instability arises from incongruity secondary to arthritis or meniscal pathology. The knee buckles due to a reflex quadriceps muscle inhibition caused by pain. Other important considerations in the history include the patient's age, vocation, activity level and expectations from treatment.

Our physical examination begins with an assessment of gait. It is important to elucidate any varus, valgus or hyperextension thrust which may be present. A thorough evaluation of alignment in both the coronal and sagittal plane is performed. It is imperative to compare the alignment of the contralateral limb. All ligaments must be assessed and instability graded by the side to side difference. Meniscal pathology must be determined and the medial, lateral and patellofemoral compartments examined for pain and crepitus.

Radiographic evaluation consists of a full leg weight bearing AP X-ray to determine alignment, a full length lateral of the tibia to assess posterior slope and our standard knee series consisting of an AP, lateral, notch and skyline view.

Treatment

The treatment of this problem is complex as many factors have to be taken into account. We believe the most important are the primary symptom, alignment, mechanical symptoms and the state of the menisci. Our approach follows as an algorithm (fig. 5).

We prefer an opening wedge osteotomy in patients with associated instability for the following reasons. The lateral collateral ligaments and posterolateral corner are re-tensioned rather than relaxed which may occur with a lateral closing wedge osteotomy, the proximal tibfib joint and common peroneal nerve do not have to be disturbed and the pathological compartment is addressed thus leaving the more normal compartment alone.

In present my technique for a combined medial opening wedge osteotomy and hamstring ACL reconstruction.

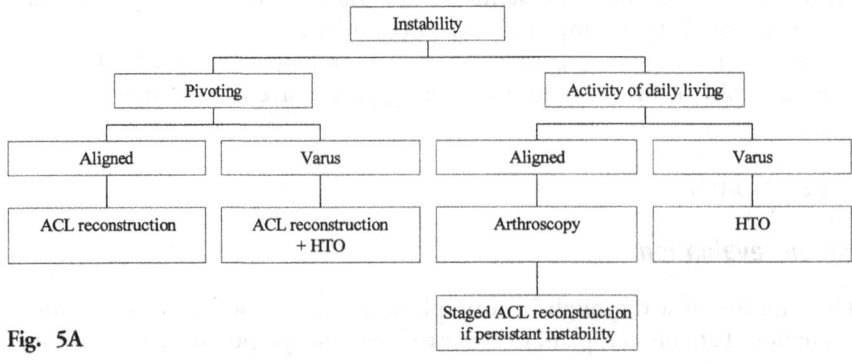

Fig. 5A

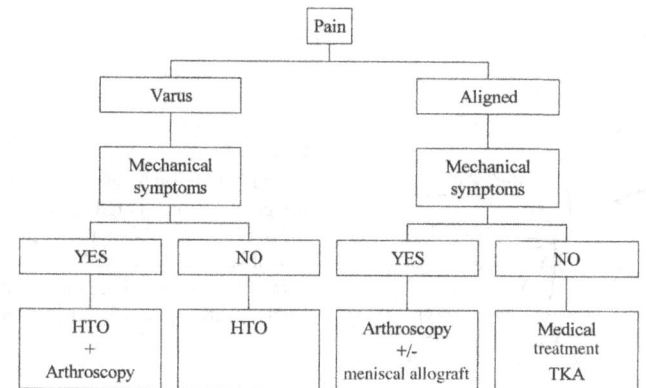

Fig. 5B

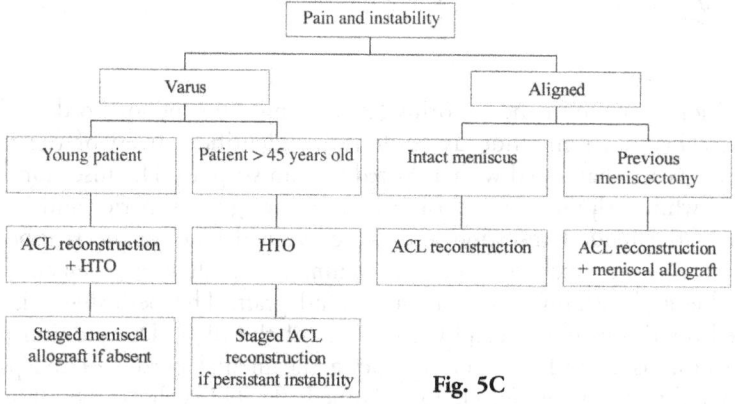

Fig. 5C

Fig. 5. – Treatment algorithm.
A: Instability as main symptom. **B:** Pain as main symptom. **C:** Pain and instability.

Preoperative templating

A long leg single stance weight bearing view is performed. The mechanical axis is determined. The new weight bearing axis is planned for at a point 62.5% along the tibial plateau in the lateral compartment. A line is drawn from the centre of the femoral head to this point and from the centre of the ankle to this point. The angle subtended is the angle of correction. This angle is then drawn at the position of the intended opening wedge osteotomy. The amount of opening required is measured. This gives the amount of opening in millimeters (fig. 6).

Operative technique

A 6cm incision is made 3cm medial to the tibial tuberosity. The superior margin of the incision is the medial joint line. Dissection is performed down to the sartorius fascia. The semitendosus and gracilis tendons are palpated.

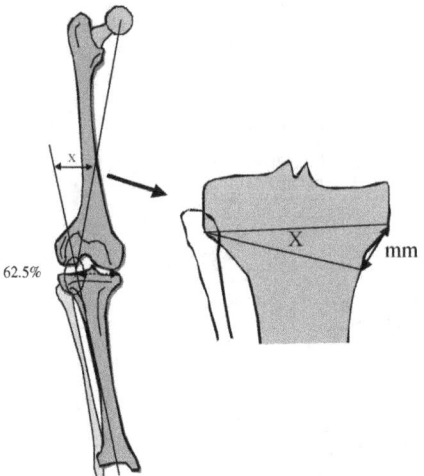

Fig. 6. – Method calculating the correction of an HTO on full length weight bearing AP radiograph (from Dugdale TW, Styer D, Noyes FR *et al*.: Preoperative planning for high tibial osteotomy (1992) The effect of lateral tibiofemoral separation and tibiofemoral length Clinical Orthopaedics and Related Research 274: 260.)

An incision is made in the sartorius fascia along the superior border of gracilis. Gracilis and semitendosus tendons are identified, freed of the fascial attachments and harvested with a slotted tendon stripper. The insertion is left attached while stripping. An incision is made along the superior and inferior border of the tendon insertion and the conjoined tendons are stripped off the bone with approx 1.5cm of periosteum. The graft is then taken to the back table and fashioned into a four strand graft. The periosteum is then stripped off the medial metaphyseal aspect of the tibia. The incision along the sartorius is extended superiorly along the medial border of the patella tendon and the tissue is reflected superomedially. This will expose the superficial medial collateral ligament. A Homan retracted is placed under the anterior margin and posterior retraction will partially strip the insertion of the MCL. A retractor is then placed under the patella tendon and a small amount of the medial insertion is released.

A guide wire is inserted along the proposed osteotomy site. It is inserted obliquely angling up approximately 30°. The lateral margin of the osteotomy is at least 2cm distal to the articular surface. I aim for the superior aspect of the fibula. The osteotomy will skirt the superior margin of the tibial tuberosity. The position is checked with fluoroscopy. The medial cortex is cut with a microsagittal saw then the osteotomy is completed with thin AO osteotomes. Care must be taken to complete the osteotomy along the posterior and anterior cortical margins and not to disrupt the lateral cortex. The position and direction of the osteotomy are frequently assessed under fluoroscopy. Once the osteotomy has been completed adequately the tuning fork is slowly inserted to the desired depth. The tuning fork is inserted as posteriorly as possible.

A slopped puddu distraction plate and screws are then inserted posteriorly (fig. 7). This will decrease the tibial slope reducing anterior tibial translation. If the plate is 7.5mm or greater a tricortical triangular iliac crest graft is inserted in the defect. If the plate is 5mm local grafting is performed from the tunnel reamings (fig. 8).

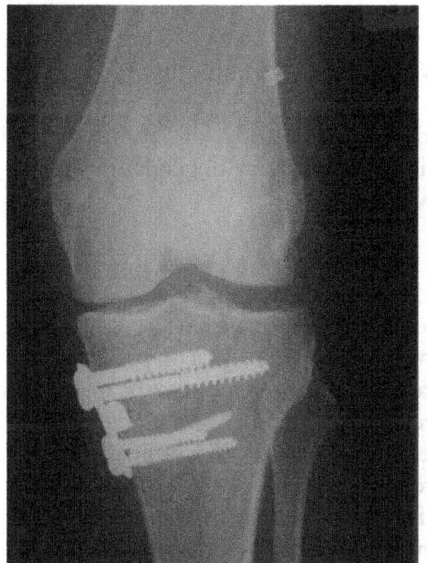
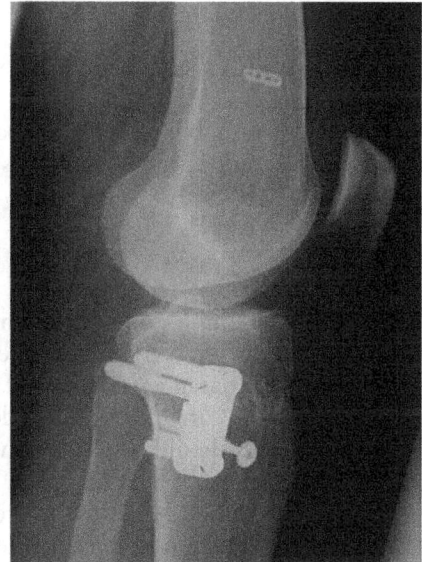

Fig. 7. – X-ray of combined ACL and HTO.

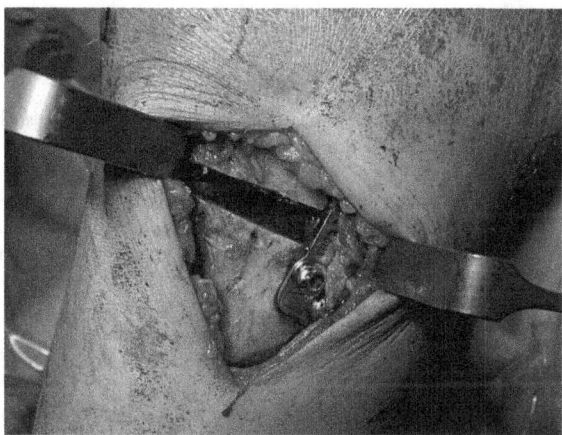

Fig. 8. – Puddu sloped plate *in situ*. Note increased opening of the osteotomy posteriorly.

An arthroscopic four strand hamstring anterior cruciate reconstruction is performed in the standard fashion. The standard endobutton 45° tibial guide is used. This should ensure the tibial tunnel exits distal to the osteotomy site. Care must be taken that the tibial tunnel does not exit proximal to the osteotomy as the tunnel may break out into the thin rim superior to the osteotomy. An Endobutton Continuous Loop is used for femoral fixation and a bioscrew backed up with a fixation post used for tibial fixation. The bioscrew is advanced up to the level of the joint to ensure aperture fixation and a good grip in the tibia proximal to the osteotomy.

Postoperative regime

The patient is placed in a ROM brace with a full range of motion for a minimum of six weeks.

The patient is mobilized with protective weight bearing for a minimum of six weeks. Weight bearing beyond this is pain and X-ray dependant.

Conclusion

A review of this complex problem is timely as recent papers have revealed promising reports on the surgical treatment of the ACL deficient patient with arthritis. It is encouraging that we are able to improve the quality of life of these patients. The current dilemma is deciding which procedure is appropriate.

Further studies should help us resolve these dilemmas. We hope to further confirm that early ACL reconstruction reduces the incidence of the post ACL arthritic knee, further define the role of meniscal transplants and determine whether early correction of malalignment in the ACL deficient knee will halt arthritis.

References

1. Aglietti P, Rinonapoli E, Stringa G *et al.* (1983) Tibial osteotomy for the varus osteoarthritic knee. Clin Orthop: 239-51
2. Ahmed AM, Burke DL (1983) *In vitro* measurement of static pressure distribution in synovial joints. Part I: Tibial surface of the knee. J Biomech Eng 105: 216-25
3. Allen PR, Denham RA, Swan AV (1984) Late degenerative changes after meniscectomy. Factors affecting the knee after operation. J Bone Joint Surg [Br] 66: 666-71
4. Alm A, Gillquist J (1974) Reconstruction of the anterior cruciate ligament by using the medial third of the patellar ligament. Treatment and results. Acta Chir Scand 140: 289-96
5. Arnold JA, Coker TP, Heaton LM *et al.* (1979) Natural history of anterior cruciate tears. Am J Sports Med 7: 305-13
6. Baratz ME, Fu FH, Mengato R (1986) Meniscal tears: the effect of meniscectomy and of repair on intra-articular contact areas and stress in the human knee. A preliminary report. Am J Sports Med 14: 270-5
7. Beynnon BD, Pope MH, Wertheimer CM *et al.* (1992) The effect of functional knee-braces on strain on the anterior cruciate ligament *in vivo.* J Bone Joint Surg Am 74: 1298-312
8. Bonnin M (1990) La subluxation tibiale antérieure en appui monopodal dans les ruptures du ligament croisé antérieur. Étude clinique et biomécanique. Thèse Med. Lyon, Ref Type: Thesis/Dissertation
9. Boss A, Stutz G, Oursin C *et al.* (1995) Anterior cruciate ligament reconstruction combined with valgus tibial osteotomy (combined procedure). Knee Surg Sports Traumatol Arthrosc 3: 187-91
10. Bourne RB, Finlay JB, Papadopoulos P *et al.* (1984) The effect of medial meniscectomy on strain distribution in the proximal part of the tibia. J Bone Joint Surg [Am] 66: 1431-7
11. Brandt KD, Myers SL, Burr D *et al.* (1991) Osteoarthritic changes in canine articular cartilage, subchondral bone, and synovium fifty-four months after transection of the anterior cruciate ligament. Arthritis Rheum 34: 1560-70
12. Brown TD, Shaw DT (1984) *In vitro* contact stress distribution on the femoral condyles. J Orthop Res 2: 190-9

13. Cameron JC, Saha S (1997) Meniscal allograft transplantation for unicompartmental arthritis of the knee. Clin Orthop: 164-71
14. Cameron M, Buchgraber A, Passler H et al. (1997) The natural history of the anterior cruciate ligament-deficient knee. Changes in synovial fluid cytokine and keratan sulfate concentrations. Am J Sports Med 25: 751-4
15. Cameron ML, Fu FH, Paessler HH et al. (1994) Synovial fluid cytokine concentrations as possible prognostic indicators in the ACL-deficient knee. Knee Surg Sports Traumatol Arthrosc 2: 38-44
16. Clark CR, Ogden JA (1983) Development of the menisci of the human knee joint. Morphological changes and their potential role in childhood meniscal injury. J Bone Joint Surg [Am] 65: 538-47
17. Coventry MB (1979) Upper tibial osteotomy for gonarthrosis. The evolution of the operation in the last 18 years and long term results. Orthop Clin North Am 10: 191-210
18. Coventry MB (1985) Upper tibial osteotomy for osteoarthritis. J Bone Joint Surg [Am] 67: 1136-40
19. Daniel DM, Stone ML, Dobson BE et al. (1994) Fate of the ACL-injured patient. A prospective outcome study [see comments]. Am J Sports Med 22: 632-44
20. Deehan DJ, Salmon LJ, Webb VJ et al. (2000) Endoscopic reconstruction of the anterior cruciate ligament with an ipsilateral patellar tendon autograft. A prospective longitudinal five-year study [In Process Citation]. J Bone Joint Surg Br 82: 984-91
21. De Jour H, Neyret P, Boileau P et al. (1994) Anterior cruciate reconstruction combined with valgus tibial osteotomy. Clin Orthop: 220-8
22. De Jour H, Neyret P, Bonnin M (1994) Instability and Osteoarthritis in Knee Surgery. Fu FH, Harner CD, Vince KG. 1[1], 859-875. Williams & Wilkins. Ref Type: Serial (Book, Monograph)
23. Eriksson K, Anderberg P, Hamberg P et al. (2001) A comparison of quadruple semitendinosus and patellar tendon grafts in reconstruction of the anterior cruciate ligament. J Bone Joint Surg Br 83: 348-54
24. Faber KJ, Dill JR, Amendola A et al. (1999) Occult osteochondral lesions after anterior cruciate ligament rupture. Six-year magnetic resonance imaging follow-up study. Am J Sports Med 27: 489-94
25. Fairbank TJ. Knee joint changes after meniscectomy. J Bone Joint Surg [Br.] 30B: 664-70. 1948. Ref Type: Journal (Full)
26. Feagin JAJ, Cabaud HE, Curl WW (1982) The anterior cruciate ligament: radiographic and clinical signs of successful and unsuccessful repairs. Clin Orthop: 54-8
27. Ferretti A, Conteduca F, De CA et al. (1991) Osteoarthritis of the knee after ACL reconstruction. Int Orthop 15: 367-71
28. Finsterbush A, Frankl U, Matan Y et al. (1990) Secondary damage to the knee after isolated injury of the anterior cruciate ligament. Am J Sports Med 18: 475-9
29. Friederich NF., O'Brien WR (1993) Gonarthrosis after injury of the anterior cruciate ligament: a multicenter, long-term study. Z Unfallchir Versicherungsmed 86: 81-9
30. Fukubayashi T, Kurosawa H (1980) The contact area and pressure distribution pattern of the knee. A study of normal and osteoarthrotic knee joints. Acta Orthop Scand 51: 871-9
31. Graf BK, Cook DA, De SA et al. (1993) Bone bruises on magnetic resonance imaging evaluation of anterior cruciate ligament injuries. Am J Sports Med 21: 220-3
32. Healy W, Barber TC (1990) The role of osteotomy in the treatment of osteoarthritis of the knee. Am J Knee Surg 3: 97-109
33. Hernigou P, Medevielle D, Debeyre J et al. (1987) Proximal tibial osteotomy for osteoarthritis with varus deformity. A ten to thirteen-year follow-up study. J Bone Joint Surg [Am] 69: 332-54
34. Holden DL, James SL, Larson RL et al. (1988) Proximal tibial osteotomy in patients who are fifty years old or less. A long-term follow-up study [see comments]. J Bone Joint Surg [Am] 70: 977-82
35. Indelicato PA, Bittar ES (1985) A perspective of lesions associated with ACL insufficiency of the knee. A review of 100 cases. Clin Orthop: 77-80

36. Insall JN, Joseph DM, Msika C (1984) High tibial osteotomy for varus gonarthrosis. A long-term follow-up study. J Bone Joint Surg [Am] 66: 1040-8
37. Irvine GB, and Glasgow MM (1992) The natural history of the meniscus in anterior cruciate insufficiency. Arthroscopic analysis. J Bone Joint Surg [Br] 74: 403-5
38. Ivarsson I, Myrnerts R, Gillquist J (1990) High tibial osteotomy for medial osteoarthritis of the knee. A 5 to 7 and 11 year follow-up. J Bone Joint Surg [Br] 72: 238-44
39. Jacobsen K (1977) Osteoarthrosis following insufficiency of the cruciate ligaments in man. A clinical study. Acta Orthop Scand 48: 520-6
40. Jarvela T, Nyyssonen M, Kannus P et al. (1999) Bone-patellar tendon-bone reconstruction of the anterior cruciate ligament. A long-term comparison of early and late repair. Int Orthop 23: 227-31
41. Johnson RJ, Eriksson E, Haggmark T et al. (1984) Five- to ten-year follow-up evaluation after reconstruction of the anterior cruciate ligament. Clin Orthop: 122-40
42. Jomha NM, Borton DC, Clingeleffer AJ et al. (1999) Long-term osteoarthritic changes in anterior cruciate ligament reconstructed knees. Clin Orthop: 188-93
43. Kannus P, Jarvinen M (1987) Conservatively treated tears of the anterior cruciate ligament. Long-term results. J Bone Joint Surg [Am] 69: 1007-12
44. Kaplan PA, Walker CW, Kilcoyne RF et al. (1992) Occult fracture patterns of the knee associated with anterior cruciate ligament tears: assessment with MR imaging. Radiology 183: 835-8
45. Krause WR, Pope MH, Johnson RJ et al. (1976) Mechanical changes in the knee after meniscectomy. J Bone Joint Surg [Am] 58: 599-604
46. Kullmer K, Letsch R, Turowski B (1994) Which factors influence the progression of degenerative osteoarthritis after ACL surgery? Knee Surg Sports Traumatol Arthrosc 2: 80-4
47. Lam SJ. Reconstruction of the anterior cruciate ligament using the Jones procedure and Guys Hospital modification. J Bone Joint Surg. [Am.] 50: 1213-24. 1968. Ref Type: Journal (Full)
48. Lattermann C, Jakob RP (1996) High tibial osteotomy alone or combined with ligament reconstruction in anterior cruciate ligament-deficient knees. Knee Surg Sports Traumatol Arthrosc 4: 32-8
49. Levy IM, Torzilli PA, Warren RF (1982) The effect of medial meniscectomy on anterior-posterior motion of the knee. J Bone Joint Surg [Am] 64: 883-8
50. Lindenfeld TN, Hewett TE, Andriacchi TP (1997) Joint loading with valgus bracing in patients with varus gonarthrosis. Clin Orthop: 290-7
51. Lipke JM, Janecki CJ, Nelson CL et al. (1981) The role of incompetence of the anterior cruciate and lateral ligaments in anterolateral and anteromedial instability. A biomechanical study of cadaver knees. J Bone Joint Surg [Am] 63: 954-60
52. Liu SH, Lunsford T, Gude S et al. (1994) Comparison of functional knee braces for control of anterior tibial displacement. Clin Orthop: 203-10
53. Lohmander LS, Dahlberg L, Ryd L et al. (1989) Increased levels of proteoglycan fragments in knee joint fluid after injury. Arthritis Rheum 32: 1434-42
54. Lohmander LS, Saxne T, Heinegard D (1996) Increased concentrations of bone sialoprotein in joint fluid after knee injury. Ann Rheum Dis 55: 622-6
55. Lohmander LS, Yoshihara Y, Roos H et al. (1996) Procollagen II C-propeptide in joint fluid: changes in concentration with age, time after knee injury, and osteoarthritis. J Rheumatol 23: 1765-9
56. Lynch MA, Henning CE, Glick KRJ (1983) Knee joint surface changes. Long-term follow-up meniscus tear treatment in stable anterior cruciate ligament reconstructions. Clin Orthop: 148-53
57. Markolf KL, Bargar WL, Shoemaker SC et al. (1981) The role of joint load in knee stability. J Bone Joint Surg [Am] 63: 570-85
58. Marks PH, Goldenberg JA, Vezina WC et al. J. (1992) Subchondral bone infractions in acute ligamentous knee injuries demonstrated on bone scintigraphy and magnetic resonance imaging. J Nucl Med 33: 516-20
59. Matsuno H, Kadowaki KM, Tsuji H (1997) Generation II knee bracing for severe medial compartment osteoarthritis of the knee. Arch Phys Med Rehabil 78: 745-9

60. McDaniel WJ Jr, Dameron TBJ (1983) The untreated anterior cruciate ligament rupture. Clin Orthop: 158-63
61. Murphy BJ, Smith RL, Uribe JW *et al.* (1992) Bone signal abnormalities in the postero-lateral tibia and lateral femoral condyle in complete tears of the anterior cruciate ligament: a specific sign? Radiology 182: 221-4
62. Noyes FR, Barber-Westin SD (1997) Anterior cruciate ligament reconstruction with auto-genous patellar tendon graft in patients with articular cartilage damage. Am J Sports Med 25: 626-34
63. Noyes FR, Barber-Westin SD (1997) Arthroscopic-assisted allograft anterior cruciate liga-ment reconstruction in patients with symptomatic arthrosis. Arthroscopy 13: 24-32
64. Noyes FR, Barber-Westin SD, Hewett TE (2000) High tibial osteotomy and ligament reconstruction for varus angulated anterior cruciate ligament-deficient knees. Am J Sports Med 28: 282-96
65. Noyes FR, Barber SD, Simon R (1993) High tibial osteotomy and ligament reconstruc-tion in varus angulated, anterior cruciate ligament-deficient knees. A two- to seven-year follow-up study. Am J Sports Med 21: 2-12
66. Noyes FR, Mooar PA, Matthews D *et al.* (1983) The symptomatic anterior cruciate-defi-cient knee. Part I: the long-term functional disability in athletically active individuals. J Bone Joint Surg [Am] 65: 154-62
67. Noyes FR, Schipplein OD, Andriacchi TP *et al.* (1992) The anterior cruciate ligament-deficient knee with varus alignment. An analysis of gait adaptations and dynamic joint loadings. Am J Sports Med 20: 707-16
68. Odenbring S, Tjornstrand B, Egund N *et al.* (1989) Function after tibial osteotomy for medial gonarthrosis below aged 50 years. Acta Orthop Scand 60: 527-31
69. Pattee GA, Fox JM, Del PW *et al.* (1989) Four to ten year followup of unreconstructed anterior cruciate ligament tears. Am J Sports Med 17: 430-5
70. Pelletier JP, Roughley PJ, DiBattista JA *et al.* (1991) Are cytokines involved in osteoar-thritic pathophysiology? Semin Arthritis Rheum 20: 12-25
71. Proctor CS, Schmidt MB, Whipple RR *et al.* (1989) Material properties of the normal medial bovine meniscus. J Orthop Res 7: 771-82
72. Radin EL, De LF, Maquet P (1984) Role of the menisci in the distribution of stress in the knee. Clin Orthop: 290-4
73. Rath E, Richmond JC, Yassir W *et al.* (2001) Meniscal allograft transplantation. Two- to eight-year results. Am J Sports Med 29: 410-4
74. Rosen MA, Jackson DW, Berger PE (1991) Occult osseous lesions documented by magnetic resonance imaging associated with anterior cruciate ligament ruptures. Arthroscopy 7: 45-51
75. Satku K, Kumar VP, Ngoi SS (1986) Anterior cruciate ligament injuries. To counsel or to operate? J Bone Joint Surg [Br] 68: 458-61
76. Shelbourne KD, Gray T (2000) Results of anterior cruciate ligament reconstruction based on meniscus and articular cartilage status at the time of surgery. Am J Sports Med 28: 446-52
77. Shelbourne KD, Stube KC (1997) Anterior cruciate ligament (ACL)-deficient knee with degenerative arthrosis: treatment with an isolated autogenous patellar tendon ACL recons-truction. Knee Surg Sports Traumatol Arthrosc 5: 150-6
78. Shelbourne KD, Wilckens JH (1993) Intra-articular anterior cruciate ligament recons-truction in the symptomatic arthritic knee. Am J Sports Med 21: 685-8
79. Shelton WR, Barrett GR, Dukes A (1997) Early season anterior cruciate ligament tears. A treatment dilemma. Am J Sports Med 25: 656-8
80. Sherman M., Warren RF, Marshall JL *et al.* (1988) A clinical and radiographical analysis of 127 anterior cruciate insufficient knees. Clin Orthop 227: 229-37.
81. Shino K, Inoue M, Nakamura H *et al.* (1989) Arthroscopic follow-up of anterior cruciate ligament reconstruction using allogeneic tendon. Arthroscopy 5: 165-71
82. Shoemaker SC, Markolf KL (1986) The role of the meniscus in the anterior-posterior sta-bility of the loaded anterior cruciate-deficient knee. Effects of partial versus total excision. J Bone Joint Surg [Am] 68: 71-9

83. Shrive NG, O'Connor JJ Goodfellow JW (1978) Load-bearing in the knee joint. Clin Orthop: 279-87

84. Sommerlath K, Lysholm J, Gillquist J (1991) The long-term course after treatment of acute anterior cruciate ligament ruptures. A 9- to 16-year follow-up. Am J Sports Med 19: 156-62

85. Spindler KP, Schils JP, Bergfeld JA et al. (1993) Prospective study of osseous, articular, and meniscal lesions in recent anterior cruciate ligament tears by magnetic resonance imaging and arthroscopy. Am J Sports Med 21: 551-7

86. van AE, De BH (1995) Human meniscal transplantation. Preliminary results at 2- to 5-year follow-up. J Bone Joint Surg Br 77: 589-95

87. Vikkula M, Metsaranta M, Ala-Kokko L (1994) Type II collagen mutations in rare and common cartilage diseases. Ann Med 26: 107-14

88. Voloshin AS, Wosk J (1983) Shock absorption of meniscectomized and painful knees: a comparative in vivo study. J Biomed Eng 5: 157-61

89. Williams CJ, Jimenez SA (1993) Heredity, genes and osteoarthritis. Rheum Dis Clin North Am 19: 523-43

90. Yoldas EA, Dowdy PA, Irrgang J et al. (1997) Meniscal Transplantation: University of Pittsburgh Experience. Pitt Ortho J 8: 61-6

The medical treatment of gonarthrosis*

E. Noël, M.J. Nissen

Introduction

Gonarthrosis or osteoarthritis (OA) of the knee can be the result of natural degeneration of the menisci and/or the articular cartilage, the consequence of repeated microtrauma (either occupational or sport related), or secondary to injuries, such as a ruptured anterior cruciate ligament (which is particularly arthrogenic).

While the lesions may be either meniscal or cartilaginous in origin, the modality and the rapidity of degradation of the cartilaginous structures depend largely on local mechanisms. This degradation can occur very slowly or extremely quickly in the form of an acute flare, with an alteration in the phases of stabilization and chondrolysis.

The synovial membrane intervenes in this process of degradation, by the production of intermediary substances such as cytokines and metalloprotinases, many of which are destructive to the cartilage.

The therapeutic options at our disposal are numerous, and are aimed principally at the degenerating cartilage. They must be prescribed in accordance with the age of the patient, his functional discomfort and degree of pain, with consideration also given to the stage and to the speed of evolution of the degenerative process.

In general, the two principal objectives of management are to provide effective analgesia and, if possible, to preserve the remaining cartilage. In circumstances where these objectives are not achieved, the option of surgical intervention must be considered.

Amongst the plethora of medical treatment options which exist, there are those that have been in use for a long time and are well established, and others which are relatively recent and are still undergoing evaluation.

Non-pharmacological treatments

Weight loss

Overweight patients presenting with OA of the knee are at high risk of aggravation of their arthritis, or of the development of bilateral gonarthrosis in the case of unilateral knee disease. Moreover, the loss of weight itself can have a

---

* Written in 2002.

noticeable analgesic effect on both arthritic and non-arthritic knees. For instance, an uncontrolled study of obese patients following gastric surgery
(average weight loss of 45.5kg following the intervention) demonstrated that
57% of patients had knee pain prior to the procedure, compared to only 14%
afterwards.

Physical exercise

Patients who exercise regularly live for longer and are healthier than those who
are sedentary. The aim is to maintain joint range of motion and muscle tone,
to preserve effective proprioception and to minimize the degree of force
through the joint by means of weight loss or at least the stabilization of weight.
There are numerous programs and techniques, such as isometric and isotonic
exercises of the quadriceps and the hamstrings, or walking programs consisting of, for example, three one-hourly sessions per week. The strengthening
of periarticular muscles plays a significant role in protecting the articular cartilage from damage and consequently may result, within weeks, in a reduction in joint pain, comparable to that achieved with NSAIDs. Ettinger *et al.*
(1) published a randomized study in 1997, which evaluated the impact of
different exercise programs on the functional discomfort of arthritic knees over
a period of 18 months. The first group participated in a program of walking
and aerobic exercises (10 minutes of slow walking with warm-up exercises of
the trunk and limbs, followed by 40 minutes of walking at 50-70% of their
cardiac capacity, and finally 10 minutes of slow walking and stretching). The
second group performed resistance exercises of all limbs regularly, while the
third group attended monthly education sessions of 90 minutes duration (with
brochures detailing dietary advice). After 18 months, there was a compliance
rate of 70%, and during a questionnaire evaluating the activities of daily life
(ADL), the education group had handicap scores approximately 10% higher
than the two other groups. Both the walking and resistance exercise groups
were able to walk more rapidly and for a greater distance than the education
group, as well as having better ADL scores.

Absorbent shoes or soles

Products such as Sorbothane® can reduce the force placed through a joint by
around 40%. Whereas narrow high-heeled shoes can actually increase the stress
through a joint such as the knee. Certain authors recommend the use of
plantar orthotics designed in accordance with the morphology of the lower
limbs (i.e.: varus or valgus), but to our knowledge these have never been formally evaluated.

Walking sticks and joint braces

Walking aids can be utilized during an acute flare of arthritis in conjunction
with a non-weight-bearing (NWB) period of several days, as well as for the

chronic pain of OA, provided that the methods of utilization have been well understood by the patient. The different forms of joint braces from the simplest to the most complex can often be of great benefit. Some of the stabilized joint braces set in a position of varus or valgus can assist to realign the mechanical forces through the joint and consequently may provide a remarkable analgesic effect, thus allowing the continuation of daily activities. These are particularly useful in the case of intolerance to medications or of contraindications to surgery, or merely while awaiting a procedure.

Others

There are many other treatments that can be utilized for their analgesic effect and their minimal side effects, such as thermal treatments, electrotherapy, physiotherapy and acupuncture. However, to date with regards to gonarthrosis, they have never been evaluated formally against a placebo.

Oral pharmacological therapies

Arthritis is the result of a functional disequilibrium between the anabolic and catabolic forces on cartilage, to the advantage of the latter. In the first phase, the inflamed articular cartilage synthesizes numerous substances leading to the augmented degradation of the previously healthy tissues. The chondrocytes in the articular cartilage produce specific proteoglycans and large quantities of enzymes such as the metalloprotinases which can destroy the collagen network (which provides cartilage its strength) and the proteoglycans (responsible for the elasticity of cartilage). Under the influence of pro-inflammatory cytokines, the chondrocytes produce their own cytokines (IL-1, TNF-α and IL-6) as well as growth factors opposing the action of these cytokines (TGF-β and IGF-1).

The principal pharmacologic treatments of OA aim to relieve pain and to reduce functional impairment, by influencing the pathophysiology of arthritis. Some of these medications oppose the effect of the metalloprotinases or of the pro-inflammatory cytokines, while others aim to stimulate the growth factors. The therapeutic difficulty lies in the fact that the causes of OA are multifactorial, thus complicating the task of finding one drug to target all causes.

One can classify the drugs for the treatment of OA into two groups: symptom-modifying treatments, which can be distinguished according to their clinical kinetic profile (onset of response, duration and persistence of effect) and which are generally relatively rapid-acting (e.g.: analgesics and non-steroidal anti-inflammatory drugs [NSAIDs]), from structure-modifying drugs with a more delayed effect, which target the disease process itself (preventing, delaying, reversing, or stabilizing the alteration of joint structure). Strictly speaking, it is not possible to discuss the concept of "anti-osteoarthritic medications", as no pharmacological agent in humans to date has consistently demonstrated the capacity to slow the progression of the arthritic process.

Therefore, the current therapies have essentially a symptomatic action with regard to pain and relapses of arthritis, and their combination often permits a reduction in the consumption of NSAIDs.

Rapid-acting symptomatic treatments

Analgesics as a group have a diversely variable action on the symptoms of OA depending on their class and anti-inflammatory properties. Their clinical usefulness is undeniable for the painful component of arthritis, particularly in the case of intolerance or contraindications to NSAIDs. A number of earlier studies demonstrated that acetaminophen had an efficacy identical to that of NSAIDs with regards to arthritic knees in general without specifying the inflammatory nature.

A randomized, double-blind, crossover clinical trial by Pincus *et al.* concluded that on average, NSAIDs are more efficacious than acetaminophen for the treatment of OA, especially for the moderate to severe cases (2). Therefore the current role of acetaminophen is primarily for patients with mild OA, renal disease or oedema states.

There are a huge number of different NSAIDs and many different families, each with its own specific differences. They have both analgesic and anti-inflammatory properties, and are therefore particularly efficacious for acute arthritic flares when utilized for several days or when used preventively prior to activities which commonly precipitate pain. The contraindications and problems such as gastro-intestinal (GI) intolerance of classic NSAIDs have indisputably limited their global utilization. This situation has recently changed with the arrival of a new variety of selective NSAIDs which act to inhibit the enzyme cyclo-oxygenase type II (COX II), such as Celecoxib (Celebrex®) and Rofecoxib (Vioxx®).

The efficacy of COX II inhibitors is comparable to that of the classic NSAIDs (3), however the type and frequency of secondary effects in particular on the GI tract, but as well their cardiovascular and platelet effects, are somewhat different.

Although certain authors have suggested that some of the traditional NSAIDs have a "chondroprotective" effect, this is contested by many, as adequately controlled trials in humans to support this are lacking. In all cases, excluding Indomethacin (Indocid®) which has a deleterious action compared to placebo on the structure of cartilage after several years of consumption, no harmful effects were found with the other NSAIDs, particularly Naproxen (Naprosyn®) and Diclofenac Sodium (Voltaren®).

A recent observational study by Mamdani *et al.* compared standard NSAIDs, Diclofenac plus Misoprostol, Rofecoxib and Celecoxib in approximately 45,000 patients over the age of 66 to 100,000 control patients. They demonstrated significant differences in the GI tolerance of these different agents, with standard NSAIDs alone having a 4x higher risk compared to controls of upper GI haemorrhage, NSAID plus Misoprostol 3x, Rofecoxib 1.9x and the risk for Celecoxib was found to be equivalent to that of placebo (4).

Slow-acting symptomatic treatments

There are a large number of medications on the market that fall into this class, such as Diacerhein (Art 50®), Chondroitin sulfate (Chondrosulf 400® and Structum®), Oxaceprol (Jonctum®), Glucosamine and the unsaponifiables of soya and avocado (Piascledine®). As a group, they are generally well tolerated. Their onset of effect is usually delayed for at least a few weeks (on average four weeks) and their effects persist for a prolonged period after cessation, thereby allowing intermittent administration if desired. This is particularly the case for Chondroitin sulfate which has a residual effect after two or three months.

These treatments have generally shown beneficial effects in both animal models and human studies. Amongst humans, their positive effects are manifested by a diminution of pain and functional discomfort as well as a reduction in NSAIDs consumption.

Many of these studies are beginning to demonstrate that these agents can exert a structural effect which in turn slows the progression of the arthritic process (evaluated by radiographic means) which is essentially the major objective.

A recent study with Chondroitin sulfate (5) demonstrated a beneficial structural effect on arthritic knees (with automated measure of joint-space) with a year of follow-up. However, studies with longer periods of follow-up are required.

At this stage, their use is not justified in asymptomatic patients; however this may soon change with the results of some on the studies currently in progress.

Another major agent in this group is Glucosamine, which has been the topic of many recently published articles. Its tolerance is excellent, with only minor GI tract disturbance in about 10% of patients. Like the other products in this group, it exerts an analgesic effect greater than that of placebo for lower limb arthritis as well as a chondromodulation effect *in vivo* (i.e.: the addition of Glucosamine to human chondrocytes increases their synthesis of proteoglycans in culture) (6). This recent study suggesting the concept of "chondroprotection" in man is encouraging but certainly requires further confirmation, and despite the critics of its methodology, it was the first to demonstrate the chondroprotection effect of a medication in this therapeutic class.

Intra-articular corticosteroid injection

While systemic corticosteroids (CCS) have no place in the treatment of OA, intra-articular (IA) injections of CCS have been used empirically for 20-30 years, despite having been evaluated formally only relatively recently. The pathophysiological concept is that they block the production of proteolytic enzymes by both the synovium and the cartilaginous cells. It is only in the past few years that their efficacy has been compared to that of placebo.

There are five controlled studies that have been performed on this subject, with a follow-up period of between 4 weeks and 6 months (7). The CCS show a clear benefit compared to that of placebo over a 2-4 weeks period, with efficacy varying from 36 to 81%, but over longer periods there is no difference between the two groups. These results are therefore in favor of treatment with IA CCS, if the principal objective is to assist the patient through a temporary difficult period in order to return to an asymptomatic or functional state. This is most successful amongst patients who maintain good muscle tone and strength as well as preserved joint range of motion. Such treatment is much less valuable in the situation of a rapidly progressive arthropathy.

If one analyses the above mentioned studies in more detail, several further remarks regarding the benefits of CCS injections should be added:

– the dose of CCS injected is usually relatively weak, there are no analyses comparing the type of CCS used (e.g.: rapid or delayed action) and they have generally been investigated as a single injection, which has little relevance to standard practice (where 2-3 njections administered over a 3-4 weeks period appears empirically to many practitioners to be the most efficacious approach, despite the fact that this has not been evaluated for gonarthrosis);

– in view of the pathophysiological mechanisms described, it would appear necessary to differentiate between gonarthrosis with and without an effusion. Only a single study considered this factor and demonstrated that it was beneficial to evacuate the effusion prior to infiltration with CCS;

– the final factor to mention, one often very difficult to apply in daily practice, is the duration of a NWB state following CCS injection. If we extrapolate from findings regarding rheumatoid arthritis of the knee (8), it could be recommended for the more severely symptomatic cases to observe a strict NWB period in bed of 24 hours after the injection.

Joint lavage

The standard technique (after Ayral and Doudados), is to perform a lavage with the use of 2 × 14 gauge cannulae of 2mm diameter under local anaesthesia, irrigating the knee joint with 1 litre of 0.9% normal saline solution (9). The principle of its efficacy, now described in a number of studies, results from the partial distention of the articular capsule and the elimination of harmful agents maintaining the degradation of the cartilage (e.g.: cytokines, proteolytic enzymes, cartilaginous debris, etc). However, procedures such as this are often accompanied by a large placebo effect.

One small study demonstrated that there was no difference with regards to an intra-articular evacuation with or without the injection of 10cc of physiological serum (9). Another study by Bradley et al. concluded that most of the effect of tidal irrigation of the knee joint was attributable to a "placebo response" (10).

Other retrospective studies have shown that joint lavage with follow-up of between 3 and 12 months was more efficacious than re-education alone and than medical treatment (analgesics and NSAIDs) with isometric exercises of the quadriceps, and as efficacious as arthroscopic debridement (revised at 3 and 12 months).

The French Society of Rheumatology carried out a randomized controlled prospective study with the aim of evaluating the tolerance and efficacy of articular lavage, in accordance with the procedure described above (11). The study consisted of four therapeutic groups: IA injection of placebo (1.5mL of 0.9% normal saline), IA injection of slow-acting CCS (3.75mg of Cortivazol® in 1.5mL), joint lavage plus IA placebo, and joint lavage plus IA injection of CCS. Each intervention was performed on an outpatient basis but was followed by immediate bed rest of two hours duration.

They found that at 24 weeks the patients who had undergone joint lavage had significantly improved pain "visual analogue scores", whereas those with CCS injection alone had no "long term" effect. The results of the two treatments were additive, with the joint lavage plus IA Cortivazol® achieving the best outcomes. They concluded that while IA CCS provided short-term relief of pain (up to 4 weeks), the effects of joint lavage persisted for at least 24 weeks.

It thus follows that the use of lavage may be indicated in certain situations, particularly when there is a chronic joint effusion following an arthritic flare, in which case the usual medical treatments are often poorly effective. The factors predictive of the success of lavage, which must at present be drawn from the experience of CCS injection, are thus not well known. It would appear logical to assume that the procedure is more effective when there are no major abnormalities of the lower limbs, the onset of gonarthrosis is relatively recent and there is an associated chondrocalcinosis. A formal arthroscopic lavage is of course an alternative to this less invasive technique.

Intra-articular injections with Hyaluronic Acid (HA)

Hyaluronan (Hyalgan®) was the first agent used, initially in Italy, and there are now several years of clinical experience with a regime of one injection per week over a period of five weeks. It is an HA of relatively low molecular weight (MW) (500-730kd). The aim of injecting exogenous HA is to stimulate the aggregation of proteoglycans as well as to augment the inherent properties of synovial fluid (such as viscosity and elasticity). In addition, it may also stimulate the endogenous production of HA by the cartilage.

Huskisson et al. demonstrated that Hyalgan was clearly more efficacious than placebo (12). Other studies have compared Hyalgan® to IA CSS injection and have demonstrated that their effect is at least equal to or better than CCS in the first few weeks, and after four weeks their effects are greater and persist for a much longer duration. There is also some evidence that the combination of IA CCS with the first injection of HA has an even better outcome. On a similar theme, it has been shown that the effect of Hyalgan® at six months is superior to a standard NSAID (Naprosyn® 1g daily) over the same period (13). Whilst Hyalgan® is still not commercialized in many countries, it is used frequently in others such as Italy.

Recently a large number of different forms of HA have appeared on the market (table 1), with differences in their MW, origin (animal or otherwise) and their presentation (solution or gel). Collectively, these treatments represent what is now referred to as "viscosupplementation" and are considered to be more of a medical device than a medication as such.

Table I. – The different forms of HA which appeared on the market.

Product name	Presentation	Mg/ syringe	Origin	Molecular weight	No. injections
Arthrum®	Solution	40	Non animal	2.4	3 × 2 mL
Durolane®	Gel	60	Non animal	92	1 × 3 mL
Hyalgan®	Solution	20	Animal	0.5-0.75	5 × 2 mL
Ostenil®	Solution	20	Non animal	1.2	3 × 2 mL
Supartz®	Solution	20	Animal	0.5-0.7	5 × 2 mL
Suplasyn®	Solution	20	Non animal	?	3 × 2 mL
Synvisc®	80% solution 20% gel	16	Animal	6	3 × 2 mL
Viscorneal®	Solution	20	Animal	6	3 × 2 mL

Amongst this plethora of products, it is Synvisc® (Hylan G-F 20) which has certainly been the most widely studied. As a weekly injection administered over three weeks it has shown superior results to those obtained in control populations and when compared to regular NSAID use (13).

A randomized controlled double-blinded study by Wobig *et al.* demonstrated that Hyalgan® had a greater efficacy with regards to pain than Synvisc® over a twelve weeks period (14). The addition of a joint lavage (as detailed above) one week prior to treatment with Synvisc®, augmented the benefit obtained. In general, the best results were seen with the less severely affected arthritic joints and when there was no joint effusion present. Nevertheless, it still has a useful role in the severely arthritic joints when there are few other therapeutic options available or in the presence of a contraindication to surgical intervention. Although, the benefits obtained are often after a period as long as eight or nine months.

The tolerance of Synvisc® is satisfactory, with the most frequently reported problem being that of painful reactions at the time of injection and occasionally micro-crystal reactions with swelling, erythema and rarely sepsis. Usually this resolves over several days with rest, ice and the prescription of NSAIDs.

Currently, the routine clinical use of Synvisc® is only authorized for the treatment of gonarthrosis, but this will soon extend to the treatment of arthritic hip disease. Its role and efficacy for patello-femoral arthrosis remains to be confirmed. Other studies examining its use in the shoulder and ankle joint are in progress.

Radio-active yttrium 90

Although it has never undergone placebo controlled studies or been compared to local CCS injection, certain authors recommend it for resolving chronic gonarthrosis with long-standing or recurrent effusion, those associated with a chondrocalcinosis and those complicated by a haemarthrosis.

The therapeutic indications

The classic treatments which have been utilized for many years must be implemented as first line therapy. These include the non-pharmacological treatments, the classic NSAIDs, CCS injections and also joint lavage. More recently many slow-acting symptomatic treatments have appeared, the study of which is ongoing, with the aim of proving that they actually exert a structural effect on the articular cartilage and consequently inhibit the progression of arthritis. They may be utilized continuously or non-continuously as well as in conjunction with the above mentioned more classic treatments.

The use of these treatments does not vary according to the particular arthritic joint concerned. The more modern treatments, consisting particularly of Glucosamine, the new selective COX-II inhibitors and the principle of viscosupplementation, must have their indications more precisely defined (particularly according to the stage and localization of the arthritis) with the aim of optimizing the quality of the results obtained. They represent an additional option (in the case of viscosupplementation) or an alternative (COX-II inhibitors) to the well-known usual treatments.

In the presence of damage to different structures within the joint, such as degenerative meniscal lesions (most often the medial meniscus) it is often necessary to prioritize the medical treatments, with consideration given to arthroscopic surgery.

In conclusion, it is essential to distinguish between the treatment of an acute exacerbation of arthritis (with rest, ice, a NWB state, NSAIDs and/or CCS injections), from that of chronic painful arthritis in a slow evolutionary phase, in which the other more modern treatments are likely to have a much greater clinical impact.

References

1. Ettinger H, Bums R, Messier S *et al.* (1997) A randomized trial comparing aerobic exercise and resistance exercise with a health education program in older adults with knee osteoarthritis. The fitness arthritis and seniors trials (FAST). JAMA 277: 25-31
2. Pincus T, Koch GG *et al.* (2001) A randomised, double-blind, crossover clinical trial of diclofenac plus misoprostol versus acetominophen in patients with osteoarthritis of the hip or knee. Arthritis Rheum 44: 1587-98
3. Hubbard R, Geis G, Woods E *et al.* (1998) Efficacy, tolerability of celecoxib, a specific COX-2 inhibitor, in osteoarthritis. Arthritis Rheum 41(9): S196

4. Mamdani M, Rochon PA, Juurlink DN *et al.* (2002) Observational study of upper gastro-intestinal haemorrhage in elderly patients given selective cyclo-oxygenase-2 inhibitors or conventional non-steroidal anti-inflammatory drugs. BMJ 325: 624
5. Uebelhart D, de Vathaire F, Malaise M *et al.* (2000) European multicenter Chondroitin Sulfate knee OA study: Biochemical and radiological results with a new approach in the statistical evaluation of Rx data. Paper presented during the symposium on Chondroitin Sulfate XIIth EULAR Congress. June 2000; Nice
6. Reginster JY, Deroisy R, Lee IP *et al.* (1999) Glucosamine sulfate significantly reduces progression of knee osteoarthritis over 3 years: a large randomised placebo-controlled double-blind prospective trial. Arthritis Rheum 42(supp. 9): 1975
7. Maheu E, Guillou GB (1995) Intra-articular therapy for osteoarthritis of the knee. Prescrire international 4: 26-7
8. Chakravarty K, Pharoah PDP, Scott DGI (1994) A randomized controlled study of post injection rest following intra-articular steroid therapy for knee synovitis. Br J Rheumatol 33: 464-8
9. Ayral X, Dougados M (1995) Joint lavage. Rev Rhum Engl Ed 62: 281-7
10. Bradley JD, Heilman DK, Katz BP *et al.* (2002) Tidal irrigation as treatment for knee osteoarthritis: a sham-controlled, randomized, double-blinded evaluation. Arthritis Rheum 46(1): 100-8
11. Ravaud P, Moulinier L, Giraudeau B *et al.* (1999) Effects of joint lavage and steroid injection in patients with osteoarthritis of the knee. Arthritis Rheum 42: 475-82
12. Huskisson EC, Donnelly S (1999) Hyaluronic acid in the treatment of osteoarthritis of the knee. Rheumatology (Oxford) 1999 Jul; 38(7): 602-7
13. Scale D, Wobig M, Wolpert W (1994) Viscosupplementation of osteoarthritic knees with hylan: a treatment schedule study. Curr Ther Res 55: 220-32
14. Wobig M, Bach G, Beks P *et al.* (1999) The role of elastoviscosity in the efficacy of viscosupplementation for osteoarthritis of the knee: a comparison of hylan G-F 20 and a lower-molecular-weight hyaluronan. Clin Ther 21(9): 1549-62

SURGICAL TREATMENT

Technique in high tibial osteotomy

D.A. Parker, A.J. Trivett, A. Amendola

Introduction

Proximal tibial osteotomies are an important component of the surgical treatment options in the management of knee osteoarthritis. The value of osteotomy is in the knee with localised osteoarthritis, and a corresponding malalignment that is either causative of or contributory to the arthritis. The principles of correcting malalignment, in order to transfer load to the relatively unaffected compartment of the knee to relieve symptoms and slow disease progression, is a concept that has been used for many years (1), with techniques becoming more refined with time. In addition, despite good long-term results with total knee arthroplasty, there remains a significant concern regarding the longevity of these prostheses, particularly in younger patients. In contrast, osteotomy provides an alternative that preserves the knee joint, which, when appropriately performed, should not compromise later arthroplasty, should this be necessary.

The reported results of high tibial osteotomy vary considerably across the literature, but in general the procedure provides good relief of pain and restoration of function in approximately 80 to 90% of patients at 5 years, and 50 to 65% at 10 years (2-7). In the analysis of these results, most authors have found that success is directly related to achieving optimal alignment (3, 6, 8). Accurate preoperative assessment and technical precision are therefore essential in order to achieve satisfactory outcome. Many techniques have been described for proximal tibial osteotomies. This chapter will discuss the various options available for alignment correction in the treatment of osteoarthritis using proximal tibial osteotomy, outlining the appropriate indications and surgical technique for each.

Preoperative assessment

Clinical assessment

Perhaps the most important part of achieving success with proximal tibial osteotomy is selection of the appropriate patient. A thorough clinical assessment requires a detailed history and physical examination, followed by appropriate imaging. Specific analysis of this information will help determine whether or not a patient is likely to benefit from osteotomy.

Important aspects of a patient's general history include age, occupation, activity level, and medical and surgical history. Particularly significant are the expectations that the patient has for activity postoperatively. Questions specific to the knee include previous injury and surgery, as well as other treatments and their effectiveness. The patient may have noticed an increasing deformity or a static long-term malalignment. Pain history should focus on the site and severity, as well as aggravating and relieving factors. History of locking, catching or instability may point to a mechanical source of symptoms, and the specific details of each of these symptoms should be sought to determine if other procedures, such as arthroscopy, may be beneficial as an adjunct to osteotomy.

Physical examination should commence with an overall impression of the patient's health and build. Lower limb alignment should be assessed at each level, and the gait should be observed for any abnormalities, particularly a thrust in the direction of the deformity, indicating a significant dynamic component. Presence of deformity in all of three planes should be assessed, particularly rotational deformity as this is more difficult to assess later radiographically. Whether or not a deformity is fixed or correctable should be determined. Patellar tracking and the presence of crepitus is observed. Presence of an effusion is assessed and location of tenderness should be recorded carefully. Range of motion is measured, particularly looking for the presence of a flexion contracture and the amount of flexion comfortably achieved. Ligaments are examined, including sagittal plane laxity and the presence of coronal plane pseudolaxity, indicating loss of effective joint space. Reproduction of clicking symptoms and pain with McMurray's test may indicate a meniscal tear. Grinding of medial and lateral compartments through the mid-flexion range may reproduce symptoms from the diseased compartment, and also roughly mimic the effect of an osteotomy by loading the unaffected compartment. Adjacent joints are examined and assessment of neurovascular function is essential.

Radiographic assessment

Knee radiographs are an essential component of preoperative assessment. The standard assessment at our institution includes four short films and one full leg alignment film. The four short films are bilateral antero-posterior weight bearing radiographs taken at full extension, bilateral postero-anterior weight bearing radiographs at 45° of flexion, and lateral and skyline films of the affected leg. Full length alignment films can be either single leg standing, double leg standing or supine, and the various advantages of each have been cited by several authors (9, 10). Whichever is used, the critical aspect is to be aware of the implications of each view. Supine views may underestimate the correction required for the weight bearing situation, and single leg films may overestimate correction due to the component of soft tissue laxity not requiring a bony correction. Unfortunately at this stage there is not a general agreement on the most accurate method of radiographic assessment. It is our practice to obtain single leg standing films from hips to ankles, and to assess the joint congruency angle as an indication of the component of deformity due to soft tissue laxity. This can then be taken into account when calculating the desired correction (9).

A number of measurements are taken from these films to help with preoperative planning. Most important are the axis of weight bearing, joint congruency angle, and the individual articular angles of tibia and femur to assess the site of the deformity. The axis of weight bearing is a straight line drawn from centre of hip to centre of ankle, showing where the weight passes through the knee joint. Mechanical and anatomical axes of the knee are also measured. Congruency angle between tibial and femoral articular surfaces is recorded, and the angle between these surfaces and the axes of the respective shafts gives an indication of degree of deformity in both tibia and femur. Lateral radiographs are assessed for sagittal plane deformity, including measurement of tibial slope.

Calculations of corrections

A number of methods have been described for measuring the required correction on preoperative radiographs (9, 11, 12). The general principle is to determine the desired postoperative location of the weight bearing line and thereby calculate the angular correction necessary to achieve this. More will be discussed under the individual procedures, but in general best results are found with overcorrection of medial compartment osteoarthrosis into slight valgus alignment, whereas lateral compartment osteoarthrosis is best corrected to a more neutral alignment. Depending on the procedure the required wedge to create or remove can be calculated preoperatively, as will be discussed below.

Correcting the varus knee

The varus knee with medial compartment osteoarthrosis is certainly the most common scenario for which osteotomy has been used. As Coventry (11) advocated, the results of high tibial osteotomy in this scenario have been best when the anatomical axis is corrected to 8-10° of valgus (3). However, too much overcorrection may yield poor results, particularly in ligamentously lax individuals, in whom minimal bony overcorrection may lead to a very significant clinical deformity. Other researchers have examined this in relation to the site of the weight bearing line, with best results seen when this passes through the lateral plateau at 62-66% of the width of the plateau (9) Preoperative assessment has therefore aimed to achieve this outcome. The traditional method is to measure the preoperative mechanical and anatomical axes and calculate the angular correction necessary to produce 2-4° of mechanical or 8-10° of anatomical valgus.

More recently, methods have been described by Dugdale et al. (9) and Miniaci et al. (12). These methods determine the angular correction necessary to place the postoperative weight bearing line at 62-66% of the width of the tibial plateau (fig. 1). The current technique used at our institution is that of

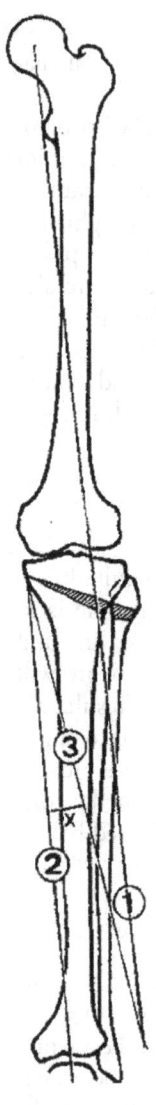

Fig. 1. – Method of preoperative calculation of correction after Miniaci *et al.* Line 1 drawn through 65% of the tibial plateau width shows the desired correction. Line 2 connects the hinge point of the osteotomy to the CTTJ. With this point as the centre and the length of line 2 as the radius, an arc is drawn from CTTJ to intersect with line 1. The angle subtended by lines 2 and 3 is the correction angle.

Dugdale *et al.* (9), calculating the correction to 62.5% of the tibial plateau width, which equates to 3-5° of mechanical valgus. Excess deformity from soft tissue laxity is accounted for by subtracting the increase in congruency angle when compared to the unaffected leg on the double leg standing film, or a non weight bearing film of the affected leg. By measuring the width of the tibia at the level of the proposed osteotomy, the angular correction can be converted into a wedge size, particularly for opening wedge osteotomies.

Lateral closing wedge osteotomy

The most commonly reported osteotomy for medial compartment osteoarthrosis is the lateral closing wedge osteotomy, popularised by Coventry (1) and Insall (13). The goal is correction of alignment as outlined above, achieved by removing a laterally based wedge of bone and closing the resultant defect (fig. 2). The main cited advantages of this procedure over the opening wedge is avoidance of need for bone graft, a more stable construct postoperatively allowing earlier weight bearing and theoretically decreased risk of non-union.

Many variations of technique have been described for this procedure (1, 2, 9, 13), even if the general principle is the same in all. The technique described herein is that used at our institution when a lateral closing wedge osteotomy is indicated. Preoperative planning is done from long leg films as described above. Traditionally an angular calculation is converted to a wedge size based on the tibial width, although newer instrument systems provide angled cutting jigs, obviating the need for this conversion. It is important when calculating a wedge size not to use the traditional rule of 1° equating to 1mm, as this will lead to an undercorrection in virtually every tibia.

The patient is positioned supine on the radiolucent operating table. Setup should allow radiographic visualisation of the lower limb from hip to ankle, with the fluoroscope coming in from the contralateral side. A foot bolster and lateral support are placed to allow the knee to rest unsupported at 90° of flexion, the position used for a significant part of the procedure. The common belief that 90° of flexion allows the posterior structures to fall away from the tibia has been shown to be unreliable (14), and care must always be taken when operating near the posterior cortex. This position does however

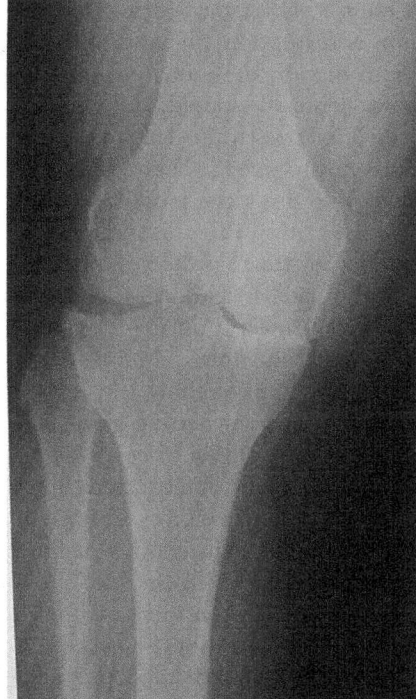

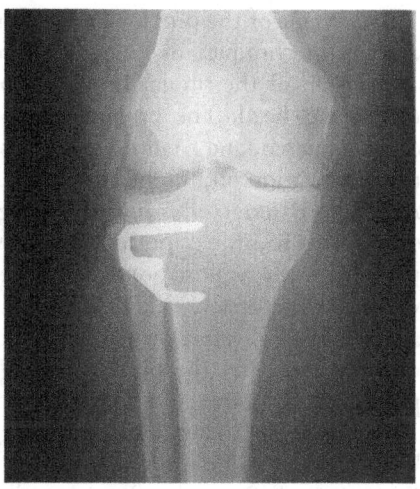

b.

a.

Fig. 2. – Preoperative and postoperative radiographs of closing wedge proximal tibial osteotomy, using staple fixation.

decrease the tension on these tissues, allowing for easier retraction. The leg is prepped and draped free, and a marking pen used to outline the fibular head, lateral joint line, patellar tendon and tibial tubercle. The limb is elevated and tourniquet inflated.

Knee arthroscopy may be required prior to commencing the osteotomy to treat mechanical symptoms. This is done on the basis of a preoperative assessment suggesting an intra-articular source of mechanical symptoms. We do not routinely perform arthroscopy to assess the lateral and patellofemoral compartments, nor if symptoms such as pain and swelling are attributable to the arthrosis, rather than arthroscopically treatable pathology such as unstable meniscal tears or loose bodies.

A multitude of skin incisions have been described, including long curved and short oblique incisions. The skin incision we use is an L-shaped one with the vertical limb along the lateral edge of the tibial tubercle and the horizontal limb parallel and 1cm distal to the lateral joint line, taken posteriorly to the anterior aspect of fibular head. Dissection is carried down to expose the fascia of the anterior compartment which is incised along the anterolateral crest of the tibia, leaving a 5mm cuff for later closure. A cobb elevator is used to elevate the muscle from the anterolateral surface of the tibia and the iliotibial tract is elevated from Gerdy's tubercle proximally, inserting a stay suture for retraction and later closure. The common peroneal nerve is not routinely exposed but is palpated and protected throughout the procedure.

Treatment of the proximal tibio-fibular joint is also characterized by many described techniques, including joint excision or disruption, fibular osteotomy, or excision of the fibular head. We prefer to disrupt the joint but preserve the fibular head. The proximal tibio-fibular joint is exposed, the anterior capsule incised, and a curved osteotome is directed posteromedially to disrupt this articulation and mobilise the fibula so as not to impede later correction. A Z-shaped retractor is placed through this joint along the posterior aspect of the tibia to protect posterior soft tissues. It is critical that this retractor be placed directly against bone along the posterior cortex to protect the neuro-vascular structures (15). The lateral edge of the patellar tendon is identified and a second Z retractor placed underneath it to protect it during the osteotomy. In this way the proximal tibia is exposed from tibial tubercle to the posterolateral cortex and is therefore prepared for the osteotomy.

In removing a laterally based wedge, either an angular cutting guide can be used or a specific size wedge can be removed. The angled cutting jig system (Intermedics®, Switzerland) was initially described by Hoffman (16), and allows for easier use of preoperative calculations and should increase the accuracy of the resultant correction. With this system, the initial step involves making two drill holes parallel to and approximately 1 cm distal to the joint line, across to but not through the medial cortex. A line drawn between these two holes should match the posterior slope of the tibia and the position is checked in both planes with the fluoroscope. These holes are the site of the final proximal fixation and serve as the reference for the remainder of the cuts. Two temporary pins are placed in these holes and a third hole is then drilled distal to these through the medial cortex and allows measurement of the tibial width to guide for depth of the saw cut. Using the jig, the proximal cut of the osteotomy is performed using a calibrated saw blade, to a depth 10 mm less than the measured tibial width. The first jig is then removed and a second jig used, which has a blade that lies in the first saw cut to its full depth and angled cutting slots of 2° increments. The second saw cut is then made through the chosen angled slot, with the jig controlling the depth of the saw cut by its position.

In performing these cuts it is important to check the position of anterior and posterior retractors, to ensure soft tissue protection, and to cut the anterior and posterior cortices fully, to within 1 cm of the medial cortex. The wedge can then be removed. If initial wedge removal is incomplete, it is important to ensure complete removal of the entire wedge using a combination of curettes, rongeurs and osteotomes before closing the osteotomy, otherwise there is a significant risk of intra-articular fracture. It is also important to ensure the wedge is complete to 1 cm from the medial cortex, or there is a chance of hinging open medially making the osteotomy unstable and potentially overcorrecting. The fluoroscope can be used to assist with assessment of completeness of wedge removal.

A three-hole L-shaped plate is then fixed to the proximal fragment using two 6.5 mm cancellous screws through the previously drilled holes. A unicortical drill hole is then made distal to the plate in the lateral cortex, serving as an anchoring point for a compression clamp which is applied to the distal hole of the plate. Using this clamp the osteotomy is closed slowly, at approximately 1mm per minute, allowing for plastic deformation of the intact medial hinge and thus a stable construct. Once done, closure of the osteotomy is confirmed with the fluoroscope and position of the weight bearing line on the tibial plateau is checked with an alignment rod centred fluoroscopically on the centres of the hip, and ankle joints. If satisfactory, the plate is secured with three 4.5mm cortical screws distally. A drain is placed against bone and closure is completed in layers. Fascial closure is interrupted and should attempt to cover the plate as much as possible without undue tension.

The more traditional method of lateral closing wedge osteotomy involves preoperative calculation of a wedge size, such that the base of the wedge on the lateral cortex is known in millimetres. The osteotomy is planned out on the lateral cortex such that the distal limb of the wedge will be just above the tibial tubercle. This maximises the size of the proximal fragment, allowing for good fixation. It is important when marking out the proposed line of the osteotomy that the plane is parallel to the joint line in the lateral plane to avoid inadvertently changing the tibial slope. Once this is done, two guide wires are passed from lateral to medial to 10mm from the medial cortex, one just above the proximal osteotomy and one just below the distal osteotomy. The two cuts of the osteotomy are then performed using an oscillating saw or osteotomes between and parallel to the placed guidewires. Same techniques as described above are used to ensure complete wedge removal before slowly closing the osteotomy using gradual valgus force in extension. Once closed, position and alignment are checked with the fluoroscope and fixation then completed, usually with two stepped staples or alternatively an ASIF L or T-shaped plate. Wound closure is the completed as described above.

Postoperative management involves use of a hinged brace for six weeks, with partial weight bearing using crutches during this time. Radiographs are taken at the 6 week mark, and if early healing of the osteotomy is evident the brace is discontinued and the patient progressed to weight bearing as tolerated. A second radiograph is done at the three month mark and if the osteotomy is united, activity level can be increased as tolerated. A long leg alignment film is taken at the six month mark to assess the accuracy of the correction.

Medial opening wedge osteotomy

Medial opening wedge osteotomy has not been as widely reported in the English-speaking literature as the closing wedge technique, but has been extensively used in Europe and is now enjoying increased popularity in North America (17, 18). The theoretical advantages of opening wedge over closing wedge include: restoration of anatomy with addition of bone to the diseased medial side, the ability to achieve predictable correction in both coronal and sagittal planes, the ability to adjust correction intraoperatively, the requirement for only one bone cut, avoidance of proximal tibiofibular joint disruption and invasion of the lateral compartment, and the relative ease of combining with other procedures such as ACL reconstruction. The disadvantages of this procedure include the creation of a defect that requires bone graft with attendant harvest morbidity, and a theoretical higher risk of non-union, as well as the longer period of restricted weight bearing postoperatively. Medial opening wedge osteotomy has been the preferred technique in our institution for the last five years for the above mentioned reasons. Graft choices include autograft, allograft or pre-prepared bone substitutes. Each option has its own advantages and disadvantages, and although iliac crest autograft probably remains the current gold standard, it has been our practice more recently to use femoral head allograft. This avoids donor site morbidity, and also decreases surgical time. This seems to result in predictable union but obviously requires a readily available bone bank facility.

The surgery is performed with the patient supine on the operating table. A radiolucent table is used with a leg extension applied to allow fluoroscopic visualisation of hip, knee and ankle joints for alignment assessment intraoperatively. A tourniquet is placed around the thigh and the involved limb is prepared and draped free. If iliac crest bone autograft is to be utilised, the ipsilateral crest is also prepared and draped. The surgeon stands with the instruments on the opposite side of the operating table to the operative leg allowing direct access to the medial side of the leg. This also allows the fluoroscopy arm to come in from the operative side.

A skin marker is used to identify the medial joint line, the tibial tubercle and patellar tendon, and the postero-medial border of the tibia (fig. 4a). The leg is elevated and the pneumatic tourniquet inflated. A 5cm longitudinal incision is created, extending from 1cm below the medial joint line midway between the medial border of the tubercle and the postero-medial border of the tibia. The sartorius fascia is exposed by sharp dissection. The superior border of the sartorius fascia is identified and the pes is then retracted distally with a blunt retractor, exposing the superficial fibres of the medial collateral ligament. The anterior border of the medial ligament is identified and this is raised with a scalpel and periosteal elevator. A blunt Hohmann retractor is then passed deep to the medial ligament, around the postero-medial corner of the proximal tibia and along the posterior cortex of the tibia to protect the posterior neurovascular structures.

The medial border of the patellar tendon is next identified. A short longitudinal incision is made to allow a second blunt lever to be placed deep to the patellar tendon just proximal to the tubercle and retract it laterally. The medial insertion of the tendon is released for a few millimetres to allow clear identification of the antero-superior corner of the tubercle. The residual retinaculum and periosteum between these anterior and posterior retractors is then elevated toward the joint line creating a proximally based flap. This gives a subperiosteal exposure of the tibia from the tibial tubercle around to its posteromedial corner.

A guidewire is then inserted along the line of the proposed osteotomy (fig. 4b). Accurate positioning of this guide wire is critical to the success of the operation. The two points of the supero-medial corner of the tibial tubercle and the tip of the head of the fibula laterally are identified. The guide wire starting point on the antero-medial tibia is the direct continuation of a straight line between these two points, which usually gives a start point on the medial tibia approximately 3-4cm distal to the medial joint line. Guide wire obliquity can be altered somewhat depending on the size of the tibia and the required size of correction (a more oblique osteotomy will allow for only a small angle of correction). Fixation failure and intra-articular fracture is more likely with increased obliquity of the osteotomy (19). The guidewire should be placed about 2mm proximal and parallel to the proposed osteotomy as the osteotomy is performed on the distal side of the guidewire.

The obligatory requirements for wire position include: osteotomy placed above the patellar tendon insertion, medial start position distal enough to allow sufficient bone for positioning of the fixation plate on the proximal fragment, osteotomy at least 1cm distal to the tibial articular surface at its most proximal (lateral) extent, and osteotomy directed toward the upper end of the proximal tibio-fibular articulation. The tibial osteotomy is performed immediately distal to the guide pin, the pin protecting against proximal migration of the osteotomy into the joint.

The slope of the osteotomy in the sagittal plane is critical and should mimic the proximal tibial joint slope. The tendency to make the osteotomy perpendicular to the long axis of the tibia should be avoided as this will create a very thin bony fragment posteriorly due to the natural posterior tibial slope of approximately 10°. The joint line can be palpated through the incision or marked with needles, and the line of the osteotomy should be equidistant from the medial joint line anteriorly and posteriorly in order to be parallel to the tibial slope. We mark the tibia along this line with a cautery device prior to performing the osteotomy.

With the previously placed retractors protecting the soft tissues anteriorly and posteriorly, a small oscillating saw is used to cut the tibial cortex from the tibial tubercle around to the posteromedial corner under direct vision. Thin, flexible osteotomes are then used to advance the osteotomy laterally, systematically working from medial to lateral and anterior to posterior. The osteotomy should be taken to within 1cm of the lateral tibial cortex, using intermittent fluoroscopy.

As much as possible should be completed with the thin osteotomes and then this is completed using solid, broad but thin osteotomes. In our early experience with this technique, intra-articular fractures were caused by using thicker, traditional osteotomes (fig. 3). A useful technique to ensure completeness of the osteotomy is to place a broad osteotome centrally to open the osteotomy slightly, and then work with a long, thin osteotome along the anterior and posterior cortices. Whilst performing the osteotomy it is important to regularly check progress with fluoroscope to ensure the appropriate depth and direction of the cut. Calibrated guide pins and osteotomes are also available and can help keep the requirement for fluoroscopy to a minimum.

The mobility of the osteotomy is checked by gentle manipulation of the leg with a valgus force. Ensure the osteotomy opens slightly before proceeding with the wedge osteotome. If the osteotomy seems incomplete, check again with a narrow flexible osteotome anteriorly and posteriorly. Often "stacking osteotomes" can be useful in encouraging mobility in the osteotomy.

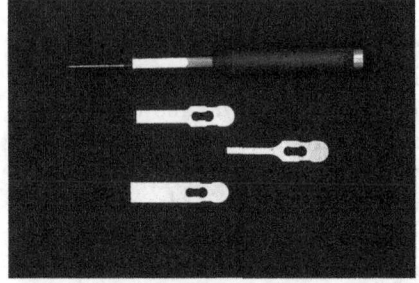

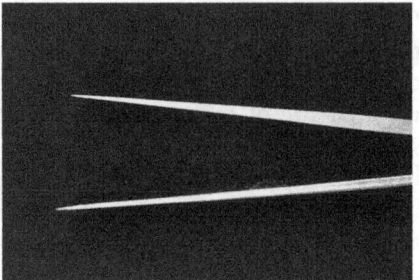

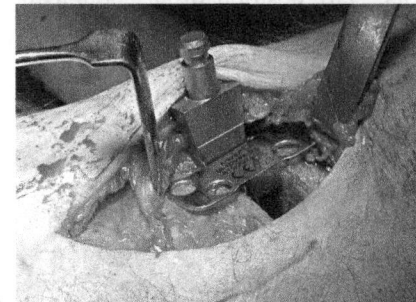

Fig. 3. – Instruments for opening wedge osteotomy.
a. Flexible osteotomes.
b. Thicker tapered osteotomes.
c. Puddu plate *in situ*.

The Puddu tapered osteotome is then engaged into the osteotomy, keeping the direction parallel to the osteotomy (fig. 4c). This is calibrated to allow assessment of the size of the opening achieved in millimetres. This should be advanced slowly to allow gradual opening of the osteotomy, with a rough guide being 5mm per minute. Fluoroscopy should be used to ensure progression of the instrument parallel to the osteotomy. Rapid advancement is likely to produce unwanted extension of the osteotomy proximally or laterally.

Alignment should be checked intermittently. Once the calculated preoperative wedge size has been reached, a long alignment rod can be used as described above with fluoroscopy. With the rod centred over the hip and ankle joints, it should lie at 62-66% of the tibial width, usually at the lateral edge of the lateral tibial spine. The sagittal plane correction should also be assessed by looking carefully at the amount of opening of the osteotomy anteriorly and posteriorly. Since the tibia is a triangular bone in cross section with apex anterior, the size of the wedge anteriorly at the tubercle should be less than that at the posteromedial corner to avoid changing tibial slope (fig. 4d). If the gap anteriorly is equal to that at the postero-medial corner, the posterior slope of the tibia will be inadvertently increased.

The sagittal alignment is also important, and the orientation of the tibial articular surface in this plane is another critical determinant of outcome. In cases of pure medial compartment osteoarthrosis in a stable knee, the normal tibial slope should be preserved, using the method described above as well as intraoperative fluoroscopy. Sagittal slope can be deliberately altered in instability patterns to decrease tibial translations and assist with knee stability (20). A decreased posterior tibial slope will decrease anterior tibial translation in

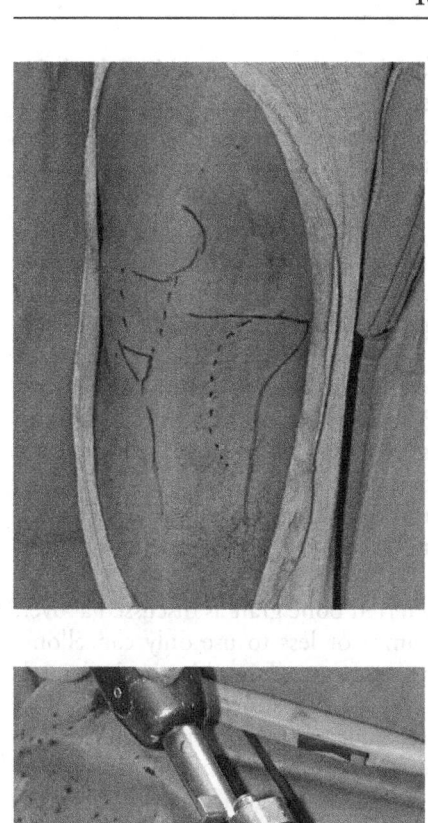

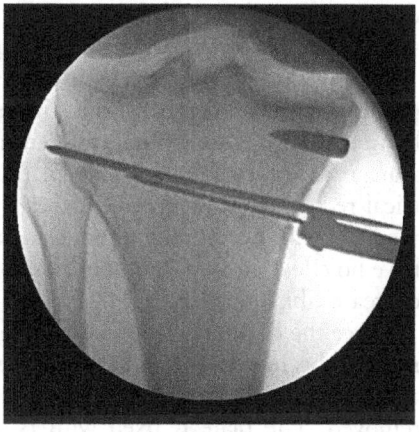

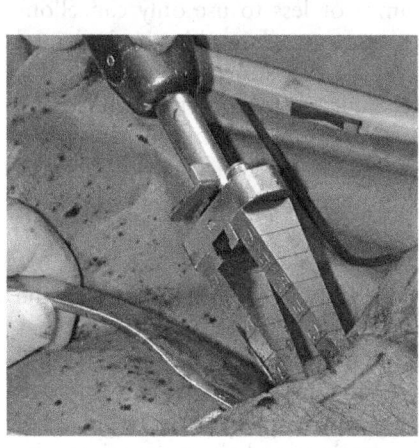

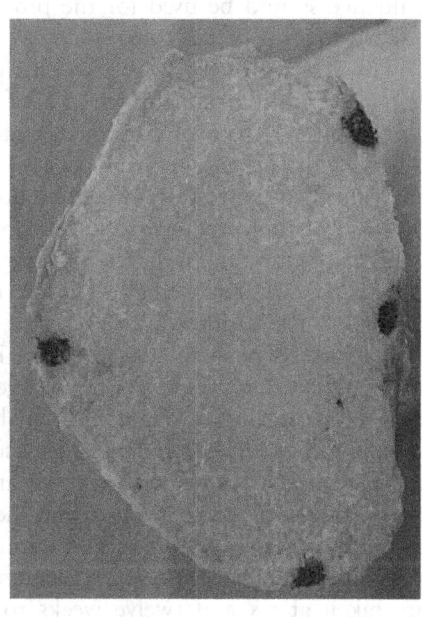

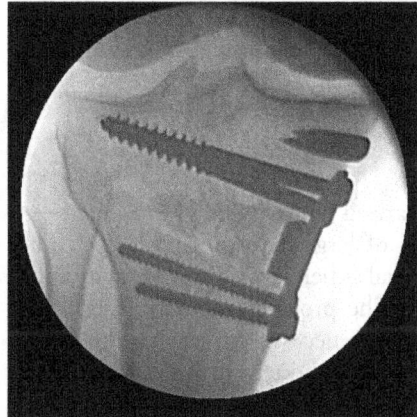

Fig. 4. – Opening wedge osteotomy.
a. Incision skin markings: incision midway between tibial tubercle and posteromedial border of tibia, in this case along a previous scar.
b. Correct guidewire placement, with flexible osteotome passing parallel and inferior to the guidewire.
c. Insertion of Puddu osteotome. Note calibrations guiding size of opening wedge.
d. Cross section of tibia at osteotomy level.
e. Completed osteotomy with bone graft filling defect.

the presence of ACL deficiency. This may be important to address both in medial compartment arthrosis subsequent to chronic ACL deficiency, and anterior instability patterns with associated varus deformity. Conversely, in the posterior cruciate deficient knee, increasing the tibial slope can be beneficial by increasing anterior tibial translation. Slope can be adjusted by the type of plate used and the positioning of the plate. Plates are available in symmetrical rectangular, or tapered shapes. Positioning a symmetrical plate anteromedially will increase the slope, using a tapered plate directly medially should have no effect on slope, and positioning a tapered plate posteromedially should decrease tibial slope.

Once the desired correction has been achieved and plate positioning determined, the insertion handle from the Puddu osteotome is removed leaving the tines *in situ*. The plate is placed between these tines which can then be removed. The plate is fixed with two partially threaded 6.5mm cancellous screws proximally and two 4.5mm fully threaded screws distally. Fluoroscopic guidance should be used for the proximal screws to avoid penetration into either the joint or the osteotomy.

The defect is then grafted using the preferred bone graft as discussed above. It has been our practice in defects of 7.5mm or less to use only cancellous chips, and in defects of 10mm or greater to use cancellous chips in the lateral aspect of the defect and two corticocancellous wedges medially, one anterior and one posterior to the plate. Final fluoroscopic assessment ensures adequate position of the osteotomy and hardware, and complete filling of the defect with bone graft (fig. 4e). The wound is irrigated and a suction drain placed against bone posteromedially. Closure is completed in layers and dry dressing applied to the wounds.

A standard postoperative regimen is followed, which is somewhat more restrive than that for the closing wedge procedure. For the first six weeks the knee is placed in a range of motion brace set at 0 to 90°, and the patient encouraged to achieve this range, particularly full extension. During this period the patient remains touch weight bearing using crutches. From week six to twelve the brace is discontinued and the weight bearing is progressed gradually to full over the six week period. From three to six months postoperatively the patient is encouraged to progress their activities as tolerated. Short radiographs are taken at six and twelve weeks to ensure maintenance of position and healing, and long leg alignment films done at six months to assess the correction achieved.

Dome osteotomy

The dome osteotomy was originally popularised by Maquet (21) and has been advocated by some authors for correction of large deformities (21-23). The osteotomy is performed proximal to the tibial tubercle with its concavity inferiorly, arcing around the tibial tuberosity. The procedure is performed on a radiolucent table with the patient supine. It is necessary to divide the fibula to allow correction to occur and this is done obliquely in the middle third of the shaft. Two Steinmann pins are then inserted into the tibia, one proximal and one distal to the proposed osteotomy, with the angle between the two pins corresponding to the proposed correction.

Through a 5cm longitudinal incision centred on the tibial tubercle the dome osteotomy is performed. This can be done using specially designed curved osteotomes, or by making multiple drill holes along a curved line marked out with the cautery and then completing the osteotomy with thin osteotomes. The fragments are then rotated until the pins are parallel and two Charnley clamps are used to fix the fragments under compression. Alternatively, a monolateral external fixator can be used on the lateral side of the tibia. Position of the osteotomy and overall alignment is checked fluoroscopically before wound closure. Range of motion is commenced immediately postoperatively and the patient is allowed to partial weight bear with crutches. Full weight bearing without crutches is commenced after eight weeks with radiological evidence of healing.

The main advantage of this procedure is that it allows essentially unrestricted correction, in contrast to the more commonly used techniques. The position of the tibial tubercle in relation to the joint line is unaffected, and Maquet actually advocated anterior displacement of the tubercle through the osteotomy. Use of an external fixator allows postoperative adjustment of alignment, which may be an advantage especially in larger corrections, although the risk of possible pin tract infection and the cumbersome nature of the treatment for patients is a potential disadvantage.

Correcting the valgus knee

Medial closing wedge osteotomy

Medial closing wedge proximal tibial osteotomy for treatment of the valgus knee with lateral compartment osteoarthritis has been the subject of very few reports in the literature (24, 25). Early experience from Coventry (24) suggested that results were not as good as those achieved with lateral closing wedge for medial compartment arthrosis. Traditionally most surgeons will use a distal femoral osteotomy in this scenario on the basis that the pathology tends to be more on the femoral side of the joint and postoperative joint obliquity is avoided. Tibial-sided surgery has been supported more recently in France by Chambat et al. (26), with the theoretical advantage over femoral osteotomy that a tibial correction will have an equal effect throughout flexion, whereas a femoral procedure may lose its effect by 90° of flexion. This is particularly relevant considering the common finding that lateral compartment arthrosis commonly appears more severe on standing radiographs with the knee at 30-45° of flexion than in full extension.

Preoperative assessment should calculate correction to a normal axis, in contrast to medial arthrosis where overcorrection is the goal, and should assess the articular angles of both femur and tibia. Creation of an obliquity in the joint line of greater than 10° of varus should be avoided. The sum of the coronal slope of the tibial articular surface and the desired correction angle should therefore not produce more than 10° of varus. The results of this procedure are also better in young patients with relatively mild arthrosis, ideally with joint space narrowing more peripherally. This procedure is therefore only indicated in a small group of patients with lateral compartment arthrosis.

The patient is set up on the operating table in the same manner as for a lateral closing wedge osteotomy described above, but with the surgeon on the contralateral side and fluoroscope coming in from the ipsilateral side. The surgical exposure is identical to that described above for medial opening wedge osteotomy. Removal of the predetermined wedge can be done using either a calibrated angular cutting jig, or by cutting between two guidewires with osteotomes as described above for the lateral closing wedge procedure. It is important to make the cuts parallel to the joint surface in the sagittal plane, and the apex of the osteotomy at the proximal tibiofibular joint to obviate the need for disrupting this articulation. In addition, note that if the two cuts are parallel to one another, the wedge should be smaller anteriorly due to the triangular shape of the tibia. Fixation can be achieved using either a plate and screws or two staples. Position of the osteotomy and leg alignment are checked with the fluoroscope prior to wound closure. Postoperative rehabilitation is the same as for the lateral closing wedge procedure described above.

Lateral opening wedge osteotomy

Another alternative for the valgus knee with lateral compartment osteoarthrosis is a lateral opening wedge tibial osteotomy (fig. 5a-c). Little has been reported about this procedure, with a recent paper by Marti *et al.* (27) reporting an 88% good or excellent outcome at an average follow-up of 11 years. They describe a lateral opening wedge osteotomy using iliac crest autograft, and conclude that the procedure is a good alternative for the treatment of isolated lateral compartment arthrosis, with the aim being a slight overcorrection. The approach is however technically more difficult than the medial closing wedge, due to the need for exposure and disruption of the proximal tibio-fibular joint.

The surgical setup is the same as for the lateral closing wedge procedure as described above, as is the exposure and disruption of the proximal tibio-fibular joint. A guidewire is placed from lateral to medial, with the proposed line of the osteotomy passing just superior to the tibial tubercle and ending 1.5cm distal to the medial joint line at the medial tibial cortex. This gives a slight obliquity from inferolateral to superomedial. The osteotomy is made 1-2mm distal to and parallel to the guidewire, in the same fashion as for the medial opening wedge osteotomy and finishing 1cm from the medial tibial cortex. The same system is used to open the osteotomy to the desired width, and the position is checked with fluoroscopy before inserting the appropriate size Puddu plate and fixing this with screws. As with the medial procedure, it is important to avoid any inadvertent change in the tibial slope. Postoperative management is the same as described for the medial procedure.

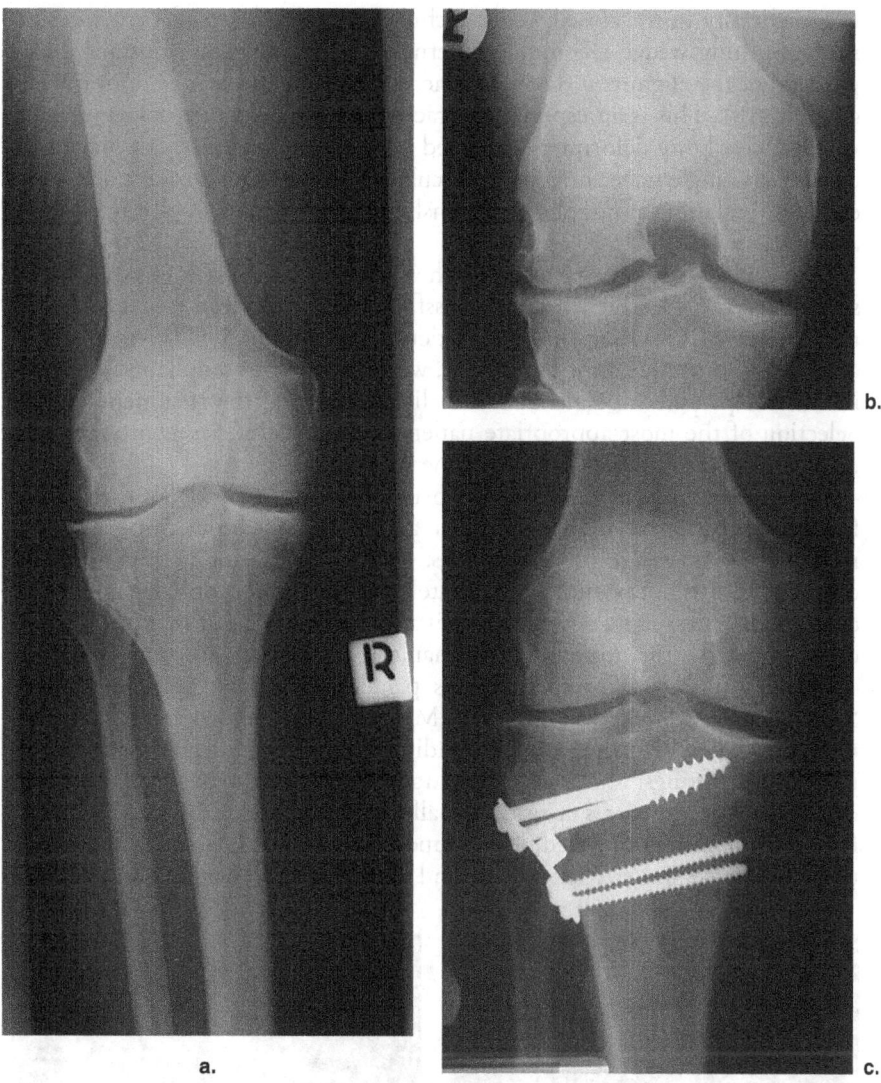

Fig. 5. – Lateral opening wedge osteotomy.
a. Preoperative AP radiograph.
b. Preoperative intercondylar radiograph demonstrating lateral compartment arthrosis.
c. Postoperative radiograph.

Gradual correction – external fixators

Use of an external fixator to achieve a gradual correction has a number of potential advantages over a single stage correction, with many authors reporting good results with this technique (18, 28-30). Firstly, large corrections may be technically impossible with standard closing or opening wedge techniques, either due to excessive bone removal compromising fixation and creating deformity in the closed wedge technique, or excessive soft tissue tension in the opening wedge technique. External fixators also allow constant manipulation of the alignment during the healing process in order to optimize alignment (18). This is an especially attractive feature for larger deformities, in which major bony deformity combined with soft tissue laxity can make prediction of a single stage correction difficult. Circular external fixators also allow easy manipulation of angular and translational correction in all three planes as necessary (28).

These advantages are balanced by the significant drawback of possible pin site infection (31), which if not successfully treated can lead to deeper infection compromising later surgery, particularly arthroplasty. The treatment is also a significant ordeal for the patient, who needs to be compliant with treatment, and prepared for alterations in lifestyle during the treatment period. Selection of the most appropriate patient for this technique is probably the most important factor in success of the procedure.

It has recently been our practice to use a circular hybrid external fixator for the correction of deformities that are technically beyond the standard medial opening wedge procedure (figs. 6a, 6b). In addition, in these larger deformities, it is not possible to accurately predict the appropriate single stage correction. The specific device we use is a hybrid ring fixator that has six obliquely oriented struts initially set to match the patient's deformity, and then gradually adjusted to bring the rings parallel. Computer software (Taylor Spatial Frame®, Smith and Nephew, Memphis, TN) allows input of deformity parameters from preoperative radiographs and subsequently calculates initial strut settings, and a correction rate set by the surgeon based on specific soft tissue structures at risk. This allows preoperative construction of the frame. It is essential to schedule a preoperative appointment with the patient to demonstrate and size the frame, and explain the procedure and postope-

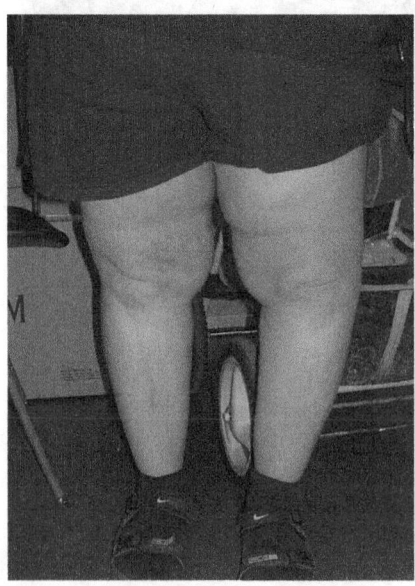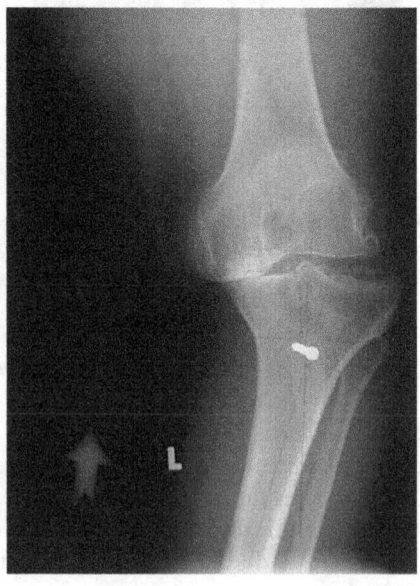

a .   b.

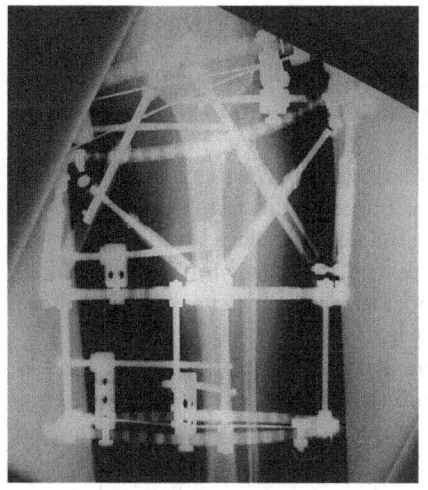

c.

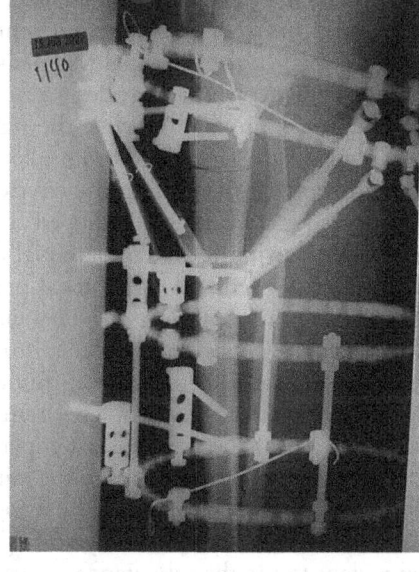

d.

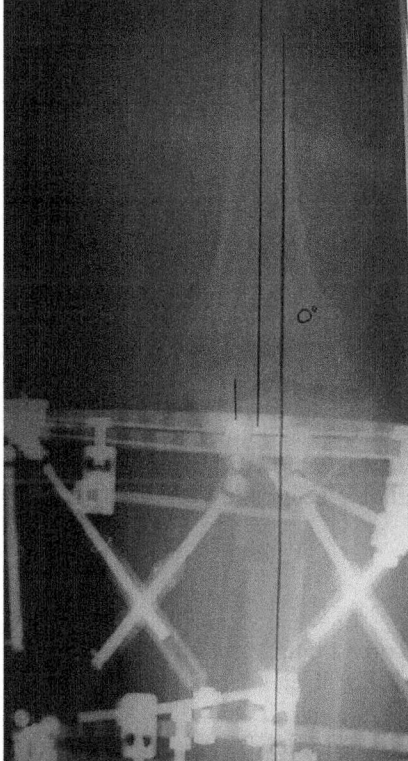

e.

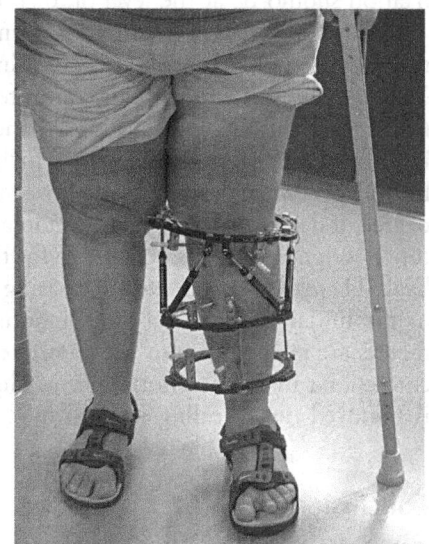

f.

Fig. 6. – Large varus deformity.
a. Preoperative clinical picture.
b. Preoperative AP radiograph, demonstrating large varus deformity with lateral tibial subluxation.
c.-d. Radiograph after initial correction: demonstrates inadequate correction, to neutral anatomic axis.
e. Radiograph after final residual correction: correction to 10° anatomic valgus and decrease in posterior tibial slope.
f. Postoperative clinical picture.

rative schedule. Ring circumference should allow for two fingerbreadths of clearance from soft tissue circumferentially. The construct we use is a single ring attached to the proximal fragment and two parallel rings attached to the distal fragment, which provides a very stable construct.

The procedure is done with the patient supine on a radiolucent table. A computer in the operating room allows adjustments in the parameters that may prove necessary during the course of frame application. A tourniquet is not necessary and the leg is draped free. Bolsters are placed under the thigh and foot allowing for circumferential access to the tibia from knee to ankle. The frame is sized and constructed preoperatively and is checked once more to ensure appropriate fit on the patient's leg.

A fine wire is passed from lateral to medial parallel to the joint surface, at least 10mm distal to the joint to minimize the risk of intrasynovial penetration with possible infection. The frame is applied to this wire and using the undersurface of the frame as a template a second fine wire is passed, taking care to keep the frame parallel to the joint surface in coronal and sagittal planes. The frame is then secured distally using a fine wire across the distal ring. The construct is then completed by adding two 5mm half pins to each ring. It is important to use the subcutaneous surface of the tibia as much as possible and avoid penetration of anterior compartment musculature. The proximal ring fixation should be at the level of, or proximal to the tibial tubercle.

The osteotomy is then done percutaneously at the lower border of the tibial tubercle, through two small incisions using a Gigli saw subperiosteally (fig. 6c-d). The two anterior struts are disconnected from the middle ring and deflected to facilitate this. Wounds are closed and pin sites dressed, and the osteotomy is left static for 10 days following which the correction is then done gradually by the patient at home, usually over a 7-14 day period depending on the degree of deformity. Range of motion as tolerated is allowed immediately and touch weight bearing is performed for the first 10 days whilst pin site wounds heal. Thereafter partial weight bearing with crutches is allowed. At the end of the initial correction a long standing weight bearing film is taken, parameters are re-entered into the computer software, and any necessary residual correction can be done until optimal alignment is achieved (figs. 6e). The frame is removed once healing is confirmed radiologically and clinically (fig. 6f).

Conclusion

Proximal tibial osteotomy can be used to correct both varus and valgus deformities in the management of isolated medial or lateral compartment osteoarthritis. There are a number of operative techniques described to achieve this goal and the relative merits of each have been outlined above. Whatever the technique used, critical to the success of the procedure are the selection of the appropriate patient, and the attainment of a precise correction without complications. If these goals are met, proximal tibial osteotomy should provide long-term relief of pain and restoration of function in patients with localised knee osteoarthritis.

References

1. Coventry MB (1984) Upper tibial osteotomy. Clin Orthop 46-52
2. Billings A, Scott DF, Camargo MP *et al.* (2000) High tibial osteotomy with a calibrated osteotomy guide, rigid internal fixation, and early motion. Long-term follow-up. J Bone Joint Surg Am 82: 70-9
3. Coventry MB, Ilstrup DM, Wallrichs SL (1993) Proximal tibial osteotomy. A critical long-term study of eighty-seven cases. J Bone Joint Surg Am 75: 196-201
4. Insall JN, Joseph DM, Msika C (1984) High tibial osteotomy for varus gonarthrosis. A long-term follow-up study. J Bone Joint Surg Am 66: 1040-8
5. Ivarsson I, Myrnerts R, Gillquist J (1990) High tibial osteotomy for medial osteoarthritis of the knee. A 5 to 7 and 11 year follow-up. J Bone Joint Surg Br 72: 238-44
6. Naudie D, Bourne RB, Rorabeck CH *et al.* (1999) The Install Award. Survivorship of the high tibial valgus osteotomy. A 10- to 22-year follow-up study. Clin Orthop 18-27
7. Rinonapoli E, Mancini GB, Corvaglia A *et al.* (1998) Tibial osteotomy for varus gonarthrosis. A 10- to 21-year followup study. Clin Orthop 185-93
8. Yasuda K, Majima T, Tsuchida T *et al.* (1992) A 10- to 15-year follow-up observation of high tibial osteotomy in medial compartment osteoarthrosis. Clin Orthop 186-95
9. Dugdale TW, Noyes FR, Styer D (1992) Preoperative planning for high tibial osteotomy. The effect of lateral tibiofemoral separation and tibiofemoral length. Clin Orthop 248-64
10. Ogata K, Yoshii I, Kawamura H *et al.* (1991) Standing radiographs cannot determine the correction in high tibial osteotomy. J Bone Joint Surg Br 73: 927-31
11. Coventry MB (1985) Upper tibial osteotomy for osteoarthritis. J Bone Joint Surg Am 67: 1136-40
12. Miniaci A, Ballmer FT, Ballmer PM *et al.* (1989) Proximal tibial osteotomy. A new fixation device. Clin Orthop 250-9
13. Insall J, Shoji H, Mayer V (1974) High tibial osteotomy. A five-year evaluation. J Bone Joint Surg Am 56: 1397-405
14. Smith PN, Gelinas J, Kennedy K *et al.* (1999) Popliteal vessels in knee surgery. A magnetic resonance imaging study. Clin Orthop 158-64
15. Georgoulis AD, Makris CA, Papageorgiou CD *et al.* (1999) Nerve and vessel injuries during high tibial osteotomy combined with distal fibular osteotomy: a clinically relevant anatomic study. Knee Surg Sports Traumatol Arthrosc 7: 15-9
16. Hofmann AA, Wyatt RW, Beck SW (1991) High tibial osteotomy. Use of an osteotomy jig, rigid fixation, and early motion versus conventional surgical technique and cast immobilization. Clin Orthop 271: 212-7
17. Hernigou P, Medevielle D, Debeyre J *et al.* (1987) Proximal tibial osteotomy for osteoarthritis with varus deformity. A ten to thirteen-year follow-up study. J Bone Joint Surg Am 69: 332-54
18. Magyar G, Ahl TL, Vibe P *et al.* (1999) Open-wedge osteotomy by hemicallotasis or the closed-wedge technique for osteoarthritis of the knee. A randomised study of 50 operations. J Bone Joint Surg Br 81: 444-8
19. Amendola A, Mrkonjic L, Clatworthy M *et al.* (1999) Opening wedge high tibial osteotomy using a Puddu distraction plate: Focus on technique, early results and complications. Presented at the International Society of Arthroscopy, Knee Surgery and Orthopaedic Sports Medicine, Washington, DC
20. Amendola A, Giffin R, Sanders D *et al.* (2001) Osteotomy for Knee Instability: The Effect of increasing Tibial Slope on Anterior Tibial Translation. Presented at Specialty Day of American Orthopaedic Society for Sports Medicine, San Francisco, March 2001
21. Maquet P (1976) Valgus osteotomy for osteoarthritis of the knee. Clin Orthop 00: 143-8
22. Takahashi T, Wada Y, Tanaka M *et al.* (2000) Dome-shaped proximal tibial osteotomy using percutaneous drilling for osteoarthritis of the knee. Arch Orthop Trauma Surg 120: 32-7
23. Sundaram NA, Hallett JP, Sullivan MF (1986) Dome osteotomy of the tibia for osteoarthritis of the knee. J Bone Joint Surg Br 68: 782-6

24. Coventry MB (1987) Proximal tibial varus osteotomy for osteoarthritis of the lateral compartment of the knee. J Bone Joint Surg Am 69: 32-8
25. Shoji H, Insall J (1973) High tibial osteotomy for osteoarthritis of the knee with valgus deformity. J Bone Joint Surg Am 55: 963-73
26. Chambat P, Ait Si Selmi T, Dejour D et al. (2000) Varus Tibial Osteotomy. Operative Techniques in Sports Medicine 8: 44-7
27. Marti RK, Verhagen RA, Kerkhoffs GM et al. (2001) Proximal tibial varus osteotomy. Indications, technique, and five to twenty-one-year results. J Bone Joint Surg Am 83: 164-70
28. Catagni MA, Guerreschi F, Ahmad TS et al. (1994) Treatment of genu varum in medial compartment osteoarthritis of the knee using the Ilizarov method. Orthop Clin North Am 25: 509-14
29. Klinger HM, Lorenz F, Harer T (2001) Open wedge tibial osteotomy by hemicallotasis for medial compartment osteoarthritis. Arch Orthop Trauma Surg 121: 245-7
30. Weale AE, Lee AS, MacEachern AG (2001) High tibial osteotomy using a dynamic axial external fixator. Clin Orthop 154-67
31 Geiger F, Schneider U, Lukoschek M et al. (1999) External fixation in proximal tibial osteotomy: a comparison of three methods. Int Orthop 23: 160-3

Opening wedge osteotomy of the distal femur in the valgus knee

G. Puddu, F. Vittorio, M. Cipolla, G. Cerullo, E. Gianni

Indications and contraindications

Osteoarthrosis of the valgus knee has many causative factors. Degenerative changes of the articular cartilage can occur through tension, compression or shear. They are highly related to the forces exerted on the bearing surfaces. The overload caused by congenital valgus deformity or secondary to articular or metaphyseal fractures and lateral meniscectomy are aetiologically important. In essence biophysical cause for osteoarthrosis is an overload or a concentration of forces beyond the ability of the cartilage and subchondral bone to cope.

In any discussion about osteoarthrosis of the knee and the possibilities of treatment, the indication of knee realignment (osteotomy) versus knee replacement (arthroplasty) is often very pertinent. It follows that alignment of the lower extremity plays an important role in osteoarthrosis of the knee. Malalignment into a valgus position will overload the lateral compartment of the joint. The rationale behind the osteotomy is to correct the angular deformity at the knee, and, therefore, decrease the excessive weight bearing load across the affected compartment which is the most involved by the degenerative process. The osteotomy is indicated for the younger, more active patients as an effective alternative to a knee replacement.

Osteotomy was popularised firstly at the tibia and only years later at the distal femur (1).

We think that the patients selected for the osteotomy should have mostly unicompartmental osteoarthrosis with axial malalignment. However, fractures and other traumas, congenital and acquired deformities, as well as idiopatic osteonecrosis are also indications for the osteotomy.

There is no definite age below which one should do an osteotomy and above which one should do an arthroplasty. The age of 65 is the most often cited, but activity level, lifestyle and general health must be considered.

The best indication is a primary lateral osteoarthritis in knees with good range of motion (ROM): at least 90° of flexion, less than 15° of extension deficit. Osteotomy should probably not be done in patients with rheumatoid arthritis, patients with very unstable knees, nor in knees with greater than

15°-20° of valgus deformity, because these knees are complicated by an associated severe ligamentous laxity and subluxation.

The overweight is a controversial topic. Obesity has a negative effect on the outcome of surgery in many orthopaedic operations. Most surgeons would agree that overweight could make a patient better candidate for osteotomy than for arthroplasty, but it is also true that obesity will increase the risk of postoperative complications.

Contraindication to the osteotomy is severe bone loss, of the tibia or femur. When the bony support is insufficient, congruent weight bearing on both tibial plateaus following the osteotomy is not possible. In this situation, tibiofemoral contact will teeter on the relatively prominent intercondylar tibial spines.

The presence of severe valgus deformity may be associated with medial subluxation of the tibia. Subluxation greater than 1cm is an absolute contraindication to osteotomy and some authors suggest that osteotomy should not be performed if any translation or subluxation is present.

Preoperative planning

The goal of the osteotomy is to realign the mechanical axis of the limb thereby shifting weight bearing forces from a diseased compartment to a more normal compartment.

The alignment of the limb is measured on full length XR of the lower extremity. The mechanical axis is a line drawn from the center of the femoral head to the center of the ankle mortise. The anatomic axis is a line drawn through the center of the shaft of the femur and through the center of the shaft of the tibia. In the normal knee the two lines cross each other in the center of the joint making an angle of 5° (physiologic valgus), and the mechanical axis passes also through the center of the knee joint, or slightly varus (about 1° medially) (fig. 1).

According to these parameters as the reference points of the "normality", the deformity is measured.

In case of valgus knee, we aim to restore the normal alignment of the limb (2, 3) with mechanical axis in neutral position (center of the knee joint).

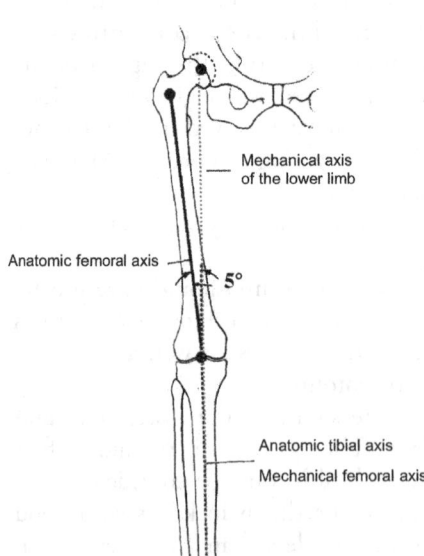

Mechanical axis
of the lower limb

Anatomic femoral axis

5°

Anatomic tibial axis

Mechanical femoral axis

Fig. 1. – In the normal knee the anatomic axes of the femur and tibia cross each other with a 5° valgus angle while the mechanical axis of the limb passes in the center of the tibial plateau, right in between the spines.

While in case of varus knee we wish to get 5° of overcorrection pushing the alignment over the physiologic 5° of valgus to the desired 9°-10°, because extensive experience has shown that overcorrection is absolutely essential if one wants to optimize a long-term result from valgus osteotomy.

The biomechanics of varus and valgus knees differ. The alignment in the normal knee creates the intrinsic valgus angle between femur and tibia and determines an asymmetric overload of the medial compartment (about 60% of the whole), then an overcorrection in a varus osteotomy can induce a catastrophic overload of the medial compartment.

In varus deformity the tibiofemoral joint line is usually parallel to the floor and proximal tibia osteotomy has been demonstrated to effectively transfer load from the medial to the lateral compartment. In valgus deformity, the joint line has a valgus tilt from supero-lateral to infero-medial direction. While tibial varus osteotomy may realign a valgus limb, it is not able to correct the joint line tilt because the procedure is performed distally to the joint. The mechanical consequence of it, in patients with severe valgus deformities (over 10°-12° according to various authors), is that the medial load transfer is limited and the resultant increased valgus tilt of the joint line increases the shear forces and the lateral subluxation during gait. In case of lateral osteoarthritis with valgus deformity, a distal femoral varus osteotomy may realign a valgus limb and correct valgus tilt of the joint line.

The preferred authors' technique is an opening wedge technique. Closing wedge technique is probably better known and certainly more diffused. It consists in taking a wedge from the medial supracondylar area of the femur leaving the lateral cortex intact and closing the osteotomy with a 90° blade plate on the medial side (4). A different technique of closing wedge, in which the fixation is achieved by a 95° condylar blade plate from lateral, analog to the osteosynthesis of a metaphysial fracture, is also described (5, 6).

The osteotomy we propose here is based on the opening wedge technique. Special plates with a spacer "tooth" (8, 9, 10) were designed for this aim. We need to know the size of the base of the wedge, calculated in millimeters, to choose the plate and fix the osteotomy at the desired correction, we have planned in angular degrees. Different widths of the femur, at the level of the osteotomy cut, correspond to different wedge sizes, for the same value of angular correction.

With the templating paper we outline the profile of the knee. After having cut the paper at the level of the osteotomy, we open a wedge until the mechanical axis we have drawn before, from the femur head to the ankle joint, passes through the center of the knee. When the axis is in this position the alignment of the limb coincide with the physiologic valgus and the base of the paper wedge corresponds to the plate with the spacer tooth of the same size (fig. 2). Taking account of the radiographic magnification (normally about 110% on the full length leg film) we plan the osteotomy and estimate in advance the plate we need during the operation.

To complete evaluation of the knee, we look at the different radiographic views including in the examination also the standard lateral and the axial of the patellofemoral joint.

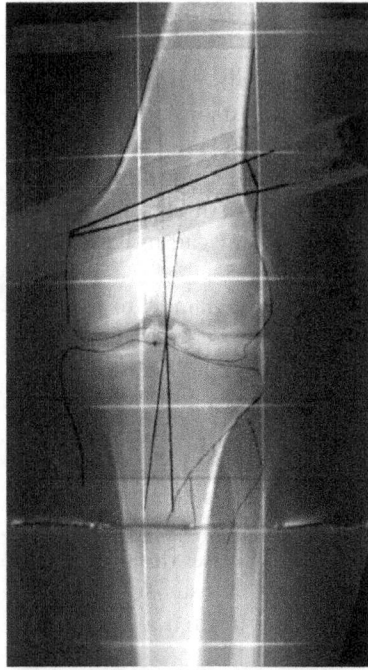

Fig. 2. – The preoperative planning is based on a drawing of the femur condyles and tibial pla-teau profiles, that permits to cut out a wedge, representing the osteotomy, from the tracing paper and calculate its size to know the plate requested for the operation.

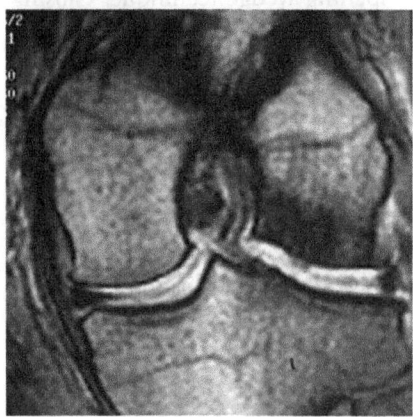

Fig. 3. – MRI can be positive for a stress reaction of the subchondral bone as the only diagnostic sign of an early degenerative process.

The Rosenberg view, comparative postero-anterior weight-bearing radiograph at 45° of knee flexion (7), facilitates the diagnose in case the standard AP view was not sensitive enough. The Rosenberg exam has a strong predictive value when the deformity is associated with a cruciate insufficiency and, therefore, the chondral wear prevails in the posterior part of the tibial plateaus.

Most of the authors don't recommend Computed Tomography (CT) scans or Magnetic Resonance Imaging (MRI) in studying a candidate for knee osteotomy, but we think that the stress reaction of the subchondral bone, detectable by MRI (fig. 3), could be the only positive sign of a degenerative process, at its earlier stage, but, already, with all the stigmates of the condemned knee.

Dedicated surgical instrumentation

The purpose of varus osteotomy is to reconduce the lower limb alignment to the physiologic 0° of the neutral mechanical axis.

We present here our technique to perform the opening wedge osteotomy and, to accomplish better reproducible results with the less technical difficulties as possible in performing the operation, the senior author developed a complete, but simple and easy, system of dedicated instruments and plates (8, 9, 10).

The plates specially designed for this osteotomy are "T" shaped with seven holes (fig. 4).

Their specificities is a spacer, a tooth as it were, available in seven different sizes from 5 to 20mm in thickness. The new plates will have the tooth increasing one size for each single millimeter more, from the thinnest to the thickest.

The tooth enters into the osteotomic line holding the position and preventing a later collapse of the bone with the recurrence of the deformity. The thickness of the spacer must coincide with the desired angle of correction, calculated in advance with the preoperative planning. The three holes of the horizontal distal arm of the plate allow the introduction of the AO 6.5mm cancellous screws, while the holes in the vertical arm are cut for the AO 4.5mm cortical screws.

The crucial point of the operation is opening the metaphysis, where the osteotomy has cut the bone, at the desired angle of correction and holding the position to allow the introduction of the plate tooth. A very simple "wedge opener" greatly facilitates this step. It looks like a fork with two wedge shaped branches, graduated to permit the opening at the correct rate (fig. 5a), and a removable handle to allow the positioning of the plate (fig. 5b).

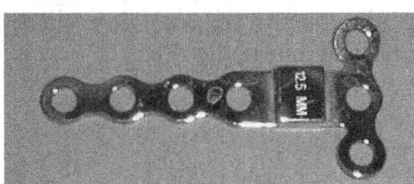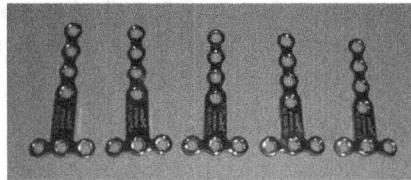

Fig. 4. – The plates are specially designed for opening wedge osteotomies in different sizes of the spacer tooth.

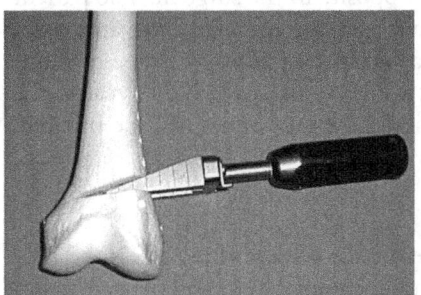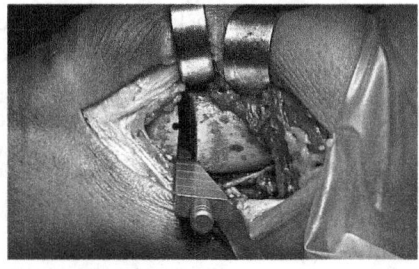

a.   b.

Fig. 5. – **a.** The "wedge opener" permits to open the osteotomy at the exact rate of correction. **b.** The removable handle allows the easy positoning of the plate.

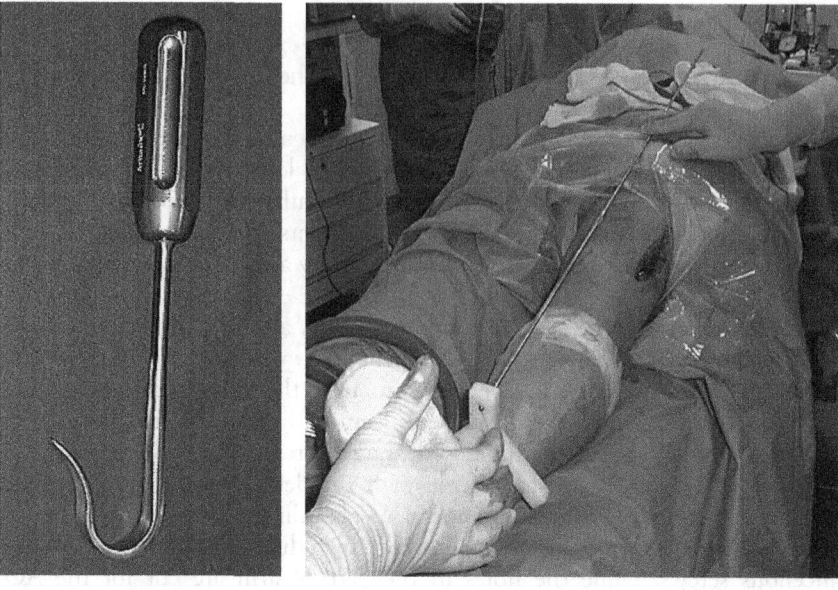

Fig. 6.   **Fig. 7.**

Fig. 6. – The special Homan is designed for the lateral femoral approach to retract the vastus lateralis.

Fig. 7. – The long rod guide with an ankle support is dedicated to the intraoperative check of the tibio-femoral alignment after the osteotomic correction.

The other two dedicated tools are the Homan retractor, especially designed for vastus lateralis (fig. 6) and a long rod guide with an ankle support to check intra-operatively the mechanical femorotibial alignment (fig. 7).

Surgical technique

Step 1: patient position

We prefer a normal operating table with the patient in a supine position and the C-arm of an image intensifier set up opposite to the surgeon. The patient is draped as usual in knee surgery; we also prepare the iliac wing and cover the foot using a very fine stockinet and a transparent adhesive drape to minimize the bulging at the ankle so that it will be possible to better realize the femorotibial alignment after the correction. The tourniquet may be inflated.

Step 2: arthroscopy

Arthroscopy of the knee is carried out before the osteotomy to assess the relative integrity of the controlateral tibiofemoral compartment and of the patellofemoral joint and to treat any intra-articular pathology: appropriate joint surface debridment, partial meniscectomy, or loose body removal is performed if needed.

Step 3: incision and exposure

We expose the lateral aspect of the femur with a standard straight incision through the skin and the fascia starting two fingers breadth distally to the epicondyle and extending the incision about 12cm proximally (fig. 8a). The dissection is carried down to the vastus lateralis, which is retracted from the posterolateral inter-muscular septum by the special dedicated Homan retractor placed ventrally (fig. 8b). Perforating vessels are to be expected and should be controlled with ligature or electro-cautery. We leave the joint capsule intact. The lateral cortex is now exposed. The procedure is facilitated by flexion of the knee.

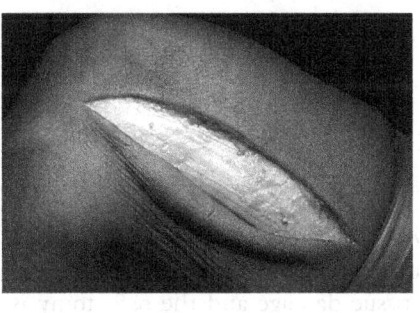
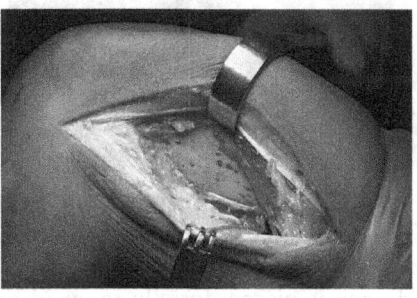

a.   b.

Fig. 8. – a. The lateral aspect of the femur is exposed with a standard straight skin incision. **b.** The dissection is carried down through the fascia to the lateral cortex, retracting the vastus lateralis with the special Homan.

Step 4: osteotomy

The authors' preferred method is a "free" technique. With the knee in extension and under fluoroscopic control, a guide pin (Steinmann) is drilled, by

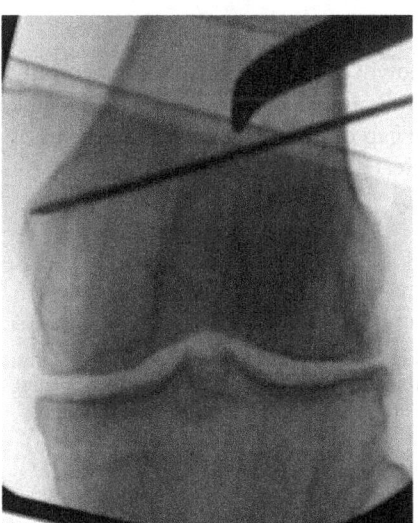

the "free hand", through the distal femur in a slightly oblique direction (about 20°), from a proximal point on the lateral cortex, three fingers breadth above the epicondyle, safely off from the throclear groove, to a distal point on the medial cortex (fig. 9).

The original instruments system also provides an Osteotomy Guide Assembly to help the surgeon in the properly placement of the guide pin and an Osteotomy Cutting Guide to facilitate the use of the oscillating saw.

Fig. 9. – The Steinmann guide pin is drilled in a slightly oblique direction from lateral to medial, safely off from the throclear groove.

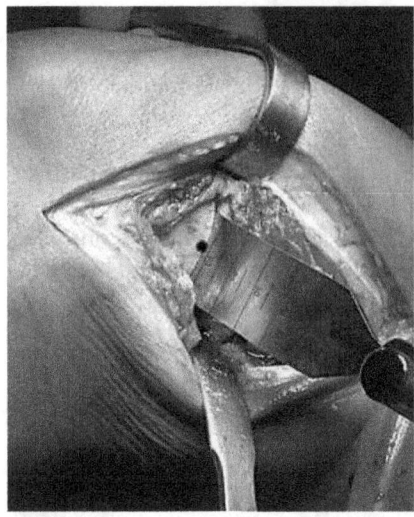

Fig. 10. – The osteotome must be kept parallel and proximal to the guide pin to help prevent intra-articular fracture.

The guide may be oriented to accommodate variations in size and anatomy and different choices in tilting the osteotomy cut is also possible. A second Homan is placed dorsally to avoid soft tissue damage and the osteotomy is started with the powered saw just to cut the cortical bone. It is very important to carry on the osteotomy with the blade, the saw and then the osteotome, parallel and proximal to the guide pin to help prevent intra-articular fracture (fig. 10). The saw is used to cut the lateral cortex only. Then a sharp osteotome is used to finish the osteotomy, making certain that all the cancellous metaphysis and, especially, the anterior and the posterior cortices are completely interrupted, but preserving a medial hinge of about 0.5cm of intact bone.

Step 5: wedge opening

The wedge opener is introduced and slowly advanced until the osteotomy has been opened to obtain the planned realignment of the knee (fig. 11). The surgeon measures the dimension of bone gap directly on the graduated limbs of the wedge opener and choose the plate.

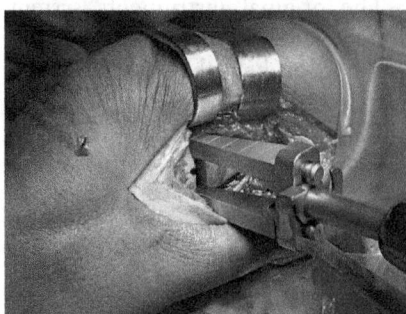

Fig. 11. – The wedge opener is inserted into the osteotomy and advanced until the opening corresponds to the planned correction.

Step 6: plate fixation

By removing the handle of the opener, the plate can be easily positioned on the lateral cortex of the femur with the spacer tooth introduced into the osteotomic line. If the plate does not fit the femur cortex properly, we must precontour it by modeling with the bending pliers. Before fixing the plate, we make an intra-operative control of the mechanical axis by means of the special guide rod, long enough to extend from the center of the femoral head to the center of the ankle, which we check under fluoroscopy at the passage on the knee joint, approximately the center of the tibial spine for neutral mechanical axis (fig. 12). When the correction is under- or oversized, we choose a different plate with a thicker or thinner tooth as needed. We then fix the plate with four cortical screws proximal to the osteotomy and two cancellous screws distally (fig. 13). A lateral plate instead of a medial one is recommended for an important biomechanical reason. When a normal knee with a valgus femoro-tibial angle is loaded in single-leg stance, the lateral femur is the tension side secondary to the extrinsic varus component of the body weight. In severe genu valgum, the mechanical axis moves laterally and, therefore, the convex medial side is subjected to tensile forces. After osteotomy, the mechanical axis is again moved medially, which returns the tension side of the knee to the lateral side. To act as a tension band, the plate must be applied to the lateral femur. Application of the plate to the medial femur after the osteotomy, as in the closing wedge osteotomy with the AO 90° angled blade plate, violates this principle and would be expected to lead to a high incidence of failure.

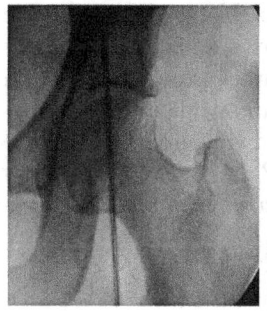
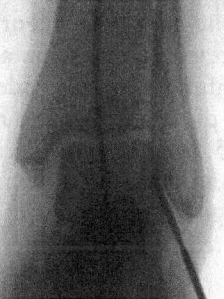
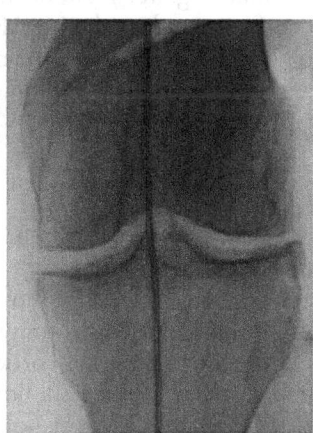

Fig. 12. – Before fixing the plate we check under fluoroscopy the mechanical axis by means of the special guide rod, long enough to extend from the center of the femoral head through the knee to the center of the ankle.

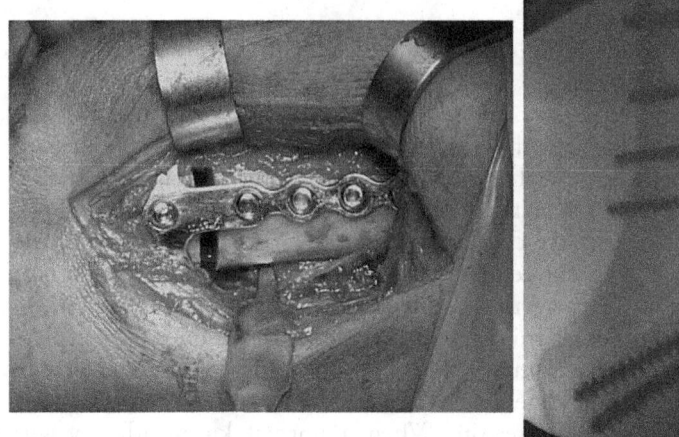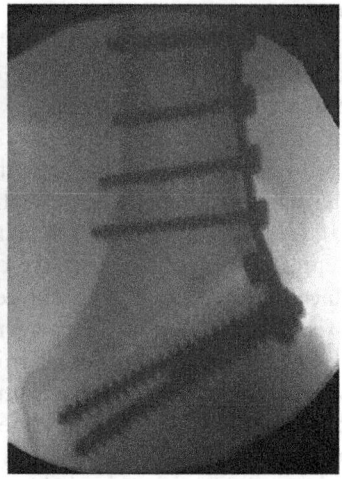

Fig. 13. – The plate is secured to the femur cortex with two (rarely three) distal cancellous screws and all the four cortical screws.

Step 7: bone grafting

With a skin incision extended from the antero-superior iliac spine 8 to 10cm above the iliac crest, we take two or three cortico-cancellous bone grafts with the same wedge shape of the osteotomy, the larger one measures the full correction, while the others are proportionately smaller. The grafts are press-fit introduced to fill the defect. It is also possible to use different grafts, such as bone from the bank or synthetic Hatric® (Arthrex Inc., Naples, FL) or bovine freeze-dried bone or, according to some other authors, no grafts at all. Bone grafting is recommended in all opening wedge osteotomies greater than 7.5mm to prevent delayed or non union and/or fixation failure, while in osteotomies 7.5, or smaller, the decision to bone graft should be individualized. The correct position of the plate and grafts is confirmed with AP and lateral radiographs (fig. 14). One or two drain(s) (the second intra-articular if needed (are) prepared and the wound is closed in a routine fashion.

Technical pitfalls and complications

The risk of intra-articular fracture is always present. This is more often due to a mistake in positioning the guide pin too close to the joint, leaving a very poor metaphysary bone stock between the osteotomy and the articular surface, or it is due to a not perfect finishing of the osteotomy without complete interruption of the anterior or, more often, posterior cortices that produces an articular fracture at the moment to varus stress the knee and open the osteotomy. The most of times it is possible, even if not easy, to fix the fracture with the distal cancellous screws introduced, as usual, through the plate.

When the hinge of intact bone is not respected by the surgeon, will the osteotomy dislocate. Checking under fluoroscopy the fixation and the align-

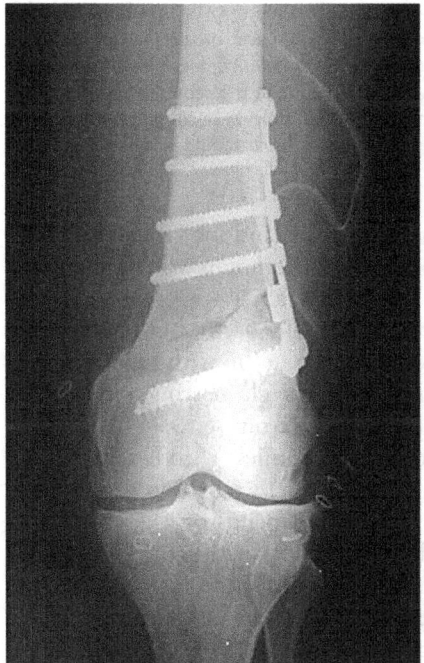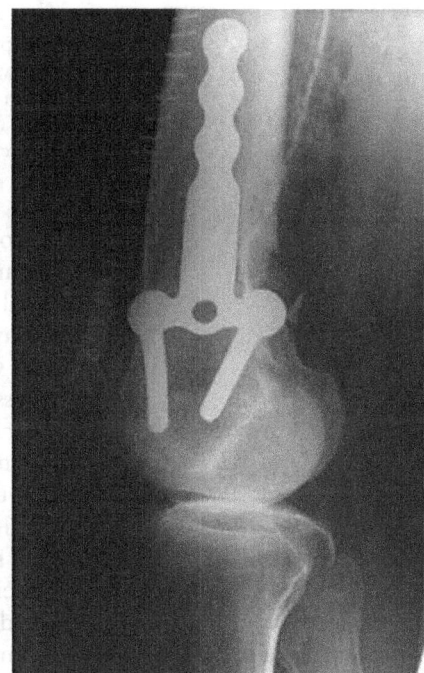

Fig. 14. – The correct position of the plate and grafts is confirmed by the postoperative radiographs.

ment of the bone, the osteotomy angle looks subluxated with the femur diaphysis slipped, medially. The trick to prevent this technical problem starts with the proper choice of the site of the osteotomy cut that should be distal enough to avoid the maximum step-off of the bone profile and address a more stable fixation, but, mainly, an intact bone hinge is essential for the stability, and this, when correctly preserved, grants the osteotomy from any possible dislocation. But if the undesired subluxation has nevertheless occurred, then a possible solution of this problem is a staple fixation by a contro-lateral incision.

The lateral position of the "T" plate is critical. The osteotomy has to be perfectly oriented in the sagittal plane, perpendicular to the longitudinal axis of the femur, to have the long arm of the plate completely lying on the bone, just in the center of the diaphysis. In fact the spacer tooth forms a right angle with the plate that prevents the correct positioning of the long arm on the bone when the osteotomy is oblique with the femur. When the vertical arm is not parallel to the diaphysis the last upper holes of the plate fall out from the bone, anteriorly or posteriorly to the cortex, and make very difficult to fix all screws properly (fig. 15).

Injuries to the vessels are not frequent. In the literature are reported accidental tears to the posterior vessels that, however, could be safely protected by correct use of a posterior Homan retractor and keeping the knee flexed during surgery. Perforating vessels are to be expected in approaching the lateral femur and should be controlled with ligature or electrocautery.

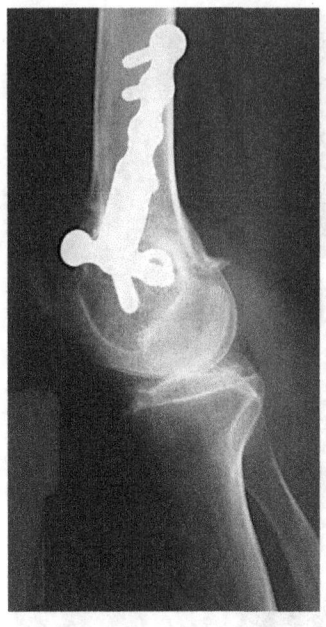

Fig. 15. – Because the osteotomy line is oblique on the sagittal plane, the tooth spacer of the plate enters into the cut with an inclination which does not allow the vertical arm of the "T" to lie in the center of the diaphysis so that the last upper hole falls too posteriorly, and makes very difficult to fix all screws properly.

Thrombophlebitis and infections are generic complications in common with all the other surgical procedures about the inferior limb.

Delayed union may occur, but most osteotomies will go on to union with time and partially assisted early weight bearing. Non union is also a possibility. In our series (44 tibial and 21 femoral osteotomies with a minimum follow-up of one year) we had no non unions and this probably depends on the systematic use of the bone grafts to fill the osteotomy.

When the osteotomy is performed in severe valgus deformities, a transitory peroneal apraxia can occur because of the overstretching of the nerve due to the correction.

It may be incorrect to include loss of the desired correction as a true complication. In opening wedge the bone collapse of the grafts might determine a decrease of the angular correction, but the new plates have been demonstrated to be effective in preventing it. Of course the continuing degenerative changes with a consequent progressive recurrence of the original deformity contribute to a gradual loss of correction as the time goes by.

Postoperative management and rehabilitation

After the operation the knee is immobilized with a range-of-motion brace in extension or at slight flexion of about 10° that allows a full range of motion when unlocked. Passive flexion-extension in a continuous passive motion device, quadriceps setting, and straight leg raising exercises are started the day after surgery. The drains are removed 48 hours later. The patients are allowed to walk with no weight bearing on the operated limb, from the second postoperative day and they are dismissed from the hospital in 4 to 5 days. Usually within the first 4 weeks, the patients are able to completely flex the knee. After 6 weeks, functional weight bearing with crutches is allowed. Full weight-bearing is normally possible after 8 to 9 weeks when the radiographs show satisfactory healing process of the bone.

References

1. Coventr, MB (1973) Osteotomy about the knee for degenerative and rheumatoid arthritis. J Bone Joint Surg [Am] 55: 23-48
2. Beaver RJ, Jinxiang-Yu, Sekyi-Otu A *et al.* (1991) Distal femoral varus osteotomy for genu valgum. A prospective review. Am J Knee Surg 1: 9-17
3. Miniaci A, Grossmann SP, JakobRP (1990) Supracondylar femoral varus osteotomy in the treatment of valgus knee deformity. Am J Knee Surg 2: 65-73
4. Marti RK, Schroder J, Witteveen A (2000) The closed varus supracondylar osteotomy. In: Operative Techniques in Sports Medicine "Osteotomies About the Athletic Knee" , vol. 8, num. 1, edited by D Drez Jr, JC De Lee, WB Saunders, Orlando Fl
5. Learmonth ID (1990) A simple technique for varus supracondylar osteotomy in genu valgum. J Bone Joint Surg Br 72: 235-7
6. Muller ME, Allgower M, Schneider R. *et al.* (1979) Manual of Internal Fixation, 2nd ed., p 376-7, Berlin, Germany, Springer-Verlag
7. RosenbergTD, Paulos LE, ParkerRD *et al.* (1988) The forty-five-degree posteroanterior weight bearing radiograph of the knee. J Bone Joint Surg [Am] 70: 1479-83
8. Puddu G, Fowler PJ, Amendola A (1998) Opening wedge osteotomy system by Arthrex. Surgical Technique. Naples, Fl., Arthrex Inc.
9. Simmons P (1999) New fixation plate improves tibial, femoral osteotomies. Orthop Today 3: 28-9
10. Puddu G, Franco V (2000) Femoral antivalgus opening wedge osteotomy. In: Operative Techniques in Sports Medicine "Osteotomies About the Athletic Knee", vol. 8, num. 1, edited by D Drez Jr, JC De Lee, WB Saunders, Orlando Fl

Unicompartmental knee arthroplasty – Results, causes of failure, indications

P. Landreau, P. Bizot

Introduction

What are the arguments to keep a place to unicompartmental knee arthroplasty (UKA) in the treatment of gonarthrosis?

This question is deliberately provocative, and current status of UKA must be questionned. UKA is an alternative to total knee arthroplasty (TKA) and to osteotomy in the treatment of gonarthrosis. Osteotomy is a conservative procedure that remains the treatment of choice in young and active patients with unicompartmental gonarthrosis. Successful outcomes have been reported for a long time in medial and lateral arthrosis with varus and valgus deformities respectively. Moreover, with improvements of prosthetic designs and surgical technique, TKA is now a predictably successful operation, and results are more reliable than those of UKA.

Based on theses data, question is to know if there is still a place for UKA in medial or lateral gonarthrosis.

The initial success of UKA was based on its simple and attractive concept. At the beginning of experience, UKA competed favourably with the first generations of TKA, which gave limited and uncertain results. However, several authors reported a high rate of early failures with UKA using early designs. Consequently, many operators switched to TKA, confirmed in their choice by the constant improvements in the results of TKA.

Nevertheless, UKA offers many advantages:

– compared to osteotomy, UKA has a higher initial success rate, a faster recovery and fewer early complications. Moreover, a preoperative loss of motion can be relieved at the time of arthrotomy by an intra-articular debridement;

– compared to TKA, UKA has a much lower morbidity, especially when using a "mini open". This is a major argument in old patients with risk factors, and also in patients with bilateral involvement which can be operated on both side in one stage procedure. The other argument over TKA is the better quality of the results in terms of mobility, proprioception, and overall function of the knee.

Controversies about the use of UKA are multifactorial:

– at the early experience, UKA suffered a high incidence of early failures. The latter were generated, however, at a time when patient selection was not clearly established, and prosthetic designs and operative technique were not yet perfected;

– many years have been necessary to clearly establish the indications and contraindications of UKA, and to define the original features of the concept. Basically, UKA should be considered as a spacer correcting the intra-articular component of the knee deformity, and not as a true hemi-arthroplasty. Consequently, deformity must be limited and all the knee ligaments must be intact;

– this original concept illustrates the technical difficulties to correctly implant a UKA. Correct positioning is more based on the experience of the operator than on the accuracy of the cutting guides.

After presenting the results of UKA, we will try to clearly define its current indications in gonarthrosis.

Results

Difficulties of objective analysis

Analysis of the results of UKA through the literature is difficult for several reasons:

– many early designs of the prosthetic components were inappropriate and suffered from, either unadapted shapes and limited sizes, either excessive constraint between the articulating surfaces, either errors in fixation methods or insufficient thickness of polyethylene (PE) (1, 2). Metal-backing of the tibial component was introduced to maximize contact area and reduce creeping of the PE. However, to preserve bone stock, thickness of PE was reduced to less than 6mm, and led to excessive PE wear and osteolysis (3);

– the operative technique and contraindications of the procedure required many years to be clearly established. Some recent series have reported discouraging results. However, the series included patients with ACL deficiency, which is known as a major pejorative factor;

– comparison of UKA with TKA requires also some cautions, especially when comparing survivorships, since the development of both implants have evolved during different periods of time.

All these parameters should be considered to objectively compare UKA to others procedures indicated in gonarthrosis, and to review the literature.

Survival analysis

Regarding the literature, there is a great variation in survivorship. The survival rates range from 67% at 10 years follow-up to 93% at 12 years (4-10), according to different prosthetic designs, indications and operative techniques.

The Symposium of the French Orthopaedic Society (Sofcot), held in Paris in 1995, has reported a survival rate for medial UKA of 67% at 10 years follow-up and 57% at 15 years if revision for any cause was the end point (11).

The survivorship was slightly better for lateral UKA. The rate of component deterioration detected on radiographs was higher than the rate of revision, probably because the majority of the patients were very old and have limited activities. Conclusions supported the results of the literature. There was no formal correlation between clinical and radiographic findings, and survivorship for UKA did remain significantly inferior to that for TKA (12, 13).

Clinical results

However, survivorship does not indicate the quality of the results. The latter may be a major argument to use UKA rather than TKA. Only few series have reported results according to the IKS score (10, 14-16). The knee score ranged from 72 to 90 and the function score varied from 57 to 84, meaning that excellent results could be obtained with UKA provided that all requirements are met. Conclusions of the French Orthopaedic Society Symposium were similar (15, 16). The multicentric series included 483 medial UKA, with 69 osteonecrosis and 414 medial gonarthrosis. The mean age at surgery was 72 years. The function score improved from 54 to 71 at 6 years of follow-up. There was no significant difference between medial and lateral UKA. Improvement of the knee score was even superior, from 32 to 76, and significantly better for the lateral UKA. Conclusion was that overall results were better in lateral UKA than in medial UKA (16).

Causes of failure

Excluding failure due to deep infection, which appears non implant-related and very unfrequent (0.7% in the series of the Softcot Symposium [15, 16]), the three main causes of UKA failure are: laxity, wear, and loosening (table I).

– Laxity may be anterior due to ACL deficiency. The latter can promote lateral subluxation of the tibia on the femur which is detrimental to the behavior of the arthroplasty and the opposite compartment as well, and preclude UKA. Laxity may also be peripheral in the convexity of the deformity. Great attention is necessary, especially in lateral gonarthrosis with valgus deformity. Stretching of the medial collateral ligament may lead to residual convex laxity, causing early failure even in the absence of associated rupture of the ACL.

– Wear and loosening are both major causes of medial UKA revision. The risk factors for loosening are often associated, and include the persistence of an impor-

Table I. – Failures in UKA according to the Symposium of the French Orthopaedic Society (Sofcot) (16).

	Revision for mechanical failure	Laxity	Wear	Loosening	Others
Lateral	8.6%	47.1%	11.8%	17.6%	23.5%
Internal	12.8%	23.7%	13.6%	50.8%	11.9%

tant postoperative varus deformity, the persistence of a residual laxity, an unsufficient PE thickness, and an incorrect positioning of the femoral component.

Other causes of failure include deterioration of the opposite tibiofemoral compartment, often promoted by an over-correction, and impingement of the femoral component with either the tibial spine or the patella.

Indications

Indications are now well established, supported by the experience of several operators who are familiar with the procedure, and also by the results of the literature, including the French Symposium of Sofcot held in Paris in 1995 (17). In medial or lateral gonarthrosis, the operator has the choice between osteotomy, UKA and TKA. However, many factors appear as essential in the quality and longevity of the results.

Patient age

It is a factor of major importance. Between 55 and 60 years of age, the choice between osteotomy and UKA is difficult, and the final decision is often made on individual case. However, in both cases, one can presume that TKA revision will be necessary at a varying delay after the initial procedure. Debate about the potential difficulties of TKA revision is still open. Some authors conclude that TKA is easier after failure of osteotomy than after UKA, the others conclude the contrary. Basically, TKA after failure of high tibial osteotomy is difficult only if the deformity of the upper tibia induced by the osteotomy is important, and the joint line of the knee is oblique. On the other hand, TKA after failure of UKA may be not so difficult, provided that the bone stock has been preserved during the first procedure.

Before 60 years of age, osteotomy is preferred in the treatment of gonarthrosis. However, UKA may be an alternative to osteotomy, only in selected patients. At the opposite, beyond 75 years of age, UKA is an excellent indication in gonarthrosis. This is supported by the low morbidity of the procedure and the limited activity of the patient. Between these two extremes, the choice will be made on individual case, according to the experience of the operator.

Patient weight

During the French symposium of Sofcot, no formal correlation between failure and patient's weight has been found. However, conclusion was to advise against UKA in obese patients and to preferentially use a tibial component with polyethylene thicker than 8mm in heavy patients, especially in active men.

Etiology

Osteonecrosis of the medial femoral condyle is an excellent indication for UKA. It is also a good indication for high tibial osteotomy. If all the requirements are met, the decision to perform an osteotomy or a UKA will be based on the age of the patient.

Inflammatory diseases of the knee are not suitable for UKA. Involvement is most often diffuse and evolutive with time. Chondrocalcinosis is also a contraindication to UKA, especially if the patellofemoral joint is altered.

Degree of joint collapse

It is measured on weighted flexed anteroposterior radiographs of the knee (Schuss). In case of a complete collapse of the joint in patient around 60 years old, UKA is preferred to osteotomy. In case of major collapse with bone loss, UKA may be insufficient to fill the bone defect and to restore the femorotibial axis, therefore TKA may be required. Varus or valgus AP stress radiographs may be necessary to detect minor narrowing of the opposite femorotibial compartment which precludes UKA, and also to eliminate a pathologic ligamenteous laxity.

ACL assessment

Deficiency of the ACL is a formal contraindication for UKA. Disruption of the ACL can be postraumatic or degenerative. Clinical examination is often sufficient to diagnose an ACL deficiency (positive Lachman test), provided that the knee deformity is mild. However, severe joint collapse with concave shape of the tibial plateau may lead to false negative test. Lateral view of the flexed knee may be useful if an anterior tibial displacement is present. Stress lateral radiographs are sometimes necessary to quantify the anterior tibial displacement. MRI may also be useful to assess the cruciate ligaments. Basically, the diagnosis is often made at arthrotomy. The first step is inspection of the ACL and the opposite femorotibial compartment. Results of this inspection will dictate the final decision between unicompartmental or total knee arthroplasty. In practice, both implants should be available in the operating room.

Mechanical axis

UKA is indicated if the deviation does not exceed 15° in varus or valgus. The objective of the procedure is to obtain an undercorrection with a final angle less than 5°, while avoiding any soft tissue release, as indicated in the guidelines. Correction of malalignment exceeding 15° is very difficult without any soft tissue release, therefore UKA is inadvisable in such knee deformities.

The bone deformity

UKA is best indicated in the absence of a so-called "epiphyseal varus", i.e., congenital varus deformity of the proximal epiphysis of the tibia. In this case, osteotomy can cause a distortion of the upper tibia giving difficulties for TKA revision, and is not recommended. UKA is still indicated if the "epiphyseal varus" does not exceed 6°, since the deformity could be easily corrected with the procedure while keeping a slight undercorrection. Beyond 6° of deformity, although UKA may be combined to an osteotomy in a one-stage procedure, UKA may be not recommended and TKA is preferable.

In lateral gonarthrosis, the valgus deformity is often related to lateral femoral condyle deficiency. UKA may be indicated, but great care should be taken to correct the deformity in the femur and not in the tibia. If not, a TKA is preferred. A thick femoral component may be necessary to compensate the lateral condyle hypoplasia and to obtain an horizontal joint axis in the frontal plane. If the deformity is corrected in the tibia, by using a thicker tibial component, obliquity of the joint axis will be obtained and detrimental for long-term results.

The femoropatellar joint

Most authors agree that any lesion of the opposite tibiofemoral compartment precludes UKA. However, there is still a debate about the indications of UKA in medial or lateral gonarthosis associated with patellofemoral joint lesions. Moderate patellofemoral lesions, found during the operation or present on preoperative radiographs, do not preclude UKA. The choice between a UKA or TKA will be first based on the presence and importance of patellofemoral clinical symptoms. In case of significant patellofemoral pains, even if the radiographs show only minor changes, primary TKA should be preferred. The efficiency of conservative procedures on the patellofemoral joint (denervation, removing of osteophytes, shaving...) remains limited and unpredictable, and these procedures are not recommended in association with UKA, except in very old patients with limited activity.

This illustrates the great importance of the history and the clinical examination of the patient in the decision for UKA in gonarthrosis. The pain must be localized to the medial or the lateral tibiofemoral compartment, and isolated. The presence of anterior knee pain, increased in stair climbing, should be carefully quantify before decision for UKA.

The preoperative range of motion

It is a major parameter in the decision for unicompartmental or total knee arthroplasty. Nowadays, the functional demand of the patient becomes higher and higher, and the patient should be informed about the expected results with both these procedures in terms of range of motion. Most authors agree that in patient with a nearly normal preoperative range of motion, the probability to conserve it after the operation will be much higher with a UKA than with a TKA. Flexion contracture is not a contraindication for UKA. Loss of extension may be related either to anterior osteophytes present in the intercondylar notch, or retraction of the posterior capsule. In the first case, anterior debridement with resection of the osteophytes will improved the motion and UKA is indicated. In the second case, posterior debridement during UKA is often difficult and limited, and TKA is preferred.

Previous surgical procedures

Previous meniscectomy or cartilage shaving do not, obviously, preclude UKA. A previous high tibial osteotomy is not a formal contraindication. However, high tibial osteotomy engenders a deformity of the upper tibia, which cannot be fully corrected by UKA. Therefore, revision of osteotomy with UKA is not recommended. The degree of deformity created by the osteotomy is of major importance in the decision. In case of undercorrection, UKA may be indicated in selected cases. However, in case of overcorrection, lesions are often bi- or tri-compartmental, and TKA is preferred.

Conclusion

With more than twenty years of experience, the place of UKA in the treatment of gonarthrosis may be currently defined, as a conservative arthroplasty possibly functioning as a nearly normal knee. However, indications are limited, and prosthetic design and patient selection are critical to the success of the procedure.

References

1. Hodge WA, Chandler HP (1992) Unicompartmental knee replacement: a comparison of constrained and unconstrained designs. J Bone Joint Surg 74-A: 877-83
2. Marmor L (1979) Marmor modular knee in unicompartmental disease. J Bone Joint Surg 61-A: 347-53
3. Engh GA, Dwyer KA, Hanes CK (1992) Polyethylene wear of metal-backed tibial components in total and unicompartmental knee prostheses. J Bone Joint Surg 74-B: 9-17
4. Cartier P, Sanouiller JL, Grelsamer RP (1996) Unicompartmental knee arthroplasty surgery. 10-year minimum follow-up period. J Arthroplasty 11: 782-8
5. Hernigou P, Goutallier D (1988) Guepar unicompartmental Lotus prosthesis for single-compartment femorotibial arthrosis. A five- to nine-year follow-up study. Clin Orthop 230: 186-95
6. Scott RD, Cobb AG, McQueary FG et al. (1991) Unicompartmental knee arthroplasty. Eight- to twelve-year follow-up evaluation with survivorship analysis. Clin Orthop 271: 96-100
7. Witvoet J, Peyrache MD, Nizard R (1993) Single-compartment "Lotus" type knee prosthesis in the treatment of lateralized gonarthrosis: results in 135 cases with a mean follow-up of 4.6 years. Rev Chir Orthop 79: 565-76
8. Lindstrand A, Stenstrom A, Lewold S (1992) Multicenter study of unicompartmental knee revision. PCA, Marmor, and St Georg compared in 3,777 cases of arthrosis. Acta Orthop Scand 63: 256-9
9. Murray DW, Goodfellow JW, O'Connor JJ (1998) The Oxford medial unicompartmental arthroplasty: a ten-year survival study. J Bone Joint Surg 80-B: 983-9
10. Koshino T, Morii T, Wada J et al. (1991) Unicompartmental replacement with the Marmor modular knee: operative procedure and results. Bull Hosp Jt Dis 51: 119-31
11. Hernigou P, Deschamps G (1996) Les prothèses unicompartimentales du genou. Symposium 70ᵉ réunion annuelle de la SOFCOT. Rev Chir Orthop 82 suppl I: 23-60
12. Stern SH, Insall JN (1992) Posterior stabilized prosthesis. Results after follow-up of nine to twelve years. J Bone Joint Surg 74-A: 980-6

13. Diduch DR, Insall JN, Scott WN *et al.* (1997) Total knee replacement in young, active patients. Long-term follow-up and functional outcome. J Bone Joint Surg 79-A: 575-82
14. Epinette JA, Edidin AA (1998) Hydroxyapatite et prothèse unicompartimentale du genou. Expérience à 5 ans et plus du genou Unix. In: Cartier P, Epinette JA, Deschamps G *et al.* (ed.) Prothèse unicompartimentale de genou. Cahiers d'enseignement de la SOFCOT. Expansion Scientifique Publications, Paris
15. Hernigou P, de Ladoucette A, Raou D *et al.* (1996) L'arthroplastie unicompartimentale interne dans la gonarthrose. Résultat de 483 prothèses avec un recul maximum de 20 ans. Symposium 70ᵉ réunion annuelle de la SOFCOT. Rev Chir Orthop 82 suppl I: 27-30
16. Landreau P, Cartier P (1996) Résultats des prothèses unicompartimentales externes. Symposium 70ᵉ réunion annuelle de la SOFCOT. Rev Chir Orthop 82 suppl I: 30-2
17. Deschamps G (1996) Prothèses unicompartimentales, l'indication idéale. Symposium 70ᵉ réunion annuelle de la SOFCOT. Rev Chir Orthop 82 suppl I: 53-4

Unicompartmental knee arthroplasty – Technical principles

G. Deschamps

Unicompartmental knee prostheses are intended to address single compartment gonarthrosis only.

Many factors involving both the indication and the surgical technique contribute to the success of the arthroplasty.

Thanks to recent works (in some of which we have taken part), indications are now well defined (1-4). However, the surgical technique is critical because Unicompartmental Knee Replacement (UKR) appears to be less "forgiving" than Total Knee Replacement (TKR).

In order to understand the rationale for the technical principles that will be described further on, we think it important to define the actual goals of UKA in the treatment of single compartment gonarthrosis.

Concept and philosophy of unicompartmental knee replacements

Indications

If one considers only the cases that are amenable to surgery, there are three types of indications which depend on the age of the patient, and above all, on the patient's activity level, weight, and ligamentous status (particularly the central pivot), and at last the severity of the deformity.

The ideal indication for a UKR is a low demand patient over 60 years of age; the UKR is particularly recommended in old or weak patients. The patient should weigh less than 85kg, but the Body Mass Index (BMI) also should be taken into account. The central pivot should be intact. The deformity should be moderate and, above all, reducible without overcorrection (varus-valgus shift when taking stress views). The residual deformity (if any) after correction should not exceed 5° varus in a varus knee and 5° valgus in a valgus knee.

In contrast, osteotomy is reserved for patients under 60 years of age, in whom single compartment gonarthrosis is associated with bone deformity (tibia vara or tibia valga, or excessive femoral valgus).

As regards Total Knee Arthroplasty (TKA), it can be considered in any patient with degenerative osteoarthritis, independent of the cause and the amount of bone deformity (whether it is reducible or not). Only the patient's age and level of activity can set limitations to its indications.

Goals

We shall only deal with the goals defined for correction of the deformity.

Schematically, one can say that:

– osteotomy is intended to address bone deformity, mostly in the metaphyseal region: overcorrection is necessary to achieve good results;

– TKA is intended to restore neutral axial alignment (180°) which is critical to the stability and durability of the implant;

– UKA can only correct the wear component of osteoarthritis. Its goal is the restoration of the mechanical axis that the patient had prior to the development of wear (i.e., undercorrection). UKA should only correct axial alignment up to the point where it compensates wear, which precludes any ligament release. As will be seen further on, slight retensioning of the ligaments on the concave side of the deformity is the correct criterium for a good reconstruction and proper correction of the deformity. This is why UKR is often described as a "wedge".

Philosophy

The main feature of UKA is that it is a very conservative procedure. On the other hand, it is associated with a certain risk of failure which will generally occur during the early postoperative period and is most often due to a faulty technique or incorrect indication. This explains why some inexperienced surgeons may be reluctant to use this technique. However, most of the adepts in UKA are surgeons who have understood the subtleness of the technique and, above all, the "philosophy" of the procedure. UKR must not be considered as one-half of a total knee prosthesis. It should be inserted using one of the limited approaches recently developed by anglo-saxon authors (so-called "minimally invasive arthroplasty").

The approach should extend as far as the superior margin of the patella which is retracted, and not everted and turned over as is done in TKA. The ligaments should be preserved because they will indicate whether the space created by the bone cuts has been properly filled. Dedicated instruments are indispensable; intramedullary guides should be avoided because they may not only damage the attachments of the central pivot but also increase the risk of postoperative bleeding.

Therefore, the goal of UKA is the reconstruction of the knee joint with none or hardly any of the complications usually associated with TKRs which are the main competitors to UKRs. This is the primary condition for the survival of UKRs, although improvements in the management of postoperative pain and prevention of complications have very much reduced the difference in postoperative management between a TKR and a UKR. The aim of this chapter is to emphasize a few technical principles that have proved essential in our experience.

Technical principles

General considerations

The technical principles applying to UKRs will be set, in comparison with the goals defined for TKRs, which are different.

In TKA, the bone cuts are performed perpendicular to the femoral and tibial mechanical axes. Stability of the ligaments is provided by the release procedures which are mandatory to restore correct axial alignment of the lower limb; these mainly involve the concave side of the deformity.

At the stage of the disease addressed by UKA, the deformity is reducible to an amount that is defined by the limitations of the indications (1):

– no overcorrection;
– residual deformity that does not exceed -5° for valgus and +5° for varus.

Ideally, the tibial cut should respect the natural obliquity of the joint line, both in the coronal and sagittal planes. This angle can be determined on preoperative stress views (forced valgus in medial compartment osteoarthritis, forced varus in lateral compartment osteoarthritis). The tibial slope should also be restored and measured on lateral views. We shall see further on how this can be done. What is important to understand at this stage of the discussion, is that strict adherence to this rule allows restoration of the initial joint line level, that is, before the development of wear. Trying to elevate the joint line level above this limit may result in overcorrection, with two detrimental effects:

– excessive pressure on the polyethylene (PE) of the tibial component;
– excessive pressure on the contralateral compartment that may result in opposite compartment progression of arthritis.

The best way to determine if the undercorrection rule has been respected is to check whether the joint line slightly opens on the concave side of the deformity, that is, whether there is a slight opening of the prosthetic joint line in extension during trialing; this slight opening is called "safety laxity". In practice, this precludes any ligament release because the tension on the ligaments is used to check for any overcorrection of the deformity. Thus, one will easily understand why a UKR is so forgiving in case of incorrect tibial resection in the frontal plane. Any error in the tibial resection will be well tolerated as long as it does not impose any undue ligament release to improve the conformity between the femoral and tibial components.

For instance, in a varus knee with a joint line that is inclined 4° relative to the tibial mechanical axis in the frontal plane, the tibial cut should ideally be sloped 4° downward and medially; this will ensure a perfect contact between the femoral and tibial components (fig. 1).

If the tibial cut is performed perpendicular to the tibial mechanical axis, the tibial component must be slightly lowered to meet the undercorrection requirement and maintain the joint line at the proper level. Such a resection will result in a V-shaped joint line (fig. 2), with the tibial component positioned in a step-off configuration.

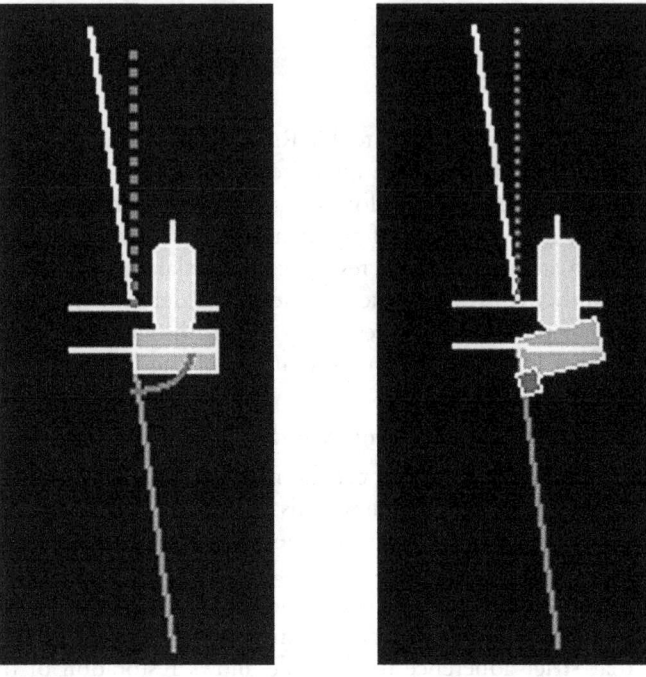

Fig. 1.   Fig. 2.

Fig. 1. – Ideal tibial cut, parallel to the joint line, that ensures full conformity between the femoral and tibial components.

Fig. 2. – Tibial cut perpendicular to the tibial mechanical axis. V-shaped joint line and lack of tibiofemoral conformity.

The only problem in this situation is the impression of nonconformity between the femoral and tibial components. But, if the surgeon readily accepts this nonconformity, which the modern femoral component designs tolerate very well, he/she can be sure that no detrimental effect will result from it. Unfortunately, it may prompt less experienced surgeons to try and correct this anomaly by inserting a thicker tibial component, which will require some release. This will result in elevation of the joint line, excessive pressure on polyethylene and excessive stresses on the lateral compartment due to over-correction of the joint line level, despite an overall neutral axis (fig. 3).

The same rules apply to the tibial slope. Performing the tibial cut at 90° in the sagittal plane may, if the operated knee had an initial slope greater than 10°, result in overloading the posterior aspect of the tibial component in flexion.

We think that such technical errors, although very mild, may explain post-operative pain, premature wear or even loosening – which is apparently unex-plained but in fact can easily be explained – in some patients.

Furthermore, obviously, one cannot be happy with a standard approximate resection both in the frontal and sagittal planes. A customized resection that

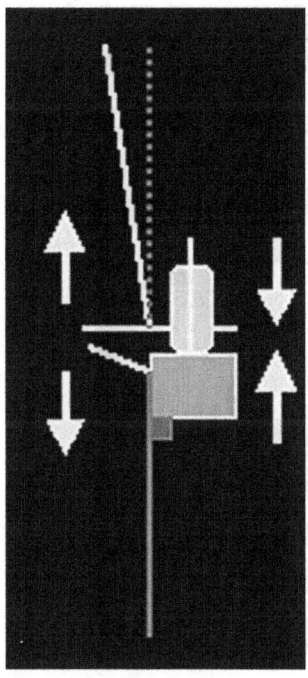

Fig. 3. – Attempt at correction of the tibiofemoral non-conformity by inserting a thicker tibial component. Over-correction with the risk of excessive pressure on the tibial component and opposite compartment progression of arthritis.

restores the patient anatomy, before wear begins to develop, appears mandatory.

In the next paragraphs, we shall see how the normal anatomy can be restored.

Medial compartment osteoarthritis (M-C OA): technical principles

The procedure consists of three main steps:

– tibial preparation;
– centering of the femoral component on the tibial component;
– checking of the absence of ligament tightness throughout the range of flexion.

Tibial preparation

The resection angle is the chief element to be determined. This is why the preoperative planning is essential to determine the coronal tibial angle formed by the joint line – less the wear which is usually minimal in the cases addressed by UKA – and the tibial mechanical axis. This angle will determine the resection angle in the frontal plane. In rare cases (straight tibia), it will be at 90° relative to the tibial mechanical axis; most often, it will lie between 2° and 5°. Beyond 5°, a wrong measurement should be suspected or a UKA is not indicated. As a matter of fact, a cut with excessive varus may result in a lateral translation of the tibial component under the femoral component, or collapse of the medial aspect of the tibia (fig. 4).

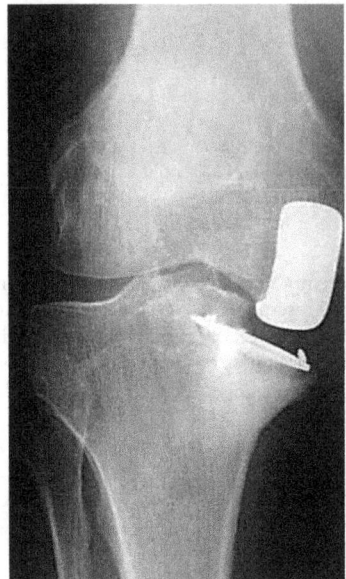

Fig. 4.

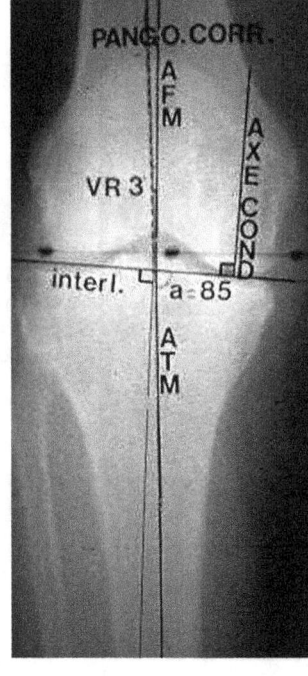

Fig. 5.

Fig. 4. – Tibial cut with excessive varus. Collapse of the medial aspect of the tibia and loosening.

Fig. 5. – Preoperative measurements taken in the frontal plane from a stress view (forced valgus). Residual 3° varus angle; the tibial cut angle in the frontal plane is 5° relative to the TMA.

Ideally, an adjustable cutting guide should be used intraoperatively to preset the inclination of the cutting block in the frontal plane, based on the angle that was preoperatively measured on the AP views (corrected AP full-length X-ray taken in forced valgus) (fig. 5).

We think that it is much more accurate and advisable to rely on the slope of the knee than to use a fixed inclination that is built into the cutting guide. The drapes may interfere with the use of the extramedullary adjustable cutting guide.

The instrument system that we have designed for the HLS® Unicompartmental Knee Prosthesis (TORNIER, Saint-Ismier, France) includes a tibial cutting guide that can be adjusted in the frontal plane and incorporates callipers to adjust the resection angle in the frontal plane (fig. 6).

Holes are designed in the cutting block for insertion of guide pins. Once the cutting guide has been adjusted in the frontal plane, a pin is inserted into the involved tibiofemoral joint line to help determine the slope (fig. 7). As osteoarthritis with anterior laxity and posterior bone loss is systematically eliminated from our indications, there is no risk of creating an excessive slope.

The upper part of the alignment guide is fixed to the tibia just a few millimetres beneath the tibial spines, using a fixation pin that is inserted through the central bushing. The distal end of the alignment guide is positioned over

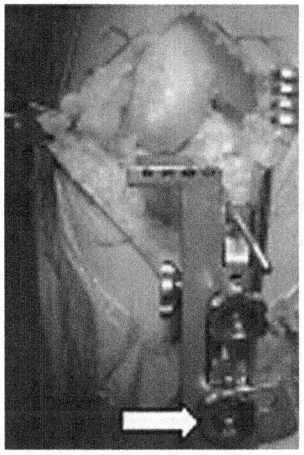

Fig. 6. – Adjustable cutting guide with callipers to adjust the inclination of the tibial cut (index).

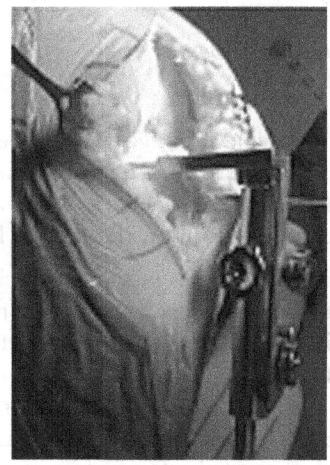

Fig. 7. – A guide pin is inserted into the joint line to allow adjustment of the slope. As this pin is tangential to the surface of the tibial plateau, it accurately defines the patient's tibial slope.

the centre of the ankle. Then, the knee is extended. The intra-articular guide pin is used to locate the reference point for determination of the tibial resection level which is the second most important step.

We consider that UKA should be a resurfacing procedure, particularly on the femoral side. The distal end of the femur should not be resected. The femoral component will fill the bone loss that is always present in the centre of the femoral condyle; in some cases, this bone loss is delimited by a ring of peripheral osteophytes which define the ideal position for the femoral component. Thus, the underlying strong dense bone will provide adequate support for the femoral component and can be used as a sound starting point for the reconstruction. Because the intra-articular guide pin rests on the damaged condylar area in extension, it can be used as a reference (zero point) for the measurement. The scale that is adjacent to the central fixation pin marks the zero point for the measurement. The intra-articular guide pin is then removed, and the scale is used to set the tibial resection level. The measurement will include the thickness of the standard femoral component (3mm), the thickness of the all-poly tibial component (as a rule, 9mm minimum), plus 2mm for the "safety laxity". Thus, for a 9mm tibial component, the central sliding tongue will be brought down to the 14mm calibration on the central scale, which corresponds to the total thickness of the tibial resection. The objective is to fill exactly the space created by the cut, without placing the ligaments under excessive tension. Any error will inevitably result in excessive pressure that may cause pain and then loosening because of the micromotions generated on the tibial component. During trialing, any excessive pressure will generally cause anterior lift-off of the trial tibial component during flexion, or loosening of the femoral component. In this case, the first thing to do is to check for any error in the posterior inclination of the tibial cut.

At last, the A/P and M/L dimensions of the tibial component are extremely important. As in TKA, optimal coverage of the resected tibial plateau is essential; however, any excessive overhang should be avoided because impingement upon the capsuloligamentous structures will cause pain.

Femoral preparation

The objective is:

– achieve correct M/L alignment of the femoral component;
– achieve correct positioning – particularly rotational positioning – of the femoral component, so as to avoid impingement of the anterior edge of the component upon the medial facet of the patella.

Generally, as previously discussed (fig. 1), high tibiofemoral conformity with the femoral component lying flat on the tibial component in the frontal plane is very much dependent on the correct inclination of the tibial cut in the frontal plane.

Thus, two things are important: select the appropriate femoral component size (sagittal radius of curvature), and achieve correct anterior-posterior positioning of the femoral component, without any anterior overhang in extension. It may be useful to mark the projection of this point with the electrocautery while the knee is extended. However, the worn area is often clearly visible and well delimited by a ring of osteophytes. This will also assist in M/L alignment and rotational positioning of the component because the "rails" created by the wear can be used as a guide.

Pitfalls may appear:

– exuberant medial osteophytes may be misleading and induce medial positioning of the femoral component;
– excessive rotation of the femoral condyle may result in malpositioning of the femoral component, with the anterior part of the component adjacent to the intercondylar notch (component externally rotated), which may cause impingement upon the medial facet of the patella in flexion, or upon the intercondylar eminence in extension.

As will be shown, these errors are more frequent in the genu valgum. The centering plate that we have included in the HLS instrument system is intended to facilitate this operative step. The second step is the posterior femoral cut to make space for the posterior part of the femoral component. As a matter of fact, in the cases addressed by UKA, the posterior condyle is always intact. Therefore, failing to resect the posterior condyle will result in considerable posterior build-up which may generate excessive pressure on the tibial component in flexion or loosening of the femoral component. As this is the second cause of component instability, it should be carefully checked during trialing. However, one thing is essential: after the resection, there must be a perfect congruity between the inner surface of the prosthetic posterior condyle and the resected surface. Any gap between the inner surface of the prosthetic posterior condyle and the cut surface may eventually result in component loosening due to "tossing" during flexion. This may explain why loosening or micromotions may go undetected on standing lateral X-rays at follow-up. When a patient presents with knee pain, only an X-ray taken in full flexion can possibly show the anterior loosening of the femoral component that generates pain (fig. 8).

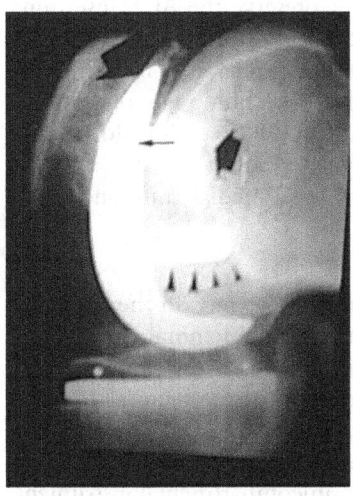

Fig. 8. – Lateral view taken in hyperflexion, showing loosening of the femoral component.

As can be seen, implantation of a medial UKR has many requirements. Several studies – which are highly controversial – show how much forgiving this type of replacement is. As far as we are concerned, we do think that minor imperfections can actually be surprisingly well tolerated, as long as they do not result in overcorrection and excessive pressure, or unbalanced alternate stresses in the flexion and extension positions. This excessive pressure, whether alternate or continuous, seems to be the main factor of early deterioration of some implants.

Lateral compartment osteoarthritis (L-C OA): technical principles

The same principles and rules apply to the lateral UKR.

However, a few points need to be stressed because this technique slightly differs from that of medial UKA.

Surgical approach

According to the UKA philosophy, an anterolateral approach is used. This avoids extended arthrotomy and reversion of the patella as would be necessary with an anteromedial approach.

This approach should be sufficiently excentric, quite limited superiorly, and should not interfere with the anterior tibial tubercle. Should conversion to TKA be necessary, a median approach may make revision difficult and carries the risk of skin necrosis.

Tibial component positioning

Positioning of the tibial component should allow for the specific anatomy of the lateral condyle which is often severely internally rotated. Therefore, the tibial component should be slightly internally rotated to avoid impingement of the anterior part of the femoral component upon the anterior aspect of the intercondylar eminence in extension. Thus, the vertical cut of the tibial plateau should be slightly medialized anteriorly, and yet preserve the ACL insertion.

In the frontal plane, the most important is to avoid directing the cut downward and medially. This natural tendency can be compensated by using the adjustable cutting guide and measuring the ideal resection angle preoperatively. With experience, one will often tilt the cutting block 2 to 3° downward and laterally.

Adjustment of the tibial slope is the same as for a medial component.

Femoral component positioning

This is the most difficult step because one is inclined to rely on the apparent obliquity of the lateral condyle in flexion. Centering the femoral component on the femoral condyle, parallel to the lateral margin of the condyle, will almost inevitably result in excessive internal rotation of the femoral component which will cause impingement of the anterior part of the component upon the intercondylar eminence in extension.

This is where the centering plate of the HLS® unicompartmental instrument system (TORNIER) proves its efficacy. It protects from this natural internal rotation tendency and assists in central positioning of the femoral component in extension. In many cases, it will result in lateral positioning of the anterior part of the femoral component. As recommended by Ph. Cartier (3), the lateral osteophytes of the femoral condyle should be retained because they are often used to support the anterior part of the femoral component (fig. 9).

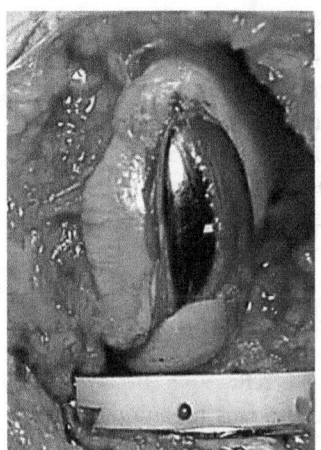

Fig. 9. – Lateral UKR: the anterior part of the femoral component rests on the lateral osteophyte.

This will often give an impression of derotation that is rather confusing in flexion. One just has to place the knee in extension to understand the special kinematics of the lateral condyle and the soundness of this choice which avoids impingement upon the intercondylar eminence in extension, and contact with the lateral facet of the patella in flexion.

It is only after the trial components have been inserted that one will decide whether a thicker femoral component (5mm) should be used, according to the location of wear. To assist in this decision, one must check whether the prosthetic condyle lies flat on the tibial component in extension, and 2 to 3mm laxity (safety laxity) persists when the knee is fully extended. This will confirm the absence of overcorrection which is particularly detrimental in the genu valgum (major risk of wear of the opposite compartment). This is the reason why we have (like Ph. Cartier – MOD III® RICHARDS) designed a special HLS® 5mm femoral component (standard thickness, 3mm) for use in L-C OA.

Conclusion

As long as the above indications and stringent technical rules are respected, the unicompartmental knee prosthesis is indeed the replacement of choice for the treatment of single compartment gonarthrosis.

The fresh interest in this type of knee replacement can be explained by the simple postoperative management. Owing to longer life expectancy, one is more and more inclined to propose surgical treatment to patients over 80 years of age with pure single compartment osteoarthritis. As a matter of fact, we think that performing a TKA in this situation is not justified. The aged are rightfully reluctant to undergo surgery and of course, the simple postoperative management for a UKR is very much attractive to these patients.

In contrast, the surgeons' apprehension about this procedure most often seems to be based on old publications which reported failures due to technical errors or wrong indications that are now well known and defined (4). We believe, without being excessively optimistic, that the future results of recent series in which all the above stringent yet simple rules have been respected, will make the UKR a most satisfactory, reliable and attractive alternative to TKR.

References

1. Deschamps G (1996) Prothèses unicompartimentales – l'indication idéale. Rev Chir Orthop 82 (suppl. 1): 53-4
2. Dejour H, Dejour D, Habi S (1997) Fate of the patellofemoral and of the opposite tibiofemoral compartment, following unicompartmental knee replacement. In: Cartier Ph, Epinette J, Deschamps G et al. (eds.). Unicompartmental Knee Arthroplasty, vol. 61. Paris: Expansion Scientifique Française: 147-50
3. Cartier Ph, Landreau Ph (1996) Technique de la prothèse unicompartimentale externe. Rev Chir Orthop (suppl. 1): 25-60
4. Deschamps G, Cartier Ph. (2001) Unicondylar Arthroplasty. In: Malek MM (eds) Knee Surgery: Complications, Pitfalls, and Salvage. NY Springer-Verlag: 364-79

Surgical indications in tibiofemoral arthrosis (TFA)

P. Chambat, N. Graveleau

Growing participation in sports activities and the overuse and injury which accompanies it, together with greater life expectancy of the population, make tibiofemoral arthrosis an increasingly frequent problem in daily orthopaedic surgery practice.

Selecting patients for surgery involves analysing the patient's functional disability, clinically and radiologically evaluating the degree of arthrosis, being familiar with the outcomes of the various alternatives available and, in the light of this information, suggesting the most appropriate solution for the patient.

To simplify the debate, we will exclude those cases of osteoarthrosis following malunion or intra-articular fractures.

Evaluation of pathology

Functional disability

Functional disability should be evaluated as objectively as possible using assessment sheets (30) that quantify a certain number of more or less objective findings.

Pain is the most important factor but also the most difficult to assess. It may evolve gradually or episodically, with phases of extreme pain alternating with calmer periods. The painful crises must be appropriately controlled before making a decision. It is the mean level of pain that must be taken into account, while being wary of patient complaints, which may appear out of proportion to the radiologic findings.

On the other hand, the walking distance, difficulty in climbing or descending stairs or getting up from a chair is more easily measured.

The patient's activity and motivation influence his or her tolerance of the disorder. Some patients refuse to accept that normal physical or sports activity may be impossible, while others are genuinely unable to carry on a comfortable daily activity, even if it is limited.

A young man who cannot run, ski or play tennis has different demands than an elderly woman who cannot go outside her home, and they must be treated accordingly. This factor allows us to put into perspective the evoked relative disability but it must be taken into account when deciding on the particular type of intervention.

Clinical examination

Clinical examination should begin by examining gait (flexion contracture, antalgia or thrust during monopodal stance) and continue with standing alignment studies in bipedal stance.

With the patient supine, we assess:

– alignment once more, along with tibial and femoral torsion;
– range of motion (limitation of flexion and extension);
– frontal plane laxity ("true medial or lateral laxity" due to ligament distension in the convexity, as opposed to "false laxity" due to wear in the concavity of the lesion, corresponding to malalignment when the two worn joint surfaces are in contact);
– possible central pivotal insufficiency in the sagittal plane;
– patellofemoral joint status, joint effusion or popliteal cyst.

Radiologic examination

Basic investigation includes frontal radiographs in extension and flexion with the patient standing on one foot (39), a lateral radiograph at 30° flexion and a sunrise view of both patellae at 30° flexion. If surgery is being considered, frontal goniometry with the patient standing on one foot, or, if technically difficult, on both feet, is indispensable.

For certain indications, notably unicompartmental prostheses, long radiographs to include the hip and the ankle in stress with correction of deformity in the frontal plane may be useful.

These images allow us to appreciate:

– femoral and tibial wear;
– possible ligament laxity in the convexity, sometimes associated with translation of the femur on the tibia;
– the tibiofemoral mechanical axis;
– the anatomic femoral axis;
– the mechanical axis of the tibia and the tibial slope;
– feasibility of correction of the deformities.

MRI is of little interest in arthritis except at an early stage, to search for intra-articular lesions. CT scan may exceptionally be necessary to assess disorders of femoral or tibial torsion, or rotation of the knee induced or not by arthritis.

In exceptional cases also, scintigraphy will show to what degree inflammation is involved in extremely painful arthritis of the knee.

These investigations make it therefore possible:

– to understand the functional disability of the patients and his or her wishes;
– to evaluate and classify the arthritis.

Treatment possibilities

The therapeutic arsenal ranges from medical treatment to total tricompart-mental knee replacement and includes arthroscopic joint debridement, osteo-tomy and unicompartmental prostheses.

Medical treatment

Medical intervention is an obligatory passage in the treatment phase. It allows us to control acute episodes of pain and to assess the pain tolerance of the patients, who should not be hurried into surgery.

Arthroscopic joint debridement

Arthroscopic joint debridement (31) is not an option if weight bearing radio-graphs show clear narrowing of the joint line or marked axis deviation (38). In the best cases lavage (30), shaving of the meniscus or cartilage if it is deta-ched may relieve pain and disability for several months, but this is a pallia-tive, temporary solution, without cartilage reconstruction (3, 40). The results of such a procedure are often unreliable (4) but they sometimes help us to be patient so as not to be precipitous with major surgery.

Osteotomy

Osteotomy, which for long was the only effective surgical procedure in arthritis, has lost its exclusivity since the advent of knee prostheses, even as we witness some renewed interest in this procedure. A distinction must be made between procedures for medial tibiofemoral arthrosis (TFA) and those for lateral TFA.

Medial TFA

With the exception of unusual morphotypes, treatment for medial TFA is not controversial. Proximal tibial metaphyseal valgus osteotomy, which relieves the load on the affected medial compartment by modifying the axis, has no harmful mechanical consequences. Because of anatomic tibial varus, which ranges between 3° and 5° (9) and medial tibial wear, a laterally oblique joint line is rarely obtained after correction. In addition, modification of the axis situated at the level of the tibia makes this osteotomy effective in flexion and in extension.

Various long-term studies

Different long-term studies (1, 8, 16, 17, 24, 25, 33) have defined the cri-teria for optimal results after osteotomy. These relate to:

– stage of arthritis. The less evolved the arthritis, the better the result (1, 8, 33). The ideal is partial or total isolated internal tibiofemoral joint line narrowing on weight bearing radiographs in extension and in 30° of flexion, with no translation in the frontal plane and no anterior translation in the sagittal plane, which would indicate preservation of the anterior cruciate ligament, and a patellofemoral joint in good condition;

– tibial morphology. Tibia varus is a positive factor likely to lead to a good result (8, 33). If the tibia is in varus, osteotomy will correct the deformity and restore a nearly normal tibia, whereas the absence of tibia vara will create malunion and possibly a laterally oblique joint line, which will be mechanically unsatisfactory;

– patient age. While it is not possible to fix a lower limit, an upper limit does exist and results differ between patients in their fifties and older patients (8). As well as chronological age, physiological age must be considered and both must be taken into account when deciding on surgery. This criterion, which is logically important for the long-term result, is also important in the short term, facilitating postoperative non weight bearing ambulation with crutches and permitting a functional recovery that should lead to a return to physical and sporting activities;

– weight. A ponderal surcharge has a negative impact (8, 16, 17, 33) on the result of osteotomy. Excess weight of the lower limbs is even more harmful as the patients stand with their feet further apart and varus constraints are increased. The constatations apply during the swing phase of the contra-lateral extremity for the monopedal stance phase of the affected extremity.

Determination of correction

Once the selection criteria for surgery have been met, the correction itself must be decided upon. Most authors use the mechanical tibiofemoral axis as reference and define the angular degree of correction (8, 9, 21, 27, 35) calculated on the main axes with weight bearing is monopedal or bipedal stance, taking into account the length of the segments and medial wear and excluding lateral laxity which increases varus. This angular correction aims to transfer the mechanical axis to the lateral plateau in an area situated between 62% and 66% (21) of the width of the knee, which corresponds to 3° to 6° valgus.

However it should be noted that taking the mechanical axis as a reference is already an approximation, as it is the centre of gravity lying at the second sacral vertebra which should be taken into account to assess strain at the knee, determining an extrinsic varus deviation (44; 45) which should theoretically be taken into account for load on the medial compartment. This is a dynamic factor, which is normally compensated for by all the lateral musculo-tendinous structures. While it can be disregarded in severe deformity, it should be taken into account for deformities of less than 5° (tibiofemoral axis). Correction in the frontal plane should not lead us to forget the sagittal plane, checking the tibial slope which should be decreased if it is in the upper range (normal values 4° to 10°) (9) or frankly abnormal.

Reaching the objective

The corrective procedure must firstly be decided upon, then performed and later checked to make sure that the goal has been reached. The distinction has then to be made between osteotomies with correction and immediate fixation by lateral closing or medial opening wedge and osteotomies with progressive correction using external fixation.

Techniques

• Osteotomies with immediate correction

– Ease of bone union is a point in favour of closing wedge high tibial osteotomies performed above the tubercle (8, 16, 17, 33). Their drawbacks are excessive bony resection which is difficult to correct as well as the problem raised by the fibula; resection at the head or release at the upper tibiofibular joint creates the risk of destabilising the lateral compartment, whereas resection in the middle part sometimes leads to delayed and even non-unions.

– Opening wedge osteotomies performed above the tubercle (22, 25) have the advantage that the correction can always be modified right up to the final decision. Their drawbacks relate to problems with bony union, which often requires a bone graft to fill the defect created by opening.

– Checking correction: whatever the method chosen, our shortcomings lie in controlling corrections during the surgery, since the techniques used (skin landmarks placed before the procedure, serial radiographs of the hip, knee and ankle using a metal bar representing the mechanical axis) are more reassuring for the surgeon than efficient in checking the angle of correction. The tibial slope must also be verified and should at least be maintained.

• Osteotomies with progressive correction and external fixation

The strong point of this technique is that correction can be checked some time after the procedure on radiographs of the entire leg. However it is used infrequently because of its disadvantages: patient discomfort, risk of short- and long-term infection.

Results of valgus tibial osteotomy

Depending on patient-related criteria and on the surgical correction, osteotomies can give good results at ten years, which should be the contract proposed by the surgeon to the patient. In another respect, this procedure gives a good quality of life, which allows sporting activity and long distances walks on uneven ground, ski, tennis and even running, though this is perhaps not advisable. However, the published long-term results concern more particularly closed osteotomies and questions remain concerning the biomechanical action of opening wedge osteotomies, which lower the patella and put tension on the medial biarticular muscles.

The results of surgical revision of failures (2, 37, 45, 46) of valgus high tibial osteotomy by total knee replacement are well known and satisfactory. Technical problems related to overcorrection or malunion of the proximal portion of the tibia with translation of the metaphysis relative to the epiphysis may arise but they often correspond to a technical error at the time of osteotomy. If the osteotomy made it possible to delay total knee replacement for ten years, we can affirm that the surgeon has fulfilled his contract, even if the procedure of implant insertion is a little difficult.

Lateral tibiofemoral arthrosis (LTFA)

For lateral tibiofemoral arthrosis (LFTA), the surgical procedure which should be performed is controversial, as no osteotomy is perfect from a biomechanical viewpoint.

– Classically, LFTA is corrected by femoral varus osteotomy (23, 36), using an open lateral supracondylar approach, which has the advantage of facility. But while this procedure effectively corrects the tibiofemoral axis in extension (13), it has no effect when the knee is at 90°. At this degree of flexion, the posterior condyles are load bearing, and their alignment has not been modified by the osteotomy. At 90° of flexion, distal femoral varus osteotomy rotates the distal femoral epiphysis internally. In order to have a varus effect it would be necessary to realize an internal rotation maneuver, the only way of modifying alignment at the level of the posterior condyles between 0° and 90°. With a femoral varus osteotomy, the varus effect progressively decreases, being maximal at 0° and nil at 90°. An osteotomy is often debated only at an early stage of LTFA, which is shown as narrowing on flexion whereas radiographs in extension are largely normal, femoral osteotomy has little effect in the ranges of motion which would be of use to the patient. It is a major procedure, which is fairly difficult to perform. The aim is to restore normal alignment but intraoperative evaluation raises the same problem as in valgus tibial osteotomy. Among the authors, the results were judged with encouragement, however those are older studies (23).

Revision of failures by total knee replacement, on the other hand, poses no particular problem apart from removal of the implant, whose imposing scar cannot be exploited for the remainder of the intervention.

– Tibial varus osteotomy is effective from 0° to 90° (13) of flexion but it has the disadvantage of creating a medially oblique joint line. The ideal criteria for this procedure is a valgus tibiofemoral alignment with a tibia with little or no varus and a lateral compartmental narrowing restricted to the meniscal region. The objective is to obtain normal alignment and if an oblique joint line angle of more than 10° is predictable preoperatively, the procedure should not be undertaken. This procedure is not technically difficult, however, controlling of correction raises the same problems as mentioned above. In the medium term, the results are not always as good as was hoped (42). They deteriorate with time and rarely last more than ten years. However revisions by total knee arthroplasty can be done without difficulty.

Unicompartmental prosthesis

The unicompartmental prosthesis was sometimes unjustly criticized for a number of years but it deserves our attention and remains an important weapon in our therapeutic arsenal for the treatment of tibiofemoral arthrosis, on the condition that the following stringent selection criteria are respected (43).

Criteria

Stage of arthrosis

It must be isolated medial or lateral tibiofemoral arthrosis with no translation in the frontal plane, an intact anterior cruciate ligament (19) and remaining range of motion.

Tibiofemoral morphology

The final aim is to retain an undercorrection (5) but there are limits to this. As the compartmental prosthesis is a wedge, which replaces worn bone, in no case can it correct excessively varus or valgus morphology, as the limit of residual varus or valgus after unicompartmental arthroplasty must not be more than 5° in order not to overload the prosthetic compartment (11, 18). Here the weight bearing radiographs are important with correction of the deformity, which according to the angle obtained will tell us whether unicompartmental prosthesis is a possibility. Postoperative alignment should never be brought to less than 5° of undercorrection by extensive release in the concavity or by excessive tensioning of the capsule, as residual physiological laxity of the revised compartment is necessary for satisfactory function (11).

Weight

As the tibial component has limited surfaces for fixation, we consider that overweight patients should not receive this type of prosthesis. Of course weight is related to the patient's height but we believe that it would be dangerous to exceed an upper limit of 80kg (11, 32).

Activity

In our experience, unicompartmental prosthesis is only possible in patients whose activity is moderate; even if sports can be practiced as long as the patient has no discomfort, this often causes pain in the prosthetic compartment and should be discouraged.

Age

Depending on the series, long-term reliability is variable. The risk is the onset of pain followed by loosening and decreased survivorship at 6 or 7 years. We believe it is preferable to propose this procedure in patients around the age of 70, who are also more likely to meet the requirement of moderate activity.

Results

In our experience, results are better with unicompartmental than with total knee prostheses. There is a good index of patient satisfaction, good pain relief and excellent range of motion, and in some series the results of lateral unicompartmental prostheses are as good as if not better than those of medial unicompartmental implants. Problems related to prosthesis design (6), polyethylene thickness and an eventual metal-backed plateau as well as insertion techniques (34) affect the results but a consensus has been reached on these points ensuring that this is a reliable procedure.

Revision

Although the revision rate is higher than for total prostheses (12, 26, 28, 29, 41, 44, 46, 47), all authors agree that replacement of a unicompartmental by a tri-compartmental prosthesis does not raise any technical problems on condition that revision is done early before loosening causes loss of bone stock. The clinical results of replacement of unicompartmental by total prostheses (10, 14, 20) are satis-factory and better even than those of replacement of one total prosthesis by another, and there should be no hesitation as to the use of a unicompartmental prosthesis to treat an arthritic knee when the selection criteria are met.

Total knee arthroplasty

Total knee arthroplasty is the extreme weapon in our therapeutic arsenal for knee arthrosis. This procedure attained its maturity some years ago and can now be proposed without hesitation. The criteria governing its use are nega-tive ones, corresponding to arthritic knees, which cannot be treated by any other technique. Age could be a criterion to be taken into account and we certainly hesitate to carry out total knee replacement in a patient younger than 50 years of age, but if that is the only reliable solution then the age argu-ment should not hold.

It is not our aim here to discuss the type of prosthesis that should be used, nor insertion techniques. At the present time a whole range of implants are available, providing solutions to all types of problem: posterior cruciate liga-ment retaining prostheses, prostheses sacrificing the posterior cruciate liga-ment with a more or less constrained stabilisation system and even hinged prostheses. These are only exceptionally indicated but may be of service in certain cases and deserve our attention, perhaps with a view towards a new design. Other controversial questions are stem length and the use or other-wise of cement. The best results allow the patient to lead a normal life and even to take some part in certain sports such as golf and cross-country skiing. On the other hand, more violent sports involving weight bearing, rapid turns, pushing off and landing on the feet may be possible but seem to us inadvi-sable because of the risk of early deterioration or periprosthetic fractures. The results of total knee replacement revision are well known but they are never as satisfactory as the results of primary implants (7).

Treatment possibilities

Medial tibiofemoral arthrosis (TFA)

Treatment indications for arthritis involving this compartment are clear. When medical treatment and possibly joint debridement are no longer effective, a more radical surgical solution has to be considered.

Tibial valgus osteotomy

This is desirable in the case of an isolated lateral FTA if the patient is in his or her fifties and in good physical condition. A lean patient with varus of tibial origin is an even better candidate especially if he or she wishes to take up regular physical activity. However, these criteria are somewhat stringent and the restrictions of the ideal schemas may be transgressed:

– if patellofemoral arthrosis is moderate, which according to some authors does not affect the final result (1, 24);

– if the anterior cruciate ligament is absent but the arthrosis too advanced for its repair to be considered. In this indication, the postoperative tibial slope is of essential importance and as long as preoperative recurvatum is not greater than 5°, surgery must aim at reducing the posterior tibial slope to less than 5°;

– if arthritis is more advanced but the patient is young, with the aim of delaying insertion of a prosthesis, even if the function obtained does not correspond to a very good clinical result;

– if the patient has passed his or her fifties, is in good physical condition and wishes to continue with intense physical activity.

The internal unicompartmental prosthesis

This is the ideal indication for isolated medial tibiofemoral arthrosis with a normal anterior cruciate ligament in a patient weighing less than 80 kilos and aged over 70 years, with only moderate activity, on condition that correction of wear by the unicompartmental prosthesis results in an undercorrection of no more than 5° varus. Patient selection criteria for a medial unicompartmental prosthesis are very restrictive but, unlike osteotomy, we believe it is dangerous to transgress them and to widen the field of application of these prostheses (11, 15).

The tricompartmental prosthesis

We consider this as an indication "by default" which applies to all patients who cannot undergo valgus tibial osteotomy or medial unicompartmental arthroplasty. The prosthetic options and insertion techniques are described elsewhere in this book.

Lateral tibiofemoral arthrosis

Management of lateral tibiofemoral arthrosis is less simple than that of medial tibiofemoral arthrosis, since femoral or tibial osteotomy creates a mechanical imperfection, which affects the result.

Femoral osteotomy

This is effective in extension and not in flexion and we consider it is justified preventively in extremely valgus knees with hypoplasia of the lateral condyle at an early stage, especially in young patients.

It can also be a salvage operation in the young patient with advanced arthrosis with joint space narrowing in extension, in order to gain time and delay the need for a prosthesis.

Tibal osteotomy

This is effective both in flexion and in extension and a good indication is early arthrosis with isolated narrowing in the meniscal area in a valgus knee with normal tibial alignment. Unfortunately it creates an oblique joint line, which limits the long-term result, and so it seems to us difficult to propose this treatment in patients younger than 55 or 60 years.

Whatever the type of osteotomy proposed, we have to recognize that it is a compromise. But even if it is easier to go straight to prosthetic insertion, honesty towards the patient, in our opinion, necessitates that osteotomy be given consideration and not eluded.

The lateral unicompartmental prosthesis

In the absolute, the same criteria as those for medial unicompartmental arthroplasty, applied to valgus, must be retained for medial unicompartmental prostheses. But where lateral compartmental arthrosis is concerned and in light of our reticence to propose an osteotomy, these rules may be transgressed if the patient is younger or if patellofemoral involvement is slight.

The tricompartmental prosthesis

As with medial compartmental arthrosis, this is an indication by default because once again in lateral tibiofemoral arthrosis osteotomy is debatable. We believe it is logical to lower the age threshold for which total knee arthroplasty is justifiable.

Conclusion

In osteoarthritis of the knee, careful consideration is required before surgery and total knee arthroplasty must not be the only solution. A surgeon in his therapeutic arsenal must be able to propose osteotomy without hesitation if this indication is justified and it is important that future generations of surgeons should be trained in these techniques. While the 1990s concentrated entirely on prostheses, now in the present decade from the year 2000 we should be able to obtain more balanced indications, on condition that we improve the quality of intra-operative evaluation of the correction obtained.

The surgical indication for arthrosis of the knee requires us to reflect and should not have, as only solution, a total knee arthroplasty. The surgeon should have in his therapeutic arsenal the possibility of offering, without second thought, an osteotomy if that indication is justified. It is also important that our future generation surgeons receive training in the decision-making and these surgical techniques. If the 1990s were totally turned towards the prosthesis, the years 2000 should permit a readjustment of indications that favors osteotomies, on condition that we gain reliability in the verification of correction process in the perioperative period.

References

1. Agglietti P, Rionapoli E, Stringa G (1983) Tibial osteotomy for the varus osteoarthritis knee. Clin Orthop 176: 239-51
2. Badet R, Aït Si Selmi T, Neyret Ph (1999) Prothèse totale du genou après ostéotomie tibiale de valgisation. In: Chambat P, Neyret Ph, Deschamp G (éd.) Chirurgie prothétique du genou. Sauramps médical, Montpellier, p. 241-57
3. Bentley G (1980) The surgical treatment of chondromalacia of the patellae. J Bone Joint Surg 52A: 221
4. Bentley G, Dowd G (1984) Current concepts of aetiology and treatment of chondromalacia of the patellae. Clin Orthop 189: 209
5. Bensadoun JL, Vidal J, Maury P (1989) Unicompartmental arthroplasty. Orthop Trans 13: 708
6. Bohm I, Landsield F (2000) Revision surgery after failed unicompartmental knee arthroplasty. J Arthroplasty 15: 982-9
7. Bonnin M, Deroche Ph, Palazzolo P (1999) Les reprises de prothèse totale du genou par prothèse totale. In: Chambat P, Neyret Ph, Deschamp G (éd.) Chirurgie prothétique du genou. Sauramps médical, Montpellier, p. 177-201
8. Bonnin M, Levigne C (1991) Ostéotomie tibiale de valgisation pour arthrose fémoro-tibiale interne. Résultat d'un échantillon de 217 ostéotomies revues avec un recul de 1 à 21 ans. 7e Journées Lyonnaises du genou, p. 142-68
9. Brown GA, Amendola A (2000) Radiographic evaluation and preoperative planning for high tibial osteotomies. Op Techn Sports Med 8: 2-14
10. Chakrabarty G, Newman J, Ackroyd C (1998) Revision of unicompartmental arthroplasty of the knee. Clinical and technical consideration. J Arthroplasty 13: 191-6
11. Cartier Ph, Deschamps G (1998) Principes techniques de l'arthroplastie unicompartimentale. In: Cartier Ph, Epinette JA, Deschamps G et al. (éd.) Prothèses unicompartimentales de genou. Cahier d'Enseignement de la SOFCOT – Expansion scientifique publication, Paris, p. 145-51
12. Cartier Ph, Sanouiller JL (1998) Prothèses unicompartimentales Marmor. Bilan clinique au recul maximal de 10 ans. In: Cartier Ph, Epinette JA, Deschamps G et al. (éd.) Prothèses unicompartimentales de genou. Cahier d'Enseignement de la SOFCOT – Expansion scientifique publication, Paris, p. 177-83
13. Chambat P, Aït Si Selmi T, Dejour D et al. (2000) Varus tibial osteotomy. Op Techn Sports Med 8: 44-7
14. Chatain F, Richard A, Deschamps G (1999) Reprise des prothèses unicompartimentale par prothèse du genou. In: Chambat P, Neyret Ph, Deschamp G (éd.) Chirurgie prothétique du genou. Sauramps médical, Montpellier, p. 159-67
15. Chesnut W (1991) Preoperative diagnostic protocol to predict candidates for unicompartmental arthroplasty. Clin Orthop 273: 146-50
16. Coventry MB (1985) Upper tibial osteotomy for osteoarthritis. J Bone Joint Surg 67A: 1136-40
17. Coventry MB Ilstrup DM, Wallrichs SL (1993) Proximal tibial osteotomy: a critical long term study of 87 cases. J Bone Joint Surg 75A: 196-201
18. Dejour D, Chatain F, Dejour H (1998) Résultats cliniques de la prothèse unicompartimentale HLS. In: Cartier Ph, Epinette JA, Deschamps G et al. (éd.) Prothèses unicompartimentales de genou. Cahier d'Enseignement de la SOFCOT – Expansion scientifique publication, Paris, p. 1226-32
19. Deschamps G, Lapeyre B (1987) La rupture du ligament croisé antérieur. Une cause d'échec souvent méconnue des prothèses unicompartimentales du genou. À propos d'une série de 79 prothèses Lotus revues au-delà de 5 ans. Rev Chir Orthop 73: 544-51
20. Deschamps G, Cartier P (2001) Unicondylar Arthroplasty. In: Malek M (ed.) Knee Surgery complications, Pitfallsand salvage. Springer Verlag, New York, p. 364-79
21. Dugdale TW, Noyes F, Styer D (1989) Preoperative planning for high tibial osteotomy. Clin Orthop 274: 248-64

22. Fowler PJ, Limtan J, Brown GA (2000) Medial open wedge high tibial osteotomy: how I do it. Op Techn Sports Med 8: 32-8
23. Healy W, Anylen J, Wasilenski S (1998) Distal femoral varus osteotomy for varus deformity of the knee. J Bone Joint Surg 70A: 111-6
24. Hernigou Ph, Goutallier D (1987) Devenir de l'articulation fémoro-patellaire du genu varum arthrosique après ostéotomie tibiale de valgisation par addition interne. Rev Chir Orthop 73: 43-8
25. Hernigou Ph, Medevielle D, Debeyre J et al. (1987) Proximal tibial osteotomy for osteoarthritis with varus deformity. A ten year follow-up study. J Bone Joint Surg 69A: 332-54
26. Hernigou Ph, Deschamps G (1996) Les prothèses unicompartimentales du genou. Symposium 70e réunion de la SOFCOT. Rev Chir Orthop 82 (suppl. I): 23-60
27. Hernigou Ph, Ovada H, Goutallier D (1992) Modélisation mathématique de l'ostéotomie tibiale d'ouverture et table de correction. Rev Chir Orthop 78: 258-63
28. Hernigou Ph, Deschamps G (1998) Prothèses unicompartimentales. Résultats de 250 prothèses Lotus avec un recul moyen de 10 ans. In: Cartier Ph Epinette JA Deschamps G et al. (ed) Prothèses unicompartimentales de genou. Cahier d'Enseignement de la SOFCOT – Expansion scientifique publication, Paris, p. 203-12
29. Insall J, Aglietti P (1980) A five to seven year follow-up of unicondylar arthroplasty. J Bone Joint Surg 62A: 1329-37
30. Insall J, Dorr LD, Scott RD et al. (1989) Rationale of the knee society clinical rating system. Clin Orthop 248: 13-4
31. Jackson RW, Marans HJ, Silver RS (1988) The arthroscopic treatment of degenerative joint disease. J Bone Joint Surg 70B: 332
32. Kozinn S, Scott R (1989) Unicondylar knee arthroplasty. J Bone Joint Surg 71A: 145-50
33. Lootvoet L, Massinon A, Rossillon R et al. (1993) Ostéotomie tibiale haute de valgisation pour arthrose sur genu varum. A propos d'une série de 193 cas revus après 6 à 10 ans de recul. Rev Chir Orthop 79: 375-84
34. Lindstrand I, Stenstrom A, Ryd L et al. S (2000) The introduction period of unicompartmental knee arthroplasty is critical. J Arthroplasty 15: 608-16
35. Miniaci A, Ballmer FT, Ballmer PM (1989) Proximal tibial osteotomy: a new fixation device. Clin Orthop 246: 250-9
36. Miniaci A, Grossman SP, Jacob RP (1990) Supra condylar femoral varus osteotomy in the treatment of varus deformity. Am J Knee Surg 2: 65-73
37. Neyret Ph, Deroche Ph, Deschamps G et al. (1992) Prothèses totales du genou après ostéotomie tibiale de valgisation. Rev Chir Orthop 78: 438-48
38. Ogilvie-Harris DJ, Fitsialos DP (1991) Arthroscopic management of the degenerative knee. J Arthroplasty 7: 151
39. Rosenberg TD, Paulos LE, Parker RD (1998) The forty-five degrees postero-anterior flexion weight bearing radiograph. J Bone Joint Surg 70A: 1479-83
40. Schmid A, Schmid F (1987) Results after cartilage shaving by electromicroscopy. Am J Sport Med 15: 386-90
41. Scott RD, Cobb AG, Mc Queary FG, et al. (1991) Unicompartmental knee arthroplasty. 8 to 12 year follow-up evaluation with survivorship analysis. Clin Orthop 271: 96-100
42. Shoji H, Insall J (1973) High tibial osteotomy for osteoarthritis of the knee with valgus deformity. J Bone Joint Surg 55A: 963-73
43. Stern SH, Becker MW, Insall JN (1993) Unicondylar knee arthroplasty. An evaluation of selection criteria. Clin Orthop 286: 143-8
44. Thomine JM, Boudjema A, Gibon Y et al. (1981) Les écarts varisants dans la gonarthrose. Fondement théorique et essai d'évaluation pratique. Rev Chir Orthop 67: 319-27
45. Torksvig-Larsen S, Magyard G, Onsten L et al. (1998) Fixation of the tibial component of total knee arthroplasty after a high tibial osteotomy: amatched radiostereometric study. J Bone Joint Surg 80B: 295-7
46. Wang M, Stulberg SD, Jigantif J et al. (1993) The natural history of unicompartmental arthroplasty: an eight year follow-up study with survivorship analysis. Clin Orthop 286: 130
47. Witwoet J, Peyrache MD, Nizard R (1993) Prothèses unicompartimentales type Lotus dans le traitement des gonarthroses. Rev Chir Orthop 79: 565-76

Points of view: What are the limits in ACL reconstruction?

V. Musahl, J.R. Giffin, F. Margheritini, F.H. Fu

Introduction

The community of middle-aged and sport-active patients is growing. There is increased interest in high-impact or high-risk sports and these activities bring with them concomitant trauma to bones, joint surfaces, and soft tissue. Epidemiological studies from the early 1990s investigated the incidence of knee ligament injuries in the United States. The average rate of knee ligament injuries was approximately 100 per 100,000 population annually (58) and can be expected to increase. Projected from this study, an estimated 70,000 isolated anterior cruciate ligament (ACL) injuries per year, 40,000 isolated medial collateral ligament (MCL) injuries per year, and 20,000 combined ACL/MCL injuries per year occur in the United States alone.

In spite of the large number of anterior cruciate ligament (ACL) reconstructions that are being performed each year around the world (estimated between 75,000 to 100,000 cases in the United States alone), the question remains: "How far can the limits in ACL reconstruction be pushed?" Independently from the selection of the graft for possible ACL reconstruction, factors like timing of the surgery, activity level of the patient, and patient expectations have to be taken into account.

Natural history of ACL deficient knees and ACL reconstructed knees

Initial injury

The classic ACL injury is a non-contact injury, which happens during cutting sport activities like football, soccer or basketball. Typically, the injury involves internal rotation, valgus stress, and/or hyperextension, whereby the patient feels a "pop", indicating that the knee has dislocated. On physical examination, an effusion (hemarthros) as well as a positive anterior drawer and Lachman test can be appreciated. The initial treatment usually includes management of the swelling and pain as well as bracing, regardless of a future operative or non-operative treatment, which is still discussed controversially.

Knee changes following ACL injury

The knee joint can be regarded as a box that transfers force from the thigh muscles to the foot, with estimated loads on the knee joint surfaces up to seven times of the body weight during normal knee activities (19). The cruciate ligaments are the main restraints to sagittal tibial translation whereby the ACL controls the anterior motion. Increased joint compression force is thereby a result of quadriceps muscle activity during normal knee function that produces a force transmitted to the tibia through the ACL, contributing to joint stability. Therefore the rupture of the ACL creates an environment where the passive sagittal motion is at least doubled and where articular contact force is unevenly distributed. The inability to compensate for joint instability during daily activities will lead to frequently repeated subluxations, with an increased risk of further joint injuries. It has been suggested that mechanoreceptors in the ACL act as detectors for the limit of motion, therefore altering joint stiffness by influencing muscle tension (41). Increased muscle tension around the knee seems to increase the ability of the ACL to sustain the load without failing. Furthermore, it is known that cytokines play an important role in joint inflammation and in the loss of articular cartilage (7, 59, 67). Recent analysis of these cytokine levels suggests that biomechanical as well as biological factors may contribute to the development of osteoarthritis (12).

Clinically, the incidence of osteoarthritis after ACL disruption is reported in several retrospective follow-up studies that are mostly based on short- to mid-term follow-up (18, 32, 55, 63). However, prediction of the individual risk of early osetoarthritic changes can only be estimated. Hertel *et al.* reported that on an average of 10.2 years after ACL reconstruction, 54% of the patients exhibited normal radiographic findings and 46% exhibited mild radiographic changes, with a joint space of more than 4mm, according to the International Knee Documentation Committee (IKDC) standard evaluation form (32). In another study, the postoperative arthrosis rate increased to 24%, when the patients were evaluated arthroscopically after ten years of follow-up (55). Of the patients from that particular study, 85% had previously undergone meniscectomy.

The meniscus lesion and subsequent medial meniscectomy is a complication of ACL rupture and influences the functional and radiologic outcome (4, 63). A study by Neyret *et al.* showed the progress of radiologic features and identified typical radiologic signs and factors influencing the development of osteoarthritis after medial meniscectomy, in an average 27-year follow-up. The course of osteoarthritic changes and possible contributing factors by meniscus lesions and meniscectomy are not well investigated (39, 42).

Postoperative osteoarthritis

On the other hand, further published works have shown that rupture of the ACL that has been reconstructed also leads to osteoarthritis (8, 15, 25, 42, 68). A study by Daniel *et al.* revealed that ACL reconstructed knees had higher levels of osteoarthritis. Their follow-up study showed radiographic evidence of increased osteoarthritis after a mean of five years in patients who had undergone ACL reconstruction regardless of acute or chronic surgery settings (15). Gillquist et al. reviewed the frequency of post-traumatic osteoarthritis of the knee. Compared with the uninjured contralateral knee, radiographic signs of osteoarthritis increased after all knee injuries. Partial or total ACL rupture without major concomitant injuries increased the risk of osteoarthritis ten fold compared to the uninjured contralateral knee (25).

In a study by Jomha et al., follow-up results of ACL deficient patients revealed that knees with chronic ACL deficiency showed early osteoarthritic changes. ACL reconstruction was shown to have a lower incidence on degenerative change (43). A study by Fink et al. compared non-operative and operative treatment using follow-up radiographs. It was found that severe osteoarthritic changes were predominant in the non-operative group, according to the Fairbank classification (21). Further support was given from a study by Shelbourne et al., who reported that ACL reconstruction could provide long-term stability and symptomatic pain relief (75). The importance of simultaneous meniscus repair in decreasing the incidence of osteoarthritis was recognized by many authors (5, 29, 77). It was thereby shown that early repair of soft tissues led to a higher return-to-sport rate, when compared to conservative treatment groups.

Long-term follow-up studies are generally a measurement for success of treatments. Professor Ejnar Eriksson from Stockholm, Sweden, stated (20): "I am waiting for the day when we can promise our ACL patients a 95-100% chance of obtaining a stable, well-functioning knee that allows them to go back to their original sport at the same level as before their injury." In the past 20 years, over 4,000 scientific research articles have been published on the ACL and related problems. The knowledge that we gained from these is an approximate failure rate of ACL reconstructions of 10-40% (60, 69), complication rates of 5-20% (2), and 75-90% of good or excellent results (32, 44).

There are several reasons for this inability to reduce the progression of osteoarthritis. The surgical trauma itself and intra-operative bleeding could act as a predisposing factor for the development of osteoarthritis. A recent study has shown that the graft selection seems to be important as well. The use of a bone-patellar tendon-bone autograft increased the risk of early osteoarthritic changes in the patellofemoral joint (40). Pretension of the graft could be another cause. It has been shown that pre-tension of the graft can cause changes in joint kinematics, that may lead to osteoarthrosis in the long term (81). Furthermore, postoperative reduction of the range of motion can increase the risk of arthrofibrosis, and eventually lead to increased production of cartilage-degrading cytokines.

Secondary injuries

Secondary injuries can occur as a result of a high impact primary injury or recurrent instability. Thereby, an isolated anterior instability can evolve towards an anteromedial or less commonly to an anterolateral instability as well as the mechanical axis can change due to loss of the menisci or cartilage.

Bone bruises

An interesting finding, which is not appreciated before MRI, is the high association of occult osseous lesions around the knee in case of ACL injury (70). The most common finding is a bone bruise, or trabecular microfracture, which has decreased signal intensity on T1-weighted images and bright signal intensity on T2-weighted images. The overlying cortical bone is intact. The most frequent injury mechanism thereby is the non-contact injury, associated with high axial compression loads. Typically, ACL injuries that occur in motor vehicle or bicycle accidents are less frequently associated with bone bruises. The lateral compartment is the most common site, usually involving the middle aspect of the lateral femoral condyle and the posterior aspect of the lateral tibial plateau. Signs of subchondral damage disappear within two to four months after an ACL injury but their final effect on long-term joint function is unclear. It has been suggested that these lesions may eventually lead to osteoarthritis (26).

Meniscal injuries

Meniscal injuries may occur from the initial injury or over time with recurrent instability (36, 55). Of these lesions, medial meniscal lesions are the most common. Secondary medial meniscal lesions occur when the medial condyle overlaps the posterior horn of the medial meniscus. The prognosis is determined by whether it is a peripheral or not-repairable tear versus a tear in the vascular or read zone that is repairable. The anterior tibial translation increases considerably not only in extension but also in flexion (4). The much more motile lateral meniscus shows tears less frequently. However, a stable and incomplete tear of the posterior horn, which is anatomically close to the tibial insertion of the ACL, is almost always seen in acute ACL disruptions.

Chondral lesions

Chondral lesions have a different etiology. These cartilaginous lesions occur at the time of secondary instabilities, especially in the medial tibiofemoral compartment. The medial tibial plateau is subluxed to the front and the posterior edge of the medial tibial plateau is impacted on the femoral condyle. The femoral condylar lesions are visible through the arthroscope on flexion and present in a radial pattern with a central ulceration. These lesions do not indicate osteoarthritis, and are true cartilaginous fractures (17). The tibial cartilaginous lesion is an overloading injury, indicating the development of osteoarthritis. It is usually seen in the posterior two-thirds of the tibial surface. These lesions are secondary to the repetition of anterior translation on unilateral weight bearing and contraction of the quadriceps muscle.

Associated ligament injuries

Several studies have investigated the relationship between the medial ligamentocapsular structures and the ACL/ACL injury (23, 31, 36, 45, 52, 84). The factors limiting the anterior tibial translation are the ACL, the posterior horn of the medial meniscus, and the posteromedial ligamentocapsular structures. Ma and coworkers could show in a goat model that the force in the ACL increased more than two fold after sectioning the MCL (52). In a further investigation, Abramowitch *et al.* showed a significant reduction in the force in the ACL after six weeks of healing of the MCL in a goat model (1).

Posterolateral corner injuries in combination with ACL injuries are extremely rare. The posterolateral corner is composed of several elements: the lateral collateral ligament, the popliteus complex as the primary restraint to external rotation, and the arcuatum complex. These lesions play no part in the anterior tibial laxity, but have an important role in the balance and anterior stability. Kanamori and coworkers reported an increased force in the LCL after sectioning the ACL by three fold (45). The posterolateral lesions are therefore one origin of osteoarthritic changes as a result of this imbalance.

Inability of current ACL replacement grafts to restore normal knee function

Normal ligament function

Anatomically, ligaments connect bones and are designed to maintain stability during normal joint motion. The functionally distinct bundles of the ACL have significantly different orientations. The AM bundle is thought to be important as a restraint to antero-posterior translation of the knee, while the PL bundle is thought to be an important restraint to rotational moments about the knee (28, 31, 73).

The complex structure of the knee includes interaction of stabilizing ligaments and muscle-force generating tendons to provide locomotive, static, and dynamic functions. These motions are combinations of 3D translations and rotations that are mediated by ligament forces, joint contact forces, externally applied forces, and musculoskeletal forces. The non-linear tensile behavior of ligaments is hereby particularly suited to guide joint motion and provide stability over a large range of motion. Because stability of the knee is maintained by this complex interaction between ligament, tendon, meniscus, capsule, and the reaction forces acting on the articulating surfaces, the disruption of any of the major ligament components causes abnormal kinematics and therefore osteoarthritis over time. For disruption of the ACL, anterior tibial translation will be increased (54). Furthermore, internal and valgus rotations will be increased, especially when the MCL is disrupted as well (27, 37). These changes in kinematics may induce modifications in some tissues around the knee in order to improve joint stability, while other tissues may experience breakdown due to excessive mechanical stress. Progressing osteoarthritis of the knee joint is then evidenced by meniscal damage, increased ligamentous laxity, and articular cartilage degeneration; e.g. for complete rupture of the ACL, it is known that functional healing will not occur (61). Therefore, various ACL reconstruction procedures have been developed to restore stability and improve function of the unstable knee joint (13, 22, 30, 71).

Normal ligament properties

The kinetic response of a joint to internal and external loads is governed by bone geometry as well as the anatomical location, morphology, and chemical composition of ligaments and other connective tissues contained within or around the joint. To understand the contribution of an individual ligament to joint kinetics, the transfer of load through a ligament's insertion, midsubstance to the opposing insertion must be considered. Physiologically, these bone-ligament complexes have been designed to transfer load uniaxially along the longitudinal direction of the ligament. Thus, tensile testing of a bone-ligament-bone complex is done to determine the structural properties. The resulting load-elongation curve reveals a non-linear, concave, upward behavior. Parameters obtained from this curve include stiffness, ultimate load, ultimate elongation, and energy absorbed at failure. From the same test, information about the mechanical properties of the ligament substance can also be obtained. This is done by normalizing the force by the cross-sectional area of the ligament and the change in elongation by the initial length of a defined region of the ligament midsubstance, defined as stress and strain, respectively (47, 85). From the stress-strain curve, the elastic modulus, ultimate tensile strength, ultimate strain, and strain energy density of the ligament substance can be determined (84) (fig. 1). To analyze the mechanical properties of the ACL, it is necessary to separate its bundles such that a more uniform orientation of fibers can be obtained. Individual units of the ACL yielded an average modulus and ultimate tensile strength of 278MPa and 35MPa, respectively (11). In a later study, non-uniform properties between bundles within the ACL were also obtained (10). The antero-medial bundle exhibited a larger modulus, ultimate stress, and strain energy density than the posterior bundle. Interestingly, most surgeons have focused on the replacement of the AM component of the ACL, respectively, during reconstruction. Ligaments are also known to process

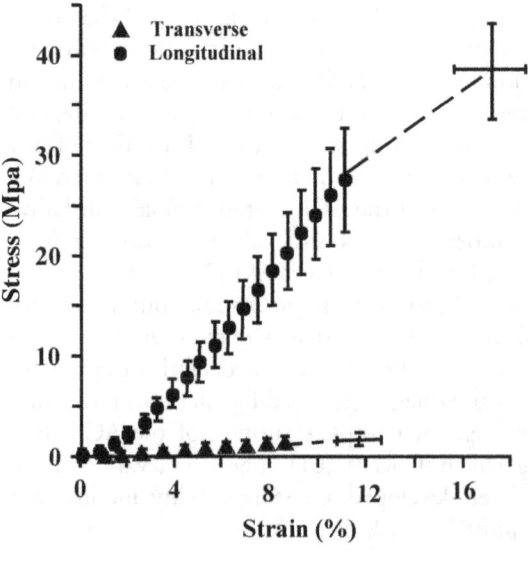

Fig. 1. – Stress-strain curves for a human ligament (i.e. MCL), longitudinal and transverse to the collagen fiber direction.

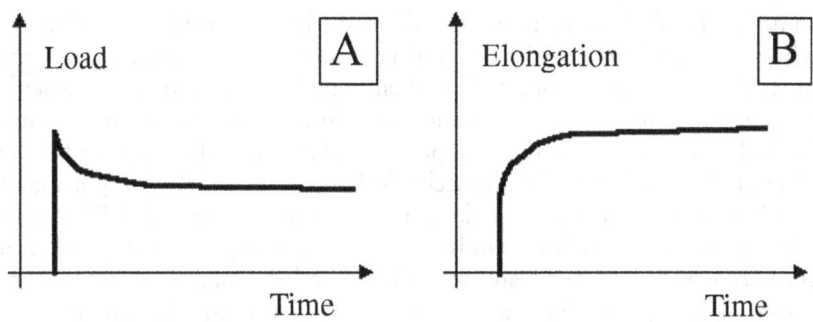

Fig. 2. – Schematic representation of (A) stress relaxation under a constant elongation, and (B) creep under a constant load.

time- and history-dependent viscoelastic properties. As a ligament is elongated, complex interactions of collagen, water, and ground substance exhibit creep or strain relaxation behaviors (fig. 2).

Ligament forces and joint kinematics

Motion of a synovial joint in response to externally applied loads is governed by a combination of joint geometry and tensile properties of ligaments. Each joint can move in six degrees of freedom (DOF): three translations and three rotations. For the knee joint, it is convenient to use three defined axes: the femoral shaft axis, the epicondylar axis, and a floating anterior-posterior axis perpendicular to these two axes to describe its motion. Translation along these three axes will lead to distraction/compression, medial-lateral translation, and anterior-posterior translation, respectively. Rotations about these three axes will lead to internal-external rotation, flexion-extension, and varus-valgus rotation respectively.

Understanding a ligament's function and its contribution to overall joint kinematics can be based on knowledge of the *in situ* forces developed in the ligament in response to external loading. The *in situ* force of the knee is an experimentally measured quantity that represents forces existing in the knee at a given position. Various devices, such as buckle transducers (3, 48), implantable force and pressure transducers and load cells (9, 53), have been used to determine the *in situ* forces and *in situ* strains in ligaments.

In our laboratory, we have successfully used a 6-degree of freedom (DOF) universal force moment sensor (UFS) in combination with a 6-DOF robotic manipulator to measure the *in situ* force of the ligament (24, 50, 72, 87). This method is based on the robot reproducing positions such that the principle of superposition can be employed to calculate changes in forces and moments of a ligament before and after it is transected. Advantages of this robotic/UFS testing system are that it does not depend on the specimen geometry or the location of the ligament to make the necessary measurements, and that the *in situ* forces in the ACL are determined without having a device physically contact the ligament. Forces and distributions in both the AM and the PL bundle of the ACL have been quantified during the anterior drawer test, Lachman test and simulated pivot shift test using human cadaveric knee specimens (73, 83). We learned that a tibial graft fixation nearest the articular surface resulted in a more stable knee and closer *in situ* forces to the intact ACL (38). We also found that the position of the tibia during graft fixation had a significant effect on the biomechanical outcome (33). Two popular grafts for ACL reconstruction, quadruple semitendinosus/gracilis and B-PT-B, were studied (86). Both were found to have little improvement over the ACL deficient knee when rotational loads were applied. Whereas an anatomical reconstruction replacing the AM and PL bundles resulted in knee kinematics significantly closer to those in the intact ACL as compared to conventional reconstruction procedures (88). Additionally, the *in situ* forces in the anatomical reconstruction were substantially closer to those of the intact ACL compared when the knee was subjected to both the Lachman and simulated pivot shift tests. However, we still consider the intact ACL as the "true gold standard" for ACL reconstruction.

Current treatment algorithm

Absolute indications for surgical treatment of an ACL injury do not clearly exist in the literature. The decision to surgically treat an acute or chronic injured knee should be based on several factors. Conservative treatment may be advisable for patients with low demand life styles, poorly motivated patients, patients who do not participate in high-risk sports, or patients with unrealistic expectations. However, patients with high functional demands may benefit from a reconstructive procedure. With excellent research in the field of rehabilitation, certain patients can acquire well functioning knees without surgical intervention (76). Age, once noted to be a relative contraindication for surgical treatment in the "older" patient, is presently less of a consideration with arthroscopic assisted techniques and accelerated rehabilitation programs. No upper age limits for ACL reconstruction have been firmly defined, and this factor does not take into consideration the status of articular cartilage nor the patient's pre-injury activity level (fig. 3).

Role of osteotomy

Historically, high tibial osteotomy (HTO) has gained acceptance and popularity as a treatment option for young patients with osseous malalignment and tibiofemoral compartment osteoarthritis (16, 46, 65). More recently, HTO with or without cruciate ligament reconstruction has been suggested for patients with malalignment, arthritis and instability, with the aim of restoring a more physiological mechanical axis, unload the degenerative compartment and when possible restore stability.

The primary indication for a valgus-producing osteotomy is the presence of medial tibiofemoral arthritis, associated pain, and functional limitations. The goal of osteotomies in these patients is to diminish symptoms, rather

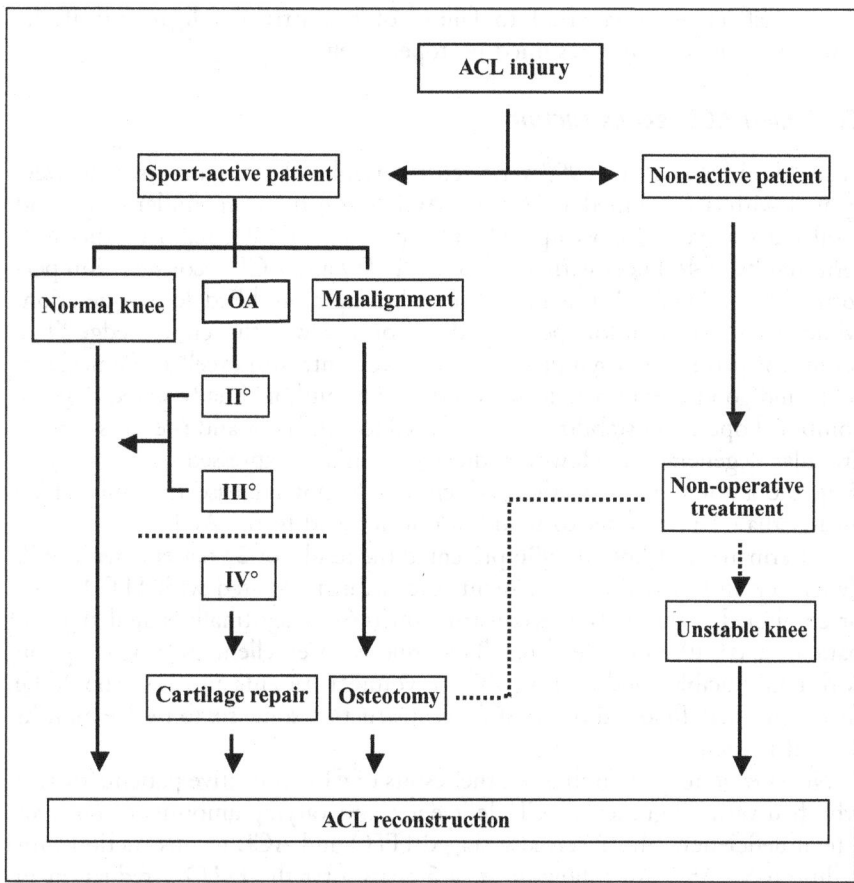

Fig. 3. – Clinical algorithm.

than a return to sports. The secondary indication is the presence of instability, without advanced osteoarthritis. The majority of these patients' knees have a deficiency in the anterior cruciate ligament with varus alignment, and ligament reconstruction is often necessary. However, data are unavailable for determining whether returning these patients to their previous sports activity level is advisable or whether this would accelerate the progression of arthritis. The osteotomy allows a more active lifestyle for short-term, with the realization that in the long-term such activities may not be possible.

Careful selection of these patients is mandatory to achieve the best results. Gait analysis has been postulated to be helpful in demonstrating abnormal knee hyperextension prior to proceeding with any ligament reconstruction and/or osteotomy (66). The thrusting hyperextension motion at the knee, which is associated with an abnormally high adduction moment that increases medial compartment compression forces and lateral distraction forces, places the ACL and any posterolateral reconstruction at risk for stretching out posteriorly. The failure to recognize these abnormal gait patterns, and the failure to retain these patients effectively, may lead to failure of reconstructed ligaments if the abnormal gait pattern is resumed postoperatively.

Combined ACL reconstruction

Neuschwander *et al.* in 1993 reported the results of five patients, who were treated with a combined HTO and ACL reconstruction, underlying good results at two-years follow-up (62). Dejour *et al.* in 1994 reported the mid-term results of 44 knees with a combined HTO and ACL reconstruction performed (16). The ACL was reconstructed using a modified Jones operation, while the most common performed osteotomy was the close wedge. The results showed marked symptomatic improvement, with excellent clinical stability and good overall patient satisfaction. The authors finally stated that the combined operation stabilizes the knee, reduces the pain and prevents further articular degeneration. However, the same authors expressed concern regarding the amount of correction, which should not increase the tibial slope greater than 10° in order to reduce a transfer load to the ACL.

Latterman and Jakob in 1996 presented the results of 27 patients with ACL deficiency and medial compartment osteoarthritis, treated with HTO alone or combined with an ACL reconstruction (46). They finally stated that, in patients aged 40 and older, an HTO alone is an excellent treatment option with reproducibly good results, while in younger patients an HTO should be first performed, followed by an ACL reconstruction some six to twelve months later, if needed.

Noyes *et al.* recently published the results of 41 consecutive patients treated who had varus alignment, ACL-deficiency, and varying amounts of posterolateral deficiency, who received a staged HTO and ACL reconstruction procedure (66). At mean follow-up of 4.5 years after the HTO a reduction in pain was found in 71%, elimination of giving-way, in 85%, and resumption of light recreational activities without problems in 66%. Correction of varus alignment was maintained in 80%. Despite all those studies reported the outcome of the HTO combined with a ligamentous reconstruction, it has to be pointed out that the first can also be performed alone. Holden in 1988 reported the results of HTO performed in a patient population less than 50 years old (34). They showed that 11 out of 14 patients with ACL deficiency at the time of the osteotomy presented excellent/good results at their longest follow-up. 6 of these 14 patients underwent an extrarticular procedure. Noyes' study compared a group of patients with HTO alone to patients with combined HTO and ACL reconstruction, and there was no significant difference in relief of symptoms or return to athletics (65). Noyes introduced the concept of the double and triple varus knee, in which the ACL deficiency is combined with severe medial arthritis and other pathologies of the posterolateral corner structures. How these combined abnormalities can be addressed to affect long-term results of these procedures will hopefully be forthcoming. Relative contraindications for HTO include symptomatic patellofemoral or lateral tibiofemoral arthritis or excessive loss of the medial tibiofemoral joint. Even loss of full extension can be considered a contraindication.

In conclusion, combined osteotomy and ACL reconstruction is a viable option in selected cases. It is important to remind that this should be seen as a salvage procedure, intended to decrease symptoms and allow activity of daily living as well as some recreational sports.

Role of meniscal transplants

With the availability of allograft materials, meniscal transplantation has become a valuable option for patients who had undergone subtotal meniscectomy and who have instability, recurrent pain, a fairly normal cartilage status and a normal alignment. Biomechanical studies by Thompson and Fu in 1991 have shown that the menisci are highly mobile structures with anterior horn segments that are more mobile than posterior horn segments bilaterally (79). Arnoczky *et al.* have shown feasibility of meniscal allografts in dogs with good function and survival after six months (6). The first reports on clinical experience came from Verdonk *et al.*, who reported of viable meniscal allografts in 54 patients after a follow-up of 1 to 8.7 years (82). The surgical technique (56) has improved over the last decade and recent short- and mid-term follow-up studies have confirmed the promising first results.

In a report on 22 patients, Milachovski *et al.* reported on sizing criteria and tissue processing of meniscal allografts (57). Noyes *et al.* reported in 1995 that the transplantation of irradiated menisci lead to a 57% failure rate (64). Fu and Harner evaluated their first patients with fresh-frozen non-irradiated transplants. Clinical outcome revealed functional restoration, meniscus revitalization and no rejections. From their first patients, 30 out of 31 felt improved after undergoing meniscus transplantation. Of these patients 88% were rated normal or nearly normal, according to the IKDC standard after a follow-up of 40 month, respectively. Radiographs revealed no progressive joint space narrowing over time and restoration of joint space in some cases (89) (fig. 4).

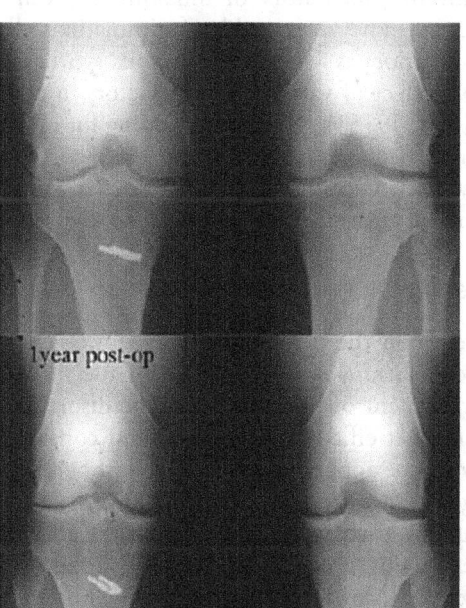

However, accelerated rehabilitation bares potential risk for failure of the transplant and one has to be aware of possible transplant ruptures, popliteal vessel injury and insufficient suturing. Overall, this procedure seems to

Fig. 4. – Bilateral p.a. radiograph. Top picture: joint space narrowing of the lateral compartment of the right knee. Bottom picture: 1year post-meniscal transplant surgery.

be successful when assembling the indications correctly and clinical outcome is very encouraging.

Future of knee ligament surgery

Limitations of ACL reconstruction

With respect to advances during the past two decades, biology, biomechanics, surgical techniques and rehabilitation protocols continue to be the limiting factors of ACL reconstruction in the osteoarthritic knee. Biologic limitations are the biological healing, graft incorporation, and regaining of neurovascular function. Furthermore, in chronic or complex cases the amount and severity of concomitant trauma to articular cartilage and secondary restraints is a determining limitation of excellent outcome. Adjusting the surgical treatment accordingly with combined surgical approaches and a customized rehabilitation protocol is crucial for the outcome and patient satisfaction. Biomechanical studies of the past decades have lead to numerous advancements in ACL reconstruction. However, *in vivo* forces in ligaments remain unknown. Perfecting postoperative rehabilitation protocols to the most effective loading of the ACL graft without exceeding the fixation strength relies on *in vivo* strain data (9) as well as the level of experience of the therapist.

The biological answers might be tissue engineering, gene therapy and cell therapy. Various growth factors have been identified to affect the healing process in tissues of the musculoskeletal system like the ACL and articular cartilage (80). Growth factors are small peptides that can be synthesized both by the resident cells at the injury site (e.g., fibroblasts, endothelial cells, mesenchymal stem cells) and by the infiltrating reparatory or inflammatory cells (e.g., platelets, macrophages, monocytes). They are capable of stimulating cell proliferation, migration and differentiation as well as the matrix synthesis (14, 74). Meanwhile, the stimulating effect of various growth factors in different tissues has been demonstrated (35, 49, 51). The gene encoding for most of the known growth factors has been determined and, using the recombinants DNA technology, we are now able to produce large quantities of these recombinant proteins for the purpose of treatment.

Gene therapy and tissue engineering

Gene therapy is a technique that relies on the delivery of therapeutic genes into cells and tissues. Originally, gene therapy was conceived for the manipulation of germ-line cells for the treatment of inheritable genetic disorders, however this method is limited to not yet efficient technology and considerable ethical concerns. Gene therapy can be applied to the field of orthopaedic surgery by transferring of defined genes encoding for growth factors or antibiotics into a target tissue (e.g., ligament, cartilage or bone). Thus, local cells at the injury site can highly and persistently produce therapeutic substances.

For gene expression, the transferred DNA material has to enter the nucleus, where it either integrates into the chromosomes of the host cells or remains

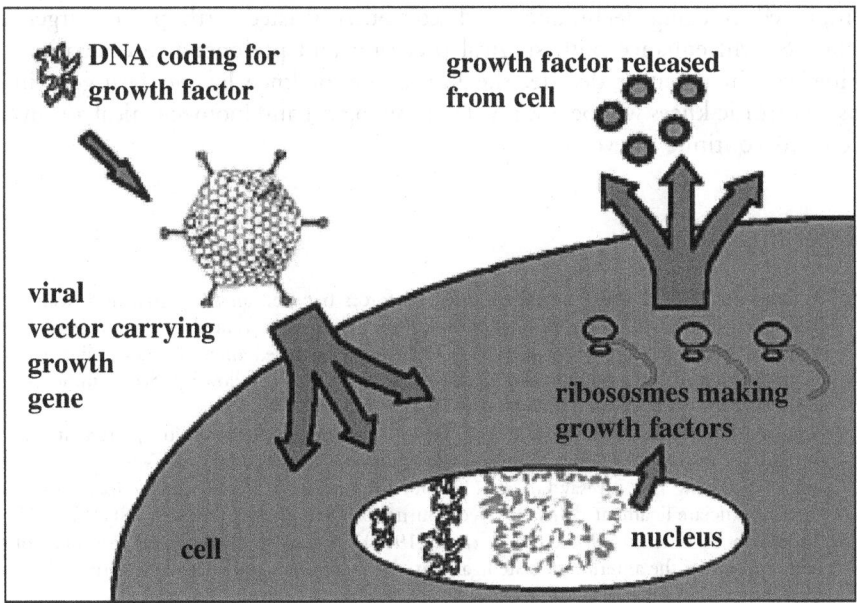

Fig. 5. – Schematic of gene transfer using a viral vector.

episomal. After transcription, the generated mRNA is then transported outside the nucleus, serving as a matrix for the production of proteins (e.g., growth factors) in the ribosomes (fig. 5). Consequently, the transduced cells become a reservoir of secreting growth factors and cytokines capable of improving the healing process. Viral (e.g., adenovirus, retrovirus) and non-viral (e.g., liposomes, gene gun) vectors can be used for delivery of generic material into cells.

Tissue engineering approaches that aim at using cells from different origin tissues (e.g., mesenchymal stem cells, muscle-derived stem cell or dermal fibroblasts) to deliver genes and might offer additional opportunities to improve the healing process (78). Selecting the appropriate gene delivery procedure depends upon various factors such as the division rate of the target cells, pathophysiology of the disorder and the accessibility of the target tissues. In summary, this section provided insight on injury and healing of biological tissues, as well as information on the basic science of treatment options. The next section will discuss biomechanical considerations in knee ligament surgery and will provide data on biomechanical properties.

Perspectives

In the future, improvement of biological incorporation of replacement grafts, gene therapy, cell therapy, and tissue engineering might be the available biological tools. A simple muscle biopsy may then be enough to provide the cell that can restore any kind of defect in the knee (cartilage) by growing the local cell line (chondrocytes). Simultaneously, a knee ligament reconstruction can be performed. Additionally, surgical techniques need to be perfected.

Improved imaging techniques and computer-assisted orthopedic surgery (CAOS) will enhance both surgical precision and pre-operative evaluation. However, in the next decade, the limitations of knee ligament surgery in osteoarthritic knees will be less pivotal as biological and biomechanical advancements continue to evolve.

References

1. Abramowitch SD (2001) The Distribution of forces between an ACL graft and healing MCL after combined injury. In Orthopaedic Research Society. Edited, San Francisco, CA

2. Aglietti P, Buzzi R, Giron F et al. (1997) Arthroscopic-assisted anterior cruciate ligament reconstruction with the central third patellar tendon. A 5-8-year follow-up (See Comments). Knee Surgery, Sports Traumatology, Arthroscopy 5(3): 138-44

3. Ahmed AM, Hyder A, Burke DL et al. (1987) In vitro ligament tension pattern in the flexed knee in passive loading. Journal of Orthopaedic Research 5(2): 217-30

4. Allen CR, Wong EK, Livesay GA et al. (2000) Importance of the medial meniscus in the anterior cruciate ligament-deficient knee. Journal of Orthopaedic Research 18(1): 109-15

5. Andersson C, Odensten M, Good L et al. (1989) Surgical or non-surgical treatment of acute rupture of the anterior cruciate ligament. A randomized study with long-term follow-up. J Bone Joint Surg Am 71(7): 965-74

6. Arnoczky SP, Warren RF, McDevitt CA (1990) Meniscal replacement using a cryopreserved allograft. An experimental study in the dog. Clinical Orthopaedics & Related Research 252: 121-8

7. Bandara G, Lin CW, Georgescu HI et al. (1992) The synovial activation of chondrocytes: Evidence for complex cytokine interactions involving a possible novel factor. Biochim Biophys Acta 1134(3): 309-18

8. Bartlett RJ, Crowe R (1984) Results in intra-articular anterior cruciate ligament reconstruction using patellar ligament. In Journal of Bone & Joint Surgery – British Volume, p. 788

9. Beynnon BD, Johnson RJ, Fleming BC et al. (1997) The strain behavior of the anterior cruciate ligament during squatting and active flexion-extension. A comparison of an open and a closed kinetic chain exercise. American Journal of Sports Medicine 25(6): 823-9

10. Butler DL, Guan Y, Kay MD et al. (1992) Location-dependent variations in the material properties of the anterior cruciate ligament. Journal of Biomechanics 25(5): 511-8

11. Butler DL, Kay MD, Stouffer DC (1986) Comparison of material properties in fascicle-bone units from human patellar tendon and knee ligaments. Journal of Biomechanics 19(6): 425-32

12. Cameron M, Buchgraber A, Passler HH et al. (1997) The natural history of the anterior cruciate ligament-deficient knee. American Journal of Sports Medicine 25(6): 751-4

13. Clancy WG Jr, Nelson DA, Reider B et al. (1982) Anterior cruciate ligament reconstruction using one-third of the patellar ligament, augmented by extra-articular tendon transfers. Journal of Bone & Joint Surgery – American Volume 64(3): 352-9

14. Collier S, Ghosh P (1995) Effects of transforming growth bactor beta on proteoglycan synthesis by cell and explant cultures derived from the knee joint meniscus. Osteoarthritis Cartilage 3(2): 127-38

15. Daniel DM, Stone ML, Dobson BE et al. (1994) Fate of the ACL-injured patient. A prospective outcome study. American Journal of Sports Medicine 22(5): 632-44

16. DeJour H, Neyret P, Boileau P and al. (1994) Anterior cruciate reconstruction combined with valgus tibial osteotomy. Clinical Orthopaedics & Related Research 220-8

17. DeJour H, Neyret P Bonnin M (1994) Instability and osteoarthritis. In Knee Surgery, p. 859-75. Edited by Fu F, Harner CD, Vince KG, Williams and Wilkins

18. DeJour H, Walch G, Deschamps G et al. (1987) Arthrosis of the knee in chronic anterior cruciate laxity. Fr J Orthop Surg 1: 85-7

19. Dye SF (1996) The Knee as a biologic transmission with an envelope of function: A theory. Clinical Orthopaedics & Related Research (325): 10-8

20. Eriksson E (1997) How good are the results of ACL reconstruction? (Editorial; Comment). Knee Surgery, Sports Traumatology, Arthroscopy 5(3): 137

21. Fink C, Hoser C, Benedetto KP (1994) Development of arthrosis after rupture of the anterior cruciate ligament. A comparison of surgical and conservative therapy. Unfallchirurg 97(7): 357-61

22. Fu FH, Bennett CH, Ma CB et al. (2000) Current trends in anterior cruciate ligament reconstruction. Part I. Operative procedures and clinical correlations. American Journal of Sports Medicine 28(1): 124-30

23. Fu FH, Harner C, Johnson D et al. (1993) Biomechanics of knee ligaments. J Bone Joint Surg 75A: 716-27

24. Fujie H, Mabuchi K, Woo SL-Y et al. (1993) The use of robotics technology to study human joint kinematics: A new methodology. Journal of Biomechanical Engineering 115(3): 211-7

25. Gillquist J, Messner K (1999) Anterior cruciate ligament reconstruction and the long-term incidence of gonarthrosis. Sports Med 27(3): 143-56

26. Graf BK, Cook DA, De Smet AA et al. (1993) "Bone bruises" on Magnetic Resonance Imaging evaluation of anterior cruciate ligament injuries. American Journal of Sports Medicine 21(2): 220-3

27. Grood GS, Noyes FR, Butler DL et al. (1981) Ligamentous and capsular restraints preventing straight medial and lateral laxity in intact human cadaver knees. J Bone and Joint Surg (Am) 63-A: 1257-69

28. Harner CD, Livesay GA, Kashiwaguchi S et al. (1995) Comparative study of the size and shape of human anterior and posterior cruciate ligaments. Journal of Orthopaedic Research 13(3): 429-34

29. Hawkins RJ, Misamore GW, Merritt TR (1986) Follow-up of the acute non-operated isolated anterior cruciate ligament tear. American Journal of Sports Medicine 14(3): 205-10

30. Hertel P (1997) Technik Der Offenen Ersatzplastik Des Vorderen Kreuzbandes Mit Autologer Patellasehne. Arthroskopie 10: 240-5

31. Hertel P (1980) Verletzung Und Spannung Von Kniebandern. Experimentelle Studie. Hefte zur Unfallheilkunde 142: 1-94

32. Hertel P, Widjaja G, Cierpinski T et al. (2000) 10 year results of a bone-patella tendon-bone press-fit fixation in ACL deficient knees. World Congress on Orthopedic Sports Trauma, April 10-13, 2000, Queensland, Australia

33. Höher J, Kanamori A, Zeminski J et al. (2000) The position of the tibia during graft fixation effects knee kinematics and graft forces for ACL reconstruction. American Journal of Sports Medicine

34. Holden D, James SL, Larson RL et al. (1988) Proximal tibial osteotomy in patients who are fifty years old or less: A long-term follow-up study. Journal of Bone & Joint Surgery – American Volume 70: 977-82

35. Hunziker EB, Rosenberg LC (1996) Repair of partial-thickness defects in articular cartilage: Cell recruitment from the synovial membrane. J Bone Joint Surg Am 78(5): 721-33

36. Indelicato P, Bittar E 1985) A perspective of lesions associated with ACL insufficient of the knee: A review of 100 cases. Clinical Orthopaedics & Related Research 198: 77-80

37. Inoue M, McGurk-Burleson E, Hollis JM et al. (1987) Treatment of the medial collateral ligament injury. I: The importance of anterior cruciate ligament on the varus-valgus knee laxity. American Journal of Sports Medicine 15: 15-21

38. Ishibashi Y, Rudy TW, Livesay GA et al. (1997) The effect of anterior cruciate ligament graft fixation site at the tibia on knee stability: Evaluation using a robotic testing system. Arthroscopy 13(2): 177-82

39. Jacobsen K (1977) Osteoarthrosis following insufficiency of the cruciate ligaments in man. A clinical study. Acta Orthop Scand 48(5): 520-6

40. Jarvela T, Paakkala T, Kannus P et al. (2001) The incidence of patellofemoral osteoarthritis and associated findings 7 years after anterior cruciate ligament reconstruction with a bone-patellar tendon-bone autograft. American Journal of Sports Medicine 29(1): 18-24

41. Johansson H, Sjolander P, Sojka P (1991) A sensory role for the cruciate ligaments. Clinical Orthopaedics & Related Research (268): 161-78
42. Johnson RJ, Kettelkamp DB, Clark W et al. (1974) Factors effecting late results after meniscectomy. J Bone Joint Surg Am 56(4): 719-29
43. Jomha NM, Borton DC, Clingeleffer AJ et al. (1999) Long-term osteoarthritic changes in anterior cruciate ligament reconstructed knees. Clinical Orthopaedics & Related Research (358): 188-93
44. Jomha NM, Pinczewski LA, Clingeleffer A et al. (1999) Arthroscopic reconstruction of the anterior cruciate ligament with patellar-tendon autograft and interference screw fixation. The results at seven years. J Bone Joint Surg Br 81(5): 775-9
45. Kanamori A, Sakane M, Zeminski J et al. (2000) The in situ forces in the medial and lateral structures of the intact and ACL deficient knee. Journal of Orthopaedic Science 5(6): 567-71
46. Lattermann C, Jakob RP (1996) High tibial osteotomy alone or combined with ligament reconstruction in anterior cruciate ligament-deficient knees. Knee Surgery, Sports Traumatology, Arthroscopy 4: 32-8
47. Lee TQ, Woo SL-Y (1988) A new method for determining cross-sectional shape and area of soft tissues. Journal of Biomechanical Engineering 110: 110-4
48. Lewis JL, Lew WD, Hill JA et al. (1989) Knee joint motion and ligament forces before and after ACL reconstruction. Journal of Biomechanical Engineering 111(2): 97-106
49. Linkhart TA, Mohan S, Baylink DJ (1996) Growth factors for bone growth and repair: Igf, Tgf Beta and Bmp. Bone 19(1 Suppl): 1S-12S
50. Livesay GA, Fujie H, Kashiwaguchi S et al. (1995) Determination of the in situ forces and force distribution within the human anterior cruciate ligament. Annals of Biomedical Engineering 23(4): 467-74
51. Luyten FP (1995) Cartilage-derived morphogenetic proteins. Key regulators in chondrocyte differentiation? Acta Orthop Scand Suppl 266: 51-4
52. Ma CB, Papageorgiou CD, Debski RE et al. (2000) Interaction between the ACL graft and MCL in a combined ACL + MCL knee injury using a goat model. Acta Orthopaedica Scandinavica 71(4): 387-93
53. Markolf KL, Gorek JF, Kabo JM et al. (1990) Direct measurement of resultant forces in the anterior cruciate ligament. An in vitro study performed with a new experimental technique. Journal of Bone & Joint Surgery – American Volume 72(4): 557-67
54. Markolf KL, Kochan A, Amstutz HC (1984) Measurement of knee stiffness and laxity in patients with documented absence of the anterior cruciate ligament. J Bone and Joint Surg [Am] 66-A(2): 242-53
55. McDaniel WJ, Dameron TB (1980) Untreated ruptures of the anterior cruciate ligament: A follow-up study. Journal of Bone & Joint Surgery – American Volume 62: 696-705
56. Menetrey J, Jones DG, Ernlund L et al. Posterior peripheral sutures in meniscal allograft replacement. Arthroscopy 15(6): 663-8
57. Milachowski KA, Weismeier K, Wirh CJ et al. Meniscus transplantation: Experimental study and first clinical report. American Journal of Sports Medicine 15: 626
58. Miyasaka KC, Daniel DM, Stone ML et al. (1991) The incidence of knee ligament injuries in the general population. American Journal of Knee Surgery 4: 3-8
59. Morales TI (1997) The role and content of endogenous insulin-like growth factor-binding proteins in bovine articular cartilage. Arch Biochem Biophys 343(2): 164-72
60. Musahl V, Cierpinski T, Hornung H et al. (1999) Sekundäe vordere Kreuzbandplastik nach Primäer Naht und Kreuzbandplastik. 63. Jahrestagung der DGU, November 1999, Berlin, Germany
61. Neurath MF (1993) Detection of luse bodies, spiralled collagen, dysplastic collagen, and intracellular collagen in rheumatoid connective tissues: An electron microscopic study. Annals of the Rheumatic Diseases 52: 278-84
62. Neuschwander DC, Drez D Jr, Paine RM (1993) Simultaneous high tibial osteotomy and ACL reconstruction for combined genu varum and symptomatic ACL tear. Orthopedics (Thorofare, NJ) 16(6): 679-84

63. Neyret P, Donell ST, DeJour D *et al.* (1993) Partial meniscectomy and anterior cruciate ligament rupture in soccer players. A study with a minimum 20-year followup. American Journal of Sports Medicine 21(3): 455-60
64. Noyes FR (1995) A histological study of failed human meniscal allografts. In Arthroscopy Association of North America Specialty Day. Edited, Orlando, FL
65. Noyes FR, Barber SD, Simon R (1993) High tibial osteotomy and ligament reconstruction in varus angulated, anterior cruciate ligament-deficient knees: A two- to seven-year follow-up study. American Journal of Sports Medicine 21: 2-12
66. Noyes FR, Barber-Westin SD, Hewett TE (2000) High tibial osteotomy and ligament reconstruction for varus angulated anterior cruciate ligament-deficient knees. American Journal of Sports Medicine 28(3): 282-96
67. Poole AR, Rosenberg LC, Reiner A *et al.* (1996) Contents and distributions of the proteoglycans decorin and biglycan in normal and osteoarthritic human articular cartilage. Journal of Orthopaedic Research 14(5): 681-9
68. Radin EL, Ehrlich MG, Chernack R *et al.* (1978) Effect of repetitive impulsive loading on the knee joints of rabbits. Clinical Orthopaedics & Related Research (131): 288-93
69. Ritchie JR, Parker RD (1996) Graft selection in anterior cruciate ligament revision surgery. Clinical Orthopaedics & Related Research (325): 65-77.
70. Rosen MA, Jackson DW (1991) Occult osseous lesions documented by Magnetic Resonance Imaging associated with anterior cruciate ligament ruptures. Arthroscopy 7(1): 45-51
71. Rosenberg TD, Deffner KT (1997) ACL reconstruction: Semitendinosus tendon is the graft of choice. Orthopedics (Thorofare, NJ) 20(5): 396
72. Rudy TW, Livesay GA, Woo SL-Y *et al.* (1996) A combined robotic/universal force sensor approach to determine *in situ* forces of knee ligaments. Journal of Biomechanics 29(10): 1357-60
73. Sakane M, Fox RJ, Woo SL *et al.* (1997) *In situ* forces in the anterior cruciate ligament and its bundles in response to anterior tibial loads. Journal of Orthopaedic Research,15(2): 285-93
74. Schmidt CC, Georgescu HI, Kwoh CK *et al.* (1995) Effect of growth factors on the proliferation of fibroblasts from the medial collateral and anterior cruciate ligaments. Journal of Orthopaedic Research 13(2): 184-90
75. Shelbourne KD, Trumper RV (1997) Preventing anterior knee pain after anterior cruciate ligament reconstruction. American Journal of Sports Medicine 25(1): 41-7
76. Snyder-Mackler L, Fitzgerald GK, Bartolozzi AR *et al.* (1997) The relationship between passive joint laxity and functional outcome after anterior cruciate ligament onjury. American Journal of Sports Medicine 25: 191-5
77. Sommerlath K, Lysholm J, Gillquist J (1991) The long-term course after treatment of acute anterior cruciate ligament ruptures. A 9 to 16 year follow-up. American Journal of Sports Medicine 19(2): 156-62
78. Stone KR, Steadman JR, Rodkey WG *et al.* (1997) Regeneration of meniscal cartilage with use of a collagen scaffold. Analysis of preliminary data. J Bone Joint Surg Am 79(12): 1770-7
79. Thompson WO, Thaete FL, Fu FH *et al.* (1993) The meniscus in the cruciate-deficient knee. Clinical Sports Medicine 12: 771-96
80. Trippel S (1997) Growth factors as therapeutic agents. Instructional Course Lectures 46: 473-6
81. van Heerwaarden RJ, Stellinga D, Frudiger AJ (1996) Effect of pretension in reconstructions of the anterior cruciate ligament with a Dacron prosthesis. A retrospective study. Knee Surgery, Sports Traumatology, Arthroscopy 3(4): 202-8
82. Verdonk R (1997) Alternative treatments for meniscal injuries. Journal of Bone & Joint Surgery – British Volume 79: 866-73
83. Wong EK, Debski RE, Yagi M *et al.* (2001) The force distribution in the bundles of the ACL during simulated joint moints: A computational approach. Journal of Biomechanical Engineering

84. Woo SL-Y, Chan SC, Yamaji T (1997) Biomechanics of knee ligament healing, repair and reconstruction. J. Biomechanics 30(5): 431-9
85. Woo SL-Y, Horibe S, Ohland KJ *et al.* (1990) The response of ligaments to injury: Healing of the collateral ligaments. In Knee Ligaments: Structure, Function, Injury, and Repair, p. 351-64. Edited by Daniel D, Raven Press, Ltd.
86. Woo SL-Y, Kanamori A, Zeminski J *et al.* (2001) The effectiveness of anterior cruciate ligament reconstruction by hamstrings and patellar tendon: A cadaveric study comparing anterior tibial load vs. rotational loads. Journal of Bone & Joint Surgery – American Volume
87. Xerogeanes JW, Takeda Y, Livesay GA *et al.* (1995) Effect of knee flexion on the *in situ* force distribution in the human anterior cruciate ligament. Knee Surgery, Sports Traumatology, Arthroscopy 3(1): 9-13
88. Yagi M, Wong EK, Fu FH *et al.* (2001) The potential advances of an anatomical ACL reconstruction. In International Society of Arthroscopy, Knee Surgery and Orthopaedic Sports Medicine, p. 4-34. Montreux, Switzerland
89. Yoldas EA, Dowdy PA, Irrgang JJ *et al.* (1998) Meniscal transplantation: University of Pittsburgh experience. In American Academy of Orthopaedic Surgeon.

TOTAL KNEE ARTHROPLASTY

Basis

Oasis

History, evolution of concepts, various current prostheses

P. Deroche

History

The total knee prosthesis did not know a linear historic evolution and numerous chronological over-lappings exist (4, 63, 75).

In the degenerative lesions of the knee, the only surgical solution was the arthodesis. Indeed, the arthroplasties by resection realized during the 19th century left persistent pain, instability and often ended with ankylosis.

The precursors

The first attempt of a knee prosthesis was that of Glück in 1890 which remained for a long time isolated. It was an ivory intra-condylar prosthesis in which the diaphysary stems were fixed by a mixture of plaster of Paris, pumice and rosin. The three surgeries he performed using this procedure ended in septic failure. Other than this attempt, one can consider that up until 1940, the knee arthroplasty was performed only with the help of autologue tissue interposition: fascia-lata or adipose tissue. So thus we see Barton's attempt of it in 1826, Ferguson (33) in 1851, Murphy in 1913, Putti in 1920, Albee in 1928 and we may also add the nylon interposition realized by Kuhan and Potter in 1950.

The partial implants

Thanks to the progress of the surgical aspesis and the bio-materials, Campbell and Boyd present to the "American Academy of Orthopaedic Surgery" in 1938 the first cases of the use of vitallium plates molded on the femoral condyles (14). The fixation is assured by hooks at the back of the condyles and by one screw at the top of the trochlea. But the anatomical restoration of the condyles is very approximate (fig. 1). Two years later, Smith Petersen will also realize a vitallium mold, mobile in an anterior-posterior direction, with regards to the femur as well as the tibia.

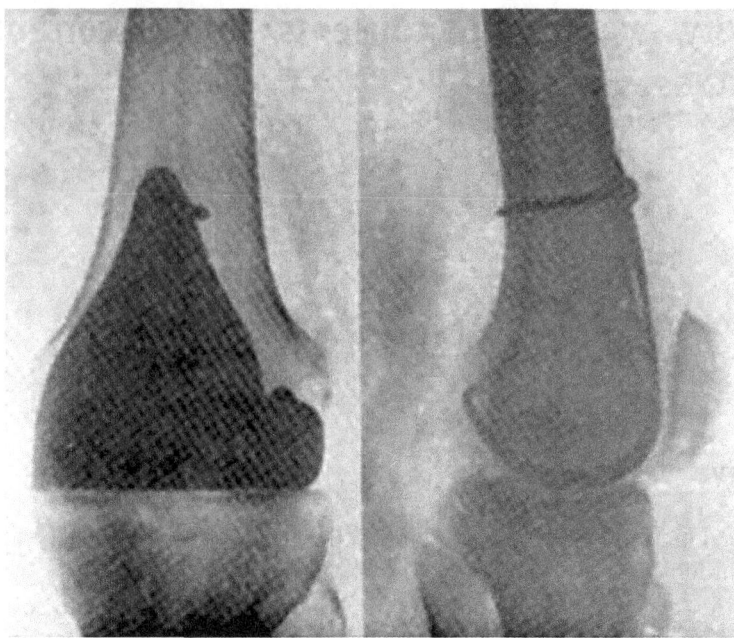

Fig. 1. – Femoral arthroplasty (Campbell, 1938).

In 1947, Delitalia realizes a femoral endoprosthesis of resection, as well as Cabitza in 1950. These two attempts will end in failure, one septic, the other mechanical.

Between 1950 and 1952, Smith Petersen improves the design of this prosthesis and adds to it an intra-medullary stem of fixation. This prosthesis will become the MGH (Massachusetts General Hospital).

In 1952, Rocher realizes a condylar arthroplasty using two Judet's acrylic femoral heads. Tran Ngoc Ninh in 1953 then Kraft and Levinthal in 1954 will use acrylic prostheses fixed to an intra-medullary metal stem.

Concomitantly to these partial femoral implants, other authors will develop tibial prosthetic implants. Burman in 1944 will use vitallium tibial trays screwed to the epiphysis.

In 1950, Mac Keever will also use a tray in vitallium but fixed with two perpendicular fins. Elliot will present in 1960 the results of 40 surgical patients with a good functioning of the knee in 39 cases.

In 1954, Mac Intosh proposes separate tibial trays in vitallium in which the innovation is to propose three different sizes with, for each size, four thicknesses. This implant is, in a sense, the close precursor of current unicompartmental prostheses.

In 1964, on the contrary, Townley will propose a single tibial tray covering the whole epiphysis but respecting the insertion of the cruciates. The fixation is realized by two screws. The first partial patellar implant is that of Mac Keever who proposes in 1955 an implant adaptable to the posterior surface of the patella and fixed by a screw (fig. 2).

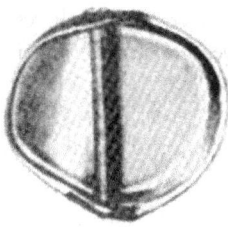 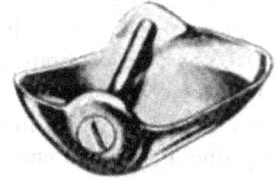

Fig. 2. – Patellar prosthesis (MacKeever, 1955).

The total prosthesis

The necessity to replace both femoro-tibial surfaces gradually became obvious. However the evolution of the various types of implants corresponds to the technological progress but also to the necessity of adapting to the various anatomical situations of knee pathology.

The hinge prostheses

In 1947, Robert and Jean Judet's prosthesis marks the beginning of the evolution of hinge prostheses (fig. 3). The principle of these prostheses is to reduce the mobility of the knee to a single movement: flexion-extension. This attempt will be fol-

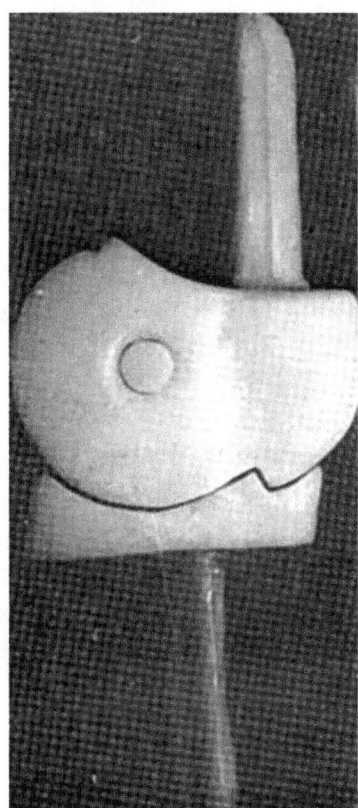

Fig. 3. – Judet prosthesis (1947).

lowed in 1951 by that of Majnoni d'Intignano who will place seven prostheses presenting cone-shaped sleeves preventing rotation. The same year, Diamant-Berger describes an acrylic cylinder fixed by tendons from kangaroos (fig. 4).

In 1953, Robert Merle d'Aubigne created a stainless steel prosthesis called *"Hirondelle"* (swallow) because it was anchored in the femoral and tibial diaphyses by means of two very fine and long stems (fig. 5).

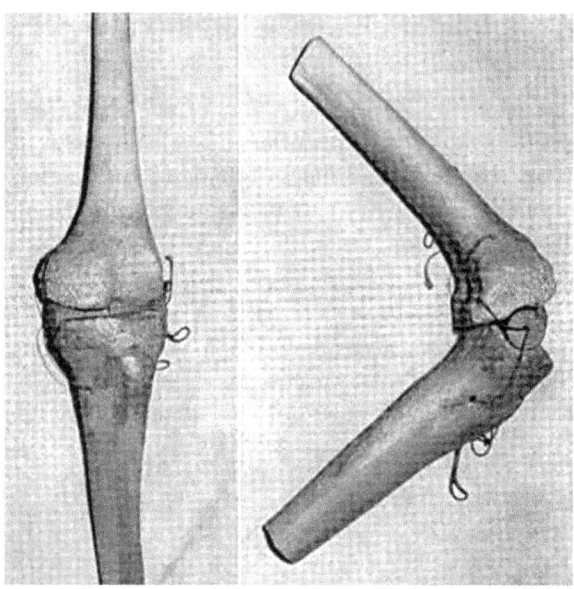

Fig. 4. – Knee prosthesis of Diamant-Berger (1951).

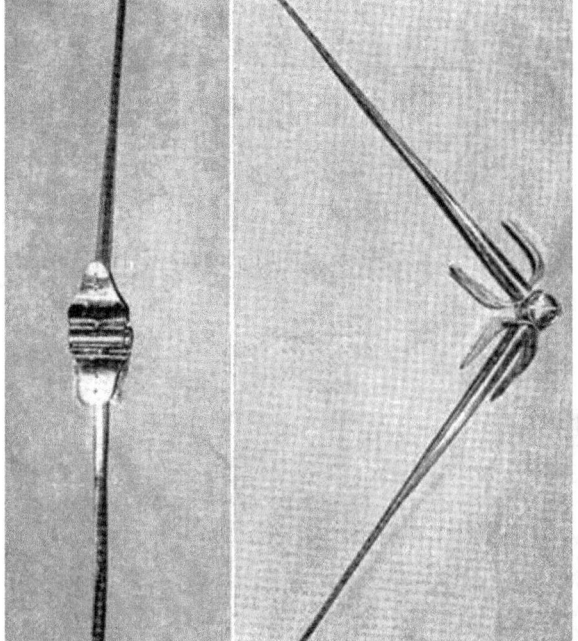

Fig. 5. – Prosthesis "Hirondelle" designed by Merle-d'Aubigné (1953).

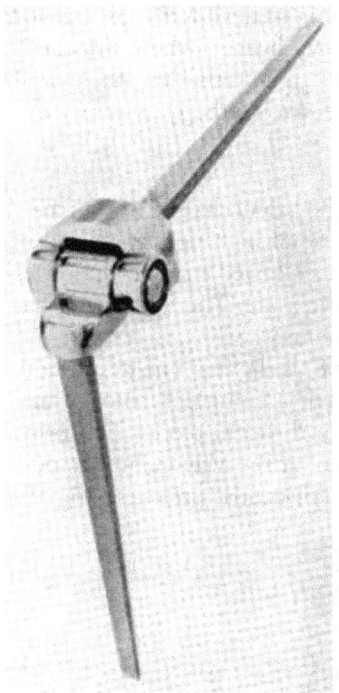

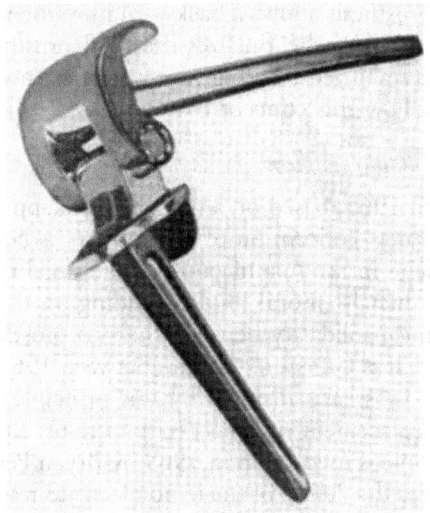

Fig. 7. – Guepar prosthesis (1970). On the picture: Guepar II (1977).

Fig. 6. – Shiers prosthesis (1954).

Walldius' prosthesis (76) in 1954 will be one of the first modern hinge prostheses as well as that of Shiers (67) which, made of stainless steel and presented the same year, will undergo numerous modifications (fig. 6). The originality of Mac Ausland's prosthesis resides in its system of fixation which consists of a perforated metal sheath which imprisons the diaphyses.

In 1963, Young introduces the femoral valgus and the blocking of the rotation is assured by points fixed to the tray. The year 1965 will see two important modifications: That brought by Jackson Burrow which consists of introducing pillow-blocks made of polyethylene in the hinge, and that of Kee whom, thanks to his experience of the total hip prosthesis, created a cemented prosthesis for the knee made of stellite.

The originality of the Guepar group will be, in 1970, to displace the axis of rotation of the prosthesis to the top and back and to provide the prosthesis with a silastic block having for role to limit the extension (5), (fig. 7). That same year, Lagrange and Letournel (54) as well as Bucholtz (12) finalize their model.

Although the hinge prostheses continue to evolve (1977: Guepar II with a reinforced stem presenting the possibility of implanting a patellar button), numerous authors reproach this prosthesis the importance of the constraints put on the stems thus causing numerous loosenings or fractures of the materials.

Semi-hinge and rotating prosthesis

It is Trillat and Bousquet (74) in 1971 who propose the first hinge prosthesis allowing an axial rotation. They are followed one year later by Devas whose prosthesis allows a backward movement of the tibia in flexion, by Gschwendt (39, 40) who finalizes the GSB prosthesis and by Sheehan whose prosthesis is stabilized by a big central ball connected to the tibia. Other prostheses will follow this concept (Attenborough [3], spherocentric Herbert).

Gliding prosthesis

In 1965, based on a more faithful approach of the biomechanics of the knee, a new conception of arthroplasty is born: The use of high density polyethylene in the manufacture of the tibial components allowed the conception of a metal femoral implant gliding on the prosthetic plate. There is no mechanical solidarity between the two prosthetic elements.

It is Gunston (4) who, between 1965 and 1968, is the first one to promote a prosthesis inspired by this principle (fig. 8). For a complete femoro-tibial replacement, it is necessary to resort to using four different pieces. This principle is used again in 1969 by Bryan Petersen who, at the Mayo Clinic, modifies the design of the femoral tray to result in the Polycentric prosthesis (fig. 9).

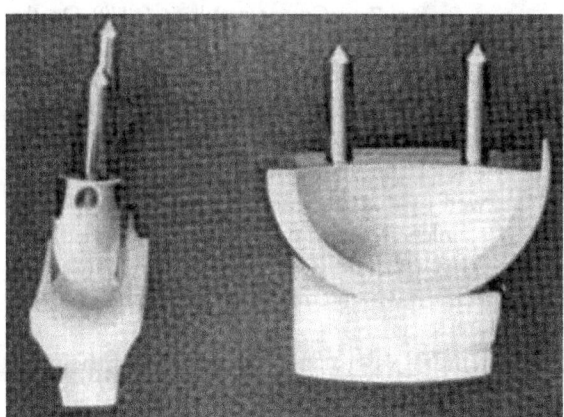

Fig. 8. – Gunston prosthesis (1965).

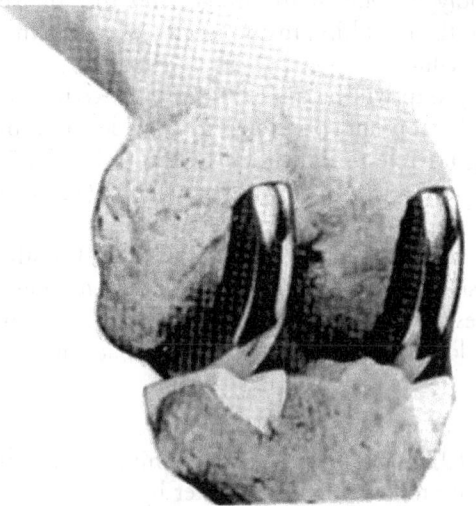

Fig. 9. – Polycentric prosthesis (1969).

This prosthesis, conceived as a double unicompartmental arthroplasty preserved the central pivot. It is the same for the Saint Georg sled prosthesis proposed by Engelbrecht in 1970, then again in 1973 of the Marmor prosthesis or Lotus prosthesis.

In 1971, Coventry, also being inspired by the Polycentric, realizes the Géomedie which will become the Anamétric in 1977 (34). This direction opened by Gunston of the non-constrained prosthesis, preserving all or some of the central pivot, will be widely used hereafter: Townley in 1972, Walker (75) with the kinematic prosthesis (1975), Cloutier (19) in 1977 and since numerous other models have appeared : PCA, Miller-Galante, Hermès, Goeland...

At the same time as these non-constrained prostheses, will develop another conception of the gliding TKR: The semi-constrained prosthesis in which the femoral and tibial components have no fixed mechanical link, but which, by their design and their kinetic conception insure a certain stability to the knee associated in a more or less important stabilizing participation of the capsulo-ligamentary and muscular formations. These prostheses function without a central pivot. This path was opened in 1970 by Freeman and Swanson, this prosthesis will evolve towards the Freeman Iclh in 1977 then towards the Freeman and Samuelson (36) in 1980 (fig. 10 and 11).

1971 marks the beginning of the series of Insall arthroplasties with the uni- and bi-condylar and the duo-condylar. From 1972, Insall and P. Walker propose the Total Condylar, then from 1975, the posterior-stabilized Total Condylar II (47, 48), then finally the Insall Burnstein prosthesis whereas Walker will propose the series of kinematic protheses.

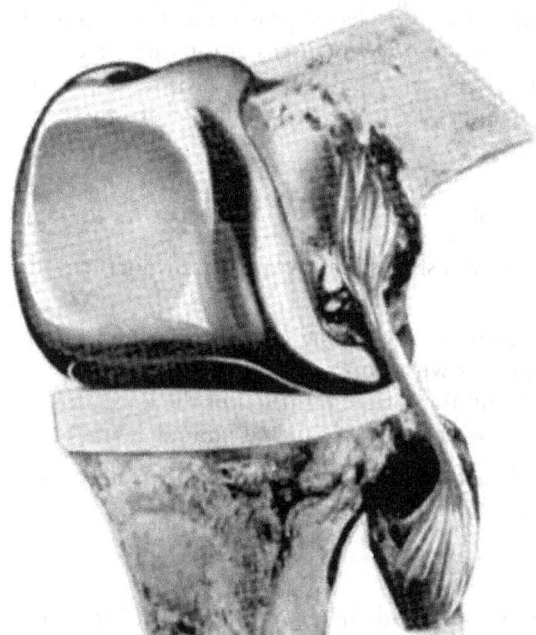

Fig. 10. – Freeman-Swanson prosthesis (1970).

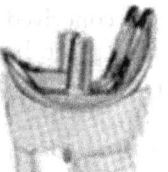

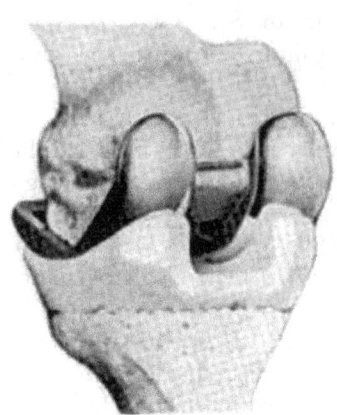

Fig. 11. – Geomedic prosthesis (1971).

In this lineage of posterior-stabilized prostheses, the HLS will be proposed from 1984 on. Its originality resides in the existence of a third condylar median which, as well as its role of posterior stabilizer, assures the neo-joint, devoid of cruciates, a femoral "roll back" during flexion, beginning at 60° of flexion in his first model and at 45° later on.

The mobile bearing total knee prostheses were introduced in order to increase the congruency of the articular surfaces without excessively soliciting the bone-implant interface. From 1977 on, Goodfellow and O'Connor (38) presented their unicompartmental prostheses "Oxford Knee", then Buechel and Pappas finalized the system of the New Jersey prostheses: Low Contant Stress (LCS), available in two versions, mobile meniscus or rotating plate. Ten years later, Polysoides and Tsakons present the Rotaglide prosthesis. At the present time, numerous manufacturers complete their range of prosthesis by a model presenting a mobile bearing surface.

The progress around the implant

The study of the evolution of the TKA shows that in fact two distinct periods exist during this evolution:

– an embryonic period of experimentation during which a few authors tried their ideas on one or several patients with unpredictable results;

– a period which marks the beginning of the diffusion of the knee arthroplasty replacement technique and which can be situated around 1965.

The knee prosthesis indeed benefited from several other advances made during these periods.

Asepsis

All surgery benefited from the progress made in the prevention of infection. Indeed, infection is facilitated by the superficial situation of the knee, by the subcutaneous complications of certain surgical approaches, as well as by the voluminous aspect of certain implants. The progress in the operating asepsis and the development of antibiotics minimized this risk.

Materials

The first prostheses, made of vitallium, acrylic, or even stainless steel are no longer used because of their fragility. Indeed after numerous fatigue fractures, particularly concerning the intra-medullary stem in the hinge prostheses, the alloys evolved towards satellite, cobalt-chrome and even more recently towards titanium and ceramic.

At the present time almost the totality of tibial trays are made of poly-ethylene because the tri-biological coefficient of the metal-polyethylene pair, also widely used in the hip, is completely favourable and the long-term studies show that wear is relatively moderate in the absence, obviously, of interposed fragments of cement.

Type of fixation of the prosthesis to the bone

Traditionally, as in the hip, the cemented prosthesis are opposed to the non-cemented prosthesis. Up until the early sixties, at which time Charnley perfected the methyl-metacrylate, all the prostheses were naturally fixed without cement. The results obtained with this mode of fixation were one of the important factors in the fast development of the TKR from this time on.

However, more and more models are conceived for a non-cemented fixation: This is particularly the case of the Freeman-Swanson prosthesis in which the tibial tray, made of polyethylene without a metal support, was directly fixed to the bone by two polyethylene pegs integral with the component, and likewise for the femoral component.

After this, the PCA prosthesis uses a porous micro-bead covering and the Miller-Galante a fibermesh for a fixation exclusively without cement.

In spite of the good results obtained with these implants, the reliability of the cement fixation in studies of long-term survival brought the manufacturers to propose almost systematically at least one cemented version on all their models.

Through clinical follow-up it became obvious that, when important stress is put on the prosthesis-bone interface, the mode of fixation does not play a determining role and that it is especially the pegs of the intra-medullary stem who effectively improve the anchoring of the prosthesis to the bone.

Biomechanics of the knee

The progress realized during these past decades concerning the knowledge of the biomechanics of the normal knee allowed to develop prostheses with a more physiological functioning.

Hinge prostheses began appearing with valgus in the femoral stem, the displacement up and back of the center of rotation, the addition of poly-ethylene at the hinge level to limit the metal-metal friction, the existence of a trochlear shield, even the possibility of cementing a patellar button and finally the increase of the anchoring surface by the longer, more massive, intra-medullary stems. From these hinge prostheses also developed prostheses with pivot allowing a certain degree of rotation.

Concerning the gliding prostheses, the evolution was made in the direction of a more physiological movement of the knee, namely respecting the femoral "roll back" in regards to the tibia, respecting the physiology of the extension system by preserving the lever function of the quadriceps, a good femoral trochlea and finally the respect of automatic rotation during the passage of flexion to extension. But the recent diffusion of the technique of TKA made necessary two other conditions for the success of the operation: the reliability of an impeccable positioning, thanks to a simplified and ever progressing instrumentation, and the adaptability of each model to the varied anatomical situations encountered in the different degenerative pathologies of the knee. The evolution of current models is towards a larger variety of sizes and thicknesses of each implant.

Instrumentation

Being the essential element in the reliability and the reproducibility of precise positioning of the total knee prosthesis, these systems are the reflection of the philosophy of the designers and the options which they wish to privilege.

They facilitate the accuracy of the bone cuts and help in the ligamentary balancing. Their precision is based on an optic either intra-or extra-medullary, usually by means of metal rods, but the current evolution of the computer navigator systems seems to increase the precision while lowering the time factor needed for its application. They can be completed or not by a robot system which realizes the cuts in place of the operator.

At the present time, these systems are operational in experimental centers which evaluate the improvement which they bring as compared to the conventional systems. The major inconvenience of these robots is their price which considerably increases the cost of the operation.

The adapted implants

The multiplication of the sizes proposed and the increasing variety of different versions of variable constraint models is the first step.

However the development of revision surgery and the extension of clinical indications for TKR to situations of more and more severe articular destruction sometimes make it necessary to use specific implants.

– The modularity. It allows, during the operation, to add stems, pegs, wedges or metal corners of various shapes and dimensions, to a standard implant in order to adapt it to a situation where the bone damage is severe, especially (but not exclusively) in cases of revision surgery (fig. 13).

– Custom made implant. In the extreme cases, particularly when severe articular damage is associated with degenerative juxta-articular bone deformations, post-traumatic or iatrogenic, these implants are made specifically

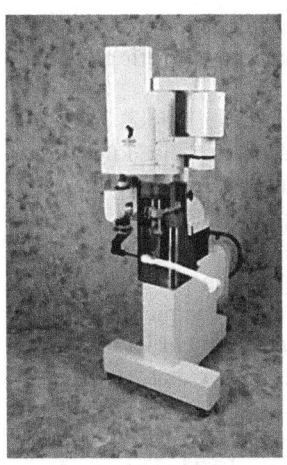
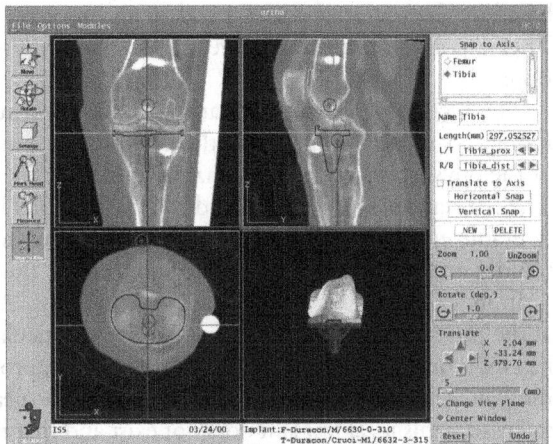

a.   b.

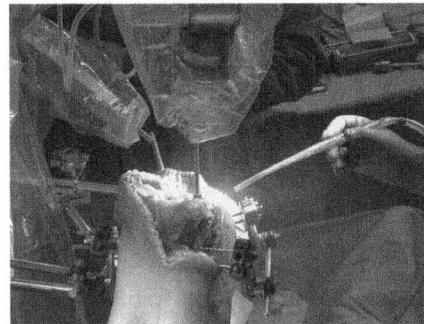
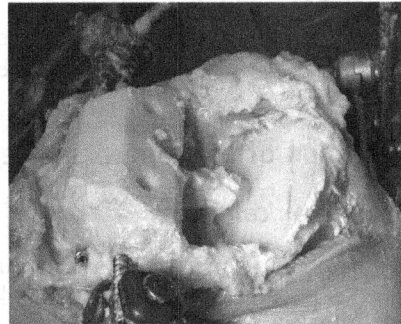

c.   d.

Fig. 12. – Robodoc system.
a. The robot. **b.** The preop planning. **c.** The bone cuts. **d.** The bone before implantation of the prosthesis.

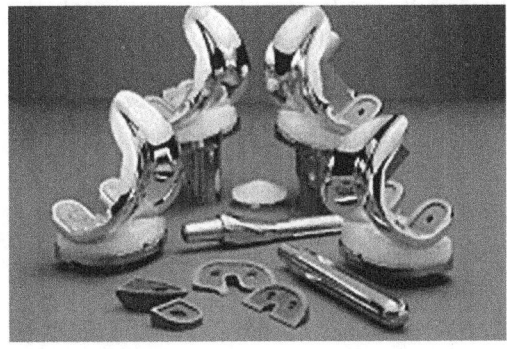
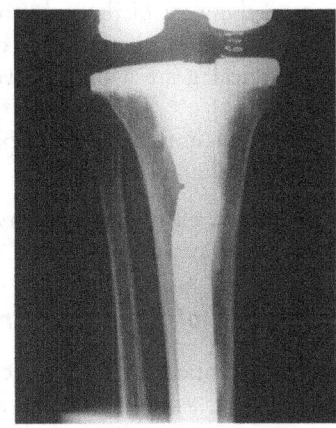

Fig. 13. – The Nexgen system adapted for revisions.

based on the pre-operative X-ray data and more often on scanographic results. They are much more expensive and so remain reserved for exceptional situations.

The technological sophistication of the present available models makes it more and more necessary for the operator to possess the precise knowledge of the physio-pathological mechanisms of the degenerative lesions of the knee. The realization of a TKA should obey a rigorous logic because the margin of tolerable error is small. Indeed, the instrumentation materiel cannot be used blindly and requires a good understanding of the operating principles.

In in 1972, Wagner and Masse (75) could say: "Although the prostheses used at the present time prove that the surgery of articular replacement has exceeded its embryonic phase, they are still really only approximate versions of the ideal implant which we might be able to use in the near future, however it seems today that this ideal implant does not exist and that the variety of existing models is only the reflection of the variety of situations encountered." The current development of revision surgery, which sometimes places the operator before very severe bone and ligament damage, often obliges him to resort to more constrained implants. This explains the renewal of interest for models considered as more rustic, made necessary by the importance of the articular destruction.

Evolution of the concepts: attempts of classification

Biomechanical basis

At the present time, a TKR should answer two objectives: restore function as close as possible to that of a normal knee (indolence, mobility, stability), and allow the most important longevity possible.

– The functional result depends:

• on the surgical technique and of its planning, taking into account the bone and ligament damage, as well as the rehabilitation;
• on the kinematics of the implant.

– The longevity depends:

• on the wear of the polyethylene itself, conditioned by the quality of the bio-materials, the congruency of the articular surfaces and to the precision of the surgical geste avoiding over-looseness of the joint (ligamentary balancing ++);
• the solicitation on the implant-bone interface: respect of the axis and the quality of the anchorage.

However, all of these factors are integrated and the final choice of a prothesis is always the result of a compromise.

Kinematics of the normal knee

It is conditioned by the presence of both cruciate ligaments making the "four-bar" system, as well as by the anatomy of the articular surfaces:

- decrease of the anterior-posterior curved radius of the femoral condyles;
- asymmetry and divergence of the condyles;
- asymmetry of the tibial plateaus and the posterior tibial sloping of 10°;
- meniscal mobility.

Thanks to the respect of these anatomical conditions, the rolling back and sliding movement of the femoral condyles on the tibial plate during the passage from flexion to extension is executed normally. The rolling movement predominates during the first 20° of flexion inducing the femoral-tibia contact point to move back, then the sliding is associated to become rapidly predominant then exclusive as the flexion progresses (27, 28, 31, 71).Because of the difference of the curved radius and of the asymmetric mobility, the back movement predominates on the outer compartment (17mm) whereas only 2.2mm on the inner side (Korosawa (52).

The constitutional or acquired lesions participate along with the degenerative modifications in the knee, candidate for a prosthesis, to move away from the normal functioning mode. If some architectural designs of total knee prostheses appear obsolete today, the complexity of the knee's articular physiology, on one hand, and the importance of the degenerative lesions bringing the patient to have surgery, on the other hand, make that several technical options are possible to respect, aid, or substitute the physiology of the normal knee.

According to the amount of damage assessed, the prosthesis used will substitute more or less for the anatomy, going from a simple resurfacing conserving the integrality of the natural system of ligament stabilization to a constrained prosthesis taking into account the entire articular stability passing as needed by all the intermediate steps.

Mechanical performances of the prostheses

They result from a balance between the constraint and the limited joint movement.

The notion of constraint

In a three dimensional space, the orthonorm reference has three axes perpendicular between them. Each point situated in this space can move in translation along each of these three axes: It therefore has 3° of freedom in translation. It can also turn over itself around each of these three axes. It therefore has 3° of freedom in rotation. Finally, a non-constrained object in a three dimensional space possesses 5° of freedom. The constraint can oppose itself to this freedom by cancelling one or several degrees, thus a sphere resting on a plane has 5° of freedom because it cannot move at all along the vertical axis. The hinge which is allowed to turn only around its own axis has only 1° of freedom. The more a system is constrained, the more it is stable (29).

Application to the knee prosthesis

The choice of the designers can go:
- either towards a constrained prosthesis less physiological, more stable,

but presenting the disadvantage of transmitting most of the stress to the bone by the intermediary of the prosthetic pieces at the anchoring point thus encouraging loosening or else requiring anchoring systems by means of voluminous stems;

– or towards a prosthesis less constrained in which the stability is assured by the ligamentary apparatus, preserved to a maximum, but with the risk of instability if this ligamentary system is not perfectly balanced or deteriorates secondarily. There is also the increased risk of wear and progressive déterioration (cold flow) because of the increased contact stress between two non-congruent surfaces. Between these two extremes, there exist several intermediary options.

Classification according to the constraints

Constrained prostheses

– The hinge prostheses are the most constrained that we can imagine because they have only one degree of liberty: flexion-extension. All the constraint and therefore the stability of the knee being assured by the prosthetic materials, it is submitted, at more or less long-term, to wear and even breakage especially at the axis level.

On the other hand, these mechanical solicitations being transmitted at the prosthesis-bone anchoring level, it is necessary that the anchoring be carried out by use of long intra-medullary stems in the tibia as well as the femur. These stems can themselves, at long-term, be the seat of fatigue fractures. In addition, the volume of the metallic implant is probably partly responsible for an infection rate apparently higher in these prostheses (5% to 8%). However in return they are privileged in indication in the degenerative lesions associated with important ligament weakness of the knee and at the present time particularly in the revision surgery after failure of a sliding prosthesis. The most utilized has been the prosthesis of the Guepar group (49), at the present time supplanted by other more elaborate models presenting a certain degree of rotation (Axel).

– One additional degree of freedom is accorded to prostheses by their authors, either, the most often, in rotation (Trillat et Bousquet (74), Lagrange et Letournel (54), or in translation (GBS prostheses (39, 40)). The functional results of these prostheses are better than those of the hinge prostheses. Nevertheless, the solicitation at the anchoring level remains important requiring, again, big encumbering prosthetic material, source of a rather high infection rate. (Link endomodel, S-ROM modular Hinge, Kinémax rotating Hinge).

Non-constrained prostheses

These are prostheses conserving the overall ligament system, meaning the collateral ligaments and the overall of the central pivot: ACL and PCL. They are represented by the Cloutier (21) prostheses, RMC, Kinématic (32) and the modular prostheses: Marmor (59, 60), Saint Georges (12), LOTUS (6).

They theoretically possess 5° of freedom.

– Technical imperatives

The design of the tibial component must spare the insertion of PCL. and ACL. Its plates must be flat to allow the rolling-sliding movement during the flexion-extension of the knee.

– The advantages:

• a minimal solicitation of the prosthetic anchoring points because the totality of the stabilization is performed by the ligaments;

• amplitudes of movement, theoretically physiological, during flexion-extension and rotation;

• an improvement of knee function, especially on the stairs;

• better proprioceptive control of the knee (1, 37).

– The disadvantages:

• a delicate implantation with difficulty of exposure and the risk of a positioning error;

• a tibial-femoral incongruence exists allowing the sliding, but the polyethylene used in the tibial plates is not very adapted for this movement and thus presents a risk of wear by "fatigue" associated with wear by abrasion;

• finally, problems due to the state of the ACL which is absent in many cases of arthritis (57%) for Cloutier (20). Certain authors have proposed to replace the absent ACL, by a prosthetic ACL however one is aware of the mechanical fragility and the absence of elasticity, not to mention the risks of postoperative knee stiffness.

In total, these prostheses only concern the knees in which the degenerative evolution is not too advanced (26), with, in particular, moderate bone axis defects. The conservation of the entire central pivot requires a very strict respect of the articular interline spacing, limiting the possibility of axis correction to the simple compensation of intra-articular wear.

The semi-constrained prostheses

They are designed to work without ACL conservation. The sacrifice is often necessary because of the severity of the arthrosis which has caused the ACL rupture. From then on, the normal kinematics is abandoned and one must opt for a compromise: The prosthesis is submitted to an anterior translation force of the tibia under the effect of the extensor system. To oppose that, it is necessary to raise up the posterior edge of the tibial plateau and the tibial sloping must be limited.

In the intermediate situation between the constrained and the non-constrained prostheses, they represent the immense majority of the prostheses put in, in Europe as well as in North America. Nevertheless, within the same group, two technical conceptions confront each other: Should the posterior cruciate ligament be retained or not?

The PCL retaining prostheses

This is the case of several models, Kinématic (32), Miller-Gallante, PCA, Kali (16, 25, 42, 62). Today most of the manufacturers propose a PCL retention possibility on their models.

The PCL is nearly always found intact: 99% for Scott (65), 100% for Hungerford (42).

The geometry of the implants must not combat the femur's posterior movement during flexion to avoid putting tension on the PCL and thus increasing the stress transmitted to the interface. Therefore the femur-tibia conformity must be low and limit the constraints:

– Lew (56) has demonstrated that on a constrained prosthesis, the forces going through the PCL reach 4.5 times the normal at 90° of flexion. This is a factor of the reduction of the flexion whereas in the case of a Kinématics prosthesis, the forces going through the PCL are comparable to those of the normal knee;

– Walker (77) shows a decrease of the rotation in the case of constrained prostheses retaining the PCL.

– Sledge (69) describes an increase of the frequency of radiolucencies in the case of concave tibial trays as compared to flat trays.

The absence of the ACL must however be palliated by posterior elevating of the tray to prevent an anterior subluxation of the tibia and this is the main problem encountered in these types of implants. This elevation is absolutely necessary, because of the existing posterior slope of the tibia which favors the flexion, but also favors the anterior translation of the tibia.

The posterior-stabilized prosthesis

The resection of the medial pivot makes necessary a posterior stabilization of the knee in two specific situations: in flexion and in the passage from flexion to extension.

Freeman (35, 36) adhering to the principal of "the roller in a non-conforming trough" realizes, in the design of his tibial component, an anterior and posterior elevated lip. The femur is held in the sagittal tibial groove by the two tensed collateral ligaments. This principle permits a flexion-extension almost free, a few degrees of rotation and AP drawer, and lateral translation motion later limited by the addition of a central tibial eminence.

The disadvantage of this system is the absence of real rolling during flexion, causing numerous femoro-patellar problems.

This system however, has the advantage of a better femur-tibia congruence, which theoretically reduces the polyethylene wear. It has since been improved, at least partially and in association with other biomechanical options (LCS [DePuy], MBK [Zimmer], Profix [Biomet], Natural Knee [Sulzer], Advanced Knee [Wright]).

This last implant reposes on the original principal of the "ball in socket": The inside tray embraces the spheric form of the condyle, while the outside tray authorizes an anatomical translation, while assuring a medial-lateral congruency (fig. 14).

Insall (47) imagined a system of posterior stabilisation which calls upon an asymmetric tibial cam which also produces a posterior rolling during flexion.

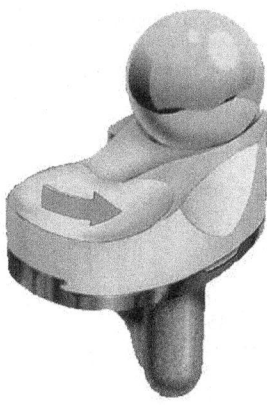

Fig. 14. – The Advanced Medial Pivot Knee (Wright Medical) is based on the "Ball in Socket" concept.

This cam produces an additional stability to the prosthesis in the sagittal plane as well as the frontal plane. The effectiveness of this system on the posterior displacement of the femur-tibia contact point permits the improvement of the lever force of the quadriceps and the correct functioning of the extensor system.

This solution permits a simplified implantation; the resection of the medial pivot gives an easy access to the posterior part of the knee permitting the eventual ablation of excess cement in the back and the correction of a flexum.

Ligamentary balancing is almost always possible even in cases of important deformation (fig. 15) and the flexion can exceed 120°.

Important constraints persist however on the tibial interface, especially A-P, because of the bearing of the femoral component on the tibial cam during flexion. This is particularly striking during the bearing when going downs-

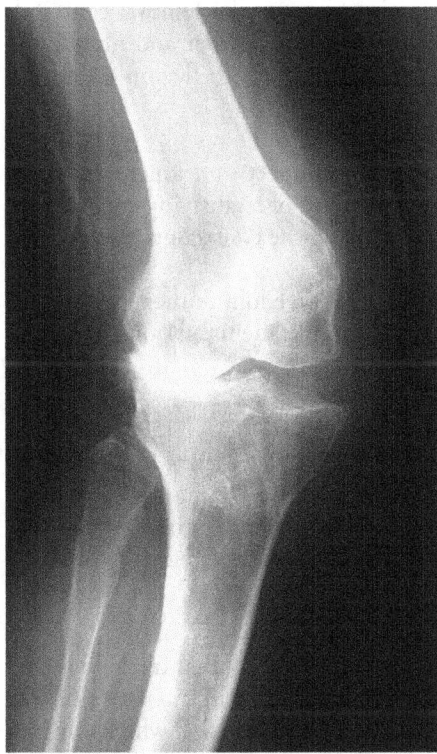
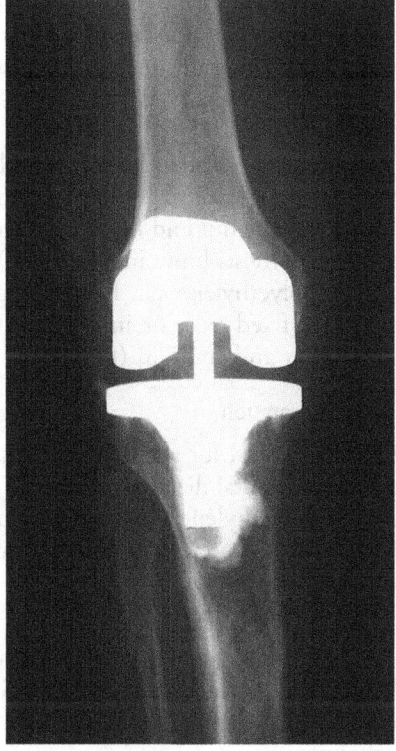

Fig. 15. – The Constrained TCIII TKA (Johnson & Johnson is a postero-stabilized TKA.

Table I. – In postero-stabilized prostheses, the cams' effect begins at various angles of flexion.

TKR	Cam Function Introduction
TRAC (Biomet)	8°
Duracon (Howmedica)	10°
AGC (Biomet)	20°
Interax (Howmedica)	< 30°
Kinematics (Howmedica)	< 30°
HLS (Tornier)	30°
Genesis (Smith Nephew)	30°
Advanced Knee (Wright)	30°
AMK (DePuy)	35°
Axiom (Wright)	35-40°
Profis (Smith Nephez)	45°
Optetrak (Exactech)	60°
Scorpio (Osteonics)	60°
PFC (DePuy)	65°
Natural Knee (Sulzer)	67°
Nexgen (Zimmer)	75°
Appolo (Sulzer)	90°

tairs. These constraints make necessary the use of a stem in the tibial component.

These constraints have been progressively reduced during the evolution of the prostheses, by lowering the contact point between the femoral cam and the tibial post on one hand, and by the introduction, earlier and more progressive, of this cam during the passage from extension to flexion (table 1).

Mobile bearing prostheses

They permit to solve the dilemma between the respect of a kinematic close to the normal knee physiology and the maintenance of a satisfying congruency between the femur and the tibia as well as reducing the constraints transmitted to the prosthesis-bone interface (55).

The polyethylene can have a single degree of freedom, either in rotation around a fixed axis, or in pure translation (mobile meniscus) or associated translation and rotation (fig. 16).

The pure rotation

Initially created for the hypercongruent designs (LCS), it finds its interest in the posterior-stabilized prostheses. The femoral cam bears on a block situated on the polyethylene tray in order to permit the backward movement of the femoro-tibial contact point during flexion. The tray must therefore by blocked antero-posteriorly.

This rotation permits:

– to compensate the rotative positioning errors of the tibial tray: Thus the fixed metallic tibial base covers maximally the bone cut with no worry of the rotation positioning of the polyethylene insert, nor the size which can be uncouple;

– to permit the automatic rotation of the tibia during flexion;

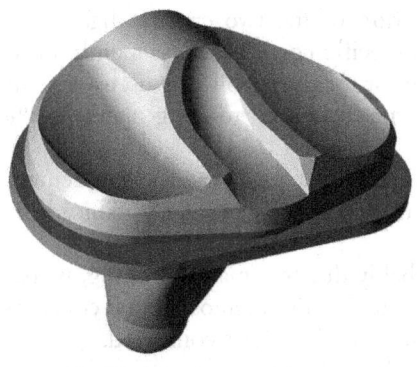

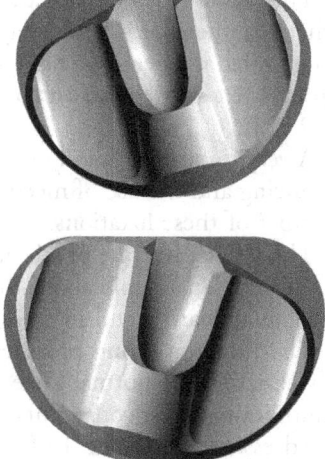

Fig. 16. – A postero-stabilized prosthesis with rotating platform: the HLS prosthesis (Tornier).

– to permit a few degrees of escaping in rotation in the very constrained prosthesis.

Translation-rotation association

Its goal is to permit the association of the CPL conservation with congruent polyethylene designs and it permits even, for some models, the conservation of the ACL.

The backward movement of the femoro-tibial contact during flexion is thus obtained by the backward sliding of the polyethylene plate.

This sliding must however by limited in the case of isolated conservation of the CPL to avoid an excessive anterior drawer leading to the luxation of the mobile tray.

Examples: MBK (Zimmer), Interax-ISA (Howmedica), Oxford 3C (Biomet), Accord, LCS APGlide (DePuy), Rotaglide (Corin), Tri CCC (SME), Seragyr (Ceraver), Sal II (Sulzer).

The major inconvenience of these implants associating A-P translation is the almost absolute obligation to obtain a perfect and physiological tension of the PCL. Indeed, if it is distended or sacrificed, as some authors recommend arguing that the anterior-posterior stabilization is obtained by the congruent design, a paradoxical movement contrary to the physiology is produced, as has been observed by Matsuda and Whiteside. This hypermobility can create such phenomena as an audible and disturbing "clicking" noise, due to the A-P stop of the polyethylene's blockage system.

Pure translation

The polyethylene plate is separate for each of the internal and external compartments and slides only anteriorly and posteriorly along a rail (New Jersey LCS meniscal [DePuy], Oxford modulaire [Biomet], Minns [Corin].

The combination of independent translations on both femoral-tibial compartments allows a rotation of the femur in regards to the tibia.

This system necessitates the conservation of the two cruciate ligaments, otherwise these prostheses may present specific complications: mainly luxations which happen either anterior-posterior for the mobile meniscus systems (from 1.3% to 7%), or in rotation for the unlimited rotating plates (0.8% to 2.2%).

A very rigorous surgical technique, particularly concerning the ligamentary balancing and the use of mechanical security systems, has largely reduced the number of these luxations.

The fatigue fracture of a bearing, probably due to a malpositioning, is specific to the LCS meniscal prosthesis (1.5% to 7.1%). It almost always concerns the lateral bearing and in cases where only the PCL was conserved.

The mobile bearing prostheses thus allow the hope of restoring kinematics closer to the normal knee and especially a more important longevity by diminution of the constraints and augmentation of the congruency as compared essentially to the TKR conserving the PCL which present an almost flat polyethylene.

The publications of recent studies, showing results at twenty years, seem to confirm this hope and explain the renewed interest in these prostheses in the last few years.

References

1. Andriacchi TP, Galante JO, Fermier RW (1982) The influence of total knee replacement design on walking and stair climbing. J Bone Joint Surg 61-A: 1328-35
2. Andriacchi TP, Galante JO, Fermier RW (1987) Supra condylar fracture of the femur after total knee arthroplasty. Clin Orthop 219: 136-9
3. Attenborough CG (1976) Total knee replacement using the stabilised gliding prosthesis. Ann R Coll Surg Engl 58: 4
4. Aubriot JH Historique et évolution des prothèses totales du genou. Cahier d'Enseignement de la SOFCOT n° 35. Paris, Expansion Scientifique Française 4
5. Aubriot JH, Deburge A, Kenesi CL *et al.* (1973) La prothèse Guepar Acta Orthop Belg 39: 257
6. Aubriot JH, Deburge A, Le Bach T et le groupe Guepar. (1998) Prothèse unicompartimentale du genou Lotus. Rev Chir Orthop Suppl. II, 74: 180
7. Becker MW, Insall JN, Faris PM (1991) Bilateral TKA. One cruciate retaining and one cruciate substituting. Clin Orthop 271: 122-4
8. Berger RA, Rosenberg AG, Barden RM. *et al.* Long-term follow-up of the Miller-Gallante total knee replacement. Clin Orthop 388: 58-67
9. Bolanos AA., Colizza WA, McCann PD *et al.*(1998) a comparison of isokinetic strength testing and gait analysis in patients with posterior cruciate-retaining and substituting knee arthroplasties J Arthroplasty 13 (8): 906-15
10. Bonnin M La prothèse totale du genou : du concept au design. In: La chirurgie prothétique du genou Sauramps Médical 95-111
11. Bousquet G, Dejesse A, Girardin P *et al.* (1989) Étude et résultats de la prothèse totale de genou vissée sans ciment. Cahier d'Enseignement de la SOFCOT n° 35 Paris, expansion scientifique française 8
12. Buchloltz HW, Kengelbrecht E, Siegel A (1973) Characteristics of the knee joint prosthesis model Saint-Georg and clinical experiences. Symposium sur les prothèses de genou, Londres
13. Buechel, Buechel JR, Pappas et al. (2001) Twenty years evaluation of meniscal bearing and rotating placement knee replacement. Clin Orthop 388

14. Campbell WC Interposition of vitallium plates in arthroplasties of the knee. Clin Orthop and Rel Res 226: 3-5

15. Cartier PH., Cheaib S, Vanvooren P (1987) Le remplacement prothétique unicomparti- mental du genou. Rev Chir Orthop Suppl II, 73: 131

16. Carlier Y, Duthoit E, Epinette JA (1989) Prothèses totales du genou de Miller-Gallante : notre expérience a 3 ans a propos de 214 cas. Cahier d'Enseignement de la SOFCOT n° 35 Paris, Expansion Scientifique Française, 9

17. Churchill DL, Incavo SJ, Jihnson CC, et al. (1998) The trans-epicondylar axis approxi- mates the optimal flexion axis of the Knee. Clin Orthop 356: 111-8

18. Clayton ML, Thompson TR, Mack RP (1986) Correction of alignment deformities during total knee arthroplasties: staged soft-tissue releases. Clin Orthop 202: 117-24

19. Cloutier JM (1983) Results of total knee arthroplasty with a non-constrained prosthesis. J Bone Joint Surg 65-A: (7) 906-19

20. Cloutier JM, Colombet P (1985) Arthroplastie totale du genou par prothèse Cloutier Acta Orthop Belg 51 (4): 498-519

21. Cloutier JM, Pilon L (1981) Arthroplastie totale du genou. une prothèse a glissement auto stable. Rev Chi. Orthop 67 Suppl. II: 114-8

22. Cloutier JM, Pilon L (1981) Total knee arthroplasty: a method of achieving stability with an unconstrained prosthesis. J Bone Joint Surg 63-B (3): 460

23. Corces A, Lotke PA, Williams JL (1989) Strain characteristics of the posterior cruciate ligament in total knee replacement. Orthop Trans 13 (3): 527

24. Deburge A Guepar hinge prosthesis complications and results with 2 years follow-up. Clin Orthop 120: 47-53

25. Deburge A la prothèse KALI. Cahier d'Enseignement de la SOFCOT n° 35 Paris, Expansion Scientifique Française 12

26. Dejour H, Chambat P Les prothèses a glissement du genou.EMC, Paris Techniques Chirurgicales

27. Denis DA, Komistek RD, Colwell CE In vivo antero-posterior femoro-tibial translation of TKA: a multicenter analysis. Clin Orthop 356: 47-57

28. Draganich LF, Andriacchi T, Andersson GBJ Interaction between intrinsic knee mecha- nics and the knee extensor mechanisms. J Orthop and Res 5: 539-47

29. Duparc J Classification des prothèses du genou. In: les prothèses du genou. Expansion Scientifique Française

30. Elias SG, Freeman MAR, Gokcay EI A correlative study of the geometry and anatomy of the distal femur. Clin Orthop 260: 98-10331. El Nahass B, Madson MM, Walter PS (1991) Motion of the knee after condylar resurfacing: an in vivo study. J Biomech 24: 1107-17

32. Ewald FC, Jacobs MA, Miegel ME et al. (1979) kinematic total knee replacement. J Bone Joint Surg 66-A, (7): 1032-40.

33. Fergusson W Excision of the knee joint: recovery with a false joint and a useful limb. Med Times Gaz. 1: 601

34. Finerman GAM, Coventry MB, Riley LH,et al. (1979) Anametric total knee arthroplasty. Clin Orthop 145: 85-90

35. Freeman MAR, Insall JN, Besser W et al.(1977) Excision of the cruciate ligaments in total knee replacement. Clin Orthop 126: 209-12

36. Freeman MAR., Samuelson KM, Bertin KC Freeman-Samuelson total arthroplasty of the knee. Clin Orthop (192): 46-58

37. Gollehon DL, Torzilli PA, Warren RF (1987) The role of the postero-lateral and cruciate ligaments in the stability of the human knee. J Bone Joint Surg 69A: 233-42

38. Goodfellow J, O'Connor J (1978) The mechanics of the knee and prosthesis design. J Bone Joint Surg 60-B (3): 358-69

39. Gschwend N, Ivosevic-Radovanovic D, Kentsch A (1985)La prothèse totale du genou GSB Acta Orthop Belg (4): 460-77

40. Gschwend N, Sheier H, Bahler A (1973) The GSB knee prosthesis. international congress of the knee Rotterdam, 261

41. Gunston FH Polycentric knee arthroplasty. J Bone Joint Surg 53-B, (2): 272-7

42. Hungerford DS, Kenna RV (1983) Preliminary experience with a total knee prosthesis with porous coating used without cement. Clin Orthop (176): 95-107
43. Incavo SJ, Johnson CC, Beynnon BD, Posterior cruciate ligament strain biomechanics in total knee arthroplasty. Clin Orthop 309: 88-93
44. Insall JN Total knee Replacement. surg of the knee, New York, Churchill Livingstone 587-695
45. Insall JN, Binazzi R, Soudry M et al. (1985) Total Knee Arthroplasty Clin Orthop 192: 13-22
46. Insall JN, Kelly M (1986) The total condylar prosthesis. Clin Orthop 205: 43-8
47. Insall JN, Rawawat CS, Scott (1976) Total condylar knee prosthesis. Preliminary report Clin Ortho 120
48. Insall JN, Scott WN, Ranawat CS (1979) The total condylar knee prosthesis.J Bone Joint Surg. 1979, 61-A, (2): 173-80
49. Jones EC, Insall JN, Inglis AE et al. (1979) Guepar knee arthroplasty results and late complications. Clin Orthop 140: 145-52
50. Julliard R. Rev Chir Orthop Suppl I 77: 161
51. Kim H, Pelker RR, Gibson DH et al. (1997) Rollback in posterior cruciate ligament-retaining total knee arthroplasty. J Arthroplasty 12 (5): 553-61
52. Kurosawa H, Walker PS, Garg A, et al. (1985) Geometry and motion of the knee for implant and orthodic design. J Biomech, 18: 4878-99
53. Krackow KA (1990) The technique of total knee arthroplasty. MOSBY, Saint-Louis
54. Lagrange J, Letournel E (1973) Principes et réalisation de la prothèse du genou "LL" Acta Orthop Belg 39: 280
55. Lemaire R (1998) Prothèses de genou a surface d'appui mobile. cahiers d'enseignement de la sofcot n° 66. Conf Enseign, 17-34. Expansion scientifique, publication
56. Lew WD, Lewis JL (1982) the effect of knee prosthesis geometry on cruciate ligament mechanics during flexion. J Bone Joint. Surg 64-A (5): 734-9
57. Lewis P, Rorabeck CH, Bourne RB et al. (1994) Posteromedial tibial polyethylene failure in total knee replacement. Clin Orthop 299: 11-7
58. Malkani AL, Rand JA, Bryan RS et al. (1995) Total knee arthroplasty with the kinematic condylar prosthesis. J Bone Joint Surg. 77A: 423-31
59. Marmor L (1988) Total knee arthroplasty in a patient with congenital dislocation of the patella. Clin. Orthop 226: 129-33
60. Marmor L (1973) The modular knee. Clin Orthop 94: 242
61. Matsuda S, Whiteside LA, White SE et al. (1997) Knee kinematics of posterior cruciate ligament sacrificed total knee arthroplasty. Clin Orthop 341: 257-66
62. Maudhuit B La prothèse PCA. Cahier d'Enseignement de la SOFCOT n° 35 Paris, Expansion Scientifique Française 10
63. Riley LH (1976) The evolution of total knee arthroplasty. Clin Orthop 120: 7-9
64. Rodriguez, Brende, Ranawat. Total condylar knee replacement. A 20 years follow-up study. Clin Orthop and Research 388: 10-7
65. Scott RD, Volatile TB (1986) Twelve years experience with posterior cruciate-retaining total knee arthroplasty. Clin Orthop 205: 100
66. Scott WN., Rubinstein M (1986) Posterior stabilized knee arthroplasty. Clin Orthop 205: 138-45
67. Shiers LGP (1954) Ecempta medica, Arthroplasty of the knee. Preliminary report of a new method. J Bone Joint Surg 36-B: 553
68. Shoji H, Yoshino S, Komagamine M (1987) Improved range of notion with the Y/S total knee arthroplasty system. Clin Orthop 218: 150-63
69. Sledge CB, Ewald EC (1979) Total knee arthroplasty experience at the Robert Breck Brigham Hospital. Clin Orthop 145: 78-84
70. Sorgel JI, Federle D, Kirk PG et al. (1997) The Posterior Cruciate Ligament in Total Knee Arthroplasty. J Arthroplasty 12, 8: 869-979
71. Sthiel JB, Dennis DA, Komitek RD, et al. (1997) In vivo kinematic analysis of a mobile bearing total knee prosthesis. Clin Orthop 345: 60-6

72. Sthiel JB, Komitek RD, Dennis DA, *et al.* (1995) Fluoroscopic analysis of kinematics after posterior cruciate retaining knee arthroplasty. J Bone Joint Surg (B) 77-B: 884-9
73. Sthiel JB, Komistek RD, Cloutier JM, *et al.* (1998) The cruciate ligaments in total knee arthroplasty: a kinematic analysis. AAOS, New Orleans, Poster
74. Trillat A, Dejour H, Bousquet G, *et al.* (1973) La prothèse rotatoire du genou. Rev Chir Orthop 59 (6): 513-22
75. Wagner J, Masse Y (1973) Historique de l'arthroplastie du genou par implants partiels et totaux. Acta. Orthop Belg 1973, 39 (1): 11-39
76. Walldius B Arthroplasty of the knee using endoprosthesis. Acta. Orthop Scand 23 (suppl.): 121
77. Walker PS (1980) Design of a knee prosthesis system. Acta Orthop Belg 45, (6): 766-75
78. Wasielewski RC, Galante JO, Leighty RM *et al.* (1994) Wear patterns on retrieved polyethylene tibial inserts and their relationship to technical consideration during TKA. Clin Orthop 299: 31-43
79. Wolf AM, Hungerford DS, Pepe CL (1991) The effect of extra-articular varus and valgus deformity on total knee arthroplasty. Clin Orthop 271: 35-51

Results of total knee arthroplasty

J. Ménétrey, R. Stern

Introduction

From the mid-1800's, orthopaedic surgeons have attempted to reconstruct the surfaces of knee joints damaged by osteoarthritis or rheumatoid arthritis (16, 27, 28, 31, 92). The goal of arthroplasty has always been the correction of deformity, restoration of joint stability, and the reduction of pain. All efforts made to improve the techniques of arthroplasty have been sound, considering that the incidence of osteoarthritis continues to increase due in large part to the number of middle-aged patients (45-65 years) suffering from osteoarthritis of the knee (1). This increase may be partly explained by a greater prevalence of risk factors such as obesity, strenuous sports activities, occupational factors, joint and limb trauma resulting in deformity, and improved diagnostic screening (1).

The surgical treatment of osteoarthritis of the knee has recent origins. The concept of debridement arthroplasty was introduced by Magnusson in 1941 (55). In 1959, Pridie advocated a more modest debridement of the knee and presented a method of resurfacing the knee joint by drilling the subchondral bone (67). The concept was further advanced by Insall (36, 37, 78). In 1974, Jackson (40) suggested that irrigation of the knee joint during arthroscopy was of benefit in the management of the osteoarthritic knee. In addition, other procedures such as high tibial osteotomy, distal femoral osteotomy, unicompartmental arthroplasty, and total knee replacement have attempted to improve the function and relieve the pain of the arthritic knee. Simple needle or arthroscopic lavage themselves have demonstrated efficacy in obtaining pain relief in the osteoarthritic knee for up until at least 1 year post-surgery (15, 20, 21, 26, 39, 52). Arthroscopic debridement of the arthritic knee provides 60-85% excellent and good results at an average follow-up of 2 years (81). The term arthroscopic debridement has included articular trimming, menisectomy, the removal of osteophytes, and articular abrasion. After such multiple arthroscopic procedures it is difficult to attribute the success or failure of the operation to any specific part of the method (34). In our experience, medial menisectomy in patients over 50 years of age suffering from osteoarthritis yields only 20% good results as regards pain relief at 6 years post-operative (60). In middle-aged patients and those involved in heavy labor or high impact sports activities, high tibial or distal femoral osteotomies yield an improvement in pain and function in 70-75% of the patients at 10 years (33, 62, 63). In the study by Naudie *et al.*, using the Kaplan-Meier method, the mean survivorship of valgus tibial osteotomy was 73% at 5 years, 51% at 10 years, 39% at 15 years and 30% at 20 years (63).

From the early 1970's, the research and development of knee implants have aimed at articular resurfacing, restoring normal kinematics, reducing debris and providing a stable fixation. The progressive achievement of these objectives has resulted in increasing successful results following total knee replacement.

The aim of this chapter is to review, in the light of recent and selected publications, the results of different types of prostheses. By "types", we mean condylar prostheses with different features. For example, a posterior cruciate ligament (PCL) substitution design is different from a posterior cruciate preserving design (fig. 1). From a definition stand point, we will use the term "postero-stabilized" for posterior cruciate ligament substitution design. Our goal is not to compare the different manufacturers' prostheses that currently exist in the marketplace. Moreover, such comparisons are difficult as one can note from a review of the literature where there are major discrepancies in the use of outcome tools to assess the results.

Other objectives of this chapter are to review the results of total knee arthroplasty performed in patients with specific conditions (post-traumatic osteoar-

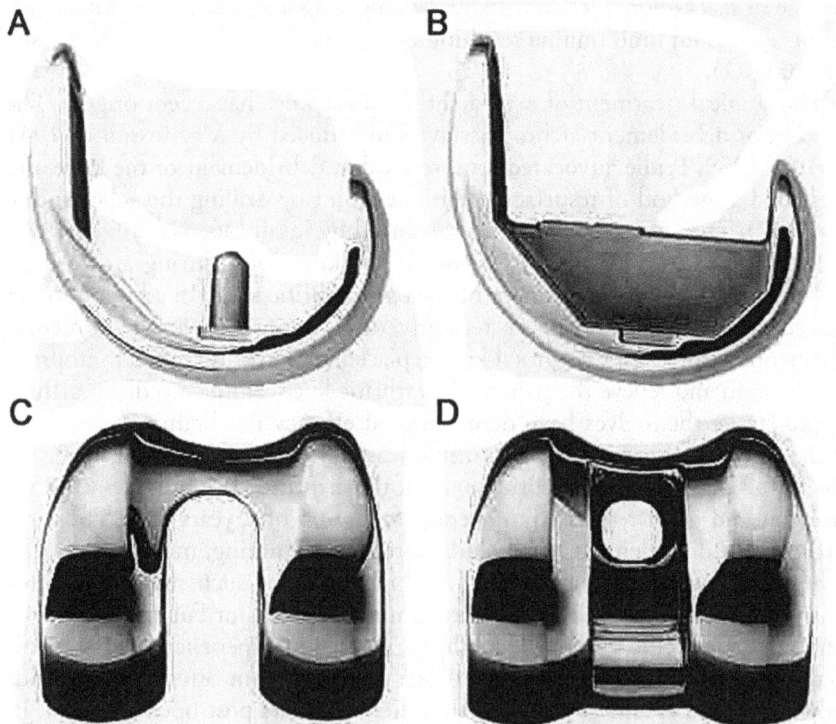

Fig. 1. – Example of PCL-retaining (A, C) and postero-stabilized (B, D) femoral designs.

thritis, a valgus knee, previous high tibial osteotomy) and specific diseases (Parkinson's disease, Charcot's disease), and as well to discuss the results of total knee replacement in young patients. Hopefully, the reader will find answers for patients when discussing possible total knee arthroplasty. Indeed, with the Internet communication, our patients' questions and concerns have become more precise and they demand a more detailed response.

Overall results

In 1991, Rand and Illstrup (71) reported the results of a survivorship analysis of 9,200 TKAs implanted between 1971 and 1987 (fig. 2). The need for revision of an implant was selected as the endpoint of survival. Among these 9,200 TKAs, 2,947 primary TKAs were performed with old designs such as the "Polycentric" and the "Geometric" knees (Howmedica, Rutherford, NJ). For this group of prostheses, the cumulative survival rate was 95% at 2 years, 89% at 5 years and 78% at 10 years. Primary total knee arthroplasty using condylar-resurfacing, PCL-retaining designs with metal-backed tibial components, were performed in 3,620 knees. These designs included the "Cruciate Condylar", "Kinematic Condylar", and "Porous-Coated Anatomic" knees (Howmedica, Rutherford, NJ), the "Townley and Cloutier" knee (De Puy, Warsaw, IN), the "Miller-Galante" knee (Zimmer, Warsaw, IN), the "PFC" knee (Johnson & Johnson Orthopaedics, Braintree, MA), and the "Orthomet" knee (Orthomet, Minneapolis, MN). The cumulative survival rate for these designs was 99% at 2 years, 98% at 5 years, and 91% at 10 years. The risks of revision were significantly greater for the older designs when compared to the condylar-resurfacing, PCL-retaining design with a metal-backed tibial component (70).

Clinical relevance: The overall results following total knee arthroplasty reveal 90% of good and excellent results at 10 years, and demonstrate that TKA is one of the most successful and satisfactory procedures in orthopaedic surgery. The analysis of these 9,200 TKAs permits the identification of four factors which diminish the likelihood of failure. These include:

– primary arthroplasty;
– rheumatoid arthritis;

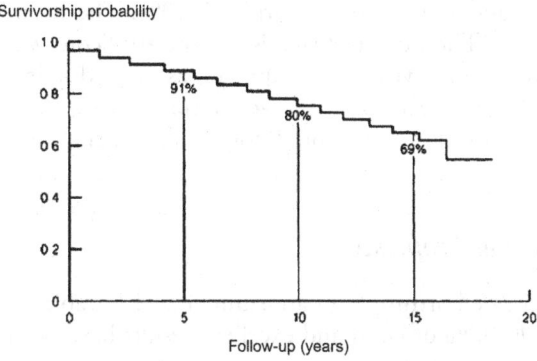

Survivorship probability

Follow-up (years)

Fig. 2. – Mean survivorship of 9,200 total knee replacements performed between 1971 and 1987. Revision or decision for revision were used as the end-point.
(From Rand JA, Ilstrup DM [1991] Survivorship analysis of total knee arthroplasty: Cumulative rates of survival of 9,200 total knee arthroplasties. J Bone Joint Surg 73-A: 397. Adapted with permission.)

– patients 60 years of age and older;

– use of a prosthesis with a metal-backed tibial component. However, it is necessary to conduct further studies to know the long-term results and benefits of modern implants.

Postero-stabilized versus PCL retaining total knee arthroplasty

There remains much controversy about the advantages and disadvantages in preserving the PCL when performing TKA. If one is going to retain the PCL, the surgeon must ensure that the knee is properly balanced. This may be technically difficult in patients with severe deformity and, in such instances, a postero-stabilized design is easier to implant properly. Furthermore, this type of prosthesis provides kinematics closer to those of a normal knee because this design demonstrates an average posterior femoral roll-back of 8mm. Posterior femoral roll-back is uncommon in PCL-retaining knees with the pathway of motion unpredictable (45, 49).

We will review the results of TKA from publications which have appeared over the last fifteen years and that report on mid- and long-term follow-up.

PCL-retaining total knee arthroplasty

The results of PCL-retaining arthroplasty are summarized in table I. With this type of prosthesis, 70-95% good and excellent results have been reported at a mean follow-up of 5 years. The re-operation rate was between 1.6% and 18% according to the different series.

Goodfellow and O'Connor (29) reviewed 125 TKAs with a mean follow-up of 4 years. 89% of the patients were painfree and the mean flexion of the knee was 99°. The same authors performed another study looking at the survivorship of 327 TKAs (30). 66% of patients were diagnosed with osteoarthritis and 32% with rheumatoid arthritis. In this series the mean survivorship at 6 years was 95% in the rheumatoid knee versus 83% in patients with osteoarthritis. Remarkably, those knees with an intact anterior cruciate ligament (ACL) at operation showed a mean survivorship of 95% at 6 years *versus* 81% in ACL-deficient knees. The failure rate was 8.3%. In another study of 473 TKAs (42) with a follow-up of 2 to 9 years, the diagnosis was osteoarthritis in 90% of the patients and rheumatoid arthritis in 10%. The mean age of the patients was 68 years. The postoperative Knee Society Score was 93 for pain and 92 for function. With revision of an implant as the end point, the mean survivorship was 95% at 8 years and the re-operation rate was 6%. 5 patients were re-operated upon for deep infection, 5 for instability, and 7 for breakage of the polyethylene.

Postero-stabilized total knee arthroplasty

The results of the postero-stabilized arthroplasty are summarized in table II. With this type of prosthesis, 90-98% of good and excellent results have been

Table 1. – Results of posterior cruciate retaining Total Knee Arthroplasty.

Authors	Number of TKA	Mean age (years)	RA (%)	OA (%)	Follow-up (years)	Good/excellent results (%)	Instability (%)	Aseptic loosening (%)	Radiolucencies (%)	Infections (%)	Re-operations/failures (%)
Goodfellow & O'Connor (1986)	125	65	40	53	4	89	–	–	96	1	7
Hungerford et al. (1987)	93	56	30	63	2-5	94.5	–	–	17	1.1	8.6
Rosenberg et al. (1989)	133	70	15	80	1-4	93	1.5	–	–	1.5	9
Buechel & Pappas (1989)	170	60	23	69	4.5	95	–	–	–	1.1	2.9
Wright et al. (1990)	112	65	32	68	2.8	93	–	–	30	1.8	3
Rand (1991)	118	66	13	62	2.8	94	–	–	75	1.8	13
Kobs et al. (1993)	41	52	49	46	3.5	88	–	–	20	2.4	10
Toksvig-Larsen et al. (1996)	106	73	–	100	6.3	87	0.7	3.5	–	–	18
Sanzen et al. (1996)	158	68	30	70	7	70	0.3	3.3	–	2	6
Knight et al. (1997)	78	72	12	85	5	89	1.2	1.2	44	1.3	8
Martin et al. (1997)	306	67	30	66	6.5	95	–	–	20	0.7	5.5

RA = Rheumatoid Arthritis
OA = Osteo-Arthritis.

Table II. – Results of postero-stabilized Total Knee Arthroplasty.

Authors	Number of TKA	Mean age (years)	RA (%)	OA (%)	Follow-up (years)	Good/excellent results (%)	PF compli-cations (%)	Aseptic loosening (%)	Radio-lucencies (%)	Infections (%)	Re-operations/failures (%)
Stern & Insall (1990)	257	–	–	–	2-6	98.5	17	–	–	0.3	0.3
Schopfer (1993)	121	72.6	17	83	7	97	–	2	12	0.1	9
Colizza & Insall (1995)	101	64	–	67	10	96	15	2.9	11	0	3.9
Scott et al. (1988)	119	67	–	74	2-8	98	–	–	–	–	–
Aglietti et al. (1988)	84	66.5	–	72	5	90	15-25	–	–	–	–
Ranawat et al. (1997)	150	70	–	83	4.8	95	8	–	–	1.3	2
Tayot et al. (1999)	376	70	22	78	11.5	92	–	2	13	3.7	6.3

RA = Rhumatoid Arthritis.
OA = Osteo-Arthritis.
PF = Patello-Femoral

reported at a mean follow-up of 6 years. The re-operation rate was between 0.3% and 4%. Several studies have commented upon anterior knee pain secondary to problems with the patello-femoral joint. The incidence of such a problem was 8-25% in the different series. Interestingly, the literature about the PCL-retaining design rarely mentioned problems with the patello-femoral joint.

The analysis of the mean survivorship of postero-stabilized arthroplasty has been done in detail by Insall's group at the Hospital for Special Surgery (HSS) (18, 88). The mean survivorship of a design with an all polyethylene tibial component was 94% at 12 years (88), and of those designs with a metal-backed tibial component, 96.4% at 11 years (18). Others authors noted a mean survivorship of 97% at 6 years (68) using a design with a metal-backed tibial component.

In 1988, Scott *et al.* (77) reported their results of 119 TKAs with a mean follow-up of 5 years. The mean age of their patients was 67 years and the diagnosis was an osteoarthritis in 74%. The mean range of motion of the knee was 107° and utilizing the HSS score, 83% of the knees were rated excellent and 15% good. After analyzing the outcome and the preoperative diagnosis, the authors demonstrated better results in those patients suffering from osteoarthritis as compared to those with rheumatoid arthritis. They also found better results in patients with a preoperative varus knee than in those with a valgus knee. The mean survivorship was 93% at 8 years.

In a long-term study, Stern *et al.* (88) reported 15% of anterior knee pain related to the patello-femoral joint. Clinical and functional examination revealed 85% of knees as grade 0 (asymptomatic), 10% grade 1 (moderate symptoms), and 5% grade 2 (severe symptoms). In his series, Ranawat *et al.* (68) noted only 8% of anterior knee pain related to the patello-femoral joint. This difference might be explained by the type of prosthesis utilized in the two series. Indeed, the "Press-Fit Condylar" system (Johnson & Johnson Orthopaedics, Braintree, MA) has a more congruent patello-femoral joint providing a symmetrical contact between the patella and the femur. This design generates a more constrained patello-femoral joint which seems to be favorable in reducing the incidence of anterior knee pain.

Clinical relevance: The various published studies do not reveal any differences in the clinical outcome between the PCL-retaining and postero-stabilized designs. No distinction can be made about the quality of the results and the survivorship of the arthroplasty. However, these statements should be viewed in light of the fact that most of the studies included a diverse group of patients without distinction as to patient age or specific conditions such as joint stiffness or major axial deformity. In fact, one might expect that a detailed analysis of these sub-groups would yield differences between both types of prostheses. Moreover, the actual data presented does not allow one to distinguish between the two prostheses with respect to the diagnosis of osteoarthritis or rheumatoid arthritis.

The difficulties of the surgical technique with a PCL-retaining design does not appear to affect either the mid-term results or the mean survivorship at

10 years. And despite concerns expressed by some regarding the inherent constraint with the postero-stabilized designs (76), there is no evidence from analysis of the survival data that long-term substitution for the PCL causes failure at the bone-cement interface.

Opinion of the authors: The concept of substitution for the PCL has proven to be versatile and durable, with excellent long-term clinical and survival results. In our university orthopaedic training program more than 200 TKAs are implanted every year, and for the past ten years we have chosen a postero-stabilized design with a metal-backed tibial component in all cases. Analysis of our current results confirms the earlier report from our institution (74) which revealed 97% of good and excellent results, comparable to the best series in the literature even with a relatively large number of different surgeons who perform such surgery in our hospital center.

Cemented versus cementless total knee arthroplasty

There are only a few studies in the literature that specifically consider the results of cemented versus cementless total knee arthroplasty. In one study of 114 hybrid TKAs (femur cementless, tibia cemented) with a follow-up of 2.8 years, the Knee Society Score was 39 before the operation and 92 postoperatively (94). Ninety-three percent of the patients were rated as having a good or excellent result. In 30% of patients radiolucencies were noted on the femur, in 30% on the tibia, and in 23% on the patella. The overall re-operation rate was 3%.

In another study comparing 59 cemented to 59 cementless TKAs (70, 71), there were 98% of good and excellent results in the cemented group and 90% in the cementless group at a mean follow-up of 2.8 years. The mobility in flexion was 103° in the cemented group and 101° in the cementless group. Complications in the cementless TKAs included 9 aseptic loosening of a metal-backed patella, 1 deep infection, 1 arthrofibrosis, and 1 deep vein thrombosis, for an overall complication rate of 20%. Complications in the cemented group consisted of 2 deep thrombosis, 1 deep infection, 1 fracture of the patella, and 1 fracture of the distal femur, for an overall complication rate of 10%. Re-operation was necessary in 7% of patients with cemented prostheses and in 19% of those in the cementless group.

Mac Caskie *et al.* (54) reported on a prospective randomized study which compared 81 cemented to 58 cementless TKAs at a 5 year follow-up. The authors did not find any difference between the two groups as regarded pain and function. When analyzed with the Nottingham Knee and the Knee Society Scores, the two groups had similar results. Only the size and the number of radiolucencies noted on the A-P tibia and lateral femur were significantly higher in the cemented group than in the cementless group. However, the authors suggested a longer period of observation to ascertain the clinical signification of such findings.

A study from the Mayo Clinic compared 51 cemented to 55 cementless TKAs at a 10 year follow-up (23). The Knee Society Score for pain and function was 92 and 72, respectively, in the cemented group and 88 and 66, respectively, in the cementless group. Joint motion was 102° in patients in the cemented group and 100° in those in the cementless group. With revision surgery as the endpoint, the mean survivorship at 10 years was 96% in the cemented group and 88% in the cementless group, and this difference was statistically significant (p = 0.05).

Clinical relevance: Our literature review does not permit us to draw any conclusions about total knee arthroplasty with or without cement. Mid-term results do not show any differences between groups, but radiolucencies were more frequently seen in the cemented group. While this might raise concerns, the long-term results do not reveal any adverse effects. Although these studies support the hypothesis that cement protects the bone from attack by polyethylene debris, thus preventing the development of aseptic loosening, once again they compare a heterogeneous patient population where the choice of the fixation was made according to the patient, and more precisely according to the bone quality.

Opinion of the authors: As mentioned previously, based upon the good results we have achieved over many years in our teaching hospital, we have opted for routine fixation by acrylic cement of the femoral, tibial, and patellar components.

Resurfacing versus non-resurfacing of the patella

The results of TKAs with or without resurfacing of the patella are comparable provided that selection criteria are carefully followed and those patients that will not benefit from resurfacing have been excluded. In a retrospective review, Picetti *et al.* (66) noted an incidence of anterior knee pain in 29% of patients who did not have patellar resurfacing, but there was no control group in this study; Boyd *et al.* (11) noted a 6% complication rate in a non-resurfacing group as compared to 4% in a resurfacing group. However, when those patients who suffered from rheumatoid arthritis were included in the study there was a 13% incidence of chronic peri-patellar pain. This difference was highly significant and the authors recommended to routinely resurface the patella in those patients with inflammatory arthritis. In two studies comparing patients who underwent patellar resurfacing with those who did not (75, 79), better functional results were noted in the resurfacing group, particularly as concerned stair-climbing.

Two studies have compared bilateral TKAs in which one group of patients underwent resurfacing and the other group did not. Keblish *et al.* (44) found no difference in outcome between the knees, while Enis *et al.* (25) concluded to a trend towards better results in those knees where the patella had been resurfaced. In a prospective randomized study, Barrack *et al.* (8) found no difference in outcome scores or patient satisfaction between a resurfacing and non-resurfacing group of patients, but reported a 10% incidence of secondary resurfacing among the original group whose patella had not been resurfaced. In another prospective randomized study, Bourne *et al.* (12) reported better results as regarded pain and force in flexion in the non-resurfacing group, as well as a revision rate of 4%.

Clinical relevance: The results of TKAs with or without resurfacing of the patella are comparable if careful patient selection is performed. A clear consensus exists that resurfacing the patella is the choice among those patients with rheumatoid arthritis, patellar deformity, primary osteoarthritis, subluxation or dislocation of the patella, patello-femoral chondropathy of grade III or more, severe dysmorphism or incongruency of the patello-femoral articulation, and in aged patients or those with a reduced life expectancy. Resurfacing of the patella should be avoided in patients with a small patella, osteopenia, normal or nearly normal cartilage surfaces, patella baja, and in young and active patients.

The decision of whether or not to resurface a patella depends upon the type of implants utilized, the patient and underlying diagnoses, and the perioperative evaluation of the patello-femoral joint and particularly its kinematics. In fact, this decision rests entirely on the experience of the surgeon.

Opinion of the author: According to Barrack (9), the expected complication rate from resurfacing the patella is 5%. He therefore believes that if one wishes to routinely resurface the patella the surgeon must ensure a rate of complication below 5%. We favor routine patella resurfacing in TKA except for the contraindications previously mentioned. In our institution, 98% of patellae are resurfaced with a complication rate far below 5%.

Specific conditions

Valgus knee

Approximately 90% of patients who present for TKA have a varus deformity of the knee and most studies are of patients of this type. Our literature review revealed only two publications that specifically reported the results of TKA in patients whose knees manifested a pre-operative alignment in greater than 10° of valgus.

Stern *et al.* (87) evaluated the results of 134 postero-stabilized TKAs implanted in patients with a pre-operative valgus alignment equal to or greater than 10°. All the components were cemented and the mean follow-up was 4.5 years. The authors noted 91% of good and excellent results, but the excellent results represented only 71% of the overall results, which is in contrast with the better outcomes achieved in other reports of TKAs with the postero-stabilized prosthesis. Remarkably, peri-operative lateral subluxation of the patella necessitated a lateral release in 76% of patients.

In a report of 51 TKAs with a mean follow-up of 6 years (4), all patients had a pre-operative valgus alignment greater than 10°. Using the Knee Society Score, the authors noted 53% excellent results, 39% of good results, and 49% of patients required a lateral release.

Clinical relevance: Total knee arthroplasty is an efficient, reliable and durable procedure in the treatment of osteoarthritis with valgus alignment. The greater complexity of the lateral compartment anatomy and the relatively rare valgus malalignment make the procedure technically more demanding, particularly with regard to obtaining the correct ligament balance. The technique for implanting a knee prosthesis in a valgus limb differs considerably from that performed in a knee with a varus deformity, specifically with regard to the bony defects present and the ligamentous releases involved (38). Valgus knees tend to present significant erosions on the lateral femoral condyle, while varus knees show a defect more likely on the tibial surface. The deformity of the lateral femoral condyle may render the external rotation positioning of the femoral component very difficult. Surgical experience has taught that if the release of the lateral capsulo-ligamentous complex starts from the femoral side, one will obtain the correct ligamentous balance and assure a satisfactory result at mid-term (87).

Opinion of the authors: Most importantly, pre-operative planning is critical especially as it concerns bone cuts and ligamentous release. We routinely sacrifice the PCL and implant a postero-stabilized design. With a valgus alignment less than 15° we advise a midline approach with a medial parapatellar arthrotomy. In those instances where the valgus deformity is greater than 15° we prefer a lateral approach, often associated with an osteotomy of the tibial tubercle. We routinely perform a lateral release. We then begin our ligamentous release by the section of the PCL followed by the postero-lateral capsule, and then if necessary, the ilio-tibial band, the popliteal tendon, and finally the lateral collateral ligament (LCL). However, section of the LCL should be avoided if possible because it may induce a pathologic lateral laxity which will certainly adversely affect the outcome of the arthroplasty (65).

Patients over 80 years old

Results of total knee arthroplasty in patients over the age of 80 years have been studied by Insall and coworkers (51). They followed 98 patients with a mean age of 82 years at the time of the operation. The mean follow-up was 4.5 years and the majority of the designs implanted were postero-stabilized (71%). Their results revealed 93% good and excellent results.

Clinical relevance: Total knee arthroplasty is an efficient and durable procedure in aged patients who suffer from osteoarthritis. In this category of patient the comorbidities determine the success of the procedure, including the occurrence of peri-operative complications and the mid-term functional outcome.

Aged patients are often less active and their prostheses are subjected to lower mechanical demands. They are therefore at less risk for developing aseptic loosening and an all-polyethylene tibial component may be implanted in such a sedentary, non-obese patient with a rate of success comparable to a metal-backed tibial component (51).

Total knee arthroplasty after high tibial osteotomy

High tibial osteotomy (HTO) has proven its value in delaying the need for a TKA, particularly in patients with high impact recreational activities or those performing heavy labor. However, controversy still exists concerning the results of TKA after HTO. While certain authors have reported less satisfactory results in TKAs after HTO than in primary TKA (43, 61), others have indicated equivalent results in patients with or without previous HTO (5, 10, 64, 91).

Meding (59) compared bilateral TKAs in an homogeneous series of 39 patients who had previously undergone a closing wedge HTO before the TKA on one side and a primary TKA on the contralateral side. The mean follow-up was 7 years, and utilizing the Knee Society Score for pain and function, no difference was found in the outcome. The mechanical axis was 6.3° valgus in the HTO group and 5.2° in the primary TKA group. In 90% of the cases, an extensive release of the lateral compartment was not necessary. To assure a quality outcome in a knee with a previous HTO, the authors recommend a minimal resection of the lateral tibial plateau and insertion of a polyethylene thicker than usual in order to restore the anatomical position of the lateral joint line (as pre-osteotomy) after implantation of the prosthesis.

A recent study of 90 TKAs after HTO revealed results similar to those following primary TKAs (7). At a mean follow-up of 6.5 years, the results of the Knee Society Score for pain and function was slightly inferior in the group undergoing TKA after HTO. Medial-lateral instability was less than 5mm in 90% of the cases and the mean survivorship at 10 years was 90%. The authors recommend that in cases of malalignment greater than 9° the TKA should be accompanied by an osteotomy that corrects the deformity.

Clinical relevance: Patients who have undergone a previous high tibial osteotomy may have important pre-operative differences from others. These include a mechanical axis in a valgus orientation, patella infera, decreased bone stock of the tibial epiphysis, instability and excessive patellar tilting due to the soft tissue retraction. These differences must be strictly analyzed during the pre-operative planning and corrected during surgery (fig. 3). If these differences are carefully considered one can expect the outcome of TKA following a HTO to be comparable to primary TKA. Nevertheless, the surgical procedure is technically more demanding and may have increased complications in patients with a previous osteotomy, and this should be considered when one discusses the indication for an osteotomy in the treatment of osteoarthritis.

Opinion of the authors: In our experience we have not found any difference in outcome between TKA after HTO and primary TKA. We insist on the importance of careful pre-operative planning and on the surgical experience necessary in these patients. Nonetheless, for the past two years, we have opted to perform an opening wedge high tibial osteotomy in indicated patients with early osteoarthritis to help prevent the difficulties that may be encountered during later implantation of a total knee prosthesis.

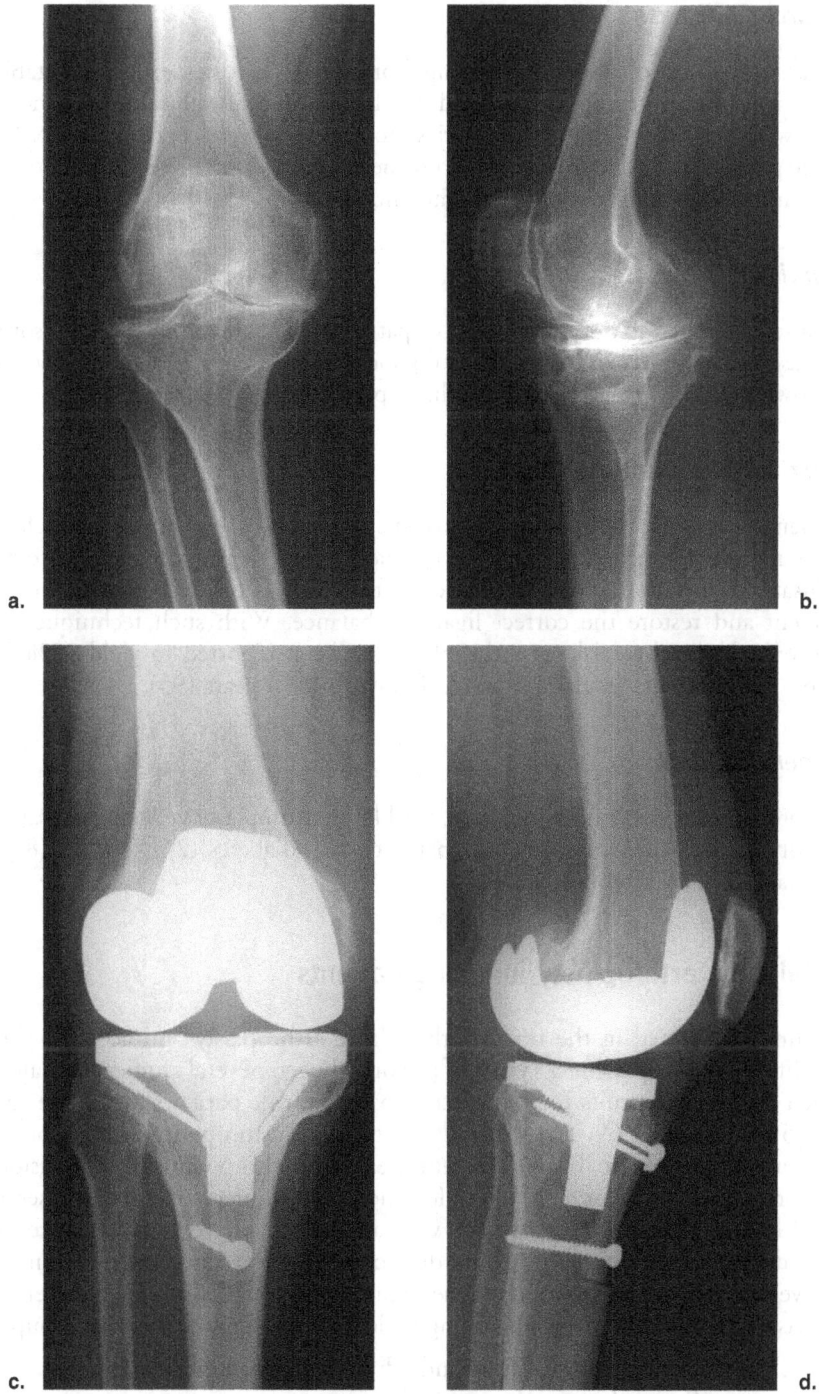

Fig. 3. – Implantation of a knee prosthesis after high tibial osteotomy may be more difficult than a primary TKA (A, B). Sometimes, it is necessary to carry out an osteotomy of the tibial tubercle to correct the malposition of the patella (C, D).

Charcot's disease

In a small series of patients suffering from Charcot's disease, postero-stabilized total knee arthroplasty yielded excellent results in all cases at a mean follow-up of 3 years (80). In this series, bone defects were corrected either by bone graft or by wedges fixed to the prosthetic components. The authors advocate meticulous balancing of the ligaments.

Parkinson's disease

In a series limited to a small number of patients who suffered from Parkinson's disease, Vince et al. (93) demonstrated good and excellent results up to 4 years following TKA with a postero-stabilized prosthesis.

Post-traumatic osteoarthritis

Patients with post-traumatic osteoarthritis present with axis and joint deformity represent a technical challenge for the surgeon. It is mandatory to compensate for any bone defect by bone graft or wedges of the prosthetic component and restore the correct ligament balance. With such techniques, a postero-stabilized total knee arthroplasty has been reported to yield 90% of good and excellent results at a mean follow-up of 4 years (95).

Other conditions

According to reports in the literature, total knee arthroplasty yields highly satisfactory results when performed in patients with diabetes (24), obesity (84), psoriasis (83) or osteonecrosis (82).

Total knee arthroplasty in young patients

"Young" is defined in the framework of knee arthroplasty and according to the literature as a patient 55 years of age or younger. Several studies have analyzed the clinical results in young active osteoarthritic patients under the age of 55 (19, 22, 53, 69, 85). Although total knee arthroplasty in the young patient has proven to be an efficient treatment, the potential for revision surgery in the course of a patient's life-time has prompted surgeons to reserve total knee replacement for patients who are at least 60 years old. Concerns regarding possible aseptic loosening due to wear debris generated by younger active patients over many years is the main reason for the limited number of TKAs performed in this group. Young patients may be divided in two groups:

  – those suffering from juvenile and adult rheumatoid arthritis;
  – those suffering from early osteoarthritis.

In a report in which 86% of the patients were diagnosed with rheumatoid arthritis, Dalury et al. (19) noted highly satisfactory results at a mean follow-up of 7.2 years. 93% of the patients were painfree and the Knee Society Score improved from 37 preoperatively to 93 post-operatively. Although radiolucencies were noted on the femur in 15% of the patients and on the tibia in 13%, no revisions were necessary at the time of the final review. In another series of 93 TKAs where the vast majority (81%) of patients had rheumatoid arthritis, the authors reported 98% of good and excellent results at a follow-up of 6 years (69). The mean postoperative Knee Society Score was 87. Radiographic analysis revealed an incidence of 30% of combined lucencies on the tibia and on the femur, and in two patients this correlated with a poor clinical result. The mean cumulative survivorship at 10 years was 96% overall. The authors concluded that TKAs in this group of young patients resulted in an outcome as durable and satisfactory as that in older patients. Moreover, the results in terms of functional recovery and implant survival were considered better than those following total hip arthroplasty in the same category of patients. However, these good results have always been explained by the low mechanical demands, that the prosthesis is subjected to in patients who suffer from multiple joint disease.

Lonner et al. (53) reported on a multi-center study from members of the Knee Society concerning 32 cemented TKAs implanted in patients under the age of 40 years suffering from osteoarthritis. The mean follow-up was 7.9 years and the analysis of these TKAs revealed 82% of good and excellent results. However, more specifically when utilizing the Knee Society Score, the authors noted only 40% of good and excellent functional results. Remarkably, if cases of pending litigation were excluded, the percentage of good and excellent overall results increased to 91% and the functional results to 50%. The failure rate in this study was 12.5% at an 8 year follow-up. It is noteworthy that 2 of the 3 aseptic loosenings occurred in patients with cementless prostheses. The authors concluded that total knee arthroplasty in young patients, whose functional expectations are much higher than those of older patients, yielded slightly inferior results to those reported in the older population. In another study of 68 cemented TKAs implanted in osteoarthritic patients under 55 years old, the authors noted 81% of excellent and 19% of good results at follow-up of 6.2 years (85). It is the authors' opinion that TKA in patients under the age of 55 years is recommended when indicated and yields mid-term results similar to those seen in older patients. However, these patients need to accept a more sedentary life-style and the limitation to low-impact activities.

The major limitation of all these studies is the absence of specific analysis of the daily and sports activities of the patients undergoing TKA. Diduch et al. (22) reported on 103 cemented postero-stabilized TKAs performed in 80 osteoarthritic patients with a mean age of 51 years (22-55 years). Mean follow-up was 8 years, but more than 35% of the patients were followed for more than 10 years, thus allowing determination of a mean survivorship. The patients were evaluated with the Knee Society Score, the HSS score and activity scores such as the Tegner and the Lysholm scores. In this series, 94% of patients had good and excellent results and the Tegner score improved from 1.3 points (range: 0-4 points) preoperatively to 3.5 points (range: 1-6 points)

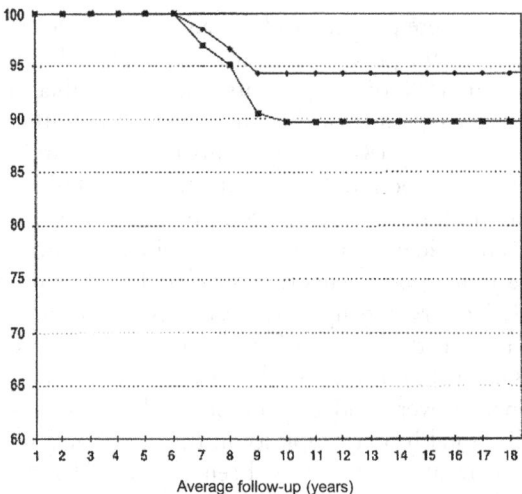

Fig. 4. – Kaplan-Meier survivorship of TKR performed in young patients (mean age 51 years). Diamonds plot the survival curve when revision of the femoral and tibial components are considered as the end-point. Squares draw the survival curve when revision of the femoral, tibial and patellar components are considered as the end-point.
(From Diduch DR, Insall JN, Scott N *et al.* [1997] Total knee replacement in young, active patients: long-term follow-up and functional outcome. J Bone Joint Surg 79-A: 575-82. Adapted with permission.)

postoperatively. The most frequent sports activity performed was walking with a mean distance of 3.2 kilometers (60% of the patients). Stationary or outdoor bicycling was the second most frequently performed activity (53% of the patients). Other activities included golfing (24% of the patients) and running on a treadmill (20% of the patients). Additional patients performed aerobic or stair-master exercises, tennis, trekking or hunting, construction or farm work, and alpine skiing. At last follow-up, 9% of the TKAs revealed radio-lucencies on the femoral and tibial sides. Utilizing revision of the femur and/or tibial component as the end-point, the mean survivorship of these TKA was 94% at 18 years follow-up. Three patients underwent revision of the patellar component only, and if these three revisions were included in the calculation of survival data, the mean survivorship was 90% (fig. 4).

As we have already discussed, the expected benefits of an arthroplasty are the reduction of pain, correction of malalignment, and functional improvement. While twenty years ago the major objective of the arthroplasty was to dramatically reduce pain, young patients actually believe that the gain in function is as important as the decrease in pain. Thus, sports activities following TKA have been studied by several authors. Bradbury *et al.* (13) assessed 160 patients (208 TKAs) as regarded their participation in sports postoperatively. Of 79 patients (45%) who had participated at least once a week in a sport activity prior to surgery, 45 (65%) still participated at the same level post arthroplasty. Of this group, 20% had resumed high impact activities such as tennis, but the majority (91%) had opted for low impact activities such as walking or bowling. Laporte *et al.* (50) reviewed 11 patients (18 TKAs) with a mean age of 72 years (47-89 years) who had played tennis preoperatively, and at a mean follow-up of 3.2 years all the patients were very satisfied with their operation. Two studies conducted with members of the Knee Society (56, 57) specifically looked at golfers and TKA. 93% of the surgeons questioned recommended, or at least did not discourage, that their patients play golf. 96% of the surgeons estimated that golf practice was not responsible for increasing the rate of complications among their patients. 60% of surgeons recommended the use of a golf cart after knee replacement. The same authors studied a separate cohort of 83 recreational golf players. Of this group, 84% had no pain while playing golf, but 35% noted moderate pain in the operated knee afterwards. Players complained more often of pain in the operated left knee than in the operated right knee.

The level of pre-operative athletic activity is an important factor in recommending athletic activity after joint replacement. Patients who have achieved high levels of skill in specific athletic events have the best chance of safely resuming these activities (32). The best example of this is skiing. Expert skiers can usually resume their sport safely, especially when they limit themselves to intermediate trails without moguls and with good snow conditions. One must remember that perhaps the most important determinant of whether or not a patient can participate in athletics after a joint replacement operation is the quality of the joint reconstruction. The importance of an anatomically and biomechanically accurate joint reconstruction with a well-designed implant and a properly balanced soft tissue/muscular envelope cannot be underestimated. Technically, the use of cobalt-chrome alloys and titanium alloys, polyethylene components of the appropriate thickness, and a cemented fixation will yield a high-quality result and the potential for the patient to resume athletic activities.

Patients who participate in athletic activity after joint replacement place themselves at greater risk for traumatic complications, as compared with those patients who remain more sedentary. Although dislocation is rare after TKA in general, it is more common with postero-stabilized implants. Excessive flexion of the components can cause disengagement of the tibial post from the femoral cam. Traumatic rupture of the PCL in a PCL-retaining implant may result in an anterior-posterior instability that will require revision arthroplasty. Patello-femoral problems represent 5% of all complications after TKA (6). Patello-femoral instability depends upon limb alignment, implant position, implant rotation, and soft tissue balancing. Peri-prosthetic fractures are rare (less than 1%) after primary knee replacement in the younger patient and usually occur after a severe trauma (6), in contrast to their more frequent occurrence from a low energy mechanism of injury in the older osteopenic patient.

Recommended sports after total knee arthroplasty include sailing, swimming, scuba diving, cycling, golfing, hiking, cross-country skiing and bowling. Activities that should be discouraged include running, water skiing, soccer, football, basketball, ice hockey, handball, karate, and racquetball. A study conducted by Healy (32) in collaboration with 58 surgeons and all members of the Knee Society analyzed the recommendations given to patients by different surgeons with respect to postoperative athletic activities. 42 athletic activities were presented to the surgeons who were asked to classify them into four groups, including "recommended/allowed", "allowed with experience", "not recommended", and "no opinion". The 58 responses were analyzed with a statistical program to determine a consensus recommendation (table III).

Table III. – Sport activities after Total Knee Arthroplasty (Knee Society Survey).

Recommended/ allowed	Allowed with preop experience	Not recommended	No opinion
Aerobics (low impact)	Road cycling	Racquetball	Fencing
Cycling (stationary)	Canoeing	Climbing	Rollerskating
Bowling	Trekking	Football	Alpin skiing
Golfing	Rowing	Tennis (single)	Body building
Dancing	Cross country skiing	Volleyball	
Equitation	Nordic walking	Gymnastic	
Hiking	Tennis (double)	Ice hockey	
Swimming	Low weight strengh-	Basketball	
Shooting	thening	Jogging	
Scuba diving	Ice skating	Power walking	
Sailing	Recreational dancing	handball	
		Unlimited stair climbing	
		Field hockey	
		Baseball	

From: Healy WL, Ioro R, Lemos MJ (2001) Athletic activity after joint replacement. Am J Sports 29: 377-88, with permission.

Clinical relevance: Total knee arthroplasty is a successful and long-lasting treatment in young patients who suffer from rheumatoid arthritis. The results are more controversial as regards the patient with juvenile rheumatoid arthritis. Total knee arthroplasty also appears to be a reasonable option in the treatment of a disabling osteoarthritic knee in a young patient. Nevertheless, the indication for TKA must be discussed in detail with patients under the age of 40 years whose expectations and functional demands may endanger a successful mid-term outcome of the knee replacement. And in cases of pending litigation, the situation should be clarified before the knee replacement surgery. It is not clear whether active patients are better served by a PCL-retaining or a postero-stabilized implant. Rand *et al.* (71) and Diduch *et al.* (22) have reported no difference between these two designs in young patients. While surgeons should make the choice with respect to their broader experience, it is advised that polyethylene thickness should be equal to or greater than 10mm and fixation should be with acrylic cement (22). Athletic activity increases the stresses on a prosthetic knee at the bone-cement-implant interfaces and at the joint bearing surface (32). Moreover, it has been demonstrated that cement is an excellent barrier against polyethylene debris that subsequently leads to aseptic loosening (17, 41, 46). The particular attention paid to the alignment of the prosthesis and the balancing of the ligaments and soft tissues may reduce the eccentric and shearing forces upon the implant and increase its longevity.

Low impact athletic activities (walking, swimming, cycling) can be safely recommended after total knee arthroplasty, but one must approach more strenuous activities, such as cross-country and downhill skiing, depending upon the preoperative skill of the patient.

Opinion of the authors: In young patients suffering from rheumatoid arthritis, we are now more aggressive than previously in performing a total knee arthroplasty. In contrast, we have not changed our approach for the young patient with an osteoarthritic knee. In these patients we first turn to other surgical options (osteotomy, arthroscopy) in order to defer the arthroplasty. However, we have noticed that the young patients we are used to treating are more active, appreciate outdoor activities, often in the mountains, and are skiing at an expert level. In such young patients, we favor a cemented, semi-constrained, condylar, postero-stabilized design, with a metal-backed tibial component. We do not discourage our patients from participating in reasonable low impact athletic activities when they are prepared and trained for such sport, and when they understand the risks involved. Intermediate activities such as cross-country skiing are allowed depending upon pre-operative experience and level of practice. We strongly discourage our patients from participating in high impact athletic activities. In all cases athletic activities are not permitted until the quadriceps and hamstring muscles are sufficiently rehabilitated. Only exceptionally do we allow participation in alpine skiing, because our young active patients are often expert alpine skiers using carving skis that may generate high eccentric and shearing loads and thus compromise the long-term outcome of the knee replacement.

References

1. Aglietti P (2001) Total knee replacement in the relatively young and active patient with osteoarthritis. ISAKOS book: 9-14
2. Aglietti P, Buzzi R, Gaudeni A (1988) Patello-femoral functional results and complications with the posterior stabilized total condylar knee prosthesis. J Arthroplasty 3: 17
3. Aglietti P, Buzzi R (1988) Posterior stabilized total knee replacement: Three to eight years' follow-up of 85 knees. J Bone Joint Surg Br 7 : 211
4. Aglietti P, Buzzi R, Giron F et al. (1996) The Insall-Burstein posterior stabilized total knee replacement in the valgus knee. Am J Knee Surg 9: 8
5. Amendola A, Rorabeck CH, Bourne RB et al. (1989) Total knee arthroplasty following high tibial osteotomy for osteoarthritis. J Arthroplasty 4: S11-S17
6. Ayers DC, Dennis DA, Johanson NA et al. (1997) Common complications of total knee arthroplasty . J Bone Joint Surg 79-A: 278-311
7. Badet R, Selmi TAS, Neyret P et al. Total knee arthroplasty after failed high tibial osteotomy. ISAKOS Montreux meeting book: 4.61
8. Barrack RL, Wolfe MW, Waldman DA et al. (1997) Resurfacing of the patella in total knee arthroplasty. J Bone Joint Surg 79-A: 1121-31
9. Barrack RL (2000) The patella in total knee arthroplasty. Instructional course lecture. American Academy of Orthopaedic Surgeons 67th Annual Meeting, Orlando
10. Bergenudd H, Sahlström A, Sanzen L (1997) Total knee arthroplasty after failed proximal tibial valgus osteotomy. J Arthroplasty 12: 635-8
11. Boyd AD Jr, Ewald FC, Thomas WH et al. (1993) Long-term complications after total knee arthroplasty with or without resurfacing of the patella. J Bone Joint Surg 75-A: 674-81
12. Bourne RB, Rorabeck CH, Vaz M et al. (1995) Resurfacing versus not resurfacing the patella during total knee arthroplasty. Clin Orthop 321: 156-61
13. Bradbury N, Borton D, Spoo G et al. (1998) Participation in sports after total knee replacement. Am J Sports Med 26: 530-5
14. Buechel FF, Pappas MJ (1989) New Jersey low-contact stress knee replacement system. Orthop Clin North Am 20: 147
15. Burks RT (1990) Arthroscopy of degenerative arthritis of the knee. Arthroscopy 6: 43-7
16. Campbell WC (1940) Interposition of vitallium plates in arthroplasties of the knee: Preliminary report. Am J Surg 47: 639

17. Chiba J, Schwendeman LJ, Booth RE *et al.* (1994) A biochemical, histologic, and immunohistologic analysis of membranes obtained from failed cemented and cementless total knee arthroplasty. Clin Orthop 299: 124-44

18. Colizza WA, Insall JN, Scuderi GR (1995) The posterior stabilized total knee prosthesis. Assessment of polyethylene damage and osteolysis after a ten-year minimum follow-up. J Bone Joint Surg 77-A: 1713

19. Dalury DF, Ewald FC, Christie MJ *et al.* (1995) Total knee arthroplasty in a group of patients less than 45 years of age. J Arthroplasty 5: 598-602

20. Dandy DJ, Jackson RW (1975) The diagnosis of problems after meniscectomy. J Bone Joint Surg 57-B: 349-52

21. Dandy DJ (1986) Abrasion chondroplasty. Arthroscopy 2: 51-3

22. Diduch DR, Insall JN, Scott N *et al.* Total knee replacement in young, active patients: Long term follow-up and functional outcome. J Bone Joint Surg 79-A: 575-82

23. Duffy GP, Berry DJ, Rand JA (1998) Cement *versus* cementless fixation in total knee arthroplasty. Clin Orthop 356: 66-72

24. England SP, Stern SH, Insall JN *et al.* (1990) Total knee arthroplasty in diabetes mellitus. Clin Orthop 260: 130

25. Enis JE, Gardner R, Robledo MA *et al.* (1995) Comparison of patellar resurfacing *versus* nonresurfacing in bilateral total knee arthroplasty. Clin Orthop 260: 38-42

26. Eriksson E, Haggmark T (1982) Knee pain in the middle aged runner. In: AAOS symposium; the foot and leg in running sports. St. Louis: CV Mosby, 106-8

27. Ferguson W (1861) Excision of the knee joint: Recovery with a false joint and useful limb. Med Times Gaz 1: 601

28. Freeman MAR, Swanson SAV, Todd RC (1973) Total replacement of the knee using the Freeman-Swanson knee prosthesis. Clin Orthop 94: 153

29. Goodfellow JW, O'Connor J (1986) Clinical results of Oxford knee. Clin Orthop 205: 21

30. Goodfellow JW, O'Connor J (1992) The anterior cruciate ligament in knee arthroplasty. Clin Orthop 276: 245

31. Gunston FH (1971) Polycentric knee arthroplasty: Prosthetic simulation of normal knee movement. J Bone Joint Surg Br 53: 271

32. Healy WL, Iorio R, Lemos MJ (2001) Athletic activity after joint replacement. AM J Sports Med 29: 377-88

33. Holden DL, James SL, Larson RL *et al.* (1988) Proximal tibial osteotomy in patients who are fifty years old or less. Along term follow-up study. J Bone Joint Surg 70-A: 977-82

34. Hubbard MJS (1996) Articular debridement versus washout for degeneration of the medial femoral condyle. J Bone Joint Surg 78-B: 217-9

35. Hungerford DS, Krackow KA, Kenna RV (1989) Cementless total knee replacement in patients 50 years old and under. Orthop Clin North Am 20: 131

36. Insall JN (1967) Intra-articular surgery for degenerative arthritis of the knee. A report of the work of the late K.H. Pridie. J Bone Joint Surg 49-B: 211-28

37. Insall JN (1974) The Pridie debridement operation for osteoarthritis of the knee. Clin Orthop 101: 61-9

38. Insall JN, Scott WN, Ranawat CS (1979) The total condylar knee prosthesis: A report of two hundred and twenty cases. J Bone Joint Surg 61-A: 173

39. Jackson RW, McCarthy DD (1971) Arthroscopy of the knee in osteoarthritis. Gordon DA, ed. Proceedings of the fourth Canadian conference in the rheumatic diseases. University of Toronto Press, 293

40. Jackson RW (1974) The role of arthroscopy in the management of the arthritic knee. Clin Orthop 101: 28-35

41. Jacobs JJ, Shanbhag A, Glant TT *et al.* (1994) Wear debris in total joints replacements. J Am Acad Orthop Surgeons 2: 212-20

42. Jordan LR, Olivo JL, Voorhost PE (1997) Survivorship analysis of cementless meniscal bearing total knee arthroplasty. Clin Orthop 338: 173

43. Katz MM, Hungerford DS, Krakow KA (1987) Results of total knee arthroplasty after failed proximal tibial osteotomy for osteoarthritis. J Bone Joint Surg 69-A: 225-33

44. Keblish PA, Varma AK, Greenwald AS (1994) Patellar resurfacing or retention in total knee arthroplasty. J Bone Joint Surg 76-B: 930-7
45. Kelly M (2001) Knee kinematics. In: Total knee replacement in the relatively young and active patients with osteoarthritis. ISAKOS Knee Committee, p. 25
46. Kilgus DJ, Moreland JR, Finerman GA et al. (1991) Catastrophic wear of tibial polyethylene inserts. Clin Orthop 273: 223-31
47. Knight JL, Atwater RD, Grothaus L (1997) Clinical results of the modular porous-coated anatomic (PCA) total knee arthroplasty with cement: A 5-year prospective study. Orthopedics 20: 1025
48. Kobs JK, Lackiewicz PF (1993) Hybrid total knee arthroplasty. Clin Orthop 226: 78
49. Komistek RD, Dennis DA (2001) Fluoroscopic analysis of total knee replacement. In: Surgery of the Knee. Ed. Insall & Scott, Churchill Livingston 3rd Ed, 1695-1704
50. LaPorte DM, Mont MA, Hungerford DS et al. (1999) Characterization of tennis players who have a total knee arthroplasty. Proceedings in the 66th Annual Meeting of the AAOS, p. 171
51. L'Insallata JC, Stern SH, Insall JN (1992) Total knee arthroplasty in elderly patients: Comparison of tibial component designs. J Arthroplasty 7: 261
52. Livesley PJ, Doherty M, Needoff M et al. (1991) Arthroscopic lavage of osteoarthritic knees. J Bone Joint Surg 73-B: 922-6
53. Lonner JH, Hershman S, Mont M et al. (2000) Total knee arthroplasty in patients 40 years of age and younger with osteoarthritis. Clin Orthop 380: 85-90
54. McCaskie AW, Dechan DJ, Green TP et al. (1998) Randomized, prospective study comparing cemented and cementless total knee replacement. J Bone Joint Surg 80-B: 971-5
55. Magnusson PB (1941) Joint debridement: Surgical treatment of degenerative arthritis. Surg Gynecol Obstet 73: 1-4
56. Mallon WJ, Callaghan JJ (1993) Total knee arthroplasty in active golfers. J Arthroplasty 8: 299-306
57. Mallon WJ, Liebelt RA, Mason JB (1996) Total joint replacement and golf. Clin Sports Med 15: 179-90
58. Martin SD, McManus JL, Scott RD et al. (1997) Press-fit condylar total knee arthroplasty. J Arthroplasty 12: 203
59. Meding JB, Keating EM, Ritter MA et al. (2000) Total knee arthroplasty after high tibial osteotomy: A comparison study in patients who had bilateral total knee replacement. J Bone Joint Surg 82-A: 1252-9
60. Ménétrey J, Siegrist O, Fritschy D et al. (2001) Medial meniscectomy in patients over the age of fifty: A six year follow-up study. Submitted Swiss Surgery
61. Mont MA, Antonaides S, Krackow KA et al. (1994) Total knee arthroplasty after failed high tibial osteotomy : a comparison with a matched group. Clin Orthop 299: 125-30
62. Morrey BF (1989) Upper tibial osteotomy for secondary osteoarthritis of the knee. J Bone Joint Surg 71-A: 554-9
63. Naudie D, Bourne RB, Rorabeck CH et al. (1999) The Insall Award. Survivorship of the high tibial osteotomy. A 10- to 22-year follow-up study. Clin Orthop 367: 18-27
64. Nizard RS, Cardinne L, Bizot P et al. (1998) Total knee replacement after failed tibial osteotomy : results of a matched-pair study. J Arthroplasty 13: 847-53
65. Peters CL, Mohr RA, Bachus KN (2001) Primary total knee arthroplasty in the valgus knee creating a balanced soft tissue envelope. Trans Orthop Res 47: 1105, San Francisco
66. Picetti GD III, McGann WA, Welch RB (1990) The patellofemoral joint after total knee arthroplasty without patellar resurfacing. J Bone Joint Surg 72-A: 1379-82
67. Pridie KH (1959) A method of resurfacing osteoarthritic knee joints. J Bone Joint Surg 41-B: 618-9
68. Ranawat CS, Luessenhop CP, Rodriguez JA (1997) The press-fit condylar modular total knee system. Four-to-six-year results with a posterior-cruciate-substituting design. J Bone Joint Surg 79-A: 342
69. Ranawat CS, Padgett DE, Ohashi Y (1989) Total knee arthroplasty for patients younger than 55 years. Clin Orthop 248: 27-33

70. Rand JA, Ilstrup DM (1991) Survivorship analysis of total knee arthroplasty: Cumulative rates of survival of 9200 total knee arthroplasties. J Bone Joint Surg 73-A: 397
71. Rand JA (19991) Cement or cementless fixation in total knee arthroplasty? Clin Orthop 273: 168
72. Rosenberg AG, Barden R, Galante JO (1989) A comparison of cemented and cementless fixation with the Miller-Galante total knee arthroplasty. Orthop Clin North Am 20: 97
73. Sansén L, Sahlström A, Gentz CF et al. (1996) Radiographic wear assessment in a total knee prosthesis. J Arthroplasty 11: 738
74. Schopfer A (1993) L'arthroplastie totale du genou à Genève de 1979 à 1987. Thèse de doctorat # 9455 de la Faculté de Médecine de l'Université de Genève
75. Schroeder-Boersch H, Scheller G, Fischer J et al. (1998) Advantages of patellar resurfacing in total knee arthroplasty. Two year results of a prospective randomized study. Arch Orthop Trauma Surg 117: 73-8
76. Scott RD, Volatile TB (1986) Twelve years' experience with posterior cruciate retaining total knee arthroplasty. Clin Orthop 205: 100
77. Scott WN, Rubinstein M, Scuderi G (1988) Results after knee replacement with a posterior cruciate substituting prosthesis. J Bone Joint Surg 70-A: 1163
78. Scott WN, Insall JN, Kelly MA (1993) Arthroscopy and Meniscectomy: Surgical Approaches, Anatomy and Techniques. In: Surgery of the knee, Insall JN (ed). New York, Churchill Livingstone, p. 165-216
79. Shoji J, Yoshino S, Kajino A (1989) Patellar replacement in bilateral total knee arthroplasty. J Bone Joint Surg 71-A: 853-6
80. Soudry M, Binazzi R, Johansson NA et al. (1986) Total knee arthroplasty in Charcot and Charcot-like joints. Clin Orthop 208: 1999
81. Sprague NF (1981) Arthroscopic debridement for degenerative knee joint disease. Clin Orthop 160: 118-23
82. Stern SH, Insall JN, Windsor RE (1988) Total knee arthroplasty in osteonecrotic knees. Orthop Trans 12: 722
83. Stern SH, Insall JN, Windsor RE et al. (1989) Total knee arthroplasty in patients with psoriasis. Clin Orthop 248: 108
84 Stern SH, Insall JN (1990) Total knee arthroplasty in obese patients. J Bone Joint Surg 72-A: 1400
85. Stern SH, Insall JN (1990) Posterior stabilized prosthesis: Total knee arthroplasty in obese patients. J Bone Joint Surg 72-A: 1400
86. Stern SH, Bowen MK, Insall JN et al. (1990) Cemented total knee arthroplasty for gonarthrosis in patients 55 years old or younger. Clin Orthop 260: 124-9
87. Stern SH, Moeckel BH, Insall JN (1991) Total knee arthroplasty in valgus knees. Clin Orthop 273: 5
88. Stern SH, Insall JN (1992) Posterior stabilized prosthesis: Results after 9-12 years follow-up of nine to twelve years. J Bone Joint Surg 74-A: 980
89. Tayot O, Adam Ph, Neyret Ph (1999) Résultats des prothèses totales du genou HLS-1. In: La chirurgie prothétique du genou et de l'épaule. 9e Journées Lyonnaises. Edit. Chambat P, Walch G, Neyret Ph et al. :115-30
90. Tocksvig-Larsen S, Ryd L, Stenström A et al. (1996) The porous-coated anatomic total knee experience. J Arthroplasty 11: 11
91. Toksvig-Larsen S, Magyar G, Önsten I et al. (1998) Fixation of the tibial component of total knee arthroplasty after high tibial osteotomy. A matched radiostereometric study. J Bone Joint Surg 80-B: 295-7
92. Verneuil A (1860) De la création d'une fausse articulation par section ou résection partielle de l'os maxillaire inférieur, comme moyen de remédier à l'ankylose vraie ou fausse de la mâchoire inférieure. Arch Gen Med 15 (ser. 5): 174
93. Vince KG, Insall JM, Bannerman CE (1989) Total knee arthroplasty in the patient with Parkinson's disease. J Bone Joint Surg 71-B: 793
94. Wright RJ et al. (1990) Two to four year results of posterior cruciate sparing condylar total knee arthroplasty with an uncemented femoral component. Clin Orthop 260: 80
95. Zelicof SB, Scuderi GR, Vince KG et al. (1988) Total knee arthroplasty in post-traumatic arthritis. Orthop Trans 12: 547

Failure mechanisms in total knee arthroplasty

M. Bonnin

Total knee replacement is now a reliable, reproducible procedure with a high survival rate. Failures may nevertheless occur because of unexplained pain, an objective mechanical problem which requires replacement of all or part of the prosthesis, or infection.

We will deal here only with problems related to objective failure of the tibiofemoral implant, such as loosening or instability, or to unexplained pain. Complications related to the extensor apparatus as well as the problem of infected implants will be addressed elsewhere.

Management of a failed total knee replacement has a double aim: Firstly diagnosis of the immediate reason for failure, such as loosening or instability, which we will call the "cause of failure", and secondly analysis of the mechanisms which led to this failure, which we will call "factors of failure". These may be surgeon-related (malpositioning, poor soft tissue balance, faulty implant fixation), implant-related (quality of the polyethylene, alloys used, design) or patient-related (concomitant arthritis in particular of the hip at a higher or the ankle at a lower level, major bone deficiency, previous knee surgery). The incidence of these "secondary" factors of failure has been assessed at 36% (surgeon), 14% (implant) and 33% (patient) (7). Analysis of failure is of fundamental importance, so that the initial underlying cause is not reproduced if the implant is replaced.

Precise, complete evaluation is a necessity in order to anticipate the technical difficulties of any revision surgery and to plan other procedures if necessary. If implant failure was related to an underlying hip disorder (hip arthrodesis, congenital subluxation) this should be treated before considering revision. At a lower level, the same applies to the knee: Valgus flat foot deformity related to degenerative posterior tibial tendon rupture may cause progressive valgus tilt of the prosthesis. The hindfoot axis must then be corrected by subtalar and mediotarsal arthrodesis before considering a new implant.

Full investigation should include:

– Study of radiographs obtained since insertion of the primary prosthesis;
– Complete clinical examination, without forgetting the adjacent joints;
– Full X-ray work-up with weight bearing views, axial views of the patella and goniometry.

In some cases more precise investigation is required: Dynamic views to search for "hidden instability", fluoroscopic views to obtain a better view of the bone/prosthesis interface, lateral views in flexion to look for a posterior drawer or tilting of the components. Comparative views performed by the same radiologist and at the same magnification may be useful to reveal an oversized prosthesis. CT scan (6) should be requested if rotational malposition is suspected, in particular in the case of patellofemoral failure or external flexion instability. Some authors consider this investigation should be routinely done before revision of total knee arthroplasty. Technetium bone scan is useful in particular if there is unexplained pain or suspicion of infection, and can be completed if necessary by a gallium or labeled neutrophil scan. A complete laboratory work-up should always be done to look for an inflammatory syndrome. Joint aspiration may be useful for diagnosis (bacterial culture, search for bacterial nucleic acids, polyethylene particles) and some authors (20) believe it should be routinely performed before total knee revision so that infection can be definitely excluded.

After these investigations, the reasons for failure are generally clear and total knee revision is then only a technical problem. In some cases, no objective cause of pain can be found and a choice must be made between systematic revision arthroplasty or surgical or arthroscopic investigation.

Aseptic loosening

Aseptic loosening is the main cause of implant failure, occurring on average seven years after the first insertion (7, 8, 13, 46). It is due to failed component fixation, generally involving the tibia and leading to revision arthroplasty. Certain authors consider that loosening is related to progressively increasing micromotion at the fixation (12). If this is in fact the case, prevention requires maximum fixation with deep penetration of the cement in the subchondral bone. Others consider it is due to the implant sinking into demineralised or necrotic bone (37, 71). On this assumption, prevention requires maximum sparing of subchondral bone, in particular by restricting the penetration of cement which could reduce its viability. Walker (85) considers that optimal penetration is 3mm. In any case, loosening generally follows excessive strain on the implant, due sometimes to faulty initial fixation, sometimes to premature polyethylene wear which causes osteolysis by release of intra-articular foreign bodies. This complication occurs in both cemented and cementless implants. The diagnosis is generally made when secondary pain appears after a pain-free interval. More rarely, the prosthesis was painful immediately after surgery, which should raise the suspicion of early infection or faulty initial fixation. Sometimes it is routine radiographic check-up which reveals signs of loosening. In all cases of loosening thorough investigation is imperative to detect latent infection.

Diagnosis relies primarily on radiography, which can reveal a radiolucent line, component displacement or osteolytic lesions and is easy when a radiolucent line and component displacement are evident (fig. 1). It may be difficult, and new images of perfect quality are required, obtained under image intensifdier with the ray perfectly parallel to the metal baseplate. A 3° deviation of the X-ray beam relative to the bone/prosthesis interface is enough to obscure a radiolucent line 2mm wide (52). The existence of a radiolucent line elsewhere is not in itself a synonym of loosening. The cement/bone interface is in fact not static and even if initially the cement penetrates the trabecular bone satisfactorily, localised bone resorption may occur and intervening fibrous tissue may be built up. This generally occurs during the first six months (81) and in order to affirm that a radiolucent line is abnormal, its gradual progression after that time is of fundamental importance. Ewald (24) codified the following definitive criteria of loosening: A radiolucent line of more than 2mm whatever its location, a radiolucent line extending over the entire surface of the tibial plateau, a radiolucent line in zones 5-6-7 or a progressive radiolucent line (fig. 2). Sometimes, particularly in cementless prostheses, indirect signs must suffice to establish a diagnosis, such as metallosis or osteolytic lesions (fig. 3).

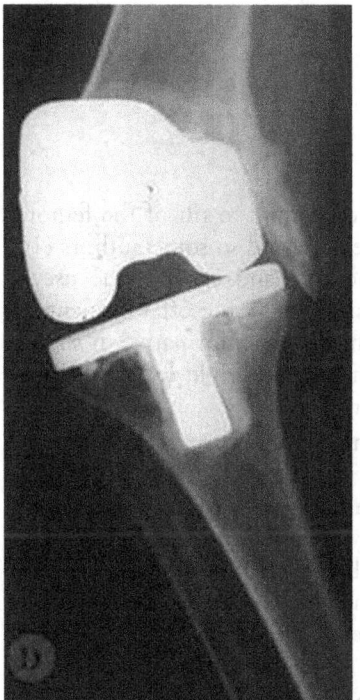

Dynamic views or fluoroscopic evaluation may sometimes be necessary to reveal minimal loosening. Fehring (27), in 20 patients with pain unaccounted for on plain radiographs, found that fluoroscopically-guided radiographs revealed a significant radiolucent line in 14 cases. Loosening was always confirmed at revision.

Routine investigation has usually included technetium 99 bone scan but its diagnostic value is limited, as increased isotope uptake, particularly in the tibia, can persist for several years after surgery. False positives are frequent (7) and it is difficult to decide on revision on bone scan arguments alone.

Isolated loosening of the femoral component is rare and difficult to demonstrate on radiographs, particularly with a cementless prosthesis (14, 44). It is asso-

Fig. 1 – Femoral loosening with migration of the implant.

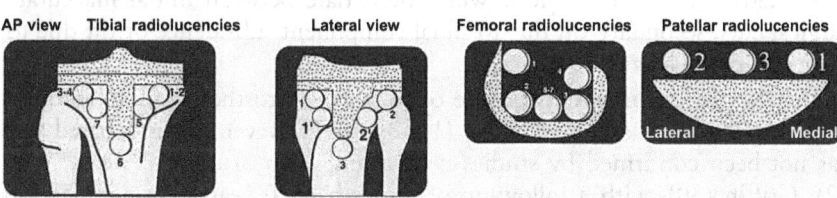

Fig. 2 – The various zones of the bone/prosthesis interface.

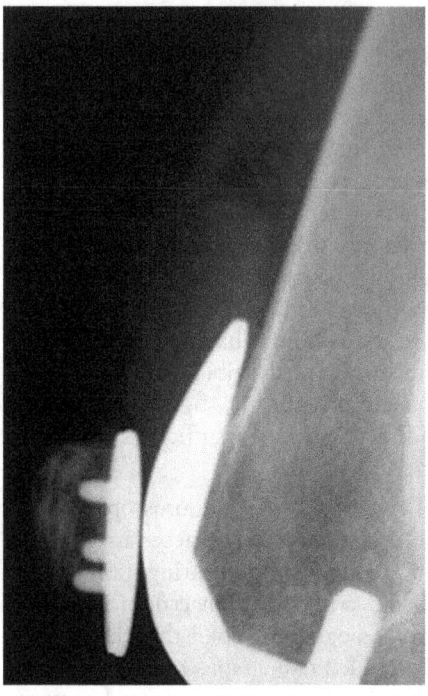

Fig. 3 – Metallosis seen as densification of the suprapatellar pouch.

ciated with osteolysis of the posterior condyles leading to tilt of the femoral component in flexion. Stresses in this area are high and so some authors (14, 44) emphasize the quality of posterior cementing and criticise the use of cementless femoral components. Isolated femoral loosening often presents as unexplained pain because standard radiographs are not informative. It should thus be carefully looked for as revision will make it possible to establish the diagnosis and change the loosened component (44).

Several causes can account for aseptic loosening, the main cause being initial malposition of the prosthesis (27% of cases) (7). This is usually tibial varus but may sometimes be an abnormality of the tibial slope or an oblique joint line on an axis which is generally satisfactory. The harmful impact of varus alignment has been stressed in several clinical (37, 40, 50, 57) and biomechanical (36) studies which have shown increased stresses on the internal compartment in varus. Others, however, found no relation between malposition and loosening (35, 73, 78)

In a varus deformity associated with loosening, study of serial radiographs, goniometry and dynamic views will differentiate between initial inaccurate surgical cuts, secondary tilt due to tibial component subsidence or tilt due to poor soft tissue balance.

Overweight is a theoretical cause of total knee prosthesis failure through loosening related to excessive strain (1, 38, 39). However, this is debated and has not been confirmed by studies with a follow-up of up to 7 years (55, 72). Griffin (30), with a follow-up of more than 10 years, did not observe more frequent loosening in overweight patients. Nevertheless, after this time,

25% of obese patients presented a radiolucent line (< 2mm) compared with 4% of non-obese patients. In this study, the criterion for obesity was a body mass index greater than 30kg/m^2, or 86.7kg for a height of 1.70m.

Implant size has been incriminated by some authors, as an implant which is too small may have a high risk of subsidence (65, 84). Deroches (17) did not corroborate this finding, and obtaining peripheral cortical support for the tibial component at any cost is not an absolute requirement.

FaultyF initial fixation (57) may be a cause of loosening for both cemented and cementless implants. Cementing must be done with meticulous care, with good preparation of the resected surfaces; these must be flat to allow homogeneous support of the tibial plate and cement penetration, which may require local preparation if there is bone condensation. If the procedure is carried out without a tourniquet, the bony surfaces must be clean and dry when cementing is done, and here a pulsed lavage gun is useful.

The patient's physical activity is a factor of loosening which should not be neglected, particularly in the young subject. In the hip, a 100% loosening rate at 10 years has been described in patients aged less than 45 years (15, 18) and the risk is increased two-fold if sports are practised (41). Some studies however found contrary results with decreased risk of loosening if patients participated in sports (19, 83). Regarding the knee, such a relation has not been clearly established and most series on total knee replacement in young subjects include a majority of cases of rheumatoid arthritis, where low activity leads to bias in the results. Lonner (49) in a series of 32 total knee arthroplasties in patients aged under 40 years observed 9.4% of mechanical loosening which had required revision at 8 years follow-up and 11.5% if radiographic loosening was taken into account. Bradbury (11) noted that 65% of patients who had previously participated in sports resumed sporting activity and at 5 years follow-up the number of revisions was not higher in this group. LaPorte (45) with a 3-year follow-up of tennis players and Healy (33) with golfers made the same observation for tennis and the same remarks concerning follow-up. However, increased sports-related risk of implant loosening only became evident after 10 years for the hip and follow-up is still too short in total knee replacement series.

Polyethylene wear is a factor in loosening as it releases particles which cause osteolysis (see below).

Theoretically, bone quality may be responsible. In rheumatoid arthritis (RA), the strength of trabecular bone is decreased and depending on the area it may be only 11% to 26% of normal values (4). However, this relative osteopenia is not reflected in a higher rate of mechanical implant loosening in RA and Ranawat (65) observed a 15-year survival rate of 95.2% in RA compared with 91.1% in arthrosis. Tayot (77) found the risk of septic loosening was higher in the first 3 years but after that time the survival curve in RA was stable and at 14 years the HLS I prosthesis had an 86% survival rate, all causes and reasons for revision included, compared with 94% in RA.

Prosthesis design plays an important role through the strain it brings to bear. If the design of the joint surfaces causes increased strain, this is transferred to the fixation, thus increasing the rate of loosening. An extreme case is the hinged implant, which has a high rate of aseptic loosening from 2 years of follow-up (3, 21, 60). On the other extremity, the use of mobile trays reduces strain on the fixation and prostheses which retain both cruciate ligaments are theoretically the ideal way of protecting the fixation (86).

Instability

Instability is a frequent cause of knee replacement failure, necessitating revision on average 4 years after the initial procedure (7, 8). The problem of knee instability in total knee prostheses may arise in two different situations.

In some cases instability is clinically evident (26): Varus tilt on walking, varus, valgus or genu recurvatum when walking, repeated episodes of instability or even tibiofemoral dislocation. Clinically, instability is easily observed by tilting while walking and laxity on full extension, usually asymmetric in varus-valgus. Dynamic views in varus-valgus or plain radiographs with the patient standing on one leg may confirm the diagnosis, showing asymmetric lift-off (fig. 4). This is instability in extension, often related to a technical error during insertion. Initial soft tissue imbalance, if substantial, is enough to cause disabling frontal instability in particular in late-stage external arthroses with internal distension. It accounts for 28% of cases of instability requiring implant revision (7).

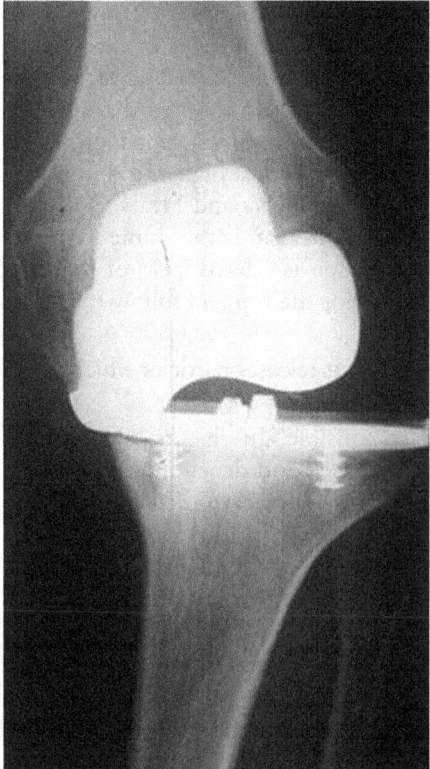

Inadequate correction of a preoperative deformity is a decisive factor. It is sufficient on its own to lead to considerable instability, particularly in genu valgum, but it generally acts as a contributory factor. Residual instability in moderate extension which could be well tolerated in a normally aligned knee will rapidly deteriorate if there is misalignment, and this represents 35% of revision procedures for instability (7).

Other aggravating factors have been noted: At a higher level, dysplasia or congenital subluxation of the hip which has not been surgically corrected or has been poorly corrected, in particular with persisting excessive femoral antever-

Fig. 4 – Lateral instability visible on a plain radiograph with the patient standing on one foot.

sion or femoral adduction due to lateralisation of the femoral head. When several factors are involved, overall reflection is required before embarking on surgery and a custom-made prosthesis which corrects malrotation may help to solve complex problems. Underlying deformities of the ankle or hindfoot, particularly in valgus, may also require correction before considering insertion of a new implant. A prosthesis which is too small may also cause instability (82).

All substantial instability requires revision, in general to replace the prosthesis, and raises the problem of correction of deformity and of any peripheral ligament lesions. If there is no deformity, some authors propose tautening (32) or ligament allografts, alone or in association with implant replacement. The main problem raised by genu recurvatum in total knee prostheses is that of its origin. It may be related to faulty quadricipital locking of mechanical origin (rupture of the patellar or quadricipital tendon) and its treatment is then difficult, ranging from simple repair to allograft (66). If there is a neurological deficiency, treatment may consist of an orthotic device, arthrodesis or for some authors a hinged implant with the risk of rupture or loosening. In general, the problem is merely ligamentous and implant replacement is required (fig. 5).

In certain cases, the prosthesis is stable in extension and instability only becomes evident in flexion. The symptoms are equivocal (effusion, knee giving way, diffuse pain) and clinical examination yields little information. Here the risk is that these "concealed" instabilities will be classified as persistent pain (61). These flexion instabilities may be of two types:

– Direct symmetric instability: too lax a flexion space in a posterior stabilized prosthesis may occur if the femoral component is too small, if posterior condylar resection is excessive or the polyethylene is not sufficiently thick. Functional disability then persists after the procedure. In posterior cruciate ligament retaining prostheses, flexion instability may appear in the immediate postoperative period if there is a technical defect (excessive release, too marked tibial slope, faulty component resection). More frequently it is due to secondary rupture or distension of the posterior cruciate ligament and the symptoms appear after a clear interval of several months or years. Diagnosis is based on precise clinical and radiographic analysis looking for anteroposterior instability with the knee in 90° flexion. Treatment generally involves implant replacement; more rarely, it may be sufficient to increase the thickness of the tibial polyethylene.

– External flexion instability: malposition of the femoral component in internal rotation may lead to an asymmetric flexion space with persistent external instability, generally manifested by pain and a poor functional result. Clinical diagnosis is difficult. It is based either on demonstration of rotational malposition itself by CT scan, or of flexion instability on dynamic views under fluoroscopic guidance (68). It is treated by implant replacement and correction of rotational malposition.

Wear and osteolysis

Tibial polyethylene wear has been variously evaluated in the various series in the literature and it is to a large degree multifactorial. It depends on the polyethylene itself (intrinsic quality, mode of sterilisation, length of storage before use), on the quality of positioning and on implant design which governs its kinematic qualities. This last factor is probably decisive since cases of catastrophic polyethylene wear (42, 48, 87) are more often seen in posterior cruciate retaining prostheses with flat trays.

Polyethylene wear is inevitable over time. It occurs at the upper surface of the polyethylene (tibiofemoral joint line) and also on the lower surface, in the case of a metal-back plateau. The degree of wear can be assessed in volumetric terms (volume of particles produced per unit of time) or linear terms (decreased thickness). Wear leads to release of polyethylene particles in the joint; these build up in the synovial fluid and gradually migrate to the bone/cement junction or the bone/prosthesis interface for cementless implants, and along the tibial screws if present. They generate a foreign-body reaction producing an afflux of osteolytic factors leading to focal osteolysis which creates the conditions for loosening.

Marked osteolysis is generally associated with loosening. In 490 total knee replacement revisions for non-septic complications (13) no case of isolated osteolysis required revision. This phenomenon, well known in the hip, has been described more recently in total knee replacement (63). This relative "protection" of knee replacements from osteolysis is related to the following (23):

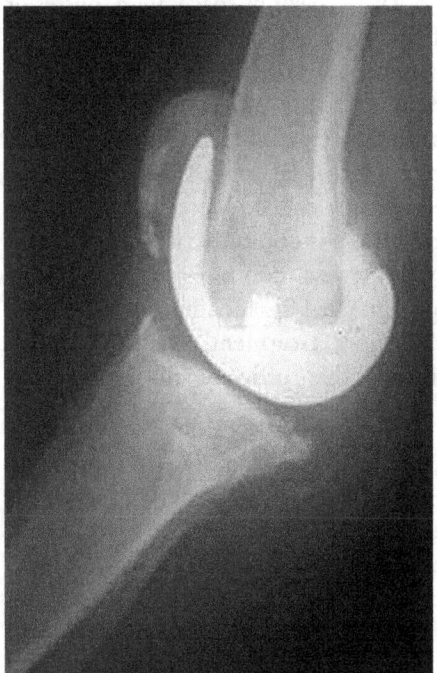

Fig. 5 – Genu recurvatum due to progressive ligament distension.

1. Greater capacity of the synovial membrane of the knee to absorb particles;

2. Better adaptation of the cement to the spongy bone in knee replacements than to the cortical bone in hip replacements, which makes for fewer fractures and fissures in the cement. Particles migrate in part through these fissures;

3. The cement forms a more hermetic compartment at the knee;

4. Polyethylene particles are smaller in hip replacements.

The last factor is an essential one, because it is the release of polyethylene microparticles (< 1µm) which stimulates the macrophage reaction which releases osteoclast recruiting factors (TNF-alpha). This effect is marked in the hip because the purely sliding movement leads to wear by abrasion which releases small-size particles. In the knee, wear is more complex because it is related to the rolling-sliding-translation movement leading to the formation of macroparticles (> 2µm) which are biologically much more inert. Schmalzreid (74) observed however that 71% of polyethylene particles released by a knee prosthesis are inferior to 1µm. This observation underlines the fact that several types of wear can occur in a knee replacement (table I), releasing particles of varying sizes. Also, the predominant type of wear can differ from one prosthesis to another.

Table I – The various types of polyethylene wear and size of particles released. From Walker (86).

Type of wear	Mechanism	Particle size
Adhesive wear (1)	Release of fibrils on asperities of the PE	2-5µm by 0.2-0.5µm
Adhesive wear (2)	Release of a PE granule	0.1-1µm
Adhesive wear (3)	Detachment of a "plaque" of PE	2-10µm
Abrasion	Release of fibrils or granules by an asperity of the metal	0.1µm-5µm
Foreign body abrasion	Foreign body (metal, cement, ceramic)	0.1µm-5µm
Pitting	Particles released by stress related to sliding	0.5mm
Delamination	Crack propagation 0.5mm below surface of PE: progressive lesion	strips of PE

The rate of osteolysis in total knee replacements is variable, ranging from 0% (89) to 30% (25) (fig. 6). The diagnosis is generally made at the loosening stage and treatment then consists of changing the prosthesis. In certain cases (23) the prosthesis is stable and some authors propose simply filling in the osteolytic areas by bone grafts. However, this situation was never observed in the Sofcot series (13)

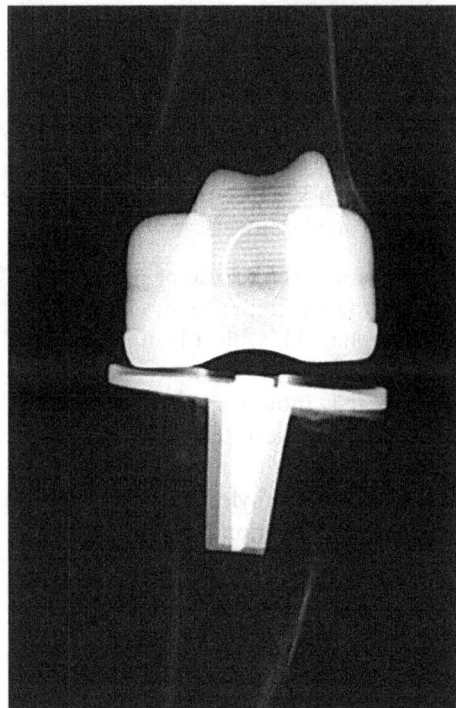

Fig. 6 – Tibial polyethylene wear.

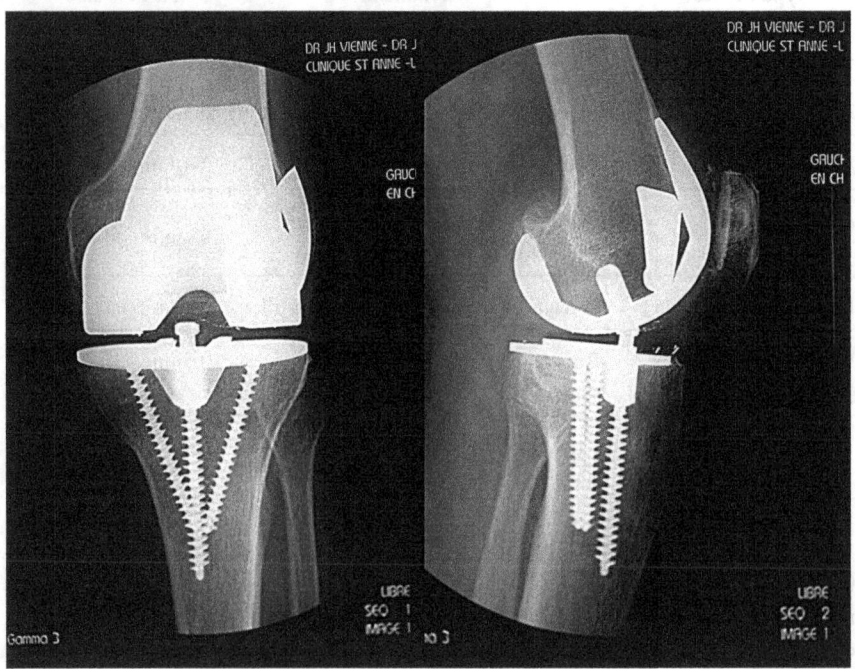

Fig. 7 – Fracture of a ceramic femoral condyle.

Mechanical failure of the implant

Implant-related problems are rare. The implant itself (tibial baseplate or condyles) or intramedullary long stems may fracture. Dislocation of the Polyethylene or fracture of a ceramic condyle can be observed (fig. 7 and 8). Prevention is a question of improving design and the biomaterials used. Whiteside (88) observed that femoral component rupture rate decreased from 0.51% to 0.0061% of cases after improvements in the covering layers. In another respect, these failures raise the issue of notification of the administrative authorities, for better collection and analysis of these rare problems. Lastly, from a technical viewpoint revision should be performed before osteolysis becomes too widespread.

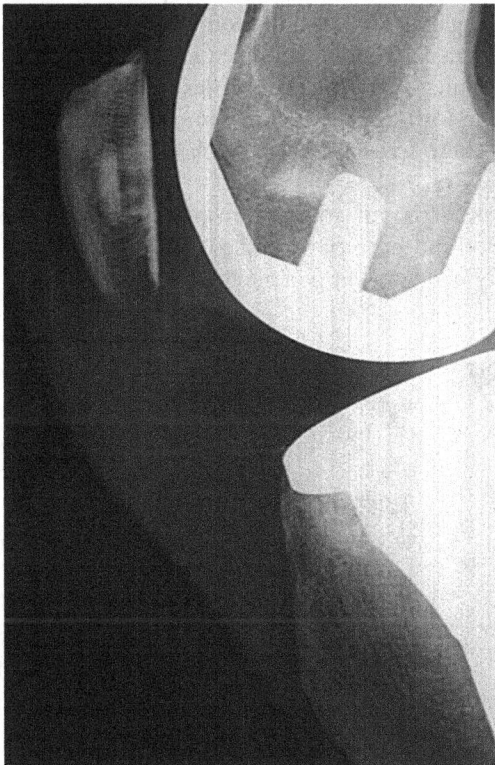

Fig. 8 – Tibial polyethylene dislocation.

Stiffness

Depending on the study, the flexion which can generally be expected after total knee replacement varies between 100° and 110° (2) and is obtained during the early months. No significant improvement can be expected later than one year (39). Inadequate flexion after total knee replacement is a frequent complication: 8% to 12% for Daluga (16), 54% to 60% for Shoji (75), 10.4% for Scranton (69). The causes of stiffness are multiple and are often interwoven with poorly-controlled factors such as patient motivation and reflex sympathetic dystrophy. Latent infection can cause stiffness and should be excluded.

Causes of stiffness after total knee replacement

Patient-related causes

The range of preoperative flexion is one of the principal factors found in most studies. A knee which is stiff preoperatively will have less good flexion after rehabilitation (31, 62, 79). However, final mobility tends to converge towards median values and patients with good preoperative mobility lose a little whereas stiff patients gain. Anouchi (2) found that patients with preoperative flexion of less than 90° gained 26° flexion more than those whose preoperative flexion was greater than 105°. In total knee replacement after ankylosis or knee arthrodesis, results vary with final flexion of 94° for Montgomery (54), 62° for Naranja (58) and 75.9° for Kim (43). The post-operative complication rate in all these series was high, with up to 53.3% of cutaneous necrosis (43).

Associated hip disorder is a risk factor for stiffness, related to quadriceps stiffness, particularly of the anterior and posterior bundles (57). Anouchi (2) observed a decreased final mobility of 11.43° in patients with several arthritic joints (fig. 9).

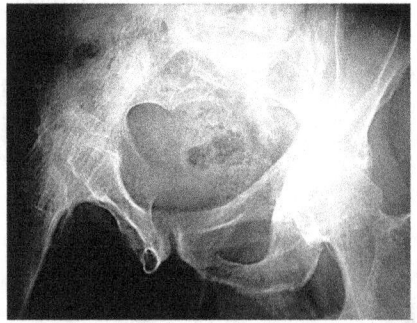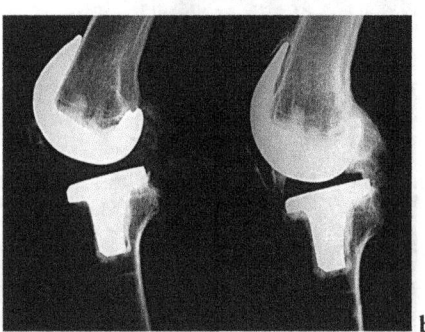

a.   b.

Fig. 9 – Failure of total knee replacement after hip arthrodesis:
a. Right hip arthrodesis; **b.** Progressive postoperative stiffening with ossification around the prosthesis. Mobility five years postoperatively: 0/20°-/30°.

A knee which has undergone several previous surgical procedures is more likely to be stiff. For Scranton (69), 77% of knees which required postoperative manipulation under anaesthesia after total knee replacement had previously undergone surgery.

Abnormal wound healing may lead to extensive intra-articular fibrosis, in particular in some cases of rheumatoid arthritis which are stiff in both flexion and extension. Ries (67) demonstrated fibrocartilaginous metaplasia in five cases of revision surgery for stiffness. In all of these, a new prosthesis brought functional improvement but only moderate gain in range of motion, suggesting some patients may be constitutionally predisposed to fibrosis (29).

Surgeon-related causes

Closure technique may influence final mobility, depending on whether it is done in flexion or in extension. Emerson (22) observed significantly better final flexion after closure in flexion (114.7° compared with 108.1°) as well as easier, shorter postoperative rehabilitation. Masri (53) did not share these conclusions and found no difference related to type of closure.

Malpositioning or bone resection errors may be responsible, in particular defective patellar resection (asymmetry, inadequate resection, lack of resurfacing). These patellar factors were found in 55% of revisions for stiffness (7, 8). Insufficient tibiofemoral resection leaves insufficient space. A reversed tibial slope, faulty alignment or rotational positioning may be responsible (59). Malpositioning of the joint line is an important factor in stiffness: An excessively low line due to excessive tibial resection, compensated for by lower femoral resection, "lengthens" the patellar track and causes excessive femoropatellar strains. An excessive rise in the joint line if stabilisation is obtained only by tibial polyethylene thickness leads to a low patella and stiffness in flexion.

Inadequate release of the posterior capsule and osteophytes or retaining too tight a posterior cruciate ligament may be responsible. Generally, any abnormality in frontal or rotational position will have an even more damaging effect on mobility if the prosthesis is one which retains one or both cruciate ligaments, as tolerance is less.

A prosthesis may be oversized in a frontal or sagittal plane or in both. Poilvache (64) has demonstrated that the ratio of the anteroposterior and transverse dimensions of the distal extremity of the femur is not the same in men and in women, as in women the knee is narrower in the frontal plane. A standard femoral component may therefore be too wide in a woman, if it is adjusted according to the anteroposterior diameter of the knee. This will cause capsular and synovial tension and impingement causing stiffness and pain (69). A femoral component which is too large in an anteroposterior dimension has an impact on both the posterior space in flexion and on the anterior femoropatellar space. If these two spaces are too constricted, flexion is limited.

The type of rehabilitation plays a part in recovery of good mobility. Too brief, inappropriate or poorly supervised rehabilitation as well as unsatisfactory postoperative pain control may lead to stiffness (see chapter on rehabilitation).

Prosthesis-related causes

Although this is not supported by objective proof, the risk of stiffness is greater in a prosthesis retaining the posterior cruciate ligament, or both cruciate ligaments (69). These prostheses make up 36% of revisions for stiffness

(7, 47). Scranton (69) considered that cementless prostheses carried a higher risk of stiffness.

Treatment

There is no single attitude to treatment of stiffness after total knee replacement. It depends on the time since surgery, cause of stiffness, type of prosthesis and functional disability of the patient. Four treatments can be considered: simple manipulation under anaesthetic, arthroscopic arthrolysis, open arthrolysis or prosthesis replacement.

Manipulation is a simple and effective procedure which results in an average gain of 42° flexion for Letenneur (47) and Scranton (69). However, its efficacy is limited in postoperative flexion contracture. The risks of manipulation (fracture, extensor apparatus rupture, wound dehiscence) are less if it is done early during the first 6 weeks. It is therefore imperative to see the patients early and to start manipulation if flexion has not reached 90° 4 to 6 weeks postoperatively. Scranton considered this time period may be extended to 10 weeks postoperatively.

Arthroscopic arthrolysis is an accessory to simple manipulation but cannot resolve major stiffness. It may be debated if the patient is seen 2 to 6 months postoperatively and time is short, or during simple manipulation if range of motion is not completely restored. Arthroscopy for resection of intra-articular fibrous bands then makes it possible to avoid dangerous forceful manipulation. Some authors consider the posterior cruciate ligament may be resected or debrided. Indelicato and Scranton (69) proposed improving this technique by "mini-invasive"arthrolysis using three limited approaches (supero-external, infero-internal and infero-lateral) and obtained a 62° increase in range of motion in four patients.

Classic open arthrolysis is technically difficult. The approach must be extremely prudent to avoid avulsion of the patellar tendon. Osteotomy of the anterior tibial tuberosity or release of the quadriceps tendon are often necessary. Removal of tibial polyethylene makes it possible to approach the posterior tibial compartment and to release the posterior capsule. This release must include the condylar gutters and above all recreate a free suprapatellar bursa. For optimal resection of fibrous tissue, Ries (67) advises removal of the femoral component at the beginning of the procedure, leaving only the metal tibial baseplate. This has the advantage of allowing replacement by a smaller component at the end of the procedure.

If a prosthesis retaining one or both cruciate ligaments is used, these are often totally or partially sacrificed during "simple" arthrolysis. This option would appear open to criticism since the design of the prosthesis is no longer appropriate to the new mode of functioning. Insertion of an entirely new implant should then be considered. Letenneur (47) found that overall open arthrolysis gives a mean improved range of motion of 20°.

Implant replacement should be considered whenever the device is malpositioned or too large. In marked stiffness, replacement gave a better range of motion than soft tissue release (47) and if flexion is less than 60° it is the treatment of choice. Mont (56) and Bonnin (8) obtained good functional results after replacement because stiffness is partially related to improved flexion but also and above all to relief from pain.

Clunk syndromes

From the early 1980s, Figgie (28) in particular stressed the problems of patellofemoral crepitation and patellar catching in total knee replacement. In 1989 Hozack (34) identified the clunk syndrome, describing 3 cases. In 1990 Thorpe (80) reported 11 cases of patellar crepitation and catching related to the development of "intra-articular fibrous bands". He described three types: type I, a transverse band above the trochlea of the implant; type II, a band extending from the superolateral angle of the patella to the patellar tendon; type III, a band extending from the distal pole of the patella to the intracondylar notch. Arthroscopic resection effected a cure in all cases. Since then, several series of clunk syndromes have been published, in particular by Lucas (51), Beight (5) and Shoji (76).

A fibrous nodule develops on the distal part of the quadricipital tendon, at its insertion on the patella; when the knee is flexed the nodule wedges into the posterior stabilising chamber of the femoral component, causing painful locking at about 40° of flexion, and suddenly dislodges on active extension (fig. 10).

This complication occurs almost exclusively in posterior stabilized prostheses and it appears to have become less frequent with improved design of the trochlear part of the femoral components. It mainly occurs when the implant has a patellar component but some authors have described clunk syndromes in knees which did not have patellar resurfacing (76). For Hozack, the main factor is a too proximal position of the patellar button, as he found this abnormality in his three first cases. However, this observation has never been made in other series of the literature.

Abnormal patellar height, whether too high or too low, is a factor which has been stressed in all published series. For Figgie (28), a patellar height of more than 30mm or less than 10mm is a risk factor. Beight, in a series of 20 clunk syndromes found patella baja in 6 knees and Lucas in 32 cases found patella alta in 8 and patella baja in 2 knees (5).

Abnormal thickness of the patella may be responsible if it differs by more than 3mm from the preoperative value, as observed by Beight in 17 of a series of 20 clunk syndromes (5). An abnormal position of the joint line is a significant risk factor if it differs by more than 8mm from the preoperative value. Beight found this factor in 14 of 20 cases and Lucas in 3 of 32 (51).

Treatment of clunk syndrome is based on surgical excision of the fibrous nodule, either by an open procedure or under arthroscopy. Good results have been obtained in the various series with both techniques (10, 51).

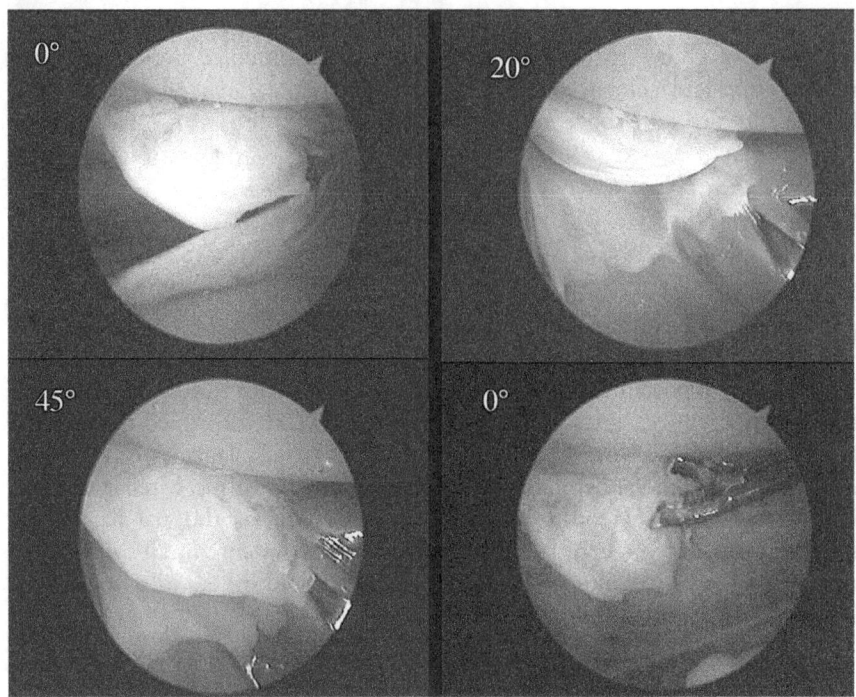

Fig. 10 – Clunk syndrome.
– In full extension, a fibrous nodule is visible between the patellar button above and the femoral component below.
– At 20° flexion, the nodule slides between the patellar and femoral components.
– At 45° flexion, the nodule is wedged into the posterior stabilizing chamber of the prosthesis.
– The nodule is removed in extension by arthroscopy, effecting a cure.

Unexplained pain without stiffness

Management of a total knee prosthesis which is painful for no evident reason starts with meticulous investigation in order to exclude infection. Chronic infection is in fact the main cause of persistent pain in total knee replacements (70).

A minor mechanical abnormality may be present and a meticulous search should be carried out for minimal or exclusively femoral loosening, wear, unsatisfactory kinematics due to poor soft tissue balance (particularly in posterior cruciate ligament retaining prostheses) or rotational malposition. An oversized prosthesis may be painful. Daluga (16) considers that an anteroposterior diameter which is increased by 12% results in significantly increased pressures. Similarly, lateral overlap of the tibial plateau may be the cause. "Hidden" instability which occurs only in flexion may account for equivocal symptoms with effusion and an impression of the knee giving way, with a clinical examination which is normal if the knee is not specifically examined in flexion.

Prosthesis replacement for persistent pain without associated stiffness generally gives poor results, less good than those of revision for other causes: 87%

of failures for Mont (56), IKS pain score on revision 15 ± 10 in a series of 8 cases (8) or 22 ± 15 in 25 cases (9). However, significantly better results are obtained in three situations: Replacement of an oversized prosthesis (pain score 28 ± 19), retaining of the posterior cruciate ligament (25 ± 17) and absence of previous surgery before the primary implant (26.5 ± 17). When these three favorable factors are combined, the pain score after revision may well be good (36 ± 12).

The second prognostic factor observed in this series (9) was the notion of a free interval. When pain appeared after a pain-free interval of some years, prosthesis replacement gave good results (pain score 39 ±11).

So in the case of a painful prosthesis with no evident anomaly on radiologic work-up or laboratory tests, care must be taken before deciding on surgical revision. The decision is generally based on a range of arguments, none of which is conclusive. The two elements in favour of revision are secondary onset of pain after a variable pain-free period and the presence of favorable prognostic factors: Replacement of an oversized primary prosthesis, a prosthesis retaining one or both cruciate ligaments, and absence of previous knee surgery.

References

1. Aglietti P, Rinonapoli E (1984) Total condylar knee arthroplasty. A five-year follow-up study of 33 knees. Clin Orthop 186: 104-11

2. Anouchi YS, McShane M, Kelly F et al. (1996) Range of motion in total knee arthroplasty. Clin Orthop 331: 87-92

3. Aubriot JH, Deburge A, Genet JP (1981) Les prothèses à charnière du genou, expérience après 5 ans. Rev Chir Orthop 67: 337-45

4. Behrens JC, Walker PS, Shoji H (1974) Variation in strength and structure of cancellous bone at the knee. J Biomech 7: 201-07

5. Beight JL, Yao B, Hozack WJ et al. (1994) The patellar "clunk" syndrome after posterior stabilized total knee arthroplasty. Clin Orthop 299: 139-42

6. Berger RA, Crossett LS, Jacobs JJ et al. (1998) Malrotation causing patellofemoral complications. Clin Orthop 356: 144-53

7. Bonnin M, Deroche P, Palazzolo P (1999) Les reprises de PTG par PTG. In: Chirurgie prothétique du genou, Chambat P, Neyret Ph, G. Deschamps G, Sauramps Médical, Montpellier, 177-201

8. Bonnin M, Deschamps G, Neyret P et al. (2000) Les changements de prothèses totales du genou non infectées. Analyse des résultats à propos d'une série continue de 69 cas. Rev Chir Orthop 86: 694-706

9. Bonnin M (2001) Les reprises de prothèses totales du genou pour clunk syndrome. Rev Chir Orthop 87, Suppl.: 1S164-6

10. Bonnin M (2001) Les reprises de prothèses totales du genou pour douleurs inexpliquées. Rev Chir Orthop 87, Suppl.: 1S166-72

11. Bradbury N, Borton D, Spoo G et al. (1998) Participation in sport after total knee replacement. Am J Sports Med 26: 530-5

12. Brassard MF, Insall JN, Scuderi (2001) Complications of total knee arthroplasty. In: Surgery of the knee. Insall JN, Scott WN. Churchill Livingstone, Philadelphia: 1801-44

13. Burdin P, Huten D (2001) Les reprises de prothèses totales du genou. Symposium de la Sofcot. Rev Chir Orthop Suppl.: 1S143-1S98

14. Campbell MD, Duffy GP, Trousdale RT (1998) Femoral component failure in hybrid total knee arthroplasty. Clin Orthop 356: 58-65
15. Chandler HP, Reineck FT, Wixson RL et al. (1981) Total hip replacement in patients younger than 30 years old. J Bone Joint Surg (Am) 63: 1426-34
16. Daluga D, Lombardi AV, Mallory TH et al. (1991) Knee manipulation following total knee arthroplasty: analysis of prognostic variables. J Arthroplasty 6: 119-28
17. Deroches P (1992) La prothèse totale à glissement du genou HLS I. Résultats d'une série de 375 cas. Thèse Med Lyon N°34
18. Dorr LD, Luckett M, Conaty JP (1990) Total hip arthroplasties in patients younger than 45 years. A nine- to ten-year follow-up study. Clin Orthop 260: 215-9
19. Dubs L, Gschwend N, Munzinger U (1983) Sport after total hip arthroplasty. Arch Orthop Trauma Surg 101: 161-9
20. Duff GP, Lachiewicz PF, Kelley SS (1996) Aspiration of the knee joint before revision arthroplasty. Clin Orthop 331: 132-9
21. Duquennoy A, Decoulx J, Epinette JA et al. (1983) Les prothèses à charnière du genou. À propos de 185 cas. Rev Chir Orthop 69: 465-74
22. Emerson RH, Ayers C, Head WC et al. (1996) Surgical closing in primary total knee arthroplasties. Clin Orthop 331: 74-80
23. Engh GA (1994) Tibial osteolysis in cementless total knee arthroplasty. A review of 25 cases treated with and without tibial component revision. Clin Orthop 309: 33-43
24. Ewald FC (1989) The Knee Society total knee arthroplasty roentgenographic evaluation and scoring system. Clin Orthop 248: 9-12
25. Ezzet KA, Garcia R, Barrack RL (1995) Effect of component fixation method on osteolysis in total knee arthroplasty. Clin Orthop 321: 86-91
26. Fehring TK, Valadie AL (1994) Knee instability after total knee arthroplasty. Clin Orthop 299: 157-62
27. Fehring TK, Mc Avoy (1996) Fluoroscopic evaluation of the painful total knee arthroplasty. Clin Orthop 331: 226-333
28. Figgie HE, Goldberg VM, Heiple KG et al. (1986) The influence of tibial-patellofemoral location on function of the knee in patients with the posterior stabilized condylar knee prosthesis. J Bone Joint Surg (Am) 68: 1035-40
29. Furia JP, Pellegrini VD (1995) Heterotopic ossification following primary total knee arthroplasty. J Arthroplasty 10: 413-9
30. Griffin FM, Scuderi GR, Insall JN et al. (1998) Total knee arthroplasty in patients who were obese with 10-years follow-up. Clin Orthop 356: 28-33
31. Harvey IA, Barry, Kirby SP et al. (1993) Factors affecting the range of movement of total knee arthroplasty. J Bone Joint Surg (Br) 75: 950-5
32. Healy WL, Iorio R, Lemos DW (1998) Medial reconstruction during total knee arthroplasty for severe valgus deformity. Clin Orthop 356: 161-9
33. Healy WL, Iorio R, Lemos MJ (2001) Athletic activity after joint replacement. Am J Sports Med 29: 377-88
34. Hozack WJ, Rothman RH, Booth RE et al. (1989) The patellar clunk syndrome. A complication of posterior stabilised total knee arthroplasty. Clin Orthop 241 203-8
35. Hsu HP, Garg A, Walker PS et al. (1989) Effect of knee component alignment on tibial load distribution with clinical correlation. Clin Orthop 248: 135-44
36. Hsu RW, Himeno S, Coventry MB et al. (1990) Normal axial alignment of the lower extremity and load bearing distribution at the knee. Clin Orthop 255: 215-27
37. Hvid I, Bentzen SM, Jorgensen J (1988) Remodelling of the tibial plateau after knee replacement. Acta Orthop Scand 59: 567-73
38. Insall JN, Hood RW, Flawn LB, Sullivan DJ (1983) The total condylar knee prosthesis in gonarthrosis. A five-to nine-year follow-up of the first hundred consecutive replacements. J Bone Joint Surg (Am) 65: 619-28
39. Insall JN, Binazzi R, Soudry M et al. (1985) Total knee arthroplasty. Clin Orthop 192: 13-22
40. Johnson F, Leitl S, Waugh W (1980) The distribution of load across the knee. A comparison of static and dynamic measurements. J Bone Joint Surg (Br) 62: 346-9

41. Kilgus DJ, Dorey FJ, Finerman GA (1991) Patient activity, sports participation and impact loading on the durability of cemented total hip replacement. Clin Orthop 269: 25-31
42. Kilgus DJ, Moreland JR, Finerman GA *et al.* (1991) Catastrophic wear of tibial polyethylene inserts. Clin Orthop 273: 223-31
43. Kim YH, Kim JS, Cho SH (2000) Total knee arthroplasty after spontaneous osseous ankylosis and takedown of formal knee fusion. J Arthroplasty 15: 453-60
44. King TV, Scott RD (1985) Femoral component loosening in total knee arthroplasty. Clin Orthop 194: 285-90
45. LaPorte DM, Mont MA, Hungerford DS (1999) Characterisation of tennis players who have a total knee arthroplasty. Proceedings of the 66th Annual Meeting of the AAOS, p. 171
46. Laskin RS (1999) The patient with a painful total knee replacement. In: Lotke PA, Garino JP (1999) Revision total knee arthroplasty. Lippincott-Raven Philadelphia: 91-106
47. Letenneur J, Guilleux Ch Gerber Ph *et al.* (2001) Les reprises de PTG pour raideur. Rev Chir Orthop 87 Suppl: 1S149-51
48. Lewis P, Rorabeck CH, Bourne RB *et al.* (1994) Posteromedial tibial polyethylene failure in total knee replacement. Clin Orthop 299: 11-7
49. Lonner JH, Hershman S, Mont M *et al.* (2000) Total knee arthroplasty in patients 40 years of age and younger with osteoarthritis. Clin Orthop 380: 85-90
50. Lotke PA, Ecker ML (1977) Influence of positioning of prosthesis in total knee replacement. J Bone Joint Surg (Am) 59: 77-9
51. Lucas TS, DeLucas PF, Nazarian DG *et al.* (1999) Arthroscopic treatment of patellar clunk. Clin Orthop 367:226-9
52. Magee FP, Weinstein AM (1986) The effect of position on the detection of radiolucent lines beneath the tibial tray. Trans Orthop Res Soc 11: 357
53. Masri BA, Laskin RS, Windsor RE *et al.* (1996) Knee closure in total knee replacement. A randomised prospective trial. Clin Orthop 331: 81-6
54. Montgomery W, Insall JN, Haas S (1998) Primary total knee arthroplasty in stiff and ankylosed knees. Am J Knee Surg 11: 20-3
55. Mont MA, Mathur SK, Krackow KA, Loewy JW *et al.* (1996) Cementless total knee arthroplasty in obese patients: a comparison with a matched control group. J Arthroplasty 11: 153-6
56. Mont MA, Serna FK, Krackow KA *et al.* (1996) Exploration of a radiographically normal total knee replacement for unexplained pain. Clin Orthop 331: 216-9
57. Moreland JR (1988) Mechanisms of failure in total knee arthroplasty. Clin Orthop 226: 49-64
58. Naranja RJ, Lotke PA, Pagano MW *et al.* (1996) Total knee arthroplasty in a previously ankylosed or arthrodesed knee. Clin Orthop 331: 234-7
59. Nicholls DW, Dorr LD (1990) Revision surgery for stiff total knee arthroplasty. J Arthroplasty 5 Suppl: S73-7
60. Nordin JY, Parent H and the Guepar Group (1989) La prothèse Guepar II scellée. Cahiers d'enseignement de la SOFCOT, 171-84
61. Pagano MW, Hanssen AD, Lewallen DG *et al.* (1998) Flexion instability after primary posterior cruciate retaining total knee arthroplasty. Clin Orthop 356: 39-46
62. Parsley BS, Engh GA, Dwyer KA (1992) Preoperative flexion. Does it influence postoperative flexion after posterior-cruciate-retaining total knee arthroplasty? Clin Orthop 275: 204-10
63. Peters PC, Engh GA, Dwyer KA *et al.* (1992) Osteolysis after total knee arthroplasty without cement. J Bone Joint Surg (Am) 74: 864-76
64. Poilvache PL, Insall JN, Scuderi GR *et al.* (1996) Rotational landmarks and sizing of the distal femur in total knee arthroplasty. Clin Orthop 331: 35-46
65. Ranawat CS, Flynn WF, Saddler S, Hansraj *et al.* (1993) Long-term results of the total condylar knee arthroplasty. A 15-year survivorship study. Clin Orthop 286: 94-102
66. Rand JA, Morrey BF, Bryan RS (1989) Patellar tendon rupture after total knee arthroplasty. Clin Orthop 244: 233-8

67. Ries MD, Badalamente M (2000) Arthrofibrosis after total knee arthroplasty. Clin Orthop 380: 177-83

68. Romero J, Binkert C, Braum V *et al.* (2001) Revision total knee arthroplasty for lateral flexion instability due to internal malrotation of the femoral component. Communication n° 402, EFORT, Rhodes, 6 June

69. Scranton PE (2001) Management of knee pain and stiffness after total knee arthroplasty. J Arthroplasty 16 :428-35

70. Scuderi GR, Insall JN (1992) Total knee arthroplasty. Current clinical perspectives. Clin Orthop 276: 26-32

71. Seitz P, Ruegsegger P, Gschwend N *et al.* (1987) Changes in local bone density after total knee arthroplasty: The use of quantitative computed tomography. J Bone Joint Surg (Br) 69: 407-11

72. Smith BE, Askew MJ Gradisar IA *et al.* (1992) The effect of patient weight on the functional outcome of total knee arthroplasty. Clin Orthop 276: 237-44

73. Smith JL, Tullos HS, Davidson JP (1989) Alignment of total knee arthroplasty. J Arthroplasty 4 Suppl: S55-61

74. Schmalzreid TP, Campbell P, Brown IC *et al.* (1995) Polyethylene wear particles generated *in vivo* by total knee replacement compared to total hip replacements. Trans Orthop Res Soc 20: 63

75. Shoji H, Yoshino S, Komagamine M (1987) Improved range of motion with the Y/S total knee arthroplasty system. Clin Orthop 218: 150-63

76. Shoji H, Shimozaki E (1996) Patellar clunk syndrome in total knee arthroplasty without patellar resurfacing. J Arthroplasty 11: 198-201

77. Tayot O, Adam Ph, Neyret Ph (1999) Résultats des prothèses totales du genou HLS 1. In: Chirurgie prothétique du genou, Sauramps Médical, Montpellier p.113-24

78. Tew M, Waugh W (1985) Tibiofemoral alignment and the results of knee replacement. J Bone Joint Surg (Br) 67: 551-6

79. Tew M, Forster IW, Wallace WA (1989) Effect of total knee arthroplasty on maximal flexion. Clin Orthop 247: 168-74

80. Thorpe CD, Bocell JR, Tullos HS (1990) Intra-articular fibrous bands. Patellar complications after total knee replacement. J Bone Joint Surg (Am) 72: 811-4

81. Uematsu O, Hsu HP, Kelley KM (1987) Radiographic study of kinematic total knee arthroplasty. J Arthroplasty 2: 317-26

82. Van de Velde D, Huten D, Bassaire M *et al.* (2001) Les reprises de prothèse totale du genou pour laxités fémoro-tibiales. Rev Chir Orthop 87 suppl: 1S158-63

83. Visuri T, Honkanen R (1980) Total hip replacement: its influence on spontaneous recreation exercise habits. Arch Phys Med Rehabil 61: 325-8

84. Walker PS, Greene D, Reilly D *et al.* (1981) Fixation of tibial component of knee prostheses. J Bone Joint Surg (Am) 63: 258-67

85. Walker PS, Soudry M, Ewald FC *et al.* (1984) Control of cement penetration in total knee arthroplasty. Clin Orthop 185: 155-64

86. Walker PS (2001) Design criteria for total knee replacement. In: Surgery of the knee. Insall JN, Scott RW. Churchill Livingstone, Philadelphia,p. 284-314

87. Wasielewski RC, Galante FO, Leighty RM *et al.* (1994) Wear pattern on retrieved polyethylene tibial inserts and their relationship to technical considerations during total knee arthroplasty. Clin Orthop 299: 31-43

88. Whiteside LA, Fosco DR, Brooks JG (1993) Fracture of the femoral components in cementless total knee arthroplasty. Clin Orthop 286: 71-7

89. Whiteside LA (1995) Effect of porous coating configuration on tibial osteolysis after total knee arthroplasty. Clin Orthop 321: 92-7

Rehabilitation after total knee arthroplasty

M. Bonnin, M. Westphal, C. Jacquemard, V. Biot, A. Giroud, J. Mathelin, J. Roberto

Since the introduction of total knee arthroplasty, rehabilitation has evolved towards accelerated protocols to help the patient become independent more rapidly. When strict immobilisation was the rule in the postoperative period, rehabilitation was laborious, requiring manipulation under anaesthetic in 20 to 30% of cases (3) and hospital stay lasted two or three weeks. The abandon of postoperative immobilisation, better management of pain and return to early weight bearing have led to a considerably shorter hospital stay, reduced manipulation under anaesthetic (14) and above all better functional recovery at the end of rehabilitation.

These advances are related to pluridisciplinary management where the surgeon, physiotherapist, anaesthetist, physical medicine specialist, nurses and patient work in close collaboration. Rehabilitation after total knee arthroplasty must be taken in its widest sense and its aims are optimal management of pain, recovery of range of motion, muscular training, detection and prevention of postoperative complications and the patient's gradual return to independence.

Rehabilitation consists of three distinct phases (table I): the postsurgical phase, the proper rehabilitation phase between postoperative days 7 to 30 and lastly the phase of readaptation-reintegration from 30 days after surgery. In some cases a preoperative rehabilitation phase may be included, which can be useful in regard to muscular training and range of motion (1, 6) and can help prepare the patient to use canes.

Immediate postoperative period (days 1 to 7)

This is the most important phase and on it depends the ulterior progress of rehabilitation and the final result. Management of pain is primordial during this period as early recovery is not possible if the patient is in too much pain. It is based on medication and loco-regional analgesia.

Principle of initial rehabilitation

Passive joint manipulation is the essential aim during this phase. It should be started as soon as possible, the goal being to obtain complete and easy extension of the knee and flexion or close to 90° before the patient is discharged.

Table I. – Phases of rehabilitation.

	D0	D1	D2	D3	D4	D5	D6	D7	D8	D15	D21	D30	D60
			Drain removal					Discharge					
Pain	LRA + morphine pump				Routinely per os				Per os ad libitum				
Flexion • aims	MAXIMUM TOLERATED FLEXION						> 90°	if < 60° return home not permitted		if < 60° manip/ GA		if < 90° manip/ GA	
Flexion • techniques	Posture cushion in bed	• Posture cushion • Manual manipulation • Edge of table • Drain removal D2-D3			• Postural exercises edge of table • Postural exercises sitting position • Manual manipulation				• SELF-REHABILITATION				
Extension	Full extension	• Postural exercises • Massages • Myorelaxant • Splint at night if required											
Walking	Standing	Walking with physiotherapist			Walking alone / Stairs				Walking permitted ad lib with two canes			Canes not needed	
Muscles		Flash contractions Patellar manipulation			• Raise stretched leg • Active extension				• Active OKC and CKC • Electrostimulation			• Proprioception • Pedalling	

LRA = loco-regional anaesthesia; OKC = open kinetic chain; CKC = closed kinetic chain; GA = general anaesthesia.

Several modes of rehabilitation may be used: manual manipulation with postural exercises and the drop-and-dangle approach or continuous passive motion (CPM) by arthromotor. The latter may be gradual, initially limited to 30° then increasing daily, or immediately as tolerated.

Continuous passive motion described by Salter in 1980 (18) was used for the first time in total knee arthroplasty by Coutts (3). The arguments in favour of CPM were:

1. recovery of better range of motion;
2. decreased pain and analgesic consumption;
3. shorter hospital stay.

Several series confirmed these advantages (2, 7, 10, 14, 17, 20, 21, 22) and some authors even added a decreased incidence of postoperative thrombosis (9).

On the other hand, other studies have stressed the disadvantages of CPM, describing increased postoperative bleeding, problems of wound healing and above all the lack of any real benefit of CPM in terms of flexion (5, 6, 8, 12, 15, 16). Maloney (12), in a retrospective study, observed 2% of cutaneous necrosis in the group without CPM compared with 12% in the group with CPM. This risk appears to be related to decreased cutaneous oxygen pressure at the wound when knee flexion is greater than 40° (5) and is thus related rather to immediate flexion than to CPM itself. Yashar (22), in a prospective study comparing progressive CPM and CPM with immediate maximal flexion at 100°, observed a serious case of cutaneous necrosis in the latter group. He considered this complication as partly related to accelerated flexion but above all to dressings which were too dry and too tight. Postoperative bleeding appears to be greater in early continuous passive motion beyond 40° flexion. Pope (15) observed 956mL total blood loss in a no-CPM patient group compared with 1,558mL in CPM with flexion over 40° and 1,017mL with 0° to 40° CPM. Yashar (22) did not observe any such negative effect of immediate maximal flexion.

The effect of CPM on the incidence of postoperative thrombosis is controversial. Some studies found decreased incidence of thrombosis with CPM (9, 21) but these results were not confirmed by other authors (6, 7, 22).

Numerous studies have sought to compare the results and risks of complications with these different modes of rehabilitation. It is difficult to compare the results as CPM protocols vary greatly, from 1 hour three times a day (7) to 20 hours a day (3), as do protocols for postoperative pain relief and thrombosis prevention. Moreover, details are often lacking on other factors influencing the results of rehabilitation, such as the mode of closure in flexion or in extension (4), preoperative flexion (1), type of prosthesis or exact rehabilitation protocol. The few randomised prospective studies which have been performed (6, 11, 22) concluded that CPM offered no benefit in terms of flexion, pain or length of hospital stay.

It is interesting to note that the duration of initial rehabilitation is important. Mauerhan (13) considered there was a clear correlation between duration of hospital stay and rate of manipulation under anaesthesia: for hospital stay durations of 6.4, 5.4 and 4.4 days, the rate of manipulation was respectively 6%, 11.3% and 12%.

Overall, the evolution of immediate postoperative rehabilitation has clearly transformed the results of total knee arthroplasty. It appears, however, that this progress is related more to overall management, including pain relief, giving the patient confidence and rapid restoration of knee function, than to the actual type of manipulation, which does not seem to be a decisive factor.

Description of our protocol

Since 1992, postoperative rehabilitation has been based on alternate postural exercises in flexion and in extension which are started as soon as the patient returns to the hospital ward. This protocol combines:

1. Pain relief by loco-regional anaesthesia by sciatic and crural block and patient-operated morphine pump. Plexus block is performed before the procedure in order to be effective as soon as the patient regains consciousness. If necessary further injections can be given via a crural catheter;

2. Manual manipulation by the physiotherapist as soon as the first postoperative day. The patella is manipulated manually in the frontal plane and vertically and horizontally. The tibiofemoral joint is mobilised in flexion, with the patient sitting on the edge of the bed or of a table, passively or actively with assistance. Manipulation in extension is essential at this stage to help prevent antalgic flexion contracture. These manipulations are preceded by massage, in particular of the sub-quadricipital recess and by passive and then active manipulation of the ankle below. Complete extension must be obtained immediately after surgery. It is essentially dependent on preoperative ligamentous balance but may be difficult to achieve in cases of marked preoperative flexion contracture or of contralateral flexion contracture. Here use of a brace support in extension during rest at night may be useful. At this stage it is essential for the patient to be involved in the effort to obtain extension;

3. Cryotherapy is routinely used. It consists of application of ice on the operated knee, preferably on its lateral aspects in order not to contribute to any delay in wound healing. It should be applied several times a day, in particular after sessions of manipulation or muscle training but should not last longer than 15 to 20 minutes;

4. Prevention of venous stasis begins as soon as the patient leaves the operating theatre. The patient, resting, is placed in a sloping position, with the legs raised and venous pressure stockings are immediately put on and worn 24 hours a day for five weeks. During this period manual lymphatic drainage is also a technique of choice. Trophic massage of the quadriceps and the lateral aspects of the knee prepare the way for manipulation. Analgesic electrotherapy can be used as an adjunct;

5. Alternate postural exercises. These follow manipulation but must be repeated several times a day. They are started as soon as the patient has left the operating theatre. During the early days, flexion exercises are carried out

on foam pads of varying angles which are placed in the bed and maintain the knee in flexion (fig. 1). Rapidly, depending on the patient's general health status, these postural exercises are carried out with the patient sitting on the edge of the bed (fig. 2). Postural exercises in extension are started immediately and no "comfort cushion" placed under the knee to relieve pain is allowed (fig. 3). These exercises are done over short periods of not more than 20 minutes and are combined with cryotherapy. As soon as the drains are removed, the patient can sit in a chair and postural exercises alternate between a position of maximum flexion with the foot on the ground and one of extension with the foot on a foot-rest (fig. 2 and 4);

6. The aim is to achieve complete extension and 90° flexion when the patient is discharged one week after surgery. If the knee is very stiff with less than 60° flexion the patient should be referred to a specialised centre and see the surgeon 15 days postoperatively for manipulation under general anaesthesia if necessary. If there is persistent flexion contracture, brace support in extension may used as night;

7. The essential aim of muscular rehabilitation is to remedy quadriceps

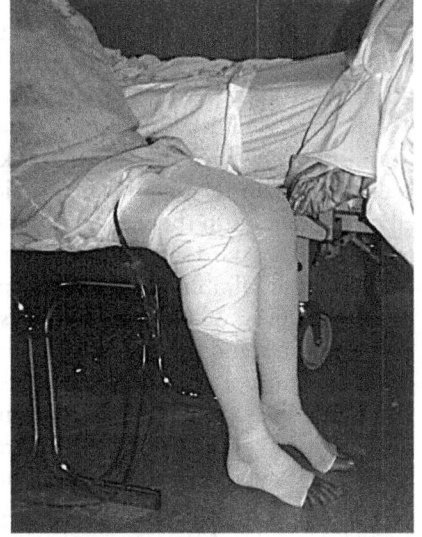

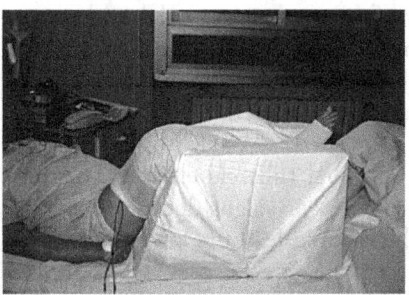

Fig. 1 – Posture in flexion on a foam pad. These postural exercises are started immediately after leaving the recovery room.

Fig. 2 – Posture in flexion as soon as the first postoperative day.

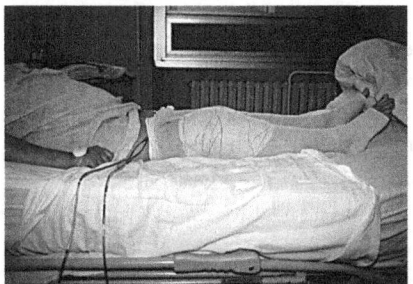

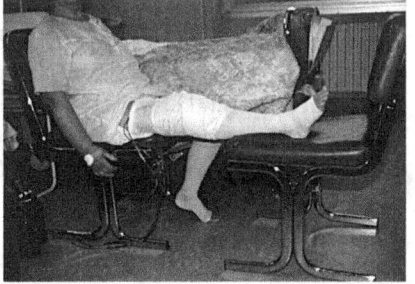

Fig. 3. – Posture in complete extension in bed, started immediately. No cushion is placed under the popliteal fossa.

Fig. 4. – Posture in extension with the patient sitting, from postoperative day 3.

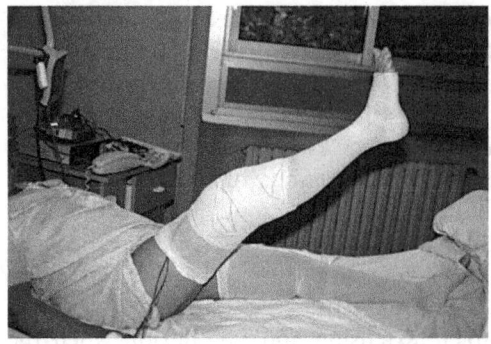

Fig. 5. – Exercise consisting of raising the stretched leg as soon as possible.

reflex inhibition, which is very often present in the early postoperative days. Open kinetic chain static, flash and held contractions are performed, to obtain active elevation of the patella, as well as elevation with the leg stretched (fig. 5). Generally at this stage of rehabilitation there is active flexion contracture of 10 to 20°, related to postoperative pain or use of a crural catheter for analgesia;

8.Recovery of walking ability. From the first postoperative day, weight bearing is allowed on the operated knee as tolerated. The patient learns to walk again with the help of the physiotherapist, with a zimmer frame or two elbow crutches. On the second day the patient is allowed to walk in the room and from the third day in the corridor if his or her general health status permits. Stair climbing is practised during the first week with the help of the physiotherapist. When going up stairs the patient leads with the healthy knee and when descending leads on the operated knee, aided by two canes or by one cane and the stair-rail.

A brace may be necessary after anterior tibial tubercle elevation or quadriceps snip if there was wide preoperative varus or valgus deviation, if there is marked quadriceps reflex inhibition which could lead the knee to give way in a standing position, or for analgesia. In the first two cases, it is removed on the surgeon's discretion, and in the last two cases when the knee is able to lock or when pain has decreased.

Results

A prospective study (19) of 58 total knee replacements identified two factors which help recovery of flexion after rehabilitation: protocols using non-constrained postural exercises rather than continuous passive motion, and prolonged loco-regional anaesthesia by crural catheter with re-injection during the first two days after surgery (fig. 6 and 7).

Supervision of wound healing

The first signs of cutaneous ischaemia appear early, between postoperative days 3 and 7, and its depth and extent cannot be assessed in the beginning. Manipulation of the joint with the dressing removed shows, by the blanching

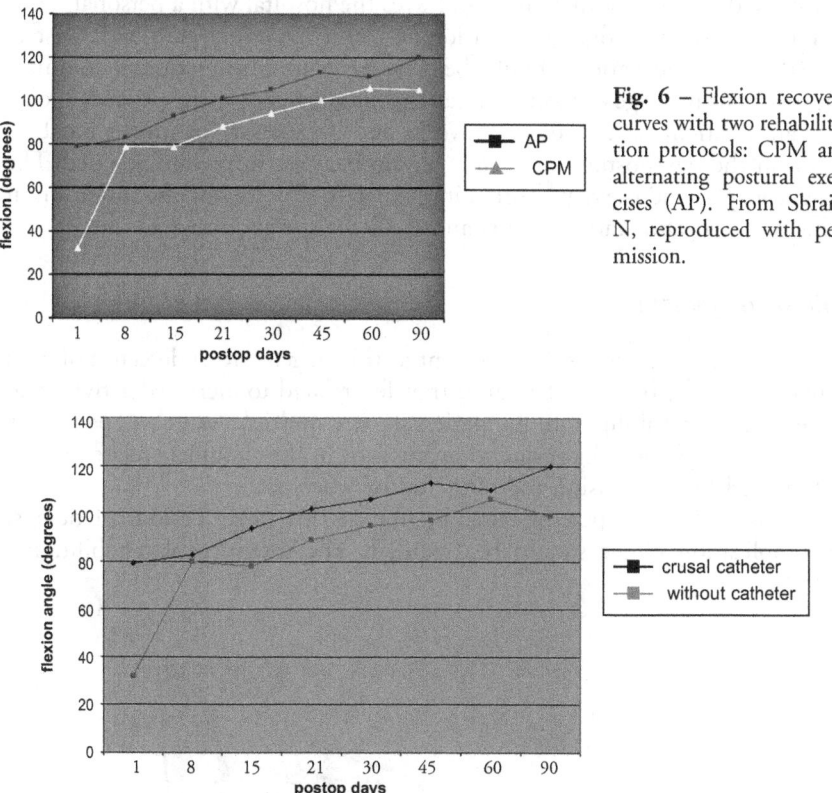

Fig. 6 – Flexion recovery curves with two rehabilitation protocols: CPM and alternating postural exercises (AP). From Sbraire N, reproduced with permission.

Fig. 7 – Flexion recovery curves with two analgesic protocols: with and without loco-regional anaesthesia (LRA) by crural catheter.
From Sbraire N, reproduced with permission.

of the cutaneous edges of the wound, the angle which must not be exceeded if healing is to be safeguarded. If there is a doubt, priority must be given to wound healing by decreasing the range of motion allowed during manipulation, because angle recovery is always possible whereas delayed healing and its accompanying risk of infection raises problems which are much more difficult to solve. Ice should never be used for more than 15 to 20 minutes and it should never be applied directly on the surgical wound, but preferably on the lateral aspects of the knee.

Rehabilitation from postoperative days 7 to 30

The patient, partially independent, is discharged from hospital to his or her home if medical factors (age, general health status, local status of the knee, absence of immediate postoperative complications) and social or logistic factors (support from family and friends, living conditions, proximity, accessibility and availability of physiotherapy in private practice) allow. The patient must be followed by a physiotherapist and leaves the hospital with a personal home exercise programme (fig. 8) and a log-book for recording pain and satisfaction (fig. 9). The patient should be seen early in consultation to monitor improvement in range of motion. In a rehabilitation centre, the patient is generally an inpatient for two or three weeks and if necessary continues rehabilitation in the day hospital or with a physiotherapist in private practice. The patient may attend the day hospital immediately after leaving the surgical unit if his or her health status permits and if all the social criteria are met.

Pain management

The treatment of pain is still important at this stage. A recrudescence of pain may occur in the first few days after transfer, related to increased activity and more intense rehabilitation. In patients with multiple arthritis, pain may appear in the opposite knee due to overuse, or in the shoulders related to use of the overhead suspension rod, crutches or wheelchair.

Rest is an integral part of rehabilitation at this stage. Periods of bedrest and application of ice should be frequent. The intensity of rehabilitation

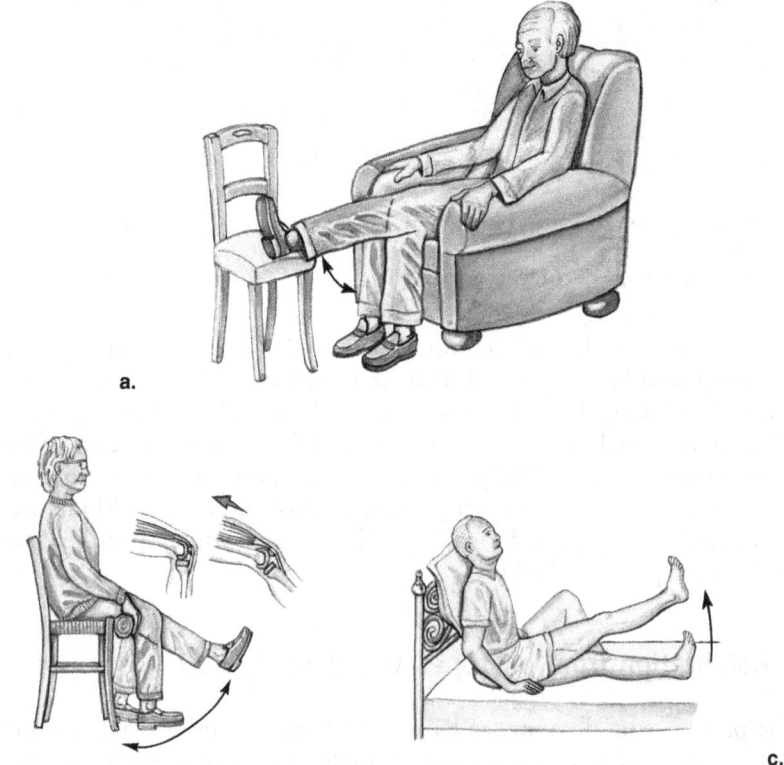

a.

b.   c.

Fig. 8. – Patient's personal home exercise programme.
a. Alternating postural exercises in flexion and in extension; **b.** Dynamic musculation of the quadriceps; **c.** Isometric exercises of the quadriceps.

should be adjusted to the patient's general health status and to the tolerance of the operated knee. A wheelchair can be used over longer distances in order to spare the recently operated joint.

Recovery of range of motion

Exercises on passive movement remain essential. The aim of this phase is conservation of complete extension and acquisition of flexion close to 110°. In all cases, the rule "never train through pain" should be respected. The patient's range of motion should improve regularly and great vigilance is required as long as the aims of this phase have not been reached.

Recovery of complete extension is essential at this stage to obtain walking without limping and above all to allow the prosthetic components to function in good mechanical conditions. Prevention of passive flexion contracture

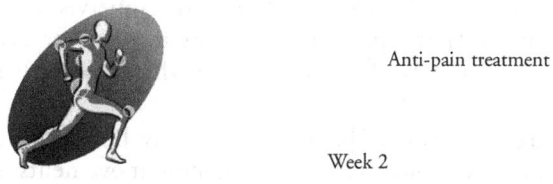

Anti-pain treatment

Week 2

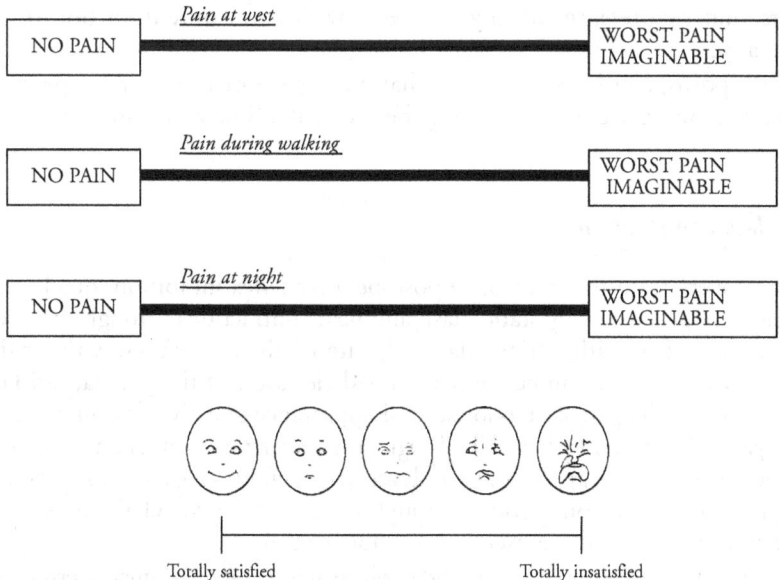

INTENSITY OF YOUR PAIN: Place a mark on the line at the level of your pain.

Pain at west

| NO PAIN | WORST PAIN IMAGINABLE |

Pain during walking

| NO PAIN | WORST PAIN IMAGINABLE |

Pain at night

| NO PAIN | WORST PAIN IMAGINABLE |

Totally satisfied   Totally insatisfied

Fig. 9. – Weekly evaluation of pain and satisfaction* using visual analog scales.
* From: Bullens PHJ, VanLoon CJM, De Waal Malefijt MC *et al.* (2001): Patient satisfaction after total knee arthroplasty. J Arthroplasty 2001; 16(6): 740-7

is all the more difficult if it was already present before the procedure and if there is also contralateral flexion contracture. Deep massage and stretching of the posterior muscle and tendon structures can be of help, as can application of relaxing currents to the posterior muscle structures. Postural exercises carried out several times a day remain the basis of work on extension.

Flexion is recovered through manipulation by the physiotherapist, but also by postural exercises carried out several times a day with the patient sitting on the edge of a table and letting the leg swinging according to the drop-and-dangle technique. Patellar manipulation is continued, insisting on its lowering in order to facilitate knee flexion and associated with massages of the subquadricipital recesses and the lateral aspects of the knee.

Progressively, we go on to active manipulation in flexion through the open kinetic chain ischial and tibial muscles then through the closed kinetic chain. Use of the arthromotor is only accessory, before or after manual manipulation. The same principles must be respected as in the immediate postoperative period: painless treatment, short sessions, no hurry, supervision by the physiotherapist and control of the patient. The joint must never become overheated and the arthromotor is of no further use when flexion is more than 90°.

When wound healing is complete, balneotherapy may be proposed for muscle relaxation, with the patient carrying out pedalling movements in the water gently and without resistance. If there is no contraindication (such as delayed healing, arteritis, phlebitis, established pulmonary embolism), pressure therapy sessions are valuable to reduce the volume of the leg. Residual painful bruising is treated by local application of creams or ointments, and by pressure therapy followed by double contention both rigid and elastic.

From postoperative day 21, lymphatic drainage of the lateral aspects of the knee (condylar convexities) may be a useful adjunct in restoring mobility.

Muscle strengthening

After recovery from the immediate postoperative reflex inhibition, quadriceps exercises are performed by static, flash and held contractions through the open kinetic chain, first with a triangular wedge under the femur then without the wedge, in order to obtain active maintained elevation of the patella, satisfactory tension of the patellar tendon and disappearance of active flexion contracture against the weight of the tibial segment; under no circumstances should additional weight be applied at the level of the ankle. As soon as possible, dynamic quadriceps contractions through the closed kinetic chain are started (type mini-squatt) if these exercises are not painful.

To strengthen the muscles, in particular if there is substantial quadriceps reflex inhibition, electrical stimulation can be used with or without biofeedback, sometimes even using a double channel to obtain more complete relaxation of the ischial and tibial muscles during quadriceps contraction (fig. 8 and 9).

Recovery of walking and independence

Recovery of walking function

From a walking distance restricted to the hospital room during the immediate postoperative stage, the patient now attains completely independent ambulation during this phase of rehabilitation. At its conclusion, walking, the most functional aspect of rehabilitation, must be possible without a limp, if not without a cane.

For correct ambulation, single foot support must be possible and therefore complete weight bearing on the operated leg. This is practised by gradually shifting the weight of the body, using scales if necessary, or on a rib stall, avoiding any excessive reliance on the pelvic or shoulder girdle.

Up to postoperative day 30, the patient walks with two elbow crutches; gait is three-time (using both crutches together for the first 10 to 15 days) and then four-time (each cane in turn). The cane on the operated side can only be abandoned when the patient has gained good walking stability and is able to lock the knee well, after postoperative day 30. For walking outside and on uneven ground, we advise the use of one or two canes, depending essentially on the patient's degree of confidence.

Ambulatory training is specially designed to eliminate any cause of limping: elevation of the hip during the swing phase of gait, heel contact in flexion contracture, walking with the knee kept stiff due to inadequate active triple flexion of the hip-knee-ankle during the swing phase, possible unequal stride length which must be compensated, hip abduction or adduction in patients who presented wide preoperative divergence in genu varum or genu valgum.

Proprioceptive training

This aims at active joint stability through the closed kinetic chain. Anteroposterior and lateral stability are taught by the physiotherapist pushing the patient off balance with the latter standing on both feet. Lateral movements towards the left and the right in turn allow work on the internal and external muscular supportive structures and ensure the lateral stability of the knee, while strengthening the periarticular muscles of the hip above.

Independence

The patient's universe immediately after surgery was restricted to the room, while during this phase he or she progresses to complete independence. Washing and dressing the legs, particularly putting on pressure stockings, may be difficult for the patient in the beginning. He or she is aided by the care staff in the early stages and then if necessary can be advised by the ergotherapist and be loaned equipment (long-handled brush and grip) which gradually help to regain independence.

Prevention and detection of local complications

These are based on weekly patient follow-up. Each week, the patient's general health status is evaluated clinically and by laboratory tests. The progress of the operated knee is monitored by a pluridisciplinary team (specialist in physical medicine and rehabilitation, physiotherapist). Skin problems and thrombophlebitis are treated elsewhere.

Hemarthrosis

This generally occurs in a context of early anti-vitamin K treatment for the prevention or cure of phlebitis and is the most painful clinical picture in total knee arthroplasty. The onset is extremely sudden, pain is severe enough to cause fainting and is accompanied by a cohort of general signs which vary from one patient to another. The patient shrinks from knee examination; when it is possible the knee is found to have very little change in volume but is very hard to the touch, unlike even marked hydarthrosis. It is mandatory to rest the joint, apply ice and give major analgesics if necessary while monitoring the patient closely. In such a context secondary flexion contracture sometimes develops which is extremely difficult to treat because of the intense pain.

Reflex sympathetic dystrophy

In this clinical picture, stiffness may develop with regression of range of motion in flexion and in extension. Pain is intense during manipulation but also during rest and at night, is refractory to analgesics and to non-steroidal anti-inflammatory agents, and may be accompanied by local vasomotor disturbances.

Rehabilitation must be adjusted in consequence, rest must be given a major place, exercises must be less demanding on the joint, aided by physiotherapy with alternate hot and cold soaks. Medical treatment must be initiated without hesitation (more powerful analgesics and calcitonin).

Stiffness

Often associated with pain in end-of-range manipulation, it appears between postoperative days 15 and 30. The joint makes no further progress and stagnates at less than 90° of flexion. There are few signs of inflammation and generally the patient makes good use when walking of the little mobility acquired. The surgeon must be informed of this interruption in progress between postoperative days 15 and 30 in order to decide whether early manipulation under general anaesthesia is required.

Readaptation and reintegration: after the first postoperative month

A number of patients still find that during this period their joint is sensitive to certain circumstances such as fatigue, prolonged standing, long car journeys or barometric pressure. They have learnt, during the preceding phases, to be attentive to their knee and to manage pain relief by themselves. If they have no other cause of pain, most patients now only use simple analgesics as required.

At the beginning of this phase flexion is generally close to 110° and it may increase slightly during the following few weeks to 120 or even 130° around 60 days postoperatively without any change in the rehabilitation methods used.

Where extension is concerned, at this period care must be taken to avoid the onset or recurrence of flexion contracture which, even if minimal, could alter the quality of ambulation and lead to excessive strain and pain of the operated joint.

The patient must be strongly and frequently encouraged to continue self-rehabilitation by postural exercises and stretching.

Muscle strengthening is continued at home with the same exercises taught by the physiotherapist: static, flash and maintained contractions with the open kinetic chain, dynamic contractions with the closed kinetic chain in the last 30° of extension.

The patient no longer needs canes for walking on an even surface; for walking outside, he or she keeps one or two canes depending on the degree of confidence. From the beginning of this phase, the walking distance may already reach or exceed one kilometre.

Up to postoperative day 6, we advise the patient to climb and *a fortiori* to descend stairs asymmetrically. Climbing can be symmetric only when the quadriceps has completely recovered its concentric strength. Going down stairs requires a quadriceps which is sufficiently strong in eccentric work and above all at least 120° knee flexion, which the patient has not necessarily acquired two months postoperatively. In addition, patients are more anxious when going down stairs, leading them to use a cane and the stair-rail.

During this phase, proprioceptive training is continued by learning to walk on uneven ground and by reintegration in local life aided by a physiotherapist in private practice. Fall prevention is taught by walking against resistance and continuation of the work with side and backward or forward pushes. Rising from a fall, particularly important for a patient who is elderly or living alone, can be learnt in a physiotherapy room making use of items of furniture, the walls or canes. Vehicle driving is allowed after 45 days for patients with a left knee replacement and after 60 days for those with a right knee replacement.

Conclusion

Early manipulation after total knee replacement has enabled fuller, more rapid recovery giving better results than in the first series. Initiation of manipulation as soon as possible and optimal management of postoperative pain appear to be the principal factors governing final mobility.

Throughout the rehabilitation process, collaboration between all those involved must be perfect in order to detect any complications and provide timely treatment for them.

References

1. Anouchi YS, McShane M, Kelly F *et al.* (1996) Range of motion in total knee replacement. Clin Orthop 331: 87-92
2. Colwell CW, Morris BA (1992) The influence of continuous passive motion on the results of total knee arthroplasty. Clin Orthop 276: 225-8
3. Coutts RD, Toth C, Kaita JH (1984) The role of continuous passive motion in the rehabilitation of the total knee patient. In: Hungerford DS, Krackow KA, Kenna RV. Total knee arthroplasty: a comprehensive approach. Williams and Wilkins, Baltimore: 126-32
4. Emerson RH, Ayers C, Head WC *et al.* (1996) Surgical closing in primary total knee arthroplasties: flexion versus extension. Clin Orthop 331: 74-80
5. Johnson DP (1990) The effect of continuous passive motion on wound-healing and joint mobility after knee arthroplasty. J Bone Joint Surg (Am) 72: 421-6
6. Kumar PJ, McPherson EJ, Dorr LD *et al.* (1996) Rehabilitation after total knee arthroplasty: a comparison of two rehabilitation techniques. Clin Orthop 331: 93-101
7. Lachiewicz PF (2000) The role of continuous passive motion after total knee arthroplasty. Clin Orthop 380: 144-50
8. Lotke PA, Faralli VJ, Orenstein EM *et al.* (1991) Blood loss after total knee replacement. Effects of tourniquet release and continuous passive motion. J Bone Joint Surg (Am) 73: 1037-40
9. Lynch AF, Bourne RB, Rorabeck CH *et al.* (1988) Deep-vein thrombosis and continuous passive motion after total knee arthroplasty. J Bone Joint Surg (Am) 70: 11-4
10. Lynch JA, Baker PL, Polly RE *et al.* (1990) Mechanical measures in the prophylaxis of postoperative thromboembolism in total knee arthroplasty. Clin Orthop 260: 24-9
11. MacDonald SJ, Bourne RB, Rorabeck CH *et al.* (2000) Prospective randomised clinical trial of continuous passive motion after total knee arthroplasty. Clin Orthop 380: 30-5
12. Maloney WJ, Schurman DJ, Hangen D *et al.* (1990) The influence of continuous passive motion on outcome in total knee arthroplasty. Clin Orthop 256: 162-8
13. Mauerhan DR, Mokris JG, Ly A *et al.* (1998) Relationship between length of stay and manipulation rate after total knee arthroplasty. J Arthroplasty 13: 896-900
14. McInnes J, Larson MG, Daltroy LH (1992) A controlled evaluation of continuous passive motion in patient undergoing total knee arthroplasty. JAMA 268: 1423-28
15. Pope RO, Corcoran S, McCaul K *et al.* (1997) Continuous passive motion after primary total knee arthroplasty. Does it offer any benefits? J Bone Joint Surg (Br) 79: 914-7
16. Ritter MA, Gandolf VS, Holston KS (1989) Continuous passive motion versus physical therapy in total knee arthroplasty. Clin Orthop 244: 239-43
17. Romness DW, Rand JA (1988) The role of continuous passive motion following total knee arthroplasty. Clin Orthop 226: 34-7
18. Salter RB, Simmonds DF, Malcolm BW *et al.* (1980) The biological effect of continuous passive motion on the healing of full thickness defects in articular cartilage. An experimental investigation in the rabbit. J Bone Joint Surg (Am) 62: 1232-51
19. Sbraire N (1999) Facteurs prédictifs de la rééducation fonctionnelle après prothèse totale du genou. MD thesis, Université de Lyon, n° 90
20. Ververeli PA, Sutton DC, Hearn SL *et al.* (1995) Continuous passive motion after total knee arthroplasty. Analysis of cost and benefits. Clin Orthop 321: 208-15
21. Vince KG, Kelly MA, Beck J *et al.* (1987) Continuous passive motion after total knee arthroplasty. J Arthroplasty 2: 281-4
22. Yashar AA, Venn-Watson E, Welsh T *et al.* (1997) Continuous passive motion with accelerated flexion after total knee arthroplasty. Clin Orthop 345: 38-43

French anesthesia for total knee arthroplasty: Medical management during the perioperative period

D. Gallet

In France in 1996, 45 000 patients had a total knee replacement (TKP) under anesthetic, which was 3% of all anesthetic procedures in France (Y. Auroy *et al.* [1]). Some patients with degenerative osteoarthropathies choose to have the operation so that they can continue with their favorite activities, but there are other patients who have serious and disabling inflammatory disease complications, or they may be elderly or obese, or they could have a complex medical history (cardiovascular disease, respiratory disease, renal disease, diabetes), and they could be subject to a variety of perioperative complications (cardiovascular, thromboembolism, infection, neuropsychological disorders and so on). Absolute contraindications to anesthesia are rare, but a benefit/risk assessment should be performed; this is done by determining the real benefit of the operation (pain, mobility, quality of life) and the perioperative risk. The specific complications will be related to the use of a tourniquet, risk of infection, risk of thromboembolism, and risk of perioperative bleeding. Risks connected with the use of acrylic cement are less important here than in total hip prosthesis (THP). Mortality at three months is estimated at 0.1% to 0.9%, pulmonary embolism caused by fibrin clots are rare at 0-0.2%, and immediate perioperative deaths can be attributed to fat embolism caused by endo-medullary surgery, which is more common with TKP than THP (2, 3). In general, patients who have had a knee prosthesis have longer life expectancy than the general population, this is especially true for women over the age of 75 years. Male gender, a history of rheumatoid polyarthritis, infection and thromboembolism complications are recognized as risk factors for earlier mortality (4). Functional disability is the most common reason for underestimating cardiac, coronary or respiratory insufficiency and the anesthesiology consultation must therefore take these factors into account. This consultation should occur at least one month before the operation, to evaluate the suitability of the patient for surgery, the risk of thrombosis, give some idea of the transfusion strategy after estimation of the risk of hemorrhage and investigate and treat any focus of infection. After patient informed and consent form signedinforming the patient and the signing of the consent form, the anesthetist will draw up an optimum anesthesia and postoperative analgesia protocol which is aimed at reducing the patient's discomfort as far as possible;

this strategy should also allow the patient to begin rehabilitation as early as possible. The anesthetist must decide on the strategy by taking into account the information from the history and clinical examination, only the patients who have the highest risk will gain any benefit from targeted supplementary tests, this will ensure that unnecessary and costly tests are avoided. Before any surgery it is vital that a preoperative assessment (5) is performed to give the patients the accurate, clear and appropriate information they require, and to develop the best ways to prevent and limit risk. The surgical course of action should only be decided after discussing the risk/benefit analysis. The entire operative procedure can turn out to be difficult and requires close coordination between the attending physician, the cardiologist, the surgeon, the anesthetist and the patient, who has been fully informed of the terms of the discussion.

Evaluation of cardiorespiratory function (6, 7)

The report produced by the American College of Cardiology and the American Heart Association (8) states that scheduled major orthopedic surgery is considered to be of intermediate cardiovascular risk; 1 to 8% of those operated on have perioperative cardiac complications (9). In all cases the cardiologist (10, 14, 15) should be consulted to coordinate the risk evaluation procedures, optimize pre-and postoperative medical treatment and, if necessary, recommend preoperative coronary revascularizsation to improve long term survival.

Strategy for minimum blood loss

Suspending treatment with platelet function inhibitors (PFI)

As the risk of hemorrhage due to treatment with PFIs has not been the subject of any studies there is little data available; however it is suggested that suspending treatment with platelet function inhibitors during the perioperative period will not increase the thrombosis risk in most cases (11). Acetylsalicylic acid, ticlopidine hydrochloride (Ticlid®) and clopidogrel bisulfate (Plavix®) must be stopped ten days before the surgical procedure otherwise there is a risk of aggravatingessential a coronary thrombotic event (12). Patients who have high risk arterial disease must be identified, as they should not have their treatment suspended or their treatment should be suspended for as short a time as possible, and a the cardiologist should be consulted.

Evaluation of transfusion requirements

At present, it is estimated that 20 to 30% of moderately anemic patients who have a surgical procedure fairly likely to cause blood loss will require a transfusion. Normally the transfusion requirements for a total knee replacement with tourniquet, 800 to 1,500mL mainly postoperatively, should be covered by 2 to 3 units of blood. Blood transfusion procedures must conform to a very complex set of regulations that ensure traceability and quality assurance programs that will deliver the best transfusion risk/benefit ratio for each patient at any given time (16). With the SFAR consensus (*Société Française d'Anesthésie et de Réanimation*, Intensive Care and Anesthesia French Society) (17) which was based on experimental and clinical studies of the peroperative and recovery metabolic requirements and critical oxygen delivery (DO2) in stress situations, the clinician now allows hemoglobin levels of between 7 and $10g/dL^{-1}$ for most stable anemic patients (hematocrit between 21% and 30%). Within these values, the decision to transfuse will rely on the clinical criteria of the patient's tolerance to the anemia, length of time the anemia has been present, the circulating blood volume, the speed rate of blood loss, the associated pathologies, the metabolic status and the body's capacity for adapting to the anemia. The a Allowable blood losses are calculated from the time of the consultation consultation according to the patient's hemoglobin volume and the acceptable minimum final hematocrit, fixed at the theoretical transfusion threshold level. The difference between the allowable and expected blood loss will determine how aggressive the preoperative strategy will be. By knowing the patient's weight and hematocrit, the total average blood loss for the operation with a given surgeon, each anesthetist can calculate the theoretic requirements between day −1 and day +5 using the formula:

$$\text{Allowable loss in mL} = \frac{\text{TBV} \times [\text{Initial hematocrit (day -1)} - \text{Final hematocrit (day +5)}]}{\text{Mean hematocrit}}$$

$$\text{TBV} = \text{total blood volume} = 70 \text{ mL/kg for men } 65 \text{ mL/kg for women}$$

$$\text{Mean hematocrit} = \frac{(\text{Initial hematocrit} + \text{Final hematocrit})}{2}$$

In homologous transfusions (18), the French current estimations of viral transmission per number of donations are in the order of 1/220,000 for hepatitis B, 1/375,000 for hepatitis C, 1/1,350,000 for HIV and 1/7,000,000 for HTLVI. Whilst the risks of immunological incompatibility are higher (1/6,000 to 1/29,000), there are still risks from bacteria (serious accident: 1/250,000), such as allergic reactions (anti-immunoglobulin A antibodies in the recipient) but there is also the possibility of transfusing non-conventional transmissible agents such as bovine spongiform encephalopathy (BSE) despite strict donor selection procedures and the removal of leucocytes, which is now standard. The most recent data in the literature gives a residual overall mortality risk of 1/100,000.

Autotransfusion

There are three main techniques used for autotransfusion, they all can be used to reduce the blood requirements without eliminating the possibility of giving a homologous transfusion if necessary.

Using planned autologous transfusion, the patients give their consent to having blood taken two or three times from the 35th to the 10th day before the operation, saving 2 to 3 units of blood. These autologous transfusion products can be stored for 6 weeks at 4°C (French government circular DGS/DH/AFS of 31/01/1997). The expected benefits will depend on the amount of red cells the patient can regenerate between the first collection and the surgical procedure after stimulation of their endogenous erythropoietin (EPO) production, insofar as this is dependent on the iron reserves. The most effective schedule seems to be starting the collections as early as possible before the operation (5 weeks) and to take the first collections fairly close together as this increases the EPO production. Patients who have received programmed autologous transfusions are 5 times less likely to be exposed to the risks of homologous transfusion (19). However, there is some disagreement over the real benefit of this technique in all cases, as it can be cumbersome, has some inherent risks and the cost effectiveness is fairly low (20). According to the French Blood Agency (AFS) and the French National Agency for Health Accreditation and Evaluation (ANAES) (21), this technique should be reserved for patients who are in good heath, are not anemic (Hb > 13g/dL^{-1}), have a life expectancy of over 10 years and have undergoing surgery having a surgical procedure where a considerable blood loss (more than 1 500mL) is expected and/or normally requires a transfusion in more than 50% of cases. The price charged by the French Blood Establishment (ETS) is 200 Euros = 1 PRC + 1 FFP compared with 165 Euros for leucocyte free PRC of homologous blood (150mL of RC). It is dangerous for patients with un decompensated cardiovascular disease, epileptic patients, patients having recently had a CVA, patients with severe liver or kidney disease, or respiratory disease. It is contraindicated if there is infection, if the hemoglobin level is less than 11g/dL^{-1}, if the patients who are known reactors to HBs markers, anti-HIV 1 and 2 antibodies, anti-HVC antibodies, anti-HTLV I and II antibodies, anti-HBc antibodies without anti-HBs, unless the patient has a rare blood group or a mix of unusual anti-red blood cell antibodies that make treatment impossible.

Planned autologous erythropheresis (red blood cell apheresis) is selective collection of 2 or 3 units of concentrated red blood cells for apheresis using a cell separator. In common with planned autologous transfusion, the French Blood Agency recommends that the blood can be stored for 42 days at 4°C. It is contraindicated when the hemoglobin level is less than 13g/dL^{-1}. The other contraindications are the same as for planned autologous transfusion, taking into account that its main drawback is that it places more strain on the patient as larger amounts of blood are exchanged. Its main advantage is that it gives better results than planned autologous transfusion for the erythropoietin production and hemoglobin levels obtained. Consequently, the cost element is not the only advantage, one serology assessment, a single visit 25 days before the operation, currently costs and a current cost of 388 Euros for 2 or 3 units of red cells. Erythropheresis performed 3 to 4 weeks before the operation on patients who are not anemic is a much more suitable procedure than standard planned autologous transfusion, as it is much more cost efficient. The number of units collected will depend on the patient's blood volume and hematocrit results on the day of collection, thus the erythropheresis session could be completed by a later planned autologous transfusion session depending on the patient's requirements. Preoperative normovolemic hemodilution (NVHD) is commonly used in the USA (22). This involves deliberate removal of whole blood before the operation, this causes the hematocrit to drop dramatically and the blood volume is replaced by infusion of crystalloids. In Europe, this technique cannot be recommended in orthopedics as the medical arguments are in favor of planned autologous transfusion. Although costs are low, there have been no reputable clinical trials that suggest that NVHD is as effective. The trial results are very mixed and the benefit risk ratio is particularly poor.

Erythropoietin

Recombinant human erythropoietin (rhEPO) is useful as it will increase the hemoglobin level if it is administered during the 3 to 5 weeks before the intervention, the blood count should be monitored during this time. Several multicenter trials (23, 24) have shown that treatment with rhEPO was beneficial in terms of increasing the number of planned autologous transfusion collections and/or reducing the requirements for homologous transfusions when the initial hemoglobin levels are between 10 and $13g/dL^{-1}$. The methods for prescribing erythropoietin (Eprex®, Recormon®) in the perioperative period are given in the latest SPC: moderate anemia between 10 and $13g/dL^{-1}$, adults without iron deficiency, planned major orthopedic surgery, moderate loss (900 to 1,800mL), administration of 600IU/kg/week in 4 subcutaneous injections, starting 3 weeks before the intervention using the Goldberg scheme (day-21, day-14, day-7 and day-1). The risk of hypertension and deep vein thrombosis has not yet been reported at these doses, but the risk factors for thromboembolism linked to the administration of EPO should be kept in mind, as well as the main contraindications: uncontrolled hypertension, unstable angina, significant carotid stenosis, history of myocardial infarct or CVA (25).

In all these cases, if the hemoglobin levels rise above $15g/dL^{-1}$ or the hematocrit above 50% the prescription must be stopped. Unfortunately use of EPO is still limited to certain regions in France as it can only be used or prescribed by hospital pharmacies.

Iron treatment

Apart from any pre-existing iron overload, iron supplements are obviously required during any programmed autologous transfusions protocols, but they are vital when EPO is used. Iron supplements are also recommended if there is iron deficiency anemia or moderate anemia of chronic inflammation. Oral iron is not particularly viable effective as only 10 to 20% of the ingested dose is absorbed, but it is still effective although it can often produce gastric problems. IM iron (Maltofer®) also has several drawbacks (pain, skin blemishes, incomplete absorption). Intravenous iron sucrose (Venofer®) (26) is released and used very effectively in the body but, like erythropoietin, it is not always available at present (27).

Perioperative blood recovery (28, 29)

The French Blood Agency recommends (circular DGS/DH/AFS of 31 January 1997) that perioperative blood recovery is only used when peroperative bleeding is above or equal to 15% of the blood volume in the first six hours after the operation (850mL for a 80kg man and 600mL for a 60kg woman). The stand-by technique is the most commonly used: collecting receptacle in place, patient receives recycled blood if required . Surgical aspiration is destructive as the blood aspirated during the intervention is lacking in hemostasis factors, contains bone particles, fat globules, cement particles, fibrin and platelet aggregates, free hemoglobin, cell debris and modified red cells. The potential risks of coagulopathy and DIVC (FDP, D-Dimers, activated factors), risks connected with the reinjection of inflammation-mediating substances (leukocytes, cytokines), the risks of fatty or bone marrow embolism and the risks of infection mean that postoperative retransfusion of large quantities of blood collected from the wound site, if not centrifuged and washed, is only recommended in extreme emergencies, and must not exceed 1 000mL. Volumes in excess of this must be centrifuged, washed and filtered. Red blood cells treated in this way can be of very high quality (ATP, 2.3 DPG) and the risks of bacterial contamination are limited. Contraindications that apply to both peroperative and postoperative blood recovery, apart from in situations of extreme emergency, are local or general infection, certain recurring cancers, use of an antiseptic product or organic glues containing thromboplastins. Any incident must be recorded and reported to the local blood monitoring representative.

Antibiotic prophylaxis (ABP)

The frequency of postoperative infection in prosthetic joint surgery is 3 to 5%. ABP should reduce the infection rate to less than 1%. It is even more beneficial if the operation cannot be performed under laminar flow conditions. In 1999 a group of French experts produced recommendations (30) stating that antibiotic prophylaxis, usually intravenous, must always be given before the surgical procedure, at a maximum time of one hour to one and a half hour before surgery, and if possible during the anesthesia induction period before inflating the tourniquet. It should be given for a brief period, usually just during the operation, occasionally for 24 hours and rarely for 48 hours. These recommendations should be followed even if there is drainage of the wound site. There is no need to prescribe repeated antibiotic injections during removal of drains, tubes or catheters. The first dose, given by weight of the patient, is usually double the standard dose. Repeated injections at the same dose will be given during the intervention procedure if the operation lasts longer than twice the half-life of the antibiotic. As with antibiotic treatment in general, antibiotic prophylaxis protocols should be established locally, after consultation with the surgeons, anesthetists and recovery staff, infections specialists, microbiologists and pharmacists. They should be displayed in the operating suite and validated by the committee dealing with nosocomial infections and the committee responsible for the establishment of drug policies. The value of local antibiotic prophylaxis by using cements impregnated with antibiotics has not been established. Early repeated operations for surgical reasons not related to infection (hematoma, dislocation, mechanical problems) will require ABP with a different antibiotic; vancomycin is recommended. The environmental conditions of the institution may also have to be taken into account (hospital acquired gram negative bacilli). High rates of operating site infections or the emergence of multi-resistant bacteria infections will require a multidisciplinary approach to combat the problem.

A straightforward knee joint prosthesis should only require antibiotic prophylaxis during the operating period. The targeted bacteria are: *S. aureus, S. epidermidis, Propionibacterium, Corynebacterium, Streptococci, E. coli, K. pneumoniae* (table I).

Anesthetic techniques

General anesthesia and regional spinal or epidural anesthesia

At the present time it is still difficult to decide between a general anesthetic and regional spinal or epidural anesthesia and the recommendations differ (21, 32, 33).

Regional nerve trunk analgesia

Postoperative pain will be at a maximum during the first 24 to 36 hours. It will persist particularly during mobilization, when regional nerve trunk analgesia is an important tool. It should be combined with the prescription of standard analgesics and morphine given as intravenous patient controlled analgesia (IVPCA); oral analgesics can then be substituted. Complete anesthesia of the knee can be produced by a combination of anterior-posterior sciatic and cutaneous nerve block posterior to the thigh arising from the sacral plexus, and the anterior nerves arising from the lumbar plexus (femoral, lateral cutaneous nerve of the thigh, obturator and saphenous). These nerve trunk blocks

Table I – ABP/1998 update of the recommendations of the 1992 SFAR Consensus Conference (30).

Orthopedic surgery: replacement material, bone graft, ligamentoplasty, closed fracture	Cefazoline	2g before surgery	Single dose (repeated injection of 1g if duration superior to 4 hours)
	Allergy: vancomycine	15mg/kg before surgery	Single dose

of the lower limb are particularly useful techniques for both the operation period and the postoperative period, as they have little effect on hemodynamics, they give a limited motor block and they are extremely effective. They are not normally used alone in major knee surgery but are combined with a general anesthetic or an epidural or spinal anesthetic to ensure the patient is calm. The nerve trunk anesthetic should preferably be given to a patient who is still awake, before anesthesia (34, 35), so that any signs of accidental nerve or intravascular injection are not masked. The patients are therefore calmed calm without their level of consciousness being altered too radically (midazolam or propofol, without morphine). By using long-acting local anesthetics (bupivacaine 0.5% or ropivacaine 0.75%) combined with low doses of clonidine (0.5mg/kg $^{-1}$) and abiding by the dosage instructions, pain relief can be prolonged postoperatively for 12 to 24 hours (36); this can be done either by single injections or it can be continued over several days by using a perineural catheter. Testing for paraesthesia while performing a peripheral block increases the risk of neurological sequela and is no longer done; neurostimulation is now the technique of choice to ensure that most blocks are successful (37). Using a neurostimulator (37, 38) (fig. 1), electrical impulses from the end of the needle produce muscle contraction specific to the nerve stimulated. The muscle response increases as the stimulus gets closer to the nerve, the intensity of the current should be reduced until the motor response is obtained at the weakest stimulation possible, usually about 0.5mA, without reducing it too much and coming too close to the nerve and damaging it. After locating the nerve with the needle a test dose of 1mL of the local anesthetic is injected so that the motor response disappears momentarily. Increasing the current will confirm that the needle is positioned properly, as the motor response will reappear. The needle must always be moved very carefully as it could cause paresthesia or searing pain. The local anesthetic solution can then be injected in divided doses, repeatedly aspirating to check that the solution is not being injected into a vessel; early discovery of a misinjection will avoid the side effects of tachycardia, discomfort, metallic taste in the mouth, convulsions, heart rate problems, that can be difficult and time-

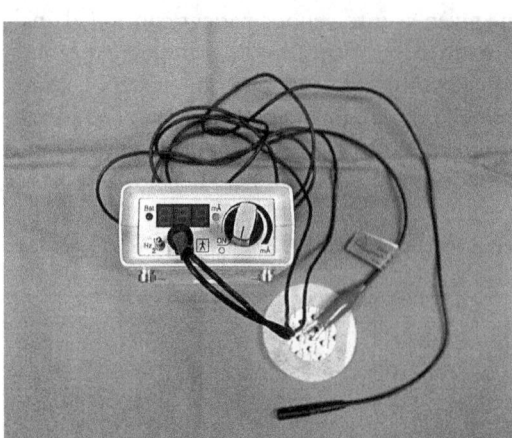

Fig. 1. – Nerve stimulator.

consuming to deal with (39, 40). The risk of a microhemotoma compressing a nerve, even after superficial nerve trunk anesthesia, cannot be ruled out; therefore anticoagulation therapy should not be started until after the injection of spinal anesthetics or peripheral nerve blocks.

As there is always a risk of sepsis, a face mask and gloves should always be worn when performing the injection, and aseptic surgical procedures used. The time required for the procedure (30 minutes) and the delay before the anesthetic is fully active is sometimes important (30 to 40 minutes for the sciatic nerve) and requires some organization. There is also a risk of sores at the distal end of the anesthesia point caused by rubbing or bad positioning if the nerve block is prolonged. Femoral or sciatic nerve and motor blocks carry with them the risk of the patients falling as their legs may buckle, this is most likely after a motor block, so the patients should walk on crutches. Postoperatively, analgesia and not anesthesia should be the rule as there is a risk of masking compartmental syndrome with anesthesia. The perineural catheter can be sealed temporarily to allow the patient to mobilize; the pump can be carried slung across the shoulder. A careful preoperative neurological assessment should be done for diabetic patients with neuropathy; in particular these patients should not be given any adrenaline-containing solutions, the minimum stimulation intensity is higher (about 1 to 1.5mA for 100µs and it is impossible to reduce this to 0.5mA) and the tourniquet will probably be more harmful than the block. In all cases, the patient must be given all the information and given the chance to talk over all the possible complications, in particular the involuntary muscle movements provoked by the nerve stimulation and the pain that may occur if a nerve is punctured. Even when everything is done strictly according to the rules, neurostimulation can cause undesirable effects, so the objective will be to avoid any immediate complications, such as intravascular injection of local anesthetics, hematoma or nerve lesions, and also delayed neurological complications. The French group SOS-ALR have published safety recommendations for risk reduction, and these are also freely available on the Internet (38, 41). They include actions to be taken in cases of neurological complications, evaluated in France in 1997 at 19/10,000 (42). Fanelli *et al.* found that the incidence of paresthesias was 14 to 23% despite neurostimulation and the overall incidence of transitory neurological disorders of 1.7%, although no definite neurological lesion was reported (43). Early clinical evaluation of the damage by a neurologist is vital for each case; the request for the neurology consultation should be accompanied by a detailed description of the problem and a discussion of the causes. Subsequent neurological evaluations should be decided case by case, early and late bilateral electrophysiological explorations (EMG, potentials produced) or imaging studies (scans or MRI) may be indicated. A detailed examination of the patient should be performed and a written report should be produced, this should include the results of any examinations, the day to day monitoring, any events that occurred and the it development, together with the ALR record. The anesthesia records must also show other possible causes of the neurological lesions, such as the use of the tourniquet, the pressure and the length of time the tourniquet was inflated, the surgical device, and the preoperative neurological examination specifying any pre-existing pain or sensitivity in the anesthetized limb and the area of surgery. In common with all anesthetic procedures, all normal precautions should be taken when performing any regional nerve block: There should be a venous access route available, the resuscitation equipment must be checked (electrocardioscope, pulse oximeter, non-invasive blood pressure monitor), careful monitoring of the patient must be performed for 30 minutes after injection of the local anesthetic, surgical cutaneous asepsismust be guaranteed (wearing sterile gown, mask and gloves).

Anesthesia and analgesia of the anterior face of the thigh and knee (fig. 2)

A single paravascular injection of femoral block, or even better a continuous block set up by placing a catheter along the femoral nerve, will anesthetize the anterior face of the thigh and the knee. Good quality postoperative analgesia in the crural region, the lateral cutaneous nerve of the thigh and the obturator nerve can be obtained with a single injection, also known as the 3 in 1 block (39) (fig. 3). Singelyn *et al.* (44), and more recently Capdevilla *et al.* (45), have shown that the analgesia obtained is better than that obtained with an IVPCA, particularly when the patient is mobilized, and the quality is comparable with that obtained with an epidural but there are less failures and undesirable effects. The femoral nerve in the psoas is formed of nerve roots anterior to L1, L2, L3, and L4. It emerges in the thigh by passing under the inguinal ligament, above the psoas, under the deep fascia of the thigh and iliac fascia, exterior to the femoral artery where it is found, in dorsal decubitus, 1cm inside the internal edge of the sartorius muscle, 2cm below the

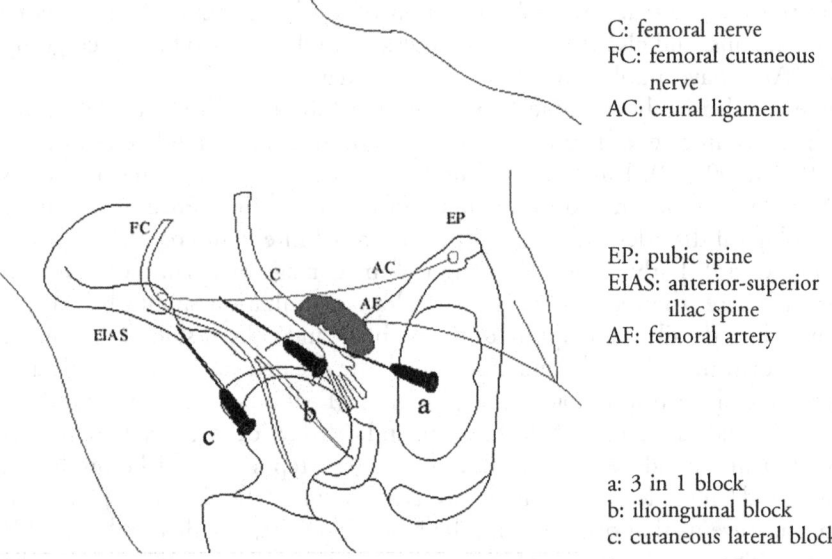

C: femoral nerve
FC: femoral cutaneous
nerve
AC: crural ligament

EP: pubic spine
EIAS: anterior-superior
iliac spine
AF: femoral artery

a: 3 in 1 block
b: ilioinguinal block
c: cutaneous lateral block

Fig. 2. – 3 in 1 block, fascia iliaca and femoral-cutaneous.

crural ligament joining with the anterior-superior iliac spine at the pubic tubercle, 1cm exterior to the femoral artery. It divides rapidly into four terminal branches, lateral and medial musculocutaneous, quadriceps femoris muscle and internal saphenous cutaneous. The needle is introduced in the cranial direction at an angle of 30° to the course of the femoral nerve, until good contraction of the quadriceps is obtained and the patellar rises. When performing local anesthesia ensure that the fascia has been penetrated - there will be a slight loss of resistance when this occurs — before injecting 0.3mL/kg of local anesthetic. The 3 in 1 block of all the branches requires some practice, a total success rate will depend on the operator's experience and also the diffusion capacity upwards towards the lumbar nerve roots (39); analgesia is usually sufficient, but will only persist postoperatively in the crural region (46). The femoral nerve is blocked correctly in 95% of cases, the lateral cutaneous nerve of the thigh in 75% of cases and the obturator in only 10% of cases.

A fascia iliac block is also possible immediately, or if the 3 in 1 block fails, this is preferable to trying to restimulate, and thus damage, a crural nerve, which is already partially anaesthetized (39). This is a multi-trunk block and is not suitable for neurostimulation. The patient is in the dorsal decubitus position; the lower limb is slightly abducted in external rotation. The needle is introduced 0.5 to 1cm below the junction of the lateral third and the medial two thirds of the crural ligament, perpendicular to the skin, until loss of resistance is felt twice as it passes through the two fascias. For continuous infusion or reinjection, the needle stylet is removed and a catheter is introduced so that is passes 1-2cm below the fascia iliaca, this is then connected to an antibacterial filter before fixing carefully to the skin. The movement of the anesthetic solution upwards in this space is rarely a reality, and the results of 3 in 1 anesthetics are as uncertain as a single injection, although it can be useful to check using an X-ray and an injection of contrast.

The obturator nerve is a terminal branch emerging from L2, L3 and L4; retained by the thickness of the psoas, it descends along the medial border of the muscle, travels along the internal border of the pelvis where it emerges through the obturator canal. A selective block of this nerve at the inguinal fold can be performed immediately or postoperatively if there is serious pain in the internal face of the knee. This will be performed by an injection located half way along a line parallel to the inguinal fold; this line is drawn between

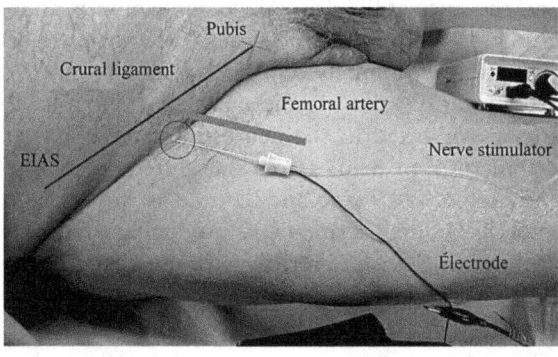

Fig. 3. – Femoral block.

the femoral artery and the internal margin of the tendon of the long adductor, externally to the spermatic cord in men, 1cm under the inguinal fold. The anterior (5mL) and then the posterior (5mL) branches can be located by neurostimulation, the contraction produced is visible on the anterior internal face and then the posterior internal face of the thigh (47). If required the lateral cutaneous nerve of the thigh or the femoral cutaneous nerve can also be blocked separately at the lateral extremity of the inguinal fold by 10mL of local anesthetic. The posterior branch supplies the motor branches for the tensor muscle of the fascia lata and participates in sensory innervation of the lateral face of the thigh. The sensory trunk can be found 2.5cm below and inside the anterior superior iliac spine by introducing the needle perpendicular to the skin until the needle is felt to "pop" through the fascia lata.

All these nerves can be blocked in one go by a posterior lumbar block (PLB) using paravertebral plexus block. When combined with a sciatic nerve block it is effective enough to dispense with a general anesthetic, but we do not have any experience of this as yet. Performing this type of block requires rigorous training. The sources of potential complications (1/500) are the proximity of the paravertebral space to the ascending lumbar vein, the ureter, the peritoneum, the kidney and the vertebral canal. The catheter should be stained and very close postoperative monitoring is required, similar to postepidural monitoring.

Anesthesia and analgesia of the posterior face of the thigh and knee

Arising from all the roots entering the sacral plexus, the sciatic nerve leaves the plexus through the greater sciatic foramen, descends the length of the posterior medial face of the femur in virtually a straight line to the apex of the popliteal fossa where it divides into its two terminal branches, the common peroneal and tibial nerves. The sciatic nerve can be blocked in the buttocks as suggested by Labat (48) by the posterior route, this is the most commonly used and is probably the most satisfactory method as it produces few problems and is extensive. The block will affect the whole area served by the sciatic nerve (49) even though it does not appear useful to block the muscles of the posterior compartment of the thigh, other than tolerating the possible use of a tourniquet. The patient is in the Sim position, lying on their healthy side, the thigh bent at 45° and the knee at 90° (fig. 4). The injection is done at the intersection of the middle of the greater trochanter (GT) – posterior superior iliac spine (PSIS) line-and the line between the GT and the sacrococcygeal hiatus (SCH) (fig. 5). After disinfecting the area and giving a local cutaneous anesthetic, the needle connected to the neurostimulator is introduced perpendicular to the skin to 6 to 8cm, across the gluteus maximus muscle. As the needle progresses the first nerve anesthetized is the inferior gluteal nerve, the motor branch of the small sciatic nerve producing rhythmic contraction of the gluteus maximus muscle. Given the size of the sciatic nerve in the buttocks (10 to 15mm), located several centimeters deeper, it is fairly easy to locate. Accurate location will give flexion of the foot (tibial nerve) or extension of the toes (deep peroneal nerve). The motor response is refined until the best muscle contraction is obtained with the least amount of electrical stimulation (0.5mA for 100µsec). This separate infiltration of the two nerve branches will give an excellent success rate but it could be pointless, or even dangerous, to relentlessly try to find both nerves, particularly if it is proving difficult. A single injection of 0.5% bupivacaine or 0.75% ropivacaine with clonidine will ensure effective postoperative analgesia by diffusion. The risks of this approach could be damage to the gluteal artery producing a perineural hematoma.

Several other techniques are described which will allow the patient to remain in the decubitus dorsal position and not block the posterior femoral cutaneous nerve. A sciatic block by the upper lateral, subtrochanterian route can be used, although this can be slightly painful as the nerve is very deep in adults. This block can inhibit nerve conduction in a line parallel to the femur, 3cm behind the GT, 5cm towards the foot. A short, sheathed, beveled 100mm neurostimulator needle is introduced perpendicular to the skin surface to find the sciatic stimulation (Plan n°3) (50).

The medial femoral route recently described appears to be of more interest as it is a shallower approach, however it does not affect the posterior face of the thigh: neurostimulation behind the femur, midway between the greater trochanter and the most prominent part of the external condyle of the femur. The 150mm sheathed needle is introduced perpendicular to the skin surface. The neurostimulator is started after the needle enters the skin with an initial intensity of 2 to 3mA. The average depth of the nerve is around 6cm (fig. 6) (51). With a single injection, no matter which technique is used, the analgesia obtained only lasts a short time, patients complain of popliteal pain when the analgesia wears off. A sciatic catheter can be suggested, using the parasacral route for example (52). However this route requires a very experienced anesthetist and cannot normally be used without the available experience and

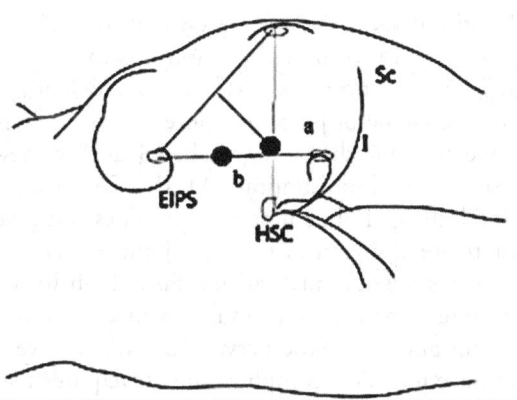

Fig. 4. – Sciatic nerve via posterior route.

Puncture points: a = posterior, b = parasacral
I: ischium
GT: greater trochanter
EIPS: posterior-superior iliac spine

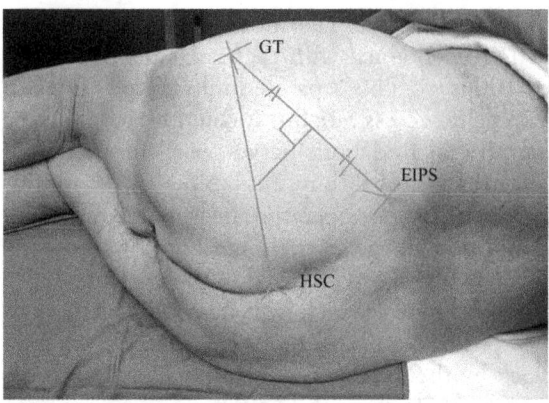

Fig. 5. – Sciatic block in the thigh.

time as it can cause complications if the lesser pelvis is penetrated close to the pelvic organs and the iliac, hypogastric or gluteal vessels. There is an additional extension of the anesthesia to the obturator nerve in 93% of cases. In the Sim position, the puncture point is located on the line between the posterior-superior iliac spine (PSIS) and the sciatic spine, 6cm below the EIPS perpendicular to the skin. Placing the catheter using the anterior approach described by Delaunay and Chelly (53) will also give a prolonged posterior analgesia. This necessitates passing through the thigh to a particularly deep nerve (10.5cm). It can also be used for a single injection, using the following anatomical markers: A line is drawn between the ASIS and the pubic symphysis, and then a perpendicular line is drawn downward from the center. The needle is introduced perpendicularly to the skin surface on this last line, 8cm from the intersection. The stimulator is adjusted to 1mA to stimulate the femoral nerve 3.5cm from the skin (the patella rises), then the intensity of the current is increased to 5mA and the needle is pushed in deeper to find the sciatic nerve which will be found between 9.5 and 13cm from the skin (foot flexion or extension). The stimulation current is decreased to less than 1mA to position the needle precisely and to limit the amount of pain, particularly if it touches the femur bone. A continuous sciatic nerve block at the level of the popliteal cavity using the lateral or posterior route is also an alternative to ensure prolonged postoperative anesthesia. It gives better quality anesthesia than that obtained with parenteral administration (IM, IVPCA) of morphine derivatives or with epidural analgesia but it sometimes does not give sufficient anesthesia of the posterolateral region of the knee joint, which has innervation from a difficult to access nerve branch arising fairly high in the popliteal cavity (44). In fact, although the use of a simultaneous continuous block of the anterior lumbar plexus and the sciatic nerve is described as very effective in the literature, it can have technical complications: It requires two infusers, it may require a high hourly dose of local anesthetic with all the accompanying toxicity risks, maintenance of the catheters, mobilization and early physiotherapy are difficult. The most commonly used technique will be a single shot sciatic block in the buttocks combined with acrural catheter and supplementary intravenous PCA.

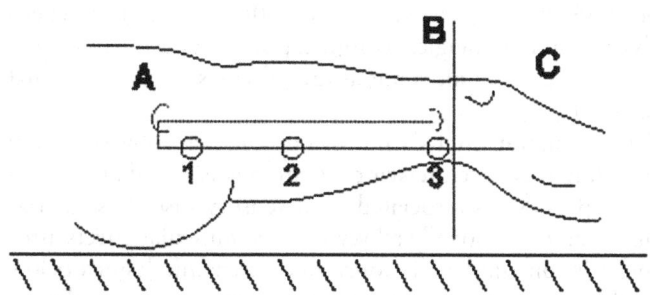

Fig. 6. – Cutaneous reference points for lateral routes (dorsal decubitus).

A: greater trochanter (GT)
B: external condyle (CE)
C: superior extremity of the patella
1: usual puncture point for the superior lateral route
2: puncture point for the medial femoral lateral route
3: puncture point for sciatic popliteal catheter by the lateral route

Postur

Complications from the dorsal decubitus position are non-specific. The patient will be monitored to ensure there are no compression points, to check the head/neck and limb line is in the proper position. Two supports are usually enough for the lower limb, one trochanter support and one plantar support will keep the knee at 90° flexion. During the operation, repeated rubbing of the heel on the pad during the hyperflexion movements should be avoided, in particular during the preparation and installation of the tibial piece.

Use of the tourniquet

An inflatable tourniquet is commonly used to obtain a bloodless surgical field, making the procedure easier and reducing the operation time. However, installing a total knee prosthesis is necessarily a hemorrhagic procedure and it seems that using a tourniquet does not alter the overall amount of bleeding, nor does it reduce a surgeon's operating time (54). Some studies report that using a tourniquet has an effect on the operating time, but it is always a modest reduction, which is largely counterbalanced by the negative effects of this technique. The quality of the bone-cement interface used to fix the prosthesis is, however, better if the bone section is not covered with blood. Esmarch bandages must not be used as they cause direct lesions by stretching, after sufficient exsanguination of the limb the tourniquet can be applied to the proximal part of the limb and inflated to not more than 300 to 350mmHg. The breadth of the tourniquet must be 0.4 time greater than the circumference of the limb. Compression and ischemia have a local effect causing cutaneous, muscular, vascular and nerve distress which delays motor healing. The most significant damage is found under the tourniquet (55). The neurological consequences are pain after 30 to 60 minutes of the tourniquet being in place, then lesions producing constant paraesthesia after 2 and a half hours

with the tourniquet at 350mmHg; pressure above 400mmHg is an independent neurological risk factor. Neurological complications can occur some time
after the operation and the causal link is not always obvious in cases of spinal
or anesthetic blocks. (56).

Fortunately, patient evaluation after six months or one year show only very
occasional sequelae. Before this time the symptomatology is varied and sometimes disabling, motor paralysis is associated with sensory disorders such as
dysesthesia, hyperalgesia and occasionally allodynia. The muscular effects associated with mechanical lesions under the tourniquet, ischemic lesions below
the tourniquet caused by necrosis after 90 minutes with or without clinical
repercussions combining a reduction in muscle strength with myodemia or
rhabdomyolysis. The vascular consequences are arterial ischemia from an *in
situ* thrombosis, atheroma embolism or venous thrombosis. Serious complications can occur if the patient has arterial disease. Cutaneous lesions under
the cuff, an inefficient or insufficiently inflated tourniquet, leaks, defective
tourniquet, sudden release or insufficient exsanguination producing copious
bleeding are just some of the undesirable effects that can occur. The hemodynamic consequences of inflating the tourniquet around the thigh produce
a sharp increase in blood volume of 400 to 500mL and an increase of 20 to
30mmHg in blood pressure causing ischemic pain. The consequences of releasing the tourniquet (54, 57) produce tachycardia and hypotension induced
by the revascularization of a vasodilated limb, by anaerobic metabolism, reduction in the pH and hyperkalemia. There is also an increase in myocardial work-
load and in oxygen consumption, hypercapnia and temporary acidosis caused
by the release of the products of anaerobic metabolism (CO_2, myoglobin,
lactates, potassium, and cell breakdown products).

Microemboli of fibrin and clotted blood, bone marrow, air and cement
constantly form emboli; the formation of a fresh thrombus in the vascular
bed of a limb that is subject to a tourniquet can produce a massive pulmonary embolism. The allergy and septic risks also increase when the tourniquet is released: bacteria, and anaphylactic mediators (58) are suddenly released
into the circulation. The anesthetist should anticipate and be immediately available at this point in the procedure. However, real contraindications to the
use of a tourniquet are uncommon: severe arterial disease of the lower limbs,
vascular bypass, arteriovenous fistula or pedicle flap, known venous thrombosis or major risk of deep vein thrombosis, progressive neuropathy, sepsis or
serious skin condition, femoral osteoma, drepanocytosis, impaired cardiovascular condition, diabetic complications. In all cases the tourniquet should not
be applied for more than two hours at 300mmHg. The equipment must be
regularly maintained and calibrated frequently.

Avoiding perioperative hypothermia from the time of induc-
tion (59, 60)

As in most interventions, even moderate unintentional hypothermia must be
avoided as it can increase postoperative morbidity: shivering, alveolar hypo-

ventilation, myocardial ischemia, bleeding (thrombopenia, reduction in platelet aggregability, fibrinolysis), somatic infections. It can cause increased hospitalization times.

Problems related to the cement

Cardiovascular manifestations occurring during the sealing procedure are more likely to be due to local impaction and external pressure and the embolic consequences than the pharmacodynamic effects of the hot acrylic cement, as the vasodilator and myocardial depressor effects of the cement have been refuted. (61). These consequences are limited by the use of the tourniquet or retarded when it is released. Circulatory collapse is rare when methyl methacrylate cement is applied, however, it does occur when long prostheses are inserted. Inserting a drain in the medullary cavity will give a reduction in embolism occurrences, although it should be remembered that neither the quality, nor the volume, nor the duration of the embolism are correlated with the clinical signs. In all cases the measures which will limit any repercussions from the use of the cement are: $FiO_2 > 40\%$, good blood volume, hemodynamic stability, analgesia.

Chronic inflammatory disease

The prevalence of rheumatoid arthritis (RA) in the general population is 1% in women, ankylosing spondylitis is less frequent (0.5% of the population, 9 times more likely in men than women). These pathologies cause problems due to general ill health: restrictive respiratory insufficiency, cardiac disorders (rheumatoid autoimmune pericarditis and myocarditis, aortic insufficiency and atrioventricular block in ankylosing spondylitis), renal disorders (amyloidosis), immunosuppression (long-term immunosuppression and corticosteroid treatment), involvement of the lumbar vertebral spine (difficulties with spinal injections) or even cervico-occipital joint (due to the medullary risks of intubation, it is sensible to monitor using dynamic X-rays of the cervical spine or MRI to look for a rheumatoid atlantoaxial lesion (62), stiffness of the cervical spine, spontaneous ankylosing spondylitis or after surgical fixation of the spine [RA]). Intubation difficulties are frequent and may be increased by temporomandibular involvement reducing opening of the mouth. Other than truncal and plexal regional anesthesia, fibroscope-guided intubation for general anesthesia is the only alternative to technical difficulties with a central neural blockade.

Using a laryngeal mask (63) under a light general anesthetic can also be suggested in cases of difficult intubation if the mouth will open sufficiently, in combination with a triple sciatic, crural and obturator block. Some maintain that antibiotic prophylaxis of these immunosuppressed patients must deal with prophylaxis against infectious endocarditis and must include cephalosporins for 48 hours and a preoperative aminoglycoside, according to the degree of renal insufficiency. In addition, auto-transfusion protocols, use of iron and EPO could also be useful for these patients (64, 65). The anesthetist must collaborate with the immunologist and rheumatologist to monitor undesirable effects of the immunosuppression treatment.

Revision of the prosthesis

Revisions of a prosthesis cause serious problems. These can be required if the prosthesis has worn out through normal use or come loose or if there have been septic complications. The surgery is usually longer, more hemorrhagic and more difficult to overcome for the eldest patients. Autotransfusion or perioperative blood retrieval are contraindicated if there is sepsis. Tolerance to acute postoperative anemia is often poor in patients whose general state is often disturbed. Postoperative pain is often worse and the rehabilitation and reeducation possibilities may be limited. If sepsis is the reason for revision, the choice of antibiotics is difficult. If the bacteria is known the antibiotic can be specifically directed against it. Otherwise, multiple preoperative samples must be taken when the patient may already be anemic. Starting with broad spectrum antibiotics targeting, in particular, methicillin resistant staphylococci, the treatment can then be adapted to the microbiology and such results as these can often take some time to come back.

The antibiotic treatment will always be for a minimum of 4 to 6 weeks, given intravenously through a central catheter or venous implant access, and then a further 3 to 6 months of oral antibiotics. This is done in close consultation with the infection-control specialists; reimplantation can then be done in one or two operations, preferably close together to limit the presence of a foreign body.

Thromboprophylaxis (67)

According to the consensus conference on prevention of thromboembolism in surgery the risks are high in TKP. This type of intervention should not be planned without giving thromboembolism prophylaxis treatment. Preventative measures have greatly reduced the rates of deep vein thrombosis, but unfortunately they have not dropped below 1% to 30% residual thrombosis threshold, and the risks of hemorrhage remain minimal. Spontaneous thromboembolic events are explained by the venous stasis and hypercoagulability, which is common to all types of surgery, they are associated with direct lesions of the vein walls in the lower limbs, an occurrence which is specific to knee and hip surgery. These risks are less frequent after knee surgery than after hip surgery, where prophylaxis is less effective. Half the events will occur before the 7th day after the operation, the other half up to the 30th day. The patient's individual risk will increase with age, obesity, cancer, history of thromboembolism, estrogen-progesterone treatment or abnormal prothrombin time results. The thrombosis begins in the perioperative period; 86 % of DVT diagnosed by phlebography performed on the 5th day are already present when immediate postoperative phlebography is performed (66). The thromboses are initially sural, subjacent to the prosthesis; this is explained by malfunction of the venous pump in the calf. They can be serious and difficult to diagnose as they are asymptomatic in 50% of cases, have the potential to cause embolism (1 to 3% of cases), and are the cause of 2/3 of the post-operative deaths after total hip prosthesis without prophylaxis. The clinical benefit of systematic screening by Doppler ultrasound in orthopedics has not been established. It has not been clearly established that the rate of clinical PE and DVT occurring within three months are the same if screening is done or not (2, 3, 68). It can be useful however if thrombosis is suspected.

Current trends are to combine several methods of prevention. Anticoagulant use is the most well known, but they must be combined with keeping the lower limbs raised, early mobilization and graduated use of elasticated stockings. Using a tourniquet seems to increase the risk slightly. A recent meta-analysis could not draw any conclusions about the real benefit of prophylaxis with low molecular weight heparin (LMWH) started on the evening before the operation, but it did point out that this could increase peroperative blood loss (69). On the other hand, real benefit was shown in bed-bound patients, who had protracted operations; often these patients also required preoperative ultrasound scans. Non-fractionated heparin (NFH) was the first anti-thrombotic treatment used but use of LMWH is more common: It is more effective, has less risk of hemorrhage and induces less thrombocytopenias. In France, in the absence of more powerful products that have as good tolerability, enoxaparin (Lovenox®) is used at a dose of 4 000 IU per day (3). Dalteparin (Fragmine®) 5 000 IU, Reviparin (Clivarine®) 3 436 IU, tinzaparin (Innohep®) 4 500 IU, nadroparin (Fraxiparine®) 0.2 to 0.6mL are also used, these require monitoring of platelet levels twice a week, as they may produce Type II heparin-induced thrombocytopenia (HIT type II), a serious condition as it can cause arterial or venous thrombosis and death.

Warfarin can be substituted to limit this rare (<0.01%) but serious sequela complication. Monitoring the warfarin using the INR is done less frequently (once a week, reduced to every two or three weeks in well-controlled patients) and is less costly. However, although warfarin is used in English-speaking countries, there are no well-conducted clinical trials that compare the tolerability and efficacy of the two methods.

Multiple controlled, randomized clinical trials have shown that extended-duration low-molecular-weight heparin therapy significantly reduces the incidence of asymptomatic venous thromboembolic events following total hip arthroplasty, although no similar benefit has been observed in patients undergoing total knee arthroplasty. There are currently no comparative studies assessing the efficacy of long-term venous thromboembolic prophylaxis with oral anti-coagulant agents. Extending low-molecular-weight heparin therapy is not associated with any increase in major bleeding complications, but it may result in more frequent minor bleeding episodes. In addition, the cost-effectiveness of prolonging low-molecular-weight heparin treatment has not yet been firmly established. Although there is evidence supporting the use of extended out-of-hospital low-molecular-weight heparin prophylaxis after total arthroplasty, this strategy has not gained widespread acceptance in North America because of concerns regarding its adverse effects, cost-effectiveness, and uncertain patient compliance. Further studies are necessary to determine the optimal duration of treatment.

Danaparoid (Orgaran®) acts like heparin by inhibiting thrombin, but does not have an antagonistic anti-Factor Xa and anti-Factor IIa effect. It induces many fewer thrombopenias and is used at doses of 750IU twice a day sub-cutaneously starting 2 to 4 hours before surgery. It is very expensive so its use is reserved for the prevention and treatment of HIT II, which is currently the reference treatment. Desirudin (Revasc®) is a specific inhibitor of thrombin, the marketing authorization indications are THP and TKP surgery and contraindications of prosthesis revisions and traumatology; the recommended dose of 15mg twice a day, should be started 15 to 30 minutes before surgery. It is not affected by antagonists, and seems to reduce the risk of thromboembolism, but its risk benefit ratio is not yet established. There are also other products in development, such as the revolutionary ximelaga-tran (70).

Support stockings, used to combat venous stasis, as long as the amount of support they provide is sufficient, will reduce the rate of DVT by 60% for moderate thrombosis risk, but their effectiveness is not shown so clearly in orthopedics practice. On the other hand, when combined with other methods of prevention these elastic stockings will give a greater reduction in the DVT levels and the indications suggested they are best used in this way. They do not have a detrimental effect on coagulation but their use is somewhat limited as they are relatively uncomfortable. Stockings are also unsuitable for the 15 to 20% of subjects whose legs are unusual size or shape. Patients tolerate wearing socks better in these indications, but in both cases patient compliance after leaving the department seems to be very random. Intermittent sequen-tial External Pneumatic Compression (IEPC) uses inflatable devices around the calf and thigh which give increasing pressure from the ankle to the thigh and reduces the number of DVT by 60% in total hip prosthesis, with even better results in total knee prosthesis, as they have a marked effect on the sural vein. AV Impulse System is a slipper which intermittently compresses the arch of the foot, mimicking the effect of walking. It has comparable effi-cacy to LMWH. These active compression methods are costly, so remain the alternative of choice when anticoagulants are contraindicated in high risk patients.

Postoperative analgesia

Pain management is fundamental and remains a priority, even though the Myles quality of postoperative recovery score, containing nine criteria scored by the patients (71), placed absence of pain in the ninth, and last, position; this was a descriptor stating absence of severe pain or moderate but prolonged pain. The seventh point related to non-specific pain: headache, backache, muscle pain. In first place was the feeling of well-being, the eighth was the absence of nausea, vomiting or retching. Points two to six were, in order, support from carers, particularly medical staff, absence of confusion and good understanding of instructions; ability to perform hygiene tasks alone; recovery of bowel and bladder movements; being able to breath easily. All these elements underline the discrepancy between the patient's and the carer's points of view; as the carer's tendency to focus exclusively on the anesthesia may alter the quality of care (45, 72). Evaluation is fundamental and must be based on consultation, clinical examination and self-assessment, which is the reference method. The aim is to measure the elements, which are sometimes difficult to interpret: intensity, type, rate, duration, causes, location, and spread radiation, affective and emotional impact. Three self-assessment methods of dynamic and rest pain measurements are found in the literature: the simple verbal scale, the simple numeric scale and the 100mm visual analog scale. The main objectives of treating the pain are to limit serious pain, limit postoperative morbidity, limit dissatisfaction, stop chronic pain appearing, due to sensitization of the central nervous system, encourage self-sufficiency and early rehabilitation to limit any complications and postoperative disability. In addition to the satisfaction and comfort that is given by the absence of postoperative pain, it also has a vital role to play in immediate post operative flexion of the knee and seems to condition the functional results in the short term (45). This type of care will also fulfill the secondary objectives: To reduce the length of time in hospital and the overall cost of care, an added benefit will be to improve the image of the care team and the establishment.

Delayed pain is mechanical and linked to rehabilitation. Immediate postoperative pain is a subjective phenomenon expressing excess nociception by hyperstimulation of the physiological systems of pain transmission (Ad et C fibers). It can lead to true hyperalgesia, even to a real chronic pain disorder and allodynia (stimuli which are ordinarily not painful can become so, conveyed by the Ab fibers). This increases, presenting with maximum intensity on the second day after the operation, improving by the third day and improving greatly with mobilization. It appears as inflammatory type pain, linked to hematoma, bone and ligament tissue destruction, and associated to muscle contraction and spasms.

Multimodal analgesia by the systemic route (73-75)

Currently this comprises a basic analgesic (paracetamol), non-steroid anti-inflammatory drugs (NSAIDs) and a patient-controlled opioid. Independent factors that significantly reduce the requirement for systemic analgesics are passive continuous postoperative mobilization of the joint using a mechanical device, daily stimulation of the quadriceps and application of ice packs on the joint.

Opioid analgesics

The preferred route is Intra-Venous Patient-Controlled Analgesia (IVPCA) (fig. 7). It is the reference method. This is permanent continuous titration of an opioid controlled by the patient; the opioid consumption is lower with this method than with SC or IM systemic routes or with pain relief on demand. However, even though patient satisfaction is increased by 90% for spontaneous pain, PCA is not effective on the intense pain occurring during the first few hours after the operation and on induced dynamic pain. Morphine is still the most commonly used product (1mg/mL of morphine hydrochlorate). Continuous administration is not recommended as there is a risk of respiratory depression. It is installed postoperatively in the recovery room after intravenous titration of the analgesic requirements and is monitored closely, regulated to use 1.5 to 2mg of morphine every 7 to 10 minutes, maximum dose of 20mg every 4 hours. It is set up to provide continuous titration of the required dose by the patient themselves at all times. It avoids the delays between the patients' requests for analgesia and the standard subcutaneous injection by the nurse, this reassures the patients, most of whom will then tolerate a certain level of residual pain (VAS = 4), thus preventing overdose. Continuous titration maintains the plasma concentration in the therapeutic region just above the minimum analgesic concentration and considerably below concentrations likely to induce excessive somnolence and respiratory depression. The system must be Y-set with an anti-reflux valve, this is vital to ensure that the opioid does not accumulate in the infusion tube if the venous access becomes occluded. Opioid consumption is higher during the first postoperative hours then reduces steadily. PCA is rarely indicated after the first 24 to 48 hours. After this time it should be replaced by an effective

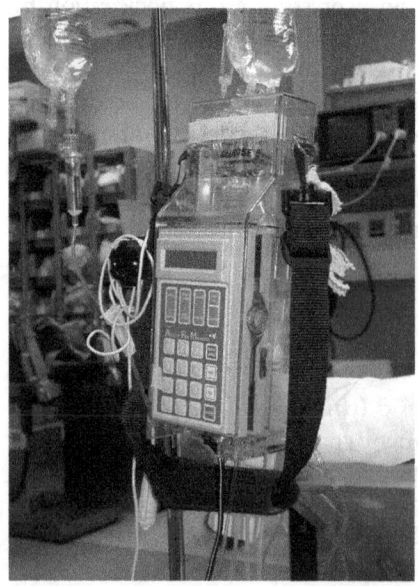

Fig. 7. – PCA.

oral analgesic, doubling the daily dosage; a patient requiring 40mg of intra-venous PCA morphine/day should have this replaced by 80mg oral morphine sulfate (Actiskénan®) in 4 divided doses, 20mg tablets, per day.

PCA has limitations however: The nurses must have regular training in opioid analgesia and PCA management and the patient must be checked regu-larly by the nurse who must be able to intervene quickly if any events occur. A monitoring protocol will be established and reviewed every 4 hours: vital signs (respiration, consciousness, heart rate, blood pressure), effectiveness para-meters (VAS pain scale), behavioral scale, quantity of opioid consumed, adverse effects (nausea, vomiting, pruritis, urine retention, constipation). Moreover the anesthetist must see the patient regularly to make any changes required to the dosage and emergency medical treatment must always be avai-lable. A respiratory event will be an air desaturation episode requiring oxygen. Excessive somnolence is a forewarning of apnea requiring an antidote, naloxone (Narcan®), and oxygen. However, the relationship between post-operative pain and postoperative nausea and vomiting (PONV) is complex as it has been established that excessive nociception, as well as its treatment by opioid agonists, are emetogenic. Tramer et al. (76) found a 67% incidence of PONV. Droperidol (Droleptan®), an anti-dopaminergic neuroleptic, is the most commonly used product to combat PONV associated with PCA mor-phine. The setrons, serotonin receptor antagonists of 5-HT3 are as effective and do not have any significant secondary effects. The ondansetron/drope-ridol combination gives very good results (77). Like naloxone (40µg) it treats the pruritus induced by opioids in 4% of patients.

Non-opioid analgesics (78)

These analgesics are useful in combination with rest and ice packs, either as an alternative treatment or in combination with opioids, they will rein-force the analgesic effects, reduce the quantities administrated and the side effects.

Intravenous propacetamol (Prodafalgan®) and Paracetamol (Perfalgan®)(79) seem likely to have a peripheral effect (anti-prostaglandin synthetase/synthase either), but their central spinal/supra-spinal anti-pyretic and analgesic effects are the most important. They give greater than 33% opioid reduction. They are, however, contraindicated in hypersensitive patients, it can cause nausea, vertigo, hot flashes and liver toxicity if an overdose of more than 12g/day is given. The standard overdose treatment is administration of N-acetyl-cysteine. The usual dosage is 30mg/kg every 4 to 6 hours. Regular dosing avoids pain and thermal variations. The analgesic peak is reached in 1 to 2 hours. Depending on the intensity of the pain, an oral codeine, dihydroco-dine or dextropropoxyphene can be given sequentially. Less opioid drugs will be given but the opioid-related undesirable effects will be increased. Oral or intravenous non-steroid anti-inflammatory drugs (NSAIDs) act on peripheral synthesis of prostaglandins by inhibition of COX 1 (continuously expressed) and COX 2 (damaged tissues) cyclo-oxygenase coenzymes (13). Their undesirable effects are mainly due to their action on COX 1 and can increase or induce renal insufficiency and gastric bleeding, and have a deleterious effect on hemostasis. They are contraindicated in patients who have hypersensitivity to NSAIDs. They should be used with care in elderly patients and patients with asthma. They must always be combined with a gastric protector product. They may have a central effect and give a synergistic ic opioid saving of 30%. Ketoprofene (Profénid®) is the most commonly used NSAID in France, it gives effective analgesia for eight hours in 60 to 70% of cases with a slow intravenous infusion at a posology of 1 to 1.5mg/kg $^{-1}$ twice a day (0.75mg/kg^1 in elderly patients). The ideal NSAID should have the lowest COX 1/COX 2 ratio possible such as meloxicam (Mobic®), rofecoxib (Viox®) or delecoxib (Celebrex®) to limit the undesirable gastric, renal and platelet effects. Unfortunately, at present there is no intravenous anti-COX 2 inducible suitable for immediate postoperative use that is effective but has no harmful side effects, in particular cardiovascular effects.

Other analgesics such as tramadol (Topalgic® or Contramal®) or nefopam (Acupan®) can also be used.

Epidural analgesia

Postoperative epidural analgesia to control postoperative pain is very effective but has harmful side effects that limit its use in orthopedics. Nevertheless, it also inhibits metabolic and neuroendocrine stress reactions when combined with local and opioid anesthetics (80). Two meta-analyses (31, 82) also confirmed the value of epidural anesthesia in reducing the incidence of postoperative respiratory and thromboembolic complications in major gastric surgery and thoracic surgery, also giving a reduction in hospitalization time. An epidural infusion of ropivacaine at an average rate of 12mg/h^{-1} over 72 hours gives effective analgesia of patients having had hip or knee prosthesis, the plasma concentrations were below toxic levels and the plateau concentration was obtained fairly rapidly (83). This technique also improves convalescence parameters and allows a more intensive rehabilitation program (81). There are also other studies showing a benefit from patient-controlled epidural analgesia (PCEA) using ropivacaine 0.2% and fentanyl 10µg/mL 5mL bolus/10 minutes. In both cases preoperative anticoagulation is contraindicated. Postoperative anticoagulation is both possible and desirable using the standard treatment regimens, but monitoring is absolutely vital and all care staff should be trained properly (84). In practice, as long as the nursing staff, rather than the specialist departments, has been trained to monitor the coagulation profiles of these patients, the literature, and experience, show that the risk is at least equivalent to using morphine in PCA. The patients must also be informed of the complications and the possible side effects (bilateral block, urine retention, problems moving with a catheter installed, risk of infection, management of the epidural catheter and the anticoagulant combination, disabling headaches, pruritis, hypotension or respiratory depression).

Multi-trunk regional analgesia

Single injections

There have been several studies comparing epidural analgesia with femoral and sciatic trunk analgesia in knee surgery; they show that, in practice, the two techniques have a comparable efficacy in this context, they also show that epidural analgesia has some side effects. The trunk analgesia seems preferable (44, 45) associated with a regular prescription of a PCA morphine pump and basic analgesics, apart from patients with the usual contraindications according to Capdevilla *et al.* (45). Patients having total knee prosthesis were operated on under general anesthetic, and then randomized to three groups according to the postoperative analgesia given for 48 hours: continuous epidural anesthetic, continuous femoral block and PCA. Pain was evaluated at regular interval at rest and during mobilization with a motorized harness that will give 40-50° flexion of the knee from the first day after the operation. The degree of flexion obtained was evaluated on the 5th and 7th day postoperatively by a surgeon, who was unaware of the analgesia technique; rehabilitation was started on the 7th day to obtain knee flexion of 110°. The VAS scores were higher in the PCA group and comparable in the other two groups but the secondary effects were more frequent in the epidural group. In the first two days, the rehabilitation objectives were more easily reached in the epidural and femoral block groups than in the PCA group, in particular the flexion angle was greater in these two groups. Average duration of rehabilitation was 37 days (30-45) in the epidural group, 40 days (31-60) in the femoral block group and 50 days (30-80) in the PCA group. At three months the functional results were the same. So pain control plays an indirect role in postoperative rehabilitation showing that active rehabilitation is vital component of pain management to achieve improvement of postoperative morbidity and produce a real influence on operative follow-up and convalescence. Effective pain control can mean considerable financial savings too, if it means that the patient only stays in hospital for 10 days instead of a month and a half. These encouraging results show that the consequences of good anesthetic care are not limited to immediate postoperative care, but have long-term effects too (74).

Perineural catheters and continuous injections (fig. 8 and 9)

A continuous peripheral neural block has the same advantages as a single injection but the effects are prolonged. It gives at least as effective postoperative analgesia as an epidural block without the central neurological inconveniences. It gives best quality analgesia, rehabilitation is clearly better and can be started more quickly in a more effective way. Postoperative management is easier than for postoperative epidural analgesia, but it requires effective staff training and information as these techniques do have some possible complications: technical difficulties and risk of failure, but also all the complications of single injection techniques such as posttraumatic nerve lesions from the needle, infection, toxicity of the local anesthetic, product errors, catheter displacement or difficulty removing the catheter (41). Both continuous and patient-controlled analgesia using perineural catheters require regular monitoring by the team; they must check the hemodynamic and respiration parameters, the resting and mobilization analgesia effectiveness (using VAS or SVS), looking for signs of local or general infection or pressure point sores, unsuitable position, compartmental syndrome, detect signs of overdose of the local anesthetics and withdraw treatment if there is any doubt at all. The normal cutaneous signs are hardened, numb skin that tingles, with slight swelling in the region of the block. The abnormal signs are parasthesia, pain, complete anesthesia and paralysis. During the analgesia maintenance period, any doubt about the integrity of the nervous system requires temporary withdrawal of the infusion so that neurology tests can be done. The outlet point of the catheter must be checked daily for leaks, displacement or signs of inflammation. The catheter is removed on the 3rd or 4th day or earlier if there is fever or inflammation at the injection point, samples should be taken and sent for culture. However, the catheter can remain *in situ* for several weeks for some cancer treatments. The solution is changed at least once every 24 hours under scrupulously aseptic conditions. There are three analgesia maintenance techniques. Repeated injections of a 20mL bolus of 0.2% ropivacaine every 6 to 8 hours give very good analgesic effect for the volume given and the patient can manage it well, but they have several inconveniences: The quality of analgesia varies over time; there is considerable motor block due to the use of concentrated solutions of local anesthetic; peak plasma levels of ropivacaine occur 30 to 60 minutes after the bolus injection, requiring patient monitoring; staff must be available to give the repeated injections. Continuous infusion with continuous mode PCA pump, standard syringe pumps or latex infuser is easier to set up. The nurse checks that the pump is working properly, monitors the patient and possibly changes the syringe or the bag. The continuous 5mL/hour dosage of 2mg/mL ropivacaine gives stable analgesia but is sometimes not suitable for variations in pain levels. The motor block is low intensity with dilute solutions of local anesthetic and guards against sudden increases in plasma levels. It does not allow for regular neurological evaluations and can delay diagnosis

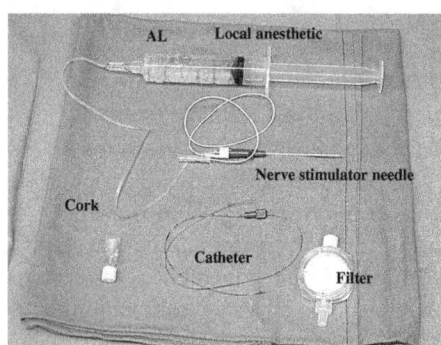

Fig. 8. – Catheter equipment.

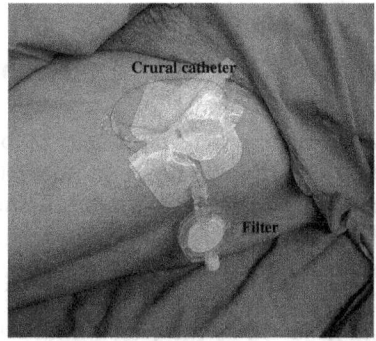

Fig. 9. – Catheter in place.

of a neurological problem (38). After several hours the nerve block is reduced on the femoral nerve, this can sometimes require additional boli and can justify the use of a perineural PCA. The patient can then alter the intensity of the analgesic effect continuously and inject supplementary boli at the rate of 5 every 45 minutes, in addition to the continuous 5mL/hour, not only when they require extra pain relief, but also during physical therapy sessions, nursing or when they are mobilizing. It is the method of choice as patient satisfaction is higher. The amount of patient information given, the patient's participation and understanding are also determinant for the success of the technique, particularly when the catheter does not cover the whole of the operation area.

Conclusion

From the time of the consultation onward, a risk/benefit evaluation of functional surgery for TKP will allow the team to foresee and therefore limit any complications. The strategies for blood saving and the prevention and treatment of thromboembolic disorders are vital. General, spinal and epidural anesthesia are available for patients. In combination with intravenous opioid PCA and standard analgesics, sciatic and femoral blocks and plexus regional analgesia, either as a continuous injection or a single injection, have become the reference technique. Although the importance of effective postoperative analgesia has been established, there is still some controversy over the overall benefits to well-being somatic benefits that can be expected: Does analgesia reduce postoperative morbidity, does it improve rehabilitation, does it really speed up convalescence and shorten hospitalization times?

References

1. Auroy Y, Clergue F, Laxenaire MC et al. (1998) Anesthetics in surgery. Ann Fr Anesth Reanim. 17: 1324-41
2. Murray DW, Britton AR, Bulstrode CJK (1996) Thromboprophylaxis and death after total hip replacement. J Bone Joint Surg 6: 863-70
3. Leclerc JR, Gent M, Hirsh J et al. (1998) The incidence of symptomatic venous thromboembolism during and after prophylaxis with enoxaparin: a multi-institutional cohort study in patients who underwent hip or knee arthroplasty. Arch Intern Med 158: 873-8
4. Perka C, Arnold U, Buttgereit F (2000) Influencing factors on perioperative morbidity in knee arthroplasty. Clin Orthop 378: 183-91
5. Ninet J, Horellou MH, Darjinoff JJ et al. (1992) Evaluation of preoperative risk factors. Ann Fr Anesth Reanim 11: 252-81
6. American society of anesthesiologists and society of cardiovascular anesthesia (1996) Guidelines for Perioperative Cardiovascular Evaluation for Non-cardiac Surgery. Circulation 93: 1280-5
7. Eagle KA and the Committee on Perioperative Cardiovascular Evaluation for Non-cardiac Surgery (1996) Executive summary of the ACC/AHA task force report: guidelines for perioperative cardiovascular evaluation for non-cardiac surgery. Anesth Analg 82 : 854-60
8. Mangano DT (1990) Perioperative cardiac morbidity. Anesthesiology 72: 153-84

9. Sirieix D, Lamonerie-Alvarez L, Olivier P *et al.* (1998) Assessment of cardiovascular perioperative risk in non-cardiac surgery. Ann Fr Anesth Réanim 17: 1225-31

10. Fleisher LA, Barash PG (1992) Preoperative cardiac evaluation for noncardiac surgery: a functionnal approach. Anesth Analg 74: 586-98

11. Patrono C, Coller B, Dalen JE (1998) Platelet-active drugs: the relationships among dose, effectiveness, and optimal therapeutic range. Chest 114: 470S-88S

12. American College of Physicians (1997) Guidelines for assessing and managing the perioperative risk from coronary artery disease associated with major non-cardiac surgery. Ann Intern Med 127: 313-28

13. Derrier M, Mercatello A (1997) Role of non-steroidal anti-inflammatory agents in the perioperative period. Usefulness and limitations. Review Ann Fr Anesth Reanim. 16: 498-520

14. Roizen MF (1994) Preoperative evaluation. In : Miller RD, ed. Anesthesia. 4th ed. New York: Churchill Livingstone p.827-82

15. Conférence d'experts (1997) Indication of the preoperative exams. In: SFAR, ed. Les référentiels en anesthésie-réanimation. Elsevier, Paris, p.131-8

16. AFS-ANAES (1998) Indications and against indications of the transfusions of unstable blood products. Recommendations for the clinical practice. (Indications et contre indications des transfusions de produits sanguins labiles. Recommandations pour la pratique clinique.) Paris, EDK, p.177

17. Conference of consensus (1995) Use of red cells for the compensation of the blood losses in surgery of the adult. Ann Fr Anesth Réanim 1: 1-107

18. McFarland JG (1999) Perioperative blood transfusions: indications and options. Chest 115: 113S-21S

19. Forgie M, Weells P, Laupacis A *et al.* International study of peri-operative transfusion (ISOPT) investigators (1998) Preoperative autologous donation decreases allogenics transfusions but increases exposure to all red blood trasfusion: result of a meta-analysis. Arch Intern Med 158: 610-6

20. Etchason J, Petz L, Keeler E *et al.* (1995) The cost effectivness of peri-operative autologous blood donations. N Engl J Med 332: 719-24

21. Conseiller C, Ozier Y, Rosencher N (1999) Compensation of the losses of red cells in surgery. In : Elsevier (Ed), Paris, Encycl Méd Chir, Anesthésie-Réanimation, 36-735-B-10, p.25

22. Goodnough LT, Despotis GJ, Merkel K *et al.* (2000) A randomized trial comparing acute normovolemic hemodilution and preoperative autologous blood donation in total hip arthroplasty Transfusion 40: 1054-7

23. Faris PM, Spence RK, Larholt KM *et al.* (1999) The predictive power of baseline hemoglobin for transfusion risk in surgery patient. Orthopedics 22: 135S-40S

24. Faris PM, Ritter MA, Abels RI (1996) The effects of recombinant erythropoïetin on perioperative transfusion requirements in patient having a major orthopaedic operation. J Bone and Joint Surg 78: 62-72

25. De Andrade J, Frei D, Guilfoyle M (1999) Integrated Analysis of Thrombotic/Vascular Event Occurence in Epoïetin Alfa-treated Patients undergoing major Elective Orthopedic Surgery. Orthopedics 22: S113-S8

26. Olijhoek G, Megens JG, Musto P *et al.* (2001) Role of oral versus IV iron supplementation in the erythropoietic response to rHuEPO: a randomized, placebo-controlled trial. Transfusion 41: 957-63

27. Weisbach V, Skoda P, Rippel R *et al.* (1999) Oral or intravenous iron as an adjuvant to autologous blood donation in elective surgery: a randomized, controlled study. Transfusion 39: 465-72

28. Williamson KR, Taswell HF (1991) Intraoperative blood salvage: a review. Transfusion 31: 662-75

29. Rosencher N, Ozier Y, Conseiller C (1999) Autotransfusion per et postopératoire. In: SFAR, ed. Conférences d'actualisation. 41e Congrès national d'anesthésie et de réanimation, Paris, Elsevier, p. 147-60

30. Group of experts (1999) Recommendations for the practice of antibioprophylaxis (ABP) in surgery. Realization of the recommendations stemming from the conference of consensus of December, 1992. In: SFAR (ed) Paris, Elsevier

31. Urwin SC, Parker MJ, Griffiths R (2000) General versus regional anaesthesia for hip fracture surgery: a meta-analysis of randomized trials. Br J Anaesth 84: 450-5

32. Rodgers A, Walker N, Schug S et al. (2000) Reduction of postoperative mortality and morbidity with epidural or spinal anaesthesia: results from overview of randomised trials. BMJ 321: 1493

33. Sorenson RM, Pace NL (1992) Anesthetic techniques during surgical repair of femoral neck fracture: a meta-analysis. Anesthesiology 77: 1095-104

34. Kadry MA, Rutter SV, Popat MT (2001) Regional anaesthesia for limb surgerybefore or after general anaesthesia. Anaesthesia 56: 450-3

35. Choquet O, Feugeas JL (1997) Neurostimulation under general anesthesia and peripheral nerve injuries. Ann Fr Anesth Reanim 16: 923-4

36. Casati A, Fanelli G, Orghi B et al. for the Study Group on Orthopedic Anesthesia of the Italian Society of Anesthesia Analgesia and Intensive Care (1999) Ropivacaine or 2% mepivacaine for lower limb peripheral nerve blocks. Anesthesiology 90: 1047-52

37. Dupré lj, Jochum D (2001) Recommendations for the practice of neurostimulation. Ann Fr Anesth Reanim 20: 307-8

38. French-Language Association for Regional Analgesia and Anaesthesia (2001) http://www.alrf.asso.org/

39. Dupré LJ (1996) Three-in-one block or femoral nerve block. What should be done and how? Ann Fr Anesth Réanim 15: 1099-106

40. Misra U, Pridie AK, McClymont C et al. (1991) Plasma concentrations of bupivacaïne following combined sciatic and femoral "3 in 1" nerve blocks in open knee surgery. Br J Anaesth 66: 310-3

41. Auroy Y, Bargue L, Benhamou D et al. (2000) Recommendations of the SOS-ALR Group on the use of locoregional anesthesia. Ann Fr Anesth Reanim 19: 621-3

42. Auroy Y, Narchi P, Messiah A, Litt L, Rouvier B, Samii K (1997) Serious complications related to regional anesthesia: results of a prospective survey in France. Anesthesiology 87: 479-86

43. Fanelli G, Casati A, Garancini P et al. for the study group on regional anesthesia (1999) Nerve stimulator and multiple injection technique for upper and lower limb blockade: failure rate, patient acceptance and neurologic complications. Anesth Analg 88: 847-52

44. Singelyn F, Gouverneur JM (1994) Continuous "3-in-1" block as postoperative pain treatment after hip, femoral shaft or knee surgery: A large scale study of efficacy and side effects. Anesthesiology 81: A1054

45. Capdevila X, Biboulet P, Bouregba M et al. (1998) Comparison of the three-in-one and fascia iliaca compartment blocks in adults: clinical and radiographic analysis. Anesth Analg 86: 1039-44

46. Vloka JD, Hadzic A, Drobnik L et al. (1999) Anatomical landmarks for femoral nerve block: a comparison of four needle insertion sites. Anesth Analg 89: 1467-70

47. Choquet O, Macaire P, Manelli JC (2001) Bloc fémoral, sciatique et obturateur au pli inguinal pour la chirurgie du genou : étude préliminaire. Ann Fr Anesth Reanim 20(S1): R307

48. Winnie AP (1975) Regional Anesthesia. Surg Clin North Am 55: 867-92

49. Bruelle P, Muller L Bassoul B et al. (1994) Block of the sciatic nerve. Cah Anesthesiol 42: 785-91

50. Guardini R, Waldron BA, Wallace WA (1985) Sciatic nerve block: the new lateral approach. Acta Anaesthesiol Scand 29: 515-9

51. Naux E, Pham-Dang C, Bodin J et al. (2000) Sciatic nerve block: a new lateral mediofemoral approach. The value of its combination with a "3 in 1" block for invasive surgery of the knee. Ann Fr Anesth Reanim 19: 9-15

52. Mansour NY (1993) Reevaluating the sciatic nerve block: another landmark for consideration. Reg Anesth 18: 322-3

53. Chelly JE, Delaunay L (1999) A new anterior approach to the sciatic nerve block. Anesthesiology 91: 1655-60
54. Abdel-Salam A, Eyres KS (1995) Effects of tourniquet during total knee arthroplasty. A prospective randomised study. J Bone Joint Surg 77: 250-3
55. Kam PC, Kavanaugh R, Yoong FF (2001) The arterial tourniquet: pathophysiological consequences and anesthetic implications. Anesthesia 56: 834-45
56. Guanche CA (1995) Tourniquet-induced tibial nerve palsy complicating anterior cruciate ligament reconstruction. Arthroscopy 11: 620-2
57. Mc Grath BJ, Hsia J, Epstein B (1991) Massive pulmonary embolism following tourniquet deflation. Anesthesiology 74: 618-20
58. Laxenaire MC, Mouton C, Frederic A et al. (1996) Anaphylactic shock after tourniquet removal in orthopedic surgery. Ann Fr Anesth Réanim 15: 179-84
59. Schmied H, Kurz A, Sessler DI et al. (1996) Mild hypothermia increases blood loss and transfusion requirements during total hip arthroplasty. Lancet 347: 289-92
60. Kurz A, Sessler DI, Lenhardt R (1996) Perioperative normothermia to reduce the incidence of surgical-wound infection and shorten hospitalization. N Engl J Med 334: 1209-15
61. Gentil B, Paugam C, Wolf C et al. (1993) Methylmetacrylate plasma level during total hip arthroplasty. Clin Ortho 287: 112-6
62. Crosby ET, Lui A (1990) The adulte cervical spine: implication for the airway management. Can J Anaesth 37: 77-93
63. Verghese C, Brimacombe JR (1996) Survey of laryngeal mask airway usage in 11,910 patients: safety and efficacity for conventional and nonconventionnal usage. Anesth Analg 82: 129-33
64. Tanaka N, Ito K, Ishii S et al. (1999) Autologous blood transfusion with recombinant erythropoietin treatment in anaemic patients with rheumatoid arthritis. Clin Rheumatol 18: 293-8
65. Goodnough LT, Marcus RE (1997) The erythropoietic response to erythropoietin in patients with rheumatoid arthritis. J Lab Clin Med 130: 381-6
66. Maynard MJ, Sculco TP, Ghelman B (1991) Progression and regression of deep vein thrombosis after total knee arthroplasty. Clin Orthop 273: 125-9
67. Pierson JL, Tavel ME (2001) Thromboembolic prophylaxis in total joint replacement. Chest 20: 302-4
68. de Thomasson E, Strauss C, Girard P et al. (2000) Detection of asymptomatic venous thrombosis after lower limb prosthetic surgery. Retrospective evaluation of a systematic approach using Doppler ultrasonography: 400 cases. Presse Med. 29: 351-6
69. Hull RD, Brandt, Pineo GF et al. (1999) Preoperative vs postoperative initiation of low-molecular-weight heparin prophylaxis against venous thromboembolism in patients undergoing elective hip replacement. Arch Int Med 159: 137-41
70. Heit JA, Colwell CW, Francis CW et al. (2001) Comparison of the oral direct thrombin inhibitor ximelagatran with enoxaparin as prophylaxis against venous thromboembolism after total knee replacement: a phase 2 dose-finding study. Arch Intern Med 161: 2215-21.
71. Myles PS, Hunt JO, Nightingale CE et al. (1999) Development of a psychometric testing of quality of recovery score after general anesthesia and surgery in adults. Anesth Analg 88: 83-90
72. Delbos (1998) Management of postoperative pain in surgical units. Ann Fr Anesth Reanim 17: 649-62
73. Practice guidelines for acute pain management in the perioperative setting (1995) A report by the American Society of Anesthesiologists Task Force on Pain Management Acute Pain Section. Anesthesiology 82: 1071-81
74. Kehlet H (1997) Multimodal approach to control postoperative pathophysiology and rehabilitation. Br J Anaesth 78: 606-17
75. Bruelle P, Viel E, Eledjam JJ (1998) Benefit-risk and monitoring modalities of different techniques and methods of postoperative analgesia. Ann Fr Anesth Reanim 17: 502-26

76. Tramer MR, Walder B (1999) Efficacy and adverse effects of prophylactic antiemetics during patient controlled analgesia therapy: a quantitative systematic review. Anesth Analg 88: 1354-61

77. Wrench IJ, Ward JE, Walder AD *et al.* (1996) The prevention of postoperative nausea and vomiting using a combination of ondansetron and droperidol. Anaesthesia 51: 776-8

78. Dahl V, Raeder JC (2000) Non-opioid postoperative analgesia. Acta Anaesthesiol Scand 44: 1191-203

79. Viel E, Langlade A, Osman M *et al.* (1999) Propacetamol: from basic action to clinical utilization. A review. Ann Fr Anesth Reanim 18: 332-40

80. Liu S, Carpenter RL, Neal JM (1995) Epidural anesthesia and analgesia. Their role in postoperative outcome. Anesthesiology 82: 1474-506

81. Williams-Russo P, Sharrock NE, Haas SB *et al.* (1996) Randomised trial of epidural verus general anesthesia. Outcomes after primary total knee replacement. Clin Orthop 331: 199-208

82. Ballantyne JC, Carr DB, DeFerranti S *et al.* (1998) The comparative effects of postoperative analgesic therapies on pulmonary outcome: cumulative meta-analyses of randomized, controlled trials. Anesth Analg 86: 598-612

83. Scott DA, Emanuelsson B-M, Mooney PH *et al.* (1997) Pharmacokinetics and efficacy of long-term epidural ropivacaine infusion for postoperative analgesia. Anesth Analg 85: 1322-30

84. Rygnestad T, Borchgrevink PC, Eide E (1997) Postoperative epidural infusion of morphine and bupivacaine is safe on surgical wards. Organisation of the treatment, effects and side-effects in 2,000 consecutive patients. Acta Anaesthesiol Scand 41: 868-76

Specialized Aspects

Total knee replacement in severe genu varum deformity

P. Neyret, O. Guyen, T. Aït Si Selmi

Introduction

In patients with osteoarthritis and severe osseous varus deformity of the knee, total knee replacement (TKR) is a major challenge. If the preoperative varus deformity exceeds 15°, restoration of the correct mechanical alignment will be difficult to achieve. Ideally, the mechanical tibiofemoral axis should be 180°, with the femoral mechanical axis, and above all the tibial mechanical axis, perpendicular to the transverse axis of the knee, and with well-balanced and stable ligaments (1-3). This will ensure a uniform stress pattern, and thus minimize polyethylene (PE) wear.

The literature on the management of osteoarthritis (OA) in knees with severe osseous varus deformities is comparatively sparse. There is virtually universal agreement that correct mechanical alignment should be obtained at TKR, in the interest of implant life. Excessive varus (either constitutional or as the result of an acquired deformity) has been considered as a possible cause of premature TKR failure (2, 4, 5). There is as yet no agreement on the policy to adopt in the management of medial compartment OA associated with a varus deformity of more than 15° (1, 3).

The first step to be taken is a detailed analysis of the deformity, to determine whether it is articular (wear, laxity) or extra-articular (constitutional or acquired bony deformity) (6).

The options open to the surgeon are:
– isolated valgus osteotomy, with TKR at a later stage;
– TKR;
– tibial or femoral valgus osteotomy plus TKR, performed in one sitting.

This chapter examines the different options, and describes the authors' preferred strategy.

Analysis of the deformity

Knees with a major varus deformity must be examined in order to establish how much of the varus is due to articular, and how much is due to extra-articular causes.

Articular deformity

Articular deformity is caused by:

– bony wear, especially of the medial tibial plateau: in advanced cases, a dished lesion will have been produced in the cartilage;

– laxity: the ligaments on the concave side will be relatively contracted. This deformity will be reducible in the early stages; later on, the medial structures (the deep and the superficial medial collateral ligament, the posteromedial capsular structures, the semimembranosus, and the posterior cruciate ligament) will be contracted. Only in very advanced cases will the structures on the convex side be stretched.

Extra-articular deformity

In the overwhelming majority of cases, the bony deformity will be constitutional. In such cases, the extra-articular part of the varus deformity will often be tibial and proximal. Acquired deformities are less frequently encountered; they tend to be associated with malunion, which may exist at a variety of levels.

Determination of the deformity

Clinical examination is not very informative (fig. 1). The deformity is assessed with the patient standing, followed by an assessment with the patient lying down. Frequently, the deformity will appear worse in the standing position. This is due to the fact that, in the recumbent patient, the articular part of the deformity will reduce (providing that the soft tissues have not contracted), while the extra-articular (constitutional or acquired) part of the deformity will not reduce.

We assess the deformity on a long-leg film (7), as well as on reduction (valgus stress) films to obtain a better view of the joint line (fig. 2). For these measurements, we use a system derived from a theoretical consideration of the tibial epiphyseal axis. For the sake of simplicity, a line is drawn tangent to the lateral tibial plateau. This line will be at right angles to the epiphyseal axis; its extension on the medial side will be representative (± 2°) of the line of the medial plateau before the onset of cartilage wear. In this way, the wear-related articular part of the deformity is readily ascertained. The extra-articular (constitutional or acquired) part of the deformity is represented by the complementary angle of the angle enclosed by the tibial mechanical axis and the straight line tangent to the lateral tibial plateau. This angle is measured on the medial side (6) (fig. 3 and 4). The extra-articular deformity must be quantitated preoperatively, since it is this value that governs the correction to be obtained with osteotomy.

Surgical strategies

To date, there is no clearly defined policy for the management of medial compartment OA associated with major varus deformity.

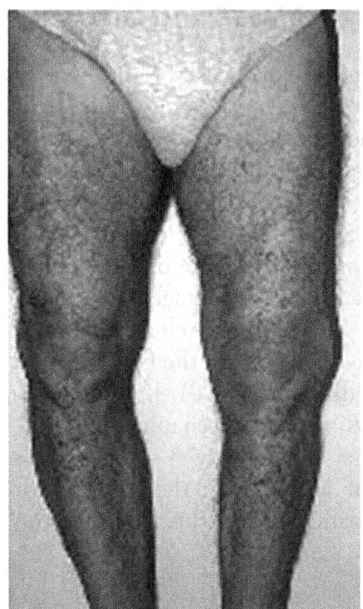

Fig. 1. – Clinical appearance of the deformity.

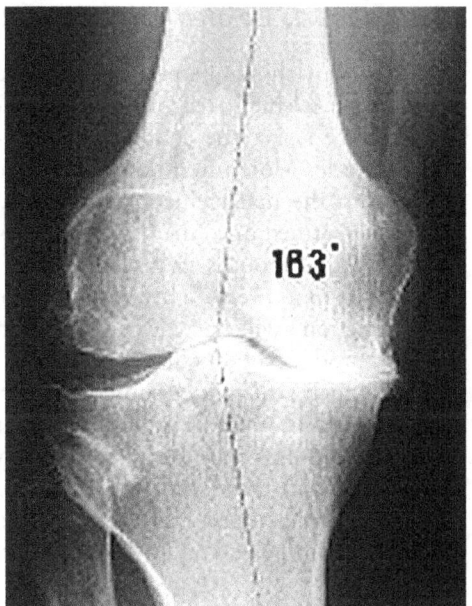

Fig. 2. – Major varus deformity in a 66-year-old male patient, with a tibiofemoral angle of the mechanical axis of 163° on the right. (By permission of Sauramps Publisher.)

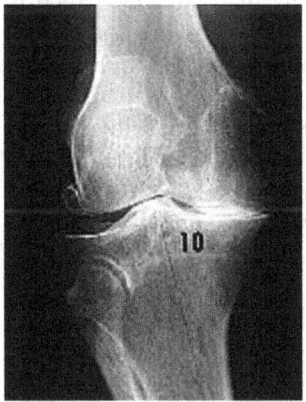

Fig. 3. – The constitutional contribution to the deformity in the tibia is 10°. (By permission of Sauramps Publisher.)

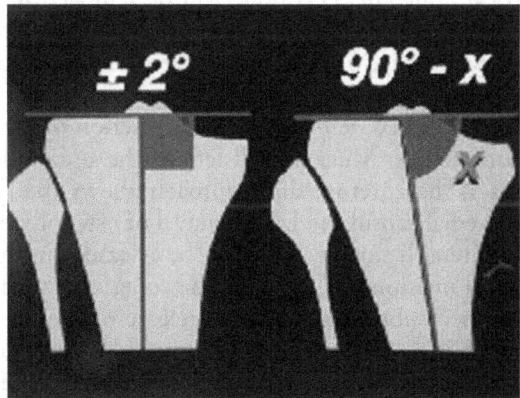

Fig. 4. – Principle of determining the constitutional contribution to the deformity. The medial tibial plateau prior to the onset of wear is a straight-line (± 2°) extension of the lateral tibial plateau (whose joint surface is always at right angles ± 2° to the epiphyseal axis). The constitutional contribution is readily calculated, as the complementary angle to the angle enclosed by the tangent to the lateral tibial plateau and the tibial mechanical axis. (By permission of Sauramps Publisher.)

Strategy no. 1: Isolated valgus osteotomy, with TKR at a later stage

The osteotomy should be performed in the segment of the lower limb (femur or tibia) that is chiefly responsible for the deformity. In the femur, the osteotomy will be above the condyles; in the tibia, it will be at the level of the tibial tubercle. More often than not, the deformity will be in the tibia. The first step in the management consists in a correction of the malalignment; TKR is performed once the osteotomy has healed (3 to 6 months later; or as late as 6 to 12 months from osteotomy, according to Cameron and Welsh [8]). In case of a severe deformity and associated advanced (stage 3 or 4) OA, "overcorrection" will be required in order to provide pain relief. This may, however, produce a bony deformity in the tibia, this time in the form of genu valgum, which will render subsequent TKR difficult (9, 10). If the correction is confined to the restoration of a physiological mechanical axis, the patient's symptoms will, in all probability, persist, and the 3 to 6 months between the two procedures will be a time of suffering for the patient. For all these reasons, we feel that there is little justification for this strategy, even though it has the backing of some authors (5, 8, 11, 12).

Strategy no. 2: Total knee replacement

Bone cuts at right angles will result in asymmetrical bone removal and cause so-called resection-related lateral laxity (relative slackening of the soft tissue restraints on the convex side of the deformity) (fig. 5). Bone cuts are referenced from the lateral side of the joint, where the ligaments are of normal length. The medial side appears to be contracted, because of the asymmetrical bone cut. Less bone will be removed medially than laterally, which is why unilateral ligament lengthening will need to be performed on the medial side (13) (fig. 6). The more severe the constitutional varus, the more extensive the medial tibial release will need to be. The sequence of steps varies in the published descriptions, as a function of the structures responsible for the contraction. Much is still left to the individual surgeon's discretion. In all cases, the anteromedial approach allows the systematic release of the anteromedial capsule and the removal of osteophytes. Where required, the medial collateral ligament may then be released (using a "checkerboard" pattern of small incisions); if need be, the superficial medial collateral ligament may be released subperiosteally. The release of the superficial medial collateral ligament is an "all-or-nothing" procedure must be performed with great care. Taking the release too far would put the patient at risk from major medial laxity, especially in flexion. (In extension, the medial collateral ligament remains in continuity with the periosteum.) In order to control this laxity, the pes anserinus tendons must be spared (fig. 7 and 8). In knees with severe constitutional varus deformity, release on the concave side must be extensive. Obviously, the release thus produced may put the knee at risk from medial laxity, and lengthen the limb by changing the surrounding ligamentous structures (13). This raises the question of how far the medial release should be allowed to go, over and above the normal length of the ligaments.

An arbitrary value of 8-12mm has been adopted, which would allow the management of an extra-articular deformity of 5°-8° (14). Any medial release beyond these limits would appear to be excessive. There are three ways in which this situation may be dealt with:

– it may be decided to accept a certain degree of laxity;
– the residual laxity may be compensated for by using a more constrained prosthesis;
– the soft tissues on the convex side may be retightened.

We prefer to do a valgus osteotomy at the time of the TKR, which avoids the excessive slackening of the medial collateral ligament.

Strategy no. 3: Valgus osteotomy and TKR in one sitting

Performing a valgus osteotomy and TKR under the same anaesthetic allows the surgeon to do a more sparing medial release. As discussed above, the valgus osteotomy is carried out either in the femur or in the tibia, depending on where the deformity is worst. Usually, the deformity will be in the tibia. The osteotomy is performed at the proximal border of the tibial tubercle, at the site of insertion of the patellar tendon.

To our way of thinking, a medial opening-wedge osteotomy is superior to a lateral closing-wedge osteotomy, for a number of reasons. Firstly, a major varus deformity should be tackled from the concave side, so as not to produce undesirable capsular or ligamentous release on the convex side. Secondly, a medial opening-wedge osteotomy allows to keep the osteotomy line away from the tibial resection line that is needed for the insertion of the knee replacement. Thirdly, as shown by Godenèche (15), opening-wedge osteotomies tend to produce significantly better long-term stability of the construct. Also, healing is thought to occur more rapidly, although this point has not as yet been proven statistically.

We decided to develop this option of tibial valgus osteotomy with a medial opening-wedge plus TKR, for the management of OA in knees with very severe constitutional varus deformity (16).

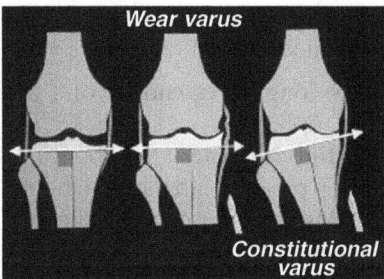

Fig. 5. – Asymmetrical tibial resection, as a result of constitutional varus, will lead to resection-related laxity. (By permission of Sauramps Publisher.)

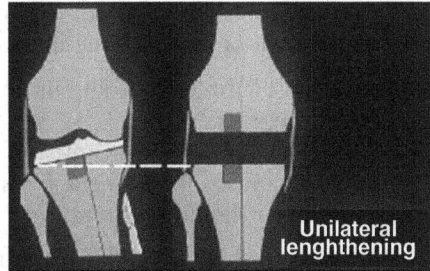

Fig. 6. – Correction of the resection-related laxity involves unilateral medial lengthening, since the normally-tensioned lateral ligaments are of normal length.

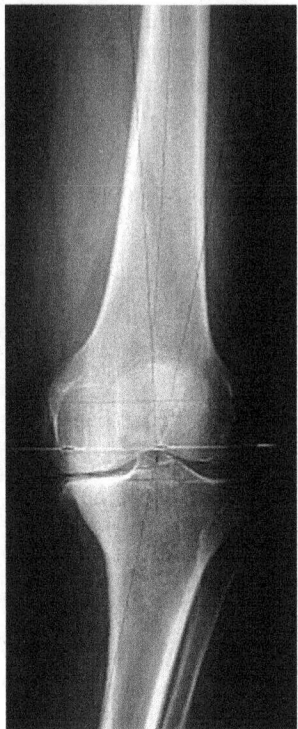

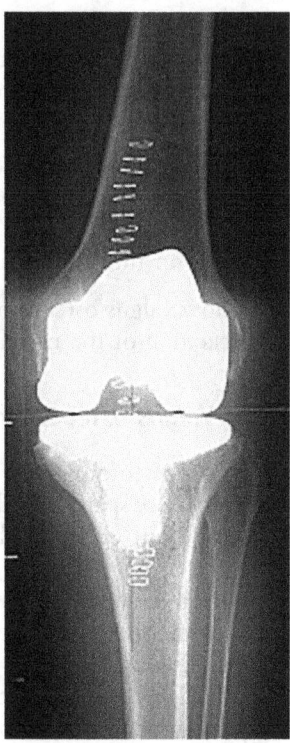

Fig. 7. – Medial compartment OA in a knee with severe varus deformity, in a 74-year-old female patient. Preoperatively, the tibio-femoral mechanical axis angle was 165°, the femoral mechanical axis angle 90°, and the tibial mechanical axis angle 80°.

Fig. 8. – Postoperative radiograph. Prior tibial osteotomy was not required for TKR. The lateral resection-related laxity produced by the asymmetrical bone resection has been perfectly balanced by a unilateral medial release (release of the anteromedial capsule, osteophyte resection, subperiosteal release of the superficial medial collateral ligament, plus division of the semimembranosus tendon). The postoperative tibiofemoral mechanical axis angle is 180°.

Surgical strategy of one-stage opening-wedge tibial valgus osteotomy and TKR

If a tibial valgus osteotomy with a medial opening-wedge and a TKR are to be performed in one sitting, the implant must meet certain criteria:

- the stem of the tibial component must be long, to extend beyond the osteotomy site;
- tibial resection must be comparatively sparing (thickness: 9mm);
- the stem must fill the metaphysis, so as to provide enhanced stability;
- the implant should not have "fins" reinforcing the stem-plateau junction.

We have opted for the HLS Evolution total knee prosthesis (Tornier, St. Ismier, France), a semiconstrained, cemented design. In this pattern, the PCL is sacrificed; however, posterior stabilization is provided by a third condyle in the midline, which engages a cam in the tibial component. The tibial stem is modular (17).

Surgical technique

Osteotomy

The approach is always via a medial parapatellar incision, without detaching the tibial tubercle (17). The soft tissues are dissected, and the tibia is prepared by releasing only the anterior portion of the joint capsule and by elevating the pes anserinus. The superficial medial collateral ligament is divided at its distal insertion, to allow the osteotomy to be performed. However, the insertion of the deep medial collateral ligament is left intact; equally, the semi-membranosus tendon and the posteromedial capsule are preserved. To guard against the risk of secondary displacement of the osteotomy site, the tibia must be dislocated forwards before the osteotomy is performed. The bone cut is slanted outwards and upwards; it remains above the level of the tibial tubercle, and as far away from the the lateral joint surface as possible, to leave sufficient bone in the tibial epiphysis to allow tibial resection and to provide a lateral bony hinge in the tibia. This means that the osteotomy line should finish up in the proximal part of the superior tibiofibular joint. The osteotomy line is fairly horizontal. The osteotomy is opened to the required extent, and temporarily held open with a Blount staple (fig. 9). The staple is not driven fully home, and care must be taken to ensure that it does not protrude into the centre of the medullary cavity, where it would interfere with the insertion of the implant stem or of the intramedullary aiming rods used for the insertion of the TKR. A small metal or cement wedge placed on the tibial periphery may also be used to prop the osteotomy open temporarily.

No intraoperative check radiographs are taken. The amount of correction to be obtained is determined from the preoperative radiographs.

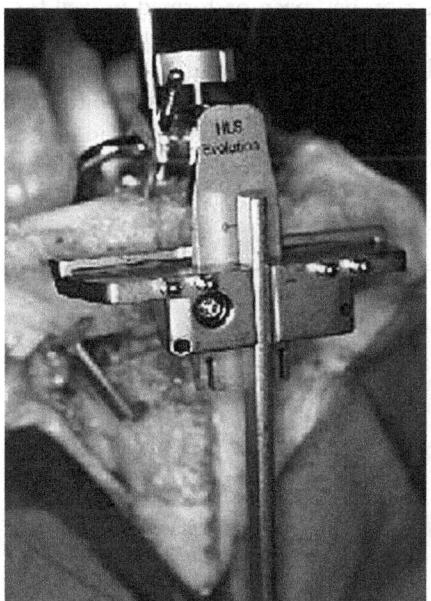

Fig. 9. – Positioning of instruments for tibial bone cuts. The previously performed tibial valgus osteotomy is held open by a staple. (Photograph used with permission from Sauramps Publisher.)

Implant insertion

Once the angular deformity has been corrected by the medial opening-wedge osteotomy, tibial resection may be proceeded with in customary fashion, using the instruments provided with the implant and taking care not to remove more than 9mm from the lateral tibial plateau. In this way, a maximum amount of bone will be left standing between the osteotomy and the resection lines.

With the joint line levelled by the osteotomy, the amount of bone to be resected from the tibia will be the same in the medial and lateral compartments, although, obviously, the resected slice will be thinner on the medial side, because of the loss engendered by OA (fig. 10). But for the prior osteotomy, the bone cut would have had to be very asymmetrical, with much more bone stock removed from the lateral than from the medial compartment. With the angular correction applied via the bone, there is no need for additional soft-tissue releases in order to balance the implant (18). The femoral component is inserted in customary fashion. The tibial component consists of a tibial plateau and a 65mm long stem that crosses the osteotomy site and ensures the stability of the implant (fig. 11). Once the trials have been removed, the definitive components are cemented. The hardware used to keep the osteotomy site open may be removed or driven home. The osteotomy defect is autografted using resection offcuts produced during the TKR part of the procedure; to prevent the collapse of the construct, a small "cortical" cement wedge is introduced (fig. 12). The patients are mobilized early, and are allowed out of bed the day after surgery. Weight bearing should be partial, with use of two walking aids for the first two months.

There are two important points to bear in mind:

The level of the osteotomy. In two of our cases, the slice of bone left standing after the osteotomy and tibial resection had been performed proved too thin, and a fracture occurred on the lateral side. Whilst this did not adversely affect the outcome, every care should be taken, in the routing of the osteotomy, to ensure that enough bone is left standing between the osteotomy and the lateral joint line. On the lateral side, the osteotomy should finish no higher than the level of the superior tibiofibular joint. This means fairly horizontal routing of the osteotomy;

The fixation of the osteotomy defect during implant insertion. Fixation with a Blount staple is a useful means of holding the osteotomy site open.

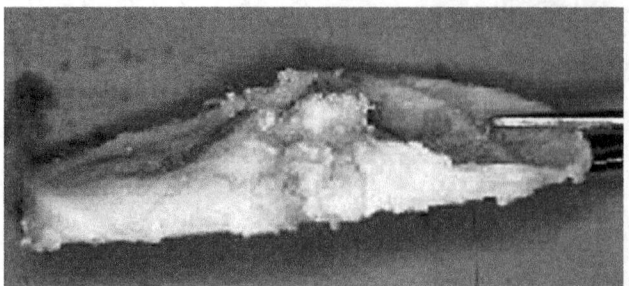

Fig. 10. – The bone slice removed is comparatively symmtrical in the two compartments, though obviously thinner on the worn side. (Photograph used with permission from Sauramps Publisher.)

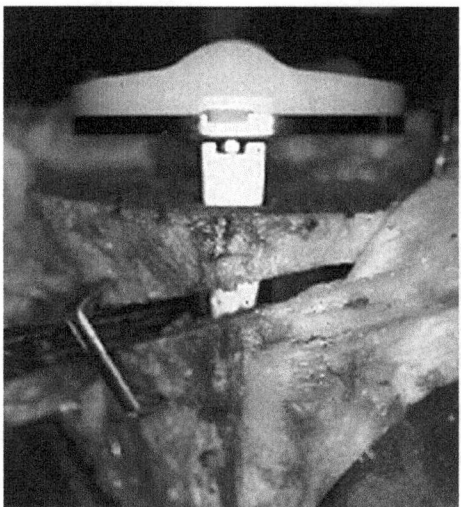 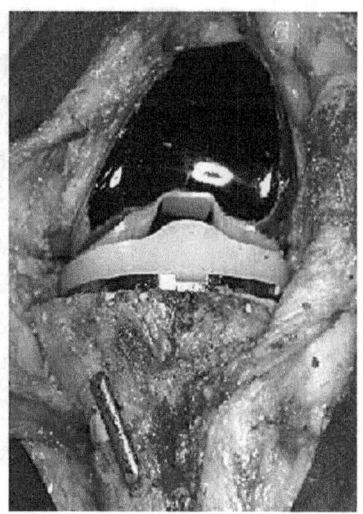

Fig. 11. – Trial of tibial component prior to cementing. The stem is seen to cross the osteotomy site. (Photograph used with permission from Sauramps Publisher.)

Fig. 12. – View at end of procedure, following the insertion of a cancellous graft obtained from resection offcuts. A small "cortical" wedge of cement is left in the osteotomy defect. (Photograph used with permission from Sauramps Publisher.)

However, the staple must be inserted with due care. It should be borne in mind that it may interfere with the insertion of the tibial stem if it protrudes into the medullary canal. This is why it should never be driven fully home at the outset. We thought, at one time, that a small metal wedge attached to a plate was a promising solution. It was fixed with unicortical screws, so as not to get in the way of the tibial stem. However, the plate did not prove superior to the Blount staple, since the screws were interfered with stem insertion, the plate was difficult to position (causing impingement on the medial collateral ligament), and would sometimes stick out under the skin. We therefore went back to the Blount staple, which we are still using today (fig. 13 and 14).

Sequence of procedures

Where the two procedures are performed in one sitting, we prefer to do the tibial valgus osteotomy first. Other authors start with the TKR. Doing the osteotomy first has the advantage of allowing the surgeon to use the customary instrumentation for the insertion of the TKR, which makes the procedure more accurate and precise. Also, the stem of the tibial component will extend beyond the osteotomy site, and patients will, therefore, be allowed immediate partial weight bearing. The hardware at the osteotomy site may be removed, to prevent skin problems. Godenèche (15) feels that the joint replacement should be performed first, with the tibial component positioned

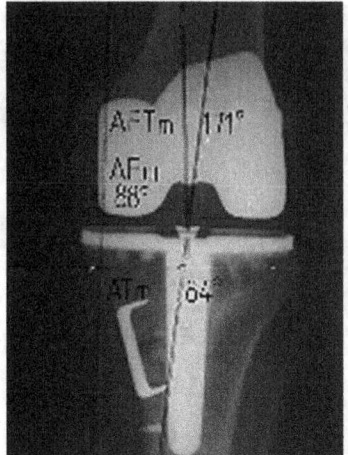 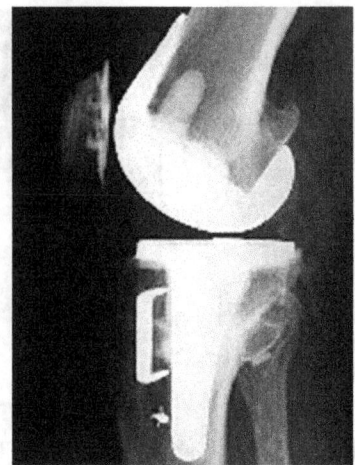

Fig. 13.-14. – Two-year radiographs. Residual varus: 6°.

parallel to the joint line, so as to leave it at right angles to the mechanical axis once the osteotomy has been performed. This makes implant positioning very awkward, since the instruments for the insertion of the device cannot be used properly. The bone cuts are made parallel to the joint line, regardless of the extra-articular deformity, and referenced from the femur, since neither the intra- nor the extramedullary rod can be used as a reference. A stemmed tibial component is ruled out by the fact that a stem would make it impossible to carry out an osteotomy below the implant. The absence of a stem means that internal fixation (stapling or plating) will need to be used at the osteotomy site, and the patient will not be allowed to weight bearing after surgery. Healing takes a long time, and non-union as well as hardware failure have been reported.

Indications

The chief indication is conditions requiring TKR: knee pain, and sometimes instability, in a sedentary or active (but not athletic) subject. TKR plus osteotomy would be indicated if the preoperative work-up suggests that the extra-articular deformity is such that resection-related laxity would cause a ligament balancing problem or excessive soft-tissue slackness (with adverse effects on the extensor mechanism, the collateral ligaments, and the level of the joint line) once the necessary bone cuts will have been made. To our way of thinking, a combined procedure would be indicated once the extra-articular deformity exceeds 8°. Our selection criteria also include "comparatively" young and active subjects (age 60-75 years); although age is not a formal criterion. With more experience, longer follow-up, and a detailed analysis of failures, we should be able, in the future, to establish more clearly the utility and the limitations of this technique.

References

1. Insall JN, Hood RW, Flawn LB et al. (1983). The total condylar knee prosthesis in gonarthrosis. A five-to nine-year follow-up of the first one hundred consecutive replacements. J Bone Joint Surg (Am) 65: 619-28
2. Tew M, Waugh W et al. (1985) Tibiofemoral alignment and the results of knee replacement. J Bone and Joint Surg (Br) 67: 551-6
3. Jonsson B, Åström J (1988) Alignment and long-term clinical results of a semiconstrained knee prosthesis. Clin Orthop 226: 124-8
4. Teeny SM, Krackow KA, Hungerford DS et al. (1991) Primary total knee arthroplasty in patients with severe varus deformity. A comparative study. Clin Orthop 273: 19-31
5. Wolff AM, Hungerford DS, Pepe CL. The effect of extraarticular varus and valgus deformity on total knee arthroplasty. Clin Orthop 271: 35-51
6. Dejour H, Neyret P, Bonnin M (1994) Instability and osteoarthritis. In: Fu FH, Harner CD, Vince GV, editors. Knee surgery. Baltimore: Williams & Wilkins: 859-75
7. Moreland JR, Basset LW, Hanker GJ (1987) Radiographic analysis of the axial alignment of the lower extremity. J Bone Joint Surg (Am) 69: 745-9
8. Cameron HU, Welsh RP (1988) Potential complications of total knee replacement following tibial osteotomy. Orthop Rev 17: 39-43
9. Neyret P, Deroche P, Deschamps G et al. (1992) Prothèses totales de genou après ostéotomie tibiale de valgisation. Rev Chir Orthop 77: 438-48
10. Karachalios T, Sarangi PP, Newman JH (1994) Severe varus and valgus deformities treated by total knee arthroplasty. J Bone and Joint Surg (Br) 76: 938-42
11. Mont MA, Alexander N, Krackow KA et al. (1994) Total knee arthroplasty after failed high tibial osteotomy. Orthop Clin North America 25: 515-25
12. Hungerford DS, Insall JN (1997) Extra-articular deformity in TKA. 14th Annual Current Concepts in Joint Replacement. Cleveland, OH. Session XVII. Papers 86 and 87
13. Rivat P, Neyret P, Ait Si Selmi T (1999) Influence de l'ordre des coupes, coupes dépendantes et indépendantes, rôle du tenseur. 9èmes Journées Lyonnaises de Chirurgie du Genou et de l'Épaule.
14. Ait Si Selmi T, Tayot O, Trojani C et al. (1999) Gestes ligamentaires dans l'équilibrage des prothèses totales du genou. 9e Journées Lyonnaises de Chirurgie du Genou et de l'Épaule.
15. Godenèche A (1998) Prothèses totales du genou et ostéotomies dans le même temps opératoire pour gonarthrose avec déviations axiales majeures (à propos de 11 cas). Comparaison avec 2 séries de 11 prothèses pour grands genu valgum et 12 prothèses sur grands genu varum. Thèse de Médecine no. 68.
16. Zanone X, Ait Si Selmi T, Neyret P (1999) Prothèse totale et ostéotomie tibiale de correction simultanées pour gonarthrose sur genu varum excessif constitutionnel. Rev Chir Orthop 85: 749-56
17. Dejour H, Deschamps G (1989) Technique opératoire de la prothèse totale à glissement du genou. Cahier Scient Paris 35: 13-23
18. Faris PM (1994) Soft tissue balancing and total knee arthroplasty. In: Fu FH, Harner CD, Vince GV, editors. Knee surgery. Baltimore: Williams & Wilkins 1385-89

Total knee replacement in the valgus knee

J.L. Lerat, A. Godenèche, B. Moyen, J.L. Besse

Total knee replacement (TKR) for treatment of osteoarthritis in a valgus knee is, in most cases, not more challenging than in a varus knee. However, in the presence of severe valgus deformity, it is more difficult to achieve good ligament balance and adequate bone coverage, despite contracture of the lateral structures. The worst case scenario is a mixed deformity which combines wear, contracture of lateral structures, slackening of medial ligamentous structures, and extra-articular bone deformity as may be seen after tibial osteotomy or post-traumatic malunion.

Anatomy/pathology of the valgus knee

Valgus deformity is accompanied by deficiency of the lateral compartment and, secondarily, by slackening of the medial ligamentous structures which further aggravates the deformity.

In the vast majority of cases, valgus knee is not more difficult to manage than varus knee. It only requires medial/lateral balancing with minimal bone resections which remove on the convex side of the deformity an amount of bone and cartilage that corresponds to the thickness of the selected components. As bone cuts are performed perpendicular to the mechanical axis of both the tibia and the femur, adequate release of soft tissues on the concave side of the deformity allows achievement of a rectangular space to accommodate the prosthetic components. Actually, release is the only tricky step of the procedure, and yet it is very simple since it generally consists in releasing the ligaments on the concave side and removing osteophytes. However, severe valgus deformities may sometimes pose some of the most difficult problems in knee arthroplasty. Often, there is external rotation of the tibia, wear that progresses towards the anterior aspect of the tibial plateau, and a bone defect into which the lateral femoral condyle sinks. With the tightening of the lateral soft tissues the valgus deformity, and external rotation become a fixed deformity. Bone loss may also be posterior or central. This asymmetric wear explains why some structures are more retracted than others, and particularly, why some structures are tighter in flexion than in extension. Release of lateral capsuloligamentous structures and tight tendons is arduous, indeed.

There is abundant published material on the subject, and many divergent opinions on how to approach the knee and perform the releases. Moreover, the order of priority of release procedures merits further discussion as no consensus has been reached yet.

The skin layer is sometimes very thin, particularly in rheumatoid patients, and it may be difficult to achieve proper coverage of the lateral stuctures after release. It may also prove very difficult to achieve perfect coverage of the prosthetic components, and skin dissection may lead to skin necrosis, especially if there is a hematoma.

Another difference with the varus knee is that there is a tendency to subluxation of the patella due to the valgus deformity and increased Q-angle. In such cases, release of the lateral retinaculum and vastus lateralis is mandatory. According to Karachalios et al. (26), clinical results are not as good in knees with a fixed valgus deformity and the rate of patellar dislocation is higher. Keblish (27) reported patellar maltracking in 8 out of 23 knees with a fixed valgus deformity greater than 15°, where a medial approach was used. Almost all authors : Stern et al. (52), Freeman et al. (16), Hungerford et al. (21), Insall et al. (23), Krackow et al. (29-31), Keblish (27), Ranawat et al. (47), Whiteside et al. (57), Dejour et al. (12), agree that a valgus knee is much more difficult to manage than a varus knee, due to the difficulty in achieving adequate soft tissue balance. Technically, there are two important issues: bone cuts, and release of lateral structures. Accurate radiological assessment is essential to plan the necessary correction and determine whether or not the deformity is correctable.

Telegoniometry in standing erect is indispensable; additionally, stress views may be taken to precisely evaluate the overall deformity, determine how much of the femur and the tibia is actually involved, evaluate ligament laxity, and determine the reducibility of the deformity.

The lateral view in extension shows the tibial slope, sagittal contour of the femoral epiphysis, and position of the patella in the femoral groove. Tangential views of the patellofemoral joint in valgus knees very often show offset positioning of the kneecap.

Surgical technique in the valgus knee

Distal femoral cut and tibial cut

Performing independent bone cuts is essential whereas the order of bone cuts is not important. To achieve a 180° axis, it is generally held (except by Hungerford et al. (21)) that the distal femoral cut and the tibial cut must be performed at 90° to the femoral and tibial mechanical axes respectively. Current instruments are designed to provide almost perfect cuts without using navigation, provided that good quality telegoniometry in standing erect has been used for preoperative planning, and that one has been careful to correct as much as possible any errors that may have been induced by flexion contracture and rotation of the knee. The distal femoral cut is performed using a cutting guide assembled to an intramedullary rod. If uncertainty exists, one can still identify the center of the femoral head radioscopically and use it as a reference to perform an accurate resection of the distal femur.

As regards the tibial cut, it is quite easy to cut the proximal tibia perpendicular to the tibial axis. Identifying the center of the ankle joint is not a problem; those who use the intramedullary alignment system also make very few errors (except in italic S-shaped tibias). Some surgeons even use a combination of the intramedullary and extramedullary alignment systems.

The posterior slope of the tibia is different whether a cruciate-retaining or a cruciate-sacrificing TKR is used. With the former design, surgeons generally agree that the average posterior tibial slope of 5° should be reproduced, because it promotes rollback of the femoral component and assists in proper tensioning of the PCL. It would seem logical to try and reproduce a near normal tibial slope in the operated knee to restore the joint line, isometric ligaments, and a normal soft tissue envelope. In reality, some knees have a posterior tibial slope $\geq 10°$; it is most hazardous to reproduce such a significant slope because of the high risk of posterior subluxation of the femur, particularly if the ACL is absent, unless a posterior lipped insert is used. Most posterior stabilized (PS) implant users favour a tibial slope of 0°.

As a rule, the distal femoral cut and the tibial cut are performed at 90° and remove from the medial femoral condyle and the medial plateau an amount of bone that corresponds to the thickness of the selected components, so that the medial ligaments will be at normal tension. Then, adequate release of the lateral ligaments will provide a balanced, rectangular space. In the vast majority of cases, no lateral release is necessary; excision of osteophytes and the limited release (10-12mm) performed to remove the resected proximal tibia are far sufficient. In our experience, further release was required in only 11% of valgus knees. Contrary to what was done in the eighties by pioneers such as Insall (23) and Freeman (16) who used to perform soft tissue balancing prior to bone cuts, we now perform bone resections first, because we found out that soft tissue balance was often naturally achieved after the cuts. Lateral soft tissue releases will be discussed further on in this article.

Anterior/posterior femoral cuts

Actually, there are two different methods: perform the anterior/posterior femoral cuts parallel to the posterior condyles, or externally rotate the femoral cuts. The authors who advocate externally rotated cuts can be classified into three categories: those who use the transepicondylar axis as a reference line, such as Berger et al. (5), those who use the anteroposterior axis as a reference line, such as Whiteside et al. (58), and those who routinely perform the femoral cuts at 3° of external rotation, such as Insall (23) and Poilvache et al. (46). This problem of posterior femoral cut in external rotation has been extensively studied. Many authors have measured the difference between the posterior condylar axis and the transepicondylar axis and have found out that it ranges from 3 to 5°, although there may be wide variations between individuals: Berger *et al* (5), Mantas *et al.* (40), Arima *et al* (4), Churchill *et al.* (10), Stiehl *et al.* (53), Elias *et al.* (14), and more recently, Boisrenoult *et al.* (6). These studies show that a significant number of knees display less than 3° difference between these two axes, and that using the transepicondylar axis in preference to the posterior condyle line seems particularly legitimate in knees with 5 to 9° difference.

An externally rotated cut may help prevent LCL laxity in flexion in the varus knee, or rather, increase the flexion gap medially. But in a valgus knee, it is exactly the opposite, which means that an internally rotated cut would be advisable. As a matter of fact, in most cases, the lateral ligament release which is intended to create a rectangular extension gap also creates a rectangular flexion gap, and the posterior cut can still be made parallel to the posterior condylar axis. However, it is as difficult to precisely identify the femoral epicondyles and materialize the epicondylar axis, as to determine the anterior-posterior axis using the Whiteside's method (58). As far as we are concerned, we think that the posterior condyle line is the most reliable landmark, except in extreme cases where the two axes are highly divergent. One may also use the Insall's method (23) and perform all bone cuts at about 3° of external rotation. But it is not more logical to perform a cut at 3° in a knee that does not need it than in a knee with 9° divergence between the two axes (Boisrenoult *et al.* [6]).

At this stage, is lateral release still necessary if the knee is tight laterally? In our experience, it was performed very exceptionally and only in severe valgus deformities with contracture. If the extension gap is correct, so will be the flexion gap. One should bear in mind that the femoral condyles are rarely worn posteriorly (except in cases of massive destruction or severe flexion contracture); this is precisely what makes the difference between a tight flexion gap and a tight extension gap: a tight extension gap is due both to condylar wear and tibial wear. Instead of using spacer blocks to measure the gap, we prefer to use trial components which provide full range of motion (ROM) and allow assessment of soft tissue tensioning at any degree of flexion/extension. It is the best way to determine whether additional release is required; should this be the case, the result can be appreciated immediately, and the release gradually completed (if necessary) with the trial components *in situ*.

What must be banned in a purely articular genu valgum deformity is performing the distal femoral cut parallel to the tibial cut after insertion of a tensioner. It is essential to perform independent cuts, after which tightness of the ligaments on the concave side can be adjusted, based on the ligaments on the convex side which are necessarily perfect if bone cuts correspond to the thickness of the selected components.

Release of lateral structures

Valgus deformity is accompanied by wear of cartilage and occasionally subchondral bone. The amount of wear varies from mild to severe, and may lead to the creation of a bone defect in the tibial plateau, into which the worn femoral condyle will sink. Genu valgum is initially a structural deformity, the cause of which is usually attributed to the femur. Many authors define it as an hypoplasia of the lateral condyle to explain the inclination of the joint line relative to the anatomic axis of the femur (F angle superior to 90°). But oftentime, the tibia also displays a few degrees of valgus. Other authors refer to it as an hypoplasia of the lateral condyle in the anterior-posterior plane which, according to them, should be considered when performing bone resections and soft tissue balance in flexion. In addition to the valgus deformity, there may be an abnormal external rotation of the tibia relative to the femur, with bone loss progressing anteriorly and resulting in a fixed rotational deformity. Sinking of the lateral condyle into this anterior bone defect promotes contracture of the ligaments, not mentioning lateral subluxation of the patella. At last, medial ligament stretch out may occur, causing the knee joint to gape medially during walking.

Several anatomic structures are retracted: iliotibial tract (ITT), LCL and popliteus muscle (tendon of which is so close to the LCL that their bony insertions can be detached as a whole during release or tightening procedures). The iliotibial tract which branches at the knee to the lateral retinaculum plays a role in the development of valgus deformity and offset position of the patella in the trochlear groove. Posterolateral structures also include the arcuate popliteal ligament and the posterior capsule.

In knees with severe valgus deformity due to wear, the PCL may be retracted and cannot always be retained if one wants to achieve full correction of the deformity and restore normal alignment (pre-OA valgus angle). It is even more difficult to retain it if one wishes to restore a 180° axis. In such cases, the PCL must be either excised or released. Normally, any contracture due to a deformity resulting from wear can be corrected, but excessive PCL tightness caused by a structural valgus deformity is obviously intractable; it can just be corrected within the limits of plastic stretching of ligaments.

If one takes care to restore the joint line, perform normal resections medially, and not increase the thickness of the tibial insert, the PCL can be retained in all cases. If the MCL is not slack, it is very simple; if it is slack, it must be tightened. But if one selects to use a thicker tibial insert to take up the slack in the MCL, further release of the lateral soft tissues will be necessary; in this case, the PCL needs to be resected or released (Whiteside *et al.* (57), Arima *et al.* (3)). Sacrificing the PCL implies further release of the lateral structures since the space to be filled is larger. It is the direct consequence of adjusting the space in reference to the slack MCL instead of the healthy central pivot. We shall see that increase of the joint space may have serious consequences.

It may even lead to extreme situations where the MCL is so overstretched that a polyethylene (PE) tibial insert of 10mm or more must be used. But the problems become really acute when the situation is aggravated by an ipsilateral extra-articular deformity (sequelae of overcorrected valgus high tibial osteotomy and malunion). These problems will be discussed further on in this article.

Standard anteromedial approach

The anteromedial approach is used by the majority of TKA surgeons, and there is no contraindication to the use of this approach in valgus knees, even in very severe cases (Scott (50), Krackow (29, 31), Laskin (34)).

The retracted structures to be released include: posterolateral structures, iliotibial tract, PCL, and sometimes vastus lateralis and biceps tendon. Release procedures are always performed in the medial-lateral direction.

LCL and popliteus ligament may be released subperiosteally to maintain a proximal attachment in continuity with the released ligaments. We prefer to move a bone block containing their combined insertion to a more distal position, and reattach it using a staple reinforced with a screw. Burdin (8) performs a real condylar osteotomy and distal fixation with two screws which likely provide better fixation than our staple reinforced with screws. This may be performed either from a medial or a lateral approach.

The disadvantage of the medial approach is that it makes it more difficult to reach the posterolateral corner. The advantage is that there is no incision on the lateral side so that component coverage is not compromised; on the other hand, repair of the released soft tissues is less easy than when a lateral approach is used. The second advantage of the medial approach is that it allows overlap repair and shortening of the medial retinaculum in cases of lateral patellar dislocation. At last, it allows for this all-important procedure: tightening of medial soft tissues in severe deformities.

The sequence of release procedures when a medial approach is used varies according to the authors. Most of them begin with femoral releases, others with release of the iliotibial tract from its tibial attachment. Insall et al. (24) follow a specific sequential order: posterolateral capsule, LCL, arcuate ligament and popliteus tendon, iliotibial tract (inferiorly from the Gerdy's tubercle), lateral intermuscular septum. PCL is routinely excised. Insall insists on release of the proximal portion of the iliotibial tract. In severe deformities, he performs releases high on the femur in spite of the risk of some devascularization. Krackow (29, 30, 31) and Hungerford (21) think that the iliotibial tract should be released first, taking care to maintain continuity with the fascia of the leg. The rest of the sequence of releases is as follows: lateral collateral ligament (LCL), posterolateral capsule (from the lateral condyle), popliteus tendon, and sometimes biceps femoris tendon.

Z-plasty lengthening of these structures is performed. These authors believe that the PCL can be retained. Healy (20) transects the iliotibial tract and releases the popliteus, but he preserves integrity of the LCL, biceps femoris, and lateral head of the gastrocnemius in cases of flexion contracture. The PCL is retained.

Ranawatt (47), Krackow (29), Karachalios (26), Whiteside (57) insist on the necessity to release the lateral retinaculum, the proximal portion of the iliotibial tract, and the posterolateral capsule-arcuate complex. Lengthening or sectioning of the vastus lateralis and biceps femoris are the final steps. For Faris (15), release of the iliotibial tract is sufficient in 75% of the cases. Where there is a valgus deformity greater than 15°, he moves the bone block containing the combined insertion of the LCL and popliteus tendon and retains the PCL. If he selects to implant a more constrained knee prosthesis, he removes the PCL and sections the popliteus and LCL. Whiteside (57) considers that if there is a lateral contracture both in flexion and extension, that is, in 80% of the cases, the LCL and popliteus, then the iliotibial tract and the posterior capsule must be released. If there is a lateral contracture only in extension, release of the iliotibial tract will be sufficient; if it is present only in flexion, he releases the LCL and rarely the popliteus, and retains the PCL. As far as we are concerned, in severe deformities, we use a medial approach with detachment of the anterior tibial tubercle and lateral dislocation of the patella (which is everted and remains pedicled to the lateral retinaculum). The patellar ligament is raised en bloc as far as the iliotibial tract which is released from its insertion on the Gerdy's tubercle, taking care to maintain continuity with the fascia of the leg (with or without a bone block).

Anterolateral approach

According to Keblish (27, 28), the lateral approach has several advantages: Lateral release and exposure can be performed in one go, access to the posterolateral structures is improved, vascularization of the medial side is maintained. Keblish performs a wide lateral arthrotomy along the lateral border of the quadriceps muscle, which is carried around the patella, taking care to leave 1cm of the lateral retinaculum. Then, he releases the iliotibial tract longitudinally from its posterior femoral insertions. All insertions must be detached without separating the ITT from the subcutaneous tissue.

Lengthening of the iliotibial tract is performed using a Z-plasty or V-Y plasty or multiple tiny incisions (like in a pie crust) that resemble stabs. These incisions are made in a medial-lateral direction, taking care not to elevate the skin. According to Keblish, release of the proximal aspect of the iliotibial tract offers several advantages: decreasing the "bow string" effect and providing slight correction of the valgus deformity prevents upward migration of the anterolateral fascia of the tibia after release, and allows maintenance of an anatomic attachment. Thus, valgus deformities of between 10 and 15°can be corrected. However, in very severe deformities, these incisions become ineffective and complete release is necessary. In deformities equal to or greater than 30°, release of the peroneal nerve must be considered. If the deformity is mild and easily correctable under anesthesia, release of the iliotibial tract is unnecessary.

A long incision is carried along the lateral border of the quadriceps muscle and around the patella, taking care to leave 1cm of the lateral retinaculum.

The incision is made from the junction between the vastus lateralis and the quadriceps tendon to the patella, through 50% of the tendon. At the upper end of the incision, the quadriceps tendon is 6-10mm thick, so that it can be split in two with a scalpel, horizontally, from the sectioning slice to the lateral margin of the patella; the deep portion is dissected free from the patella but remains attached to the deep tissue layers. Thus, the edge of the deep layer will be sutured to the free edge of the superficial layer at the end of the procedure, using a sliding plasty to improve coverage of the prosthesis at closure.

Inferiorly, Keblish releases the fibers subperiosteally from the Gerdy's tubercle, while raising the fascia of the leg and the fat pad as a single sheet as far as the tibial tuberosity. Thus, the patellar ligament is strengthened by this contiguous fascia. The patella is dislocated medially. Additionally, some authors (Hungerford (21), Whiteside (57) and Wolff (60)) perform an osteotomy of the tibial tuberosity, from medial to lateral. Then, the knee is flexed and the dislocated patella is held in this position by a retractor.

Lateral dissection which may have been initiated prior to dislocation of the patella, with the knee extended, is continued in flexion. Fibers attached to the Gerdy's tubercle are released, but continuity is maintained with the fascia of the leg. This sharp dissection is performed flush on bone and carried around the tibia to the PCL, taking care to maintain continuity between the fibers of the iliotibial tract and those of the fascia of the leg. Then, osteophytes are resected and the capsule is released from the femur. Keblish (27) recommends, in exceptional situations, that the fibular head be resected while preserving integrity of the LCL and biceps femoris. Sometimes this is sufficient to achieve the desired tibiofemoral alignment; otherwise, release of femoral attachments is necessary. It begins with release of posterolateral structures which include: LCL, popliteus, and posterolateral capsule. Proximal insertions of the LCL and popliteus are released subperiosteally.

If this approach facilitates access to these structures, it also makes preparation of the medial compartment much more difficult, even with the tibia externally rotated. If, at this stage, release is insufficient to allow insertion of a rectangular spacer block of the desired thickness, Keblish (27, 28) may want to resect the PCL, but he never tightens the medial structures (besides, this approach does not allow for it).

Now, bone cuts can be performed. The tibial cut is performed at 90° in the coronal plane, with a posterior slope (if applicable).

One may alternatively perform the femoral cut first and initiate soft tissue release, and then perform the tibial cut and complete release as needed (the space created is evaluated and checks are made using spacer blocks).

It must be pointed out that the lateral approach places the tibia in internal rotation and the medial approach in external rotation. The tibial component must be perfectly positioned in the horizontal plane; one must be very careful as tibial rotation may be misleading. The posterior margin of the tibial plateau is the most reliable landmark for correct positioning of the tibial tray.

The distal femoral cut is performed at 90° to the femoral axis. The posterior cut is internally rotated or based on the flexion gap achieved with a tensioner. Trial reductions first with the spacer blocks and then with the trials aim at achieving a rectangular space both in flexion and extension, that corresponds to the thickness of the components.

According to Keblish, it may be difficult to close the lateral compartment and technical tricks may have to be used: approximation of the infrapatellar fat pad to the patellar ligament, or separation of the vastus lateralis from the rectus femoris to subsequently suture them together in a staggered position. Z-plasty of the quadriceps tendon helps close the lateral compartment.

Variants exist, such as detachment of the Gerdy's tubercle together with the iliotibial tract, or medial shift of the tibial tuberosity. Buechel (7) described a sequential three-step lateral release that is a variant of the Keblish technique.

Tightening of medial ligaments

Medial laxity is seen in severe valgus deformities, classified as Type II by Hungerford, Krackow and Kenna (30). Mild residual medial laxity is acceptable and does not compromise the outcome, provided that a 180° tibiofemoral axis has been restored. In single leg stance, the varus stresses which are generated protect the medial ligaments.

But residual medial laxity, even mild, is badly tolerated if a valgus deviation persists postoperatively, causing instability and discomfort with weight bearing. In these conditions, medial laxity cannot but increase; in addition, external rotation occurs and the patella itself is susceptible to progressively subluxate.

Even though medial laxity is usually well tolerated in knees with correct lower limb alignment, it may be preferable to tighten the medial ligamentous structures, particularly if the PCL has been retained, because in this case, the amount of lateral release is just sufficient to correct for the valgus deformity.

Tightening may also be performed on the tibial side using transosseous sutures, after release of the ligament; this technique is very similar to that of O'Donoghue for treatment of chronic medial laxity.

One may also tighten the MCL proximally by moving a bone block with the attached MCL insertion, fixation being provided by a staple reinforced with a screw. Alternatively, the bone block may be buried in the femoral condyle and fixed with a staple reinforced with a screw, to preserve ligament isometry.

Krackow (30) described a tightening technique which consists in removing from the tibia a small bone plug with the attached insertions of the PCL and posterolateral capsule, moving it distally, and securing it with transosseous sutures. MCL tightening is achieved by moving distally a bone block with its attached tibial insertion.

Sequence of release procedures

In moderate valgus deformities, removal of osteophytes and bone resections are sufficient to correct the deformity, but in severe deformities, release of soft tissue contractures is necessary.

The iliotibial tract is always contracted. ITT is an "active" insertional structure, an extension of the fascia lata which is indispensable to control the varus stresses applied during weight bearing. The lateral intermuscular septum is contracted and needs to be released. The next most often involved elements are the LCL and the popliteus.

In the presence of a flexion contracture, the posterior capsule and popliteus must be released. The posterolateral capsule is released either from the femur or the tibia. Integrity of the biceps femoris can be preserved in all but exceptional cases.

Lateral release is ineffective in severe contractures due to combined wear and structural valgus deformity, and above all in bone deformities due to malunion or secondary to an osteotomy.

In osteoarthritis of the valgus knee, patellofemoral joint balance is the primary concern, not mentioning the problem of resurfacing/non-resurfacing of the patella which is another debate altogether and is not specific to the valgus knee. Nowadays, patella resurfacing is less and less systematic, and some authors (including ourselves) no longer resurface the patella. Let's not forget that a medialized or a lateralized patellar component may contribute to patellar instability.

Lower limb realignment which restores the Q-angle is the most important factor in stabilizing the patella. However, in some cases such as patellofemoral osteoarthritis with subluxating patella, it may be necessary to release the lateral retinaculum. One can also take advantage of elevation of the tibial tuberosity that is part of the approach, to move it slightly medially if the patella is not perfectly stable. Keblish (28) claims that his lateral approach offers a real advantage in that it preserves integrity of the medial retinaculum. A medial approach allows, in case of persistent patellar instability, overlap repair of the medial retinaculum at closure.

Other factors contribute to the stability of the patella, such as rotation of the tibial or femoral component (Yoshii and Whiteside (61)). One may wonder whether the 3-4° external rotation of the femoral component can really influence stability of the patella. The question might rather be "Does this rotation decrease the slope of the lateral trochlea, thus compromising articular conformity, instead of increasing it?"

Although the PCL can be retained in almost all valgus knees, it is important to know the possible adverse effects of excessive PCL tightening: posterior wear of the PE insert, anterior lift-off of the tibial baseplate, and restriction of flexion range of motion (ROM) (according to Ritter (48)). It is true that the PCL interferes with realignment of the lower limb, but on the other hand, it obviates the need for extensive soft tissue release and facilitates ligament balancing. Retention of the PCL allows maintenance of the joint line level. The PCL plays a major role in control of varus stresses during weight bearing by acting in synergy with peripheral ligaments, even if the ACL is absent.

Some authors claim that the PCL is never properly tensioned. According to Insall (23), proper tension is observed in only 10% of the knees. Where the PCL can be retained, a thicker PE insert is used, which affects flexion. This has been evidenced by Shoemaker (49) in a study using cadaver specimens of the knee implanted with prosthetic components.

Other authors retain the PCL without increasing PE thickness, claiming that this has some interesting advantages: more normal kinematics, improved stability, proprioceptive information. For Hungerford (21) and Whiteside (57), retention of the PCL is never a problem in the valgus knee, and we agree with them. Other authors such as Arima *et al.* (3) and Ritter *et al.* (48) selected to release the PCL when it is too tight, and perform gradual release of the PCL from its tibial insertion in 40% of their valgus knees. Krackow (29, 31) said that sometimes the PCL needs to be released and even resected; he further suggested to perform a Z-lengthening. Whiteside (57) always retains the PCL in valgus knees, but he sometimes uses a posterior stabilized knee design.

PCL sectioning is considered as a release procedure in cases where release of the peripheral ligaments failed to provide adequate balance, which, according to Delfico (13) and Ritter *et al.* (48), is always the case in valgus deformities greater than 10°. But we shall see, based on a series of patients treated for genu valgum deformity greater than 20° (purely articular deformity), that the PCL can be successfully retained.

Results of a series of TKRs implanted in patients with severe genu valgum without bone deformity

Godenèche (18), in his thesis (1998), studied 11 TKRs implanted in knees with over 20° valgus malalignment [HKA angle = 203 ± 3° (200-209)], which belonged to a consecutive series of 220 valgus TKAs performed by our team.

There were 10 females and 1 male with a mean age of 73.4 years ± 11.1 (range, 51-84 years). Etiology included: lateral tibiofemoral osteoarthritis (1 Grade III, 6 Grade IV, 4 Grade V), rheumatoid arthritis (3), patellofemoral osteoarthritis (1 Grade II, 8 Grade III, and 2 Grade IV). Both the femur and the tibia were involved: F angle = 97.3 ± 2.5° (range, 91-100°), T angle = 96.2 ± 3° (range, 92-103°), tilt = 9.8 ± 4° (range, 6-16°). Preoperative flexion was 107 ± 14° (range, 90-120°).

In all the cases, the knee was approached from the anterior aspect via a medial parapatellar arthrotomy with lateral dislocation of the patella. Elevation of the tibial tuberosity was necessary in one case only. In spite of a severe deformity, 8 out of the 11 knees did not require more extensive lateral retinacular release than that needed to perform the bone cuts and resect the osteophytes. The PCL was retained in all the knees. Lateral release was performed in 3 knees: dissection of the fascia lata which remained in continuity with the fascia of the leg, capsular release, release of the LCL and popliteus. In 2 knees, medial structures had to be tightened: decortication followed by tightening of the MCL and pes anserinus and fixation with staples onto the tibia (1), tightening of the MCL which remained attached to a bone block and fixation with a staple onto the femur (1). In 2 cases, corticocancellous grafts were used to fill a bone defect in the lateral femoral condyle. In 2 cases, 2° of residual valgus were maintained in the femur. Mean operation time was 125 ± 17.5 minutes (range, 85-65 minutes). Overall blood loss was 990 ± 408mL (range, 300-580mL, 165mm).

A few complications occurred. One female patient experienced patellar dislocation 2 months after surgery and underwent reoperation with tibial tuberosity transposition and sectioning of the lateral retinaculum. Surgical revision for valgus dislocation was performed 22 months after implantation. This patient had been treated for genu valgum with a preoperative HKA angle of 205°, F angle of 98°, T angle of 92°, and valgus tilt of 15°. She should have had tightening of the MCL or implantation of a more constrained prosthesis.

Apart from this one case, good results were achieved at an average follow-up of 17 months, with an IKS knee score of 85 ± 20 points on a 100-point scale (range, 28-98 points) and a mean gain of 60 ± 30 points (range, 11-88 points). The IKS function score was 67 ± 27 points (range, 0-100 points) with a mean gain of 33 ± 24 points (range, 15-80 points). Mean flexion was 111 ± 3.5° (range, 90-130°).

The functional results achieved in this series of TKRs implanted in knees with severe valgus deformities were similar to those in the general series of TKRs, in spite of higher technical difficulties (fig. 1). Godenèche (18) compared the functional and anatomical results achieved in these severe cases with those achieved in severe varus cases and did not note any difference either.

Conclusion regarding TKRs implanted in knees with purely articular valgus deformities

Management of soft tissues is the most challenging step in valgus total knee arthroplasty. Stability of the knee joint and patella depends on factors such as quality of bone cuts, maintenance of ligament continuity, and design of

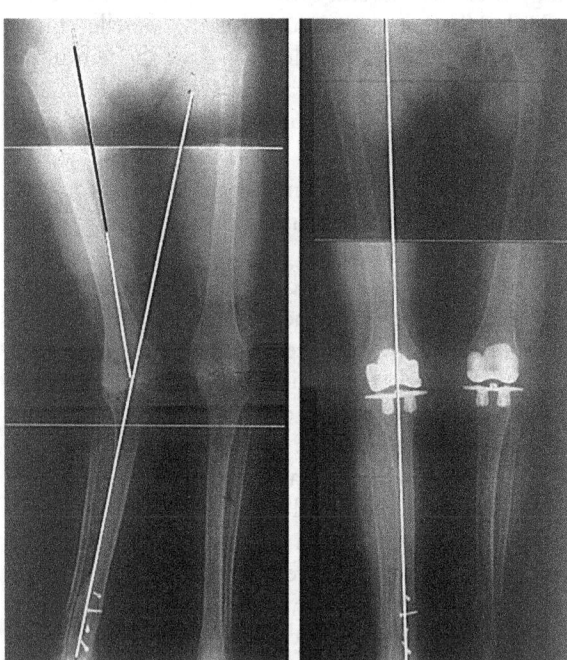

Fig. 1. – Lateral compartment osteoarthritis with 25° of valgus deformity, perfectly corrected by implantation of a cruciate-retaining total knee prosthesis and lateral release.

the prosthesis, but above all, it is the severity of the preoperative deformity that poses intraoperative technical difficulties. Fixed valgus deformity is far more difficult to correct than varus deformity which, most of the time, requires a simple release of proximal tibial attachments.

Severe genu valgum with bone deformity

Is bone deformity correctable by implantation of a total knee prosthesis? The question is not so much whether a severe bone deformity combined with advanced osteoarthritis can be corrected with TKA, but how this can be achieved.

Alignment can be restored with total knee replacement, but this implies correcting the whole deformity which is the end result of wear, ligament laxity, and extra-articular bone deformity. Wear and ligament laxity have previously been discussed. The presence of a bone deformity changes everything:

- If a non-constrained prosthesis is used: extensive ligament release must be performed on the concave side of the deformity; as a result, the joint space will dramatically gape open;
- If a hinge prosthesis is used: all deformities cannot be corrected with a hinge prosthesis. Moreover, this type of implant is known to have limited service life;
- A two-stage procedure can be performed: osteotomy, and secondarily total knee arthroplasty;
- To avoid the respective drawbacks of the above options, we have suggested a one-stage procedure in which TKA is combined with tibial or femoral osteotomy.

1st option: correct the whole deformity with total knee arthroplasty

This method relies on two cuts being performed perpendicular to the femur and the tibia, and then soft tissue balancing to restore a 180° mechanical axis. In this case, the whole deformity is corrected by a concave-side release (fig. 2).

The main advantage of this method advocated by Insall (23, 24) (and previously suggested) is that it addresses all issues in one go. The technique is simple and easily reproducible, and it allows immediate weight bearing. Unfortunately, it also has several drawbacks, beginning with stretching of neurovascular elements, particularly when there is a severe valgus deformity. Krackow (29, 31) and Ranawat (47) reported a 3-4% rate of peroneal nerve palsy. Wolff et al. (60) showed that a 3cm release is necessary to correct a 20° deformity. Moving the proximal insertion of the LCL 3cm distally would place it on the prosthesis or the joint line, or even lower! Therefore, this method is limited to correction of deformities much smaller than 20°. Furthermore, altering the length of ligaments results in loss of isometry of the stretched fibers since the size and curvature of the condyles remain unchanged. As a consequence, fibers are overly tensioned in extension and loose in flexion, which may cause instability.

Merritt *et al.* (41) reported a very high rate of instability in cases of extensive ligament release (47% versus 10% only when there was no release). Miyasaka *et al.* (42) reported 24% of instability in their series of patients treated for severe genu valgum. Lecuire *et al.* (35) published 6 cases of posterior dislocation after total condylar knee arthroplasty, including 4 knees with severe genu valgum (superior to 10°). Both the lateral/posterolateral release required for correction of these severe deformities and the difficulties to achieve correct soft tissue balance both in flexion and extension are responsible for these instabilities. In valgus knees with bone deformity, as may be seen after overcorrected valgus osteotomies, lateral release sometimes leads to dramatically increase the thickness of the polyethylene (PE) insert to fill the joint space, which has the detrimental effect of lowering both the tibial tuberosity and the patella (fig. 3).

In order to palliate this drawback, Whiteside (57) suggested to move the distal femoral cut distally in severe valgus deformities with medial laxity, by augmenting the lateral condyle (with bone grafts). In any event, this inevitably results in lengthening the lower limb.

In cases of femoral valgus malunion, one cannot expect to correct the deformity with total knee arthroplasty and simple lateral ligament release, as flexion gap balance and extension gap balance are completely different. Performing a distal femoral cut at 90° to the mechanical axis of the femur by resecting the medial condyle makes it necessary to augment the lateral condyle with a bone graft and perform extensive lateral release in order to achieve a 180° axis. In flexion, the knee will be so loose laterally that it will be impossible to cheat by performing a rotated cut; furthermore, as seen above, there would be a high risk of instability. It is still possible to compensate for it by exter-

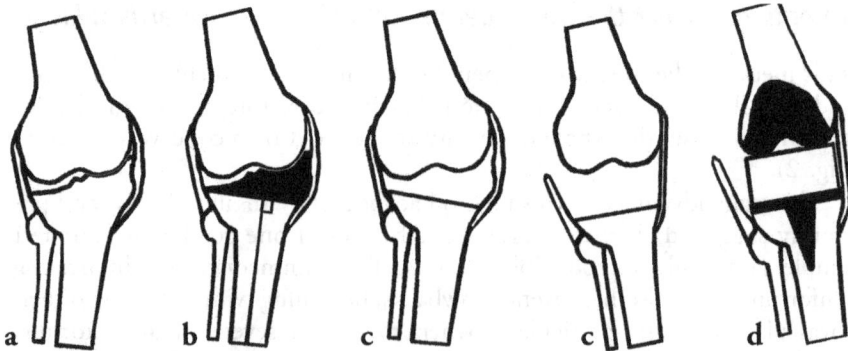

Fig. 2. – a. Typical case of overcorrected valgus osteotomy.
b. Tibial cut performed at 90° to the mechanical axis of the tibia.
c. Lateral release to create a rectangular extension gap, resection of both cruciates, and tensioning of MCL.
d. Implantation of a TKR in this situation presents some drawbacks: lenghtening of the lower limb, proximal insertion of LCL positioned too low, tension on neurovascular structures, patella baja.

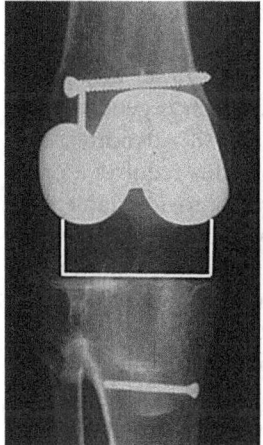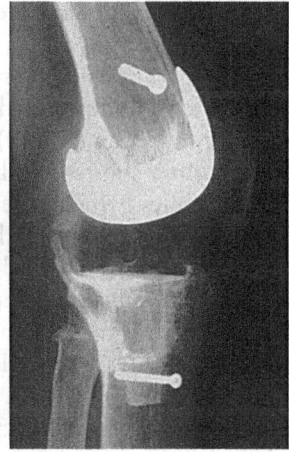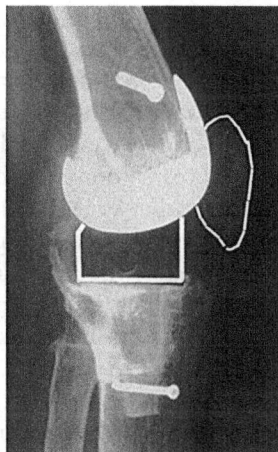

Fig. 3. – Conversion of failed osteotomy to TKR with a very thick tibial component. Detrimental effects include: lengthening, patella baja, flexion limited to 60°, pain, and peroneal nerve palsy.

nally rotating the femoral component, as recommended by Aglietti (1) (1996), but this may adversely affect the function of the patellofemoral joint. The kinematics of the knee would be very far from normal.

2ⁿᵈ option: constrained prosthesis

Sometimes, implantation of a constrained or hinge prosthesis is mandatory if soft tissue balance cannot be achieved. Stern had 8 such cases in his series (52), and Miyasaka 10 cases (42) in which he used total condylar III constrained prostheses.

With hinge prostheses, ligament problems are solved and the whole deformity can be corrected, provided that it is limited to the metaphyseal-epiphyseal region. In cases of a deformity in the metaphyseal-diaphyseal or diaphyseal region, a long stem component will not be sufficient and an osteotomy will be necessary. Besides, this type of prosthesis is associated with a higher rate of complications than unconstrained sliding prostheses. We personally used hinge prostheses in two knees because of severe ligament laxity, but the bone deformity was so severe that we also had to perform a femoral osteotomy to insert the stem and restore a normal femoral axis. This indication should remain an exception. A less constrained prosthesis must be selected whenever possible.

3ʳᵈ option: osteotomy combined with TKA

This option offers a number of advantages: osteotomy allows full correction of the bone deformity, so that the prosthesis will restore soft tissue balance, joint line, and position of the patella. One may retain the PCL and insert a non-constrained sliding prosthesis. The ACL is often intact, which allows implantation of a prosthesis that retains both cruciates, which we used to do earlier in the series.

Krackow (31) does not like this method which results in lower limb shortening when a closing-wedge osteotomy is performed, which is generally the case to correct a tibial valgus deformity. Cameron (9) (1988) advocated curviplanar osteotomy to avoid lower limb shortening, but this requires a more bulky fixation system than simple staples (which generally provide stable fixation). Alternatively, an open-wedge osteotomy may be performed. It avoids shortening of the lower limb and is commonly used to correct femoral and tibial varus deformities. However, in genu valgum, lateral open-wedge osteotomy of the proximal tibia is technically more demanding: as open-wedge osteotomy of the fibula is necessary, there is a potential risk of damage to the peroneal nerve.

In a knee with rotational malunion, Lerat *et al.* (36) consider that osteotomy is the only option available. A fibular osteotomy must be performed, particularly where rotation exceeds 20°. A CT scan is very helpful to accurately measure the amount of rotation to achieve and determine the position of the tibial tuberosity. Osteotomy and TKA can be performed as a one-stage or a two-stage procedure (osteotomy first).

Osteotomy performed prior to TKA

This operative strategy supported by Cameron (9), Wolff *et al.* (60), Krackow *et al.* (29, 31), Mont *et al.* (43) offers several advantages: it is a straightforward procedure; the osteotomy generally unites rapidly so that the second-stage total knee arthroplasty is technically very similar to a primary TKA. According to Mont (43), the osteotomy eliminated or at least delayed the need for arthroplasty in 3 patients, and according to Wolff (60) in 1 patient. A two-stage procedure was used in almost all the cases.

The main disadvantage of this strategy is that the patient must undergo two consecutive procedures. Cameron (9) insisted on the necessity of a 6- to 12-month delay between the two stages. This strategy means 2 anesthesias, 2 rehabilitation periods, and the risk of thromboembolism is multiplied by 2.

Therefore, in all such cases, should we systematically perform an osteotomy and evaluate its outcome before launching into a TKA? From a theoretical point of view, the question is at issue in patients less than 70 years of age with mild osteoarthritis, and no patellar involvement. Here, the point is not to compare the respective results of osteotomy and TKA. The patients operated on in this series were indeed standard indications for total knee replacement, considering their age and the severity of their disease. The osteotomy would not have dispensed with the need for TKA. Furthermore, one problem with performing a first-stage osteotomy is the determination of the amount of overcorrection. As a matter of fact, when a valgus osteotomy is performed as a palliative treatment, a 3 to 6° overcorrection is advisable to obtain long-term relief of pain. This is not the case when osteotomy is to be followed, a few months later, by TKA, because overcorrection may interfere with insertion of the components.

Osteotomy and TKA as a one-stage procedure

We suggested this option in 1990 and presented it during the 1991 SOFCOT Meeting (Lerat (36), within the scope of a paper about failed tibial osteotomy in which we reported the first two cases treated in 1990. Wolff and Hungerford (60) reported 2 cases in 1991, and Uchinou (56) one case in 1996. Indications were sequelae of overcorrected tibial valgus osteotomy. Hungerford (22) supported this option during the Annual Current Concepts in Joint Replacement Meeting which took place in Cleveland in December 1997. Our series consists of 19 knees operated on between 1990 and 2000; it was presented during the 2001 ISAKOS Meeting (Lerat (38)). Godenèche (18) reported the first 11 cases in his 1998 thesis. Here, we shall only present the 8 cases treated for valgus deformity.

The main advantage of this method is that everything is addressed in one go. It further allows achievement of a perfect soft tissue balance with the components *in situ*, prior to correcting the bone deformity with maximum accuracy. One of the drawbacks of this method is that some of the bone cuts cannot be performed using the dedicated instruments, due to bone deformity. Another drawback is the slow healing process, likely due to devascularization of the epiphyseal-metaphyseal segment. But these are only minor drawbacks which are greatly outweighed by the benefits to the patient.

Surgical technique

A tourniquet was systematically used. A midline skin incision was made, and the knee joint was exposed via a medial parapatellar incision in all the patients. Elevation of the anterior tibial tuberosity was performed in 5 out of 8 cases.

Initially, trial components are inserted, taking care to achieve optimal soft tissue balance (cruciate ligaments and peripheral soft tissues). In knees with a tibial deformity, the three femoral bone cuts are performed in a conventional manner, using the dedicated instruments. Then, the tibial cut is performed parallel to the posterior condyle line, in flexion, after the peripheral soft tissues and cruciate ligaments have been brought to tension (using two small retractors) (fig. 4). Extension gap is maintained with a spacer block. Then, a medial closed-wedge osteotomy is performed while maintaining a fibrous hinge, and X-rays are taken to confirm correct axial alignment of the lower limb. Then, final components are inserted; staple fixation using two staples is the last step. If pegged or short-stem components are used, the osteotomy can be performed with the prosthesis *in situ* (fig. 5). Moreover, pegs do not interfere with insertion of staples or plates (fig. 6 and 7).

In knees with a femoral deformity, the tibial cut is performed in a conventional manner, but the femoral cuts cannot be performed using the alignment

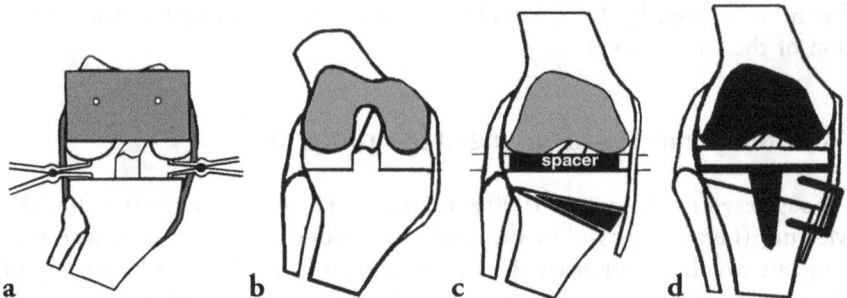

a   b   c   d

Fig. 4. – **a.** Tibial cut performed parallel to the posterior condyle line at 90° of flexion. All three femoral cuts are standard.
b. Insertion of the femoral trial.
c. Resection of a medial wedge while maintaining the joint space using a spacer block or a trial tibial component; then, alignment of the lower limb is checked with fluoroscopy.
d. Final components *in situ*; fixation achieved with staples.

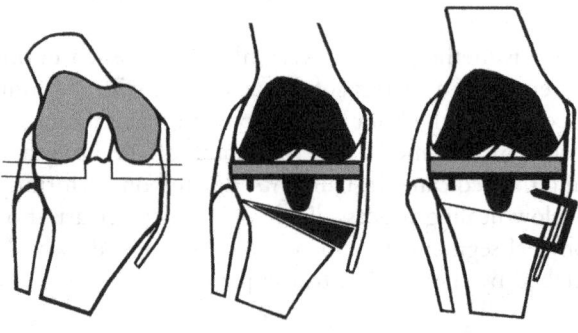

Fig. 5. – If a pegged or a short stem component is used, the final component is inserted, alignment of the lower limb is checked with fluoroscopy, and fixation is achieved with staples.

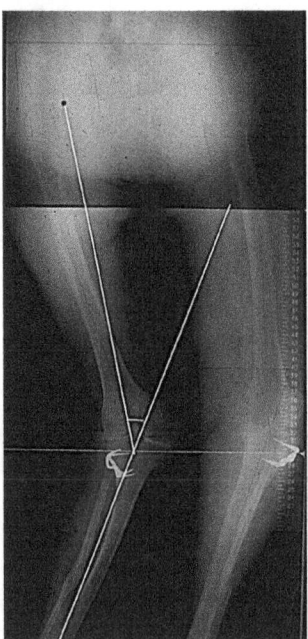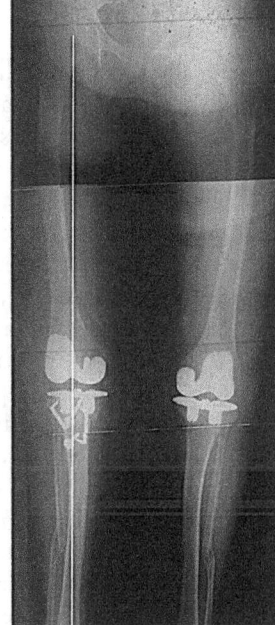

Fig. 6. – Patient with a severe valgus deformity of 30°, secondary to lateral closed-wedge osteotomy; 20° are attributable to an extra-articular bone deformity.

system. Therefore, the femoral cutting guide is applied to the femur, parallel to the resected tibial surface, in extension to perform the distal femoral cut, and in flexion to perform the anterior and posterior femoral cuts. After all bone cuts have been completed, the components are inserted (fig. 8). At this stage, there is a good soft tissue balance, but the tibiofemoral mechanical axis

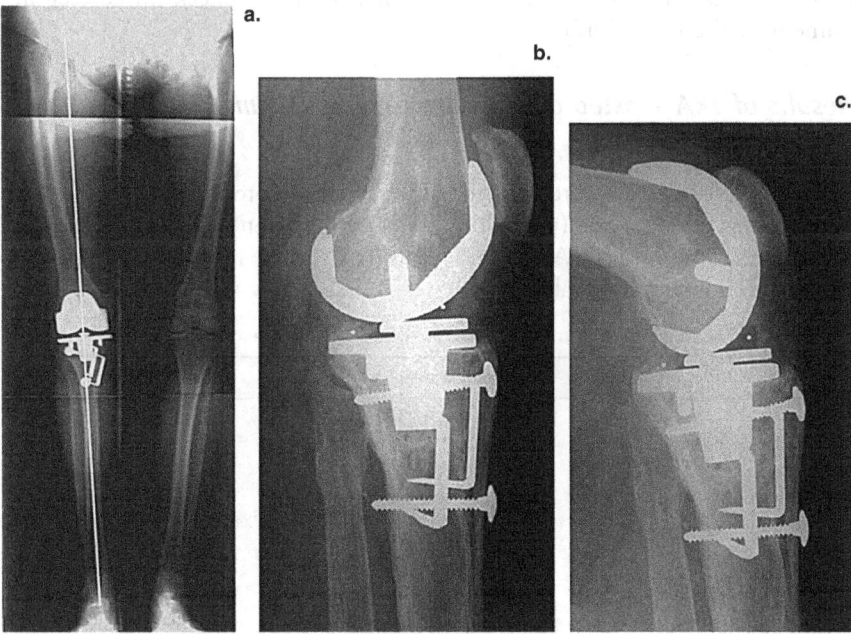

Fig. 7. – a. Short stem TKR (INNEX mobile bearing prosthesis). Osteotomy was performed as a second stage procedure. Tibial tuberosity was elevated.
b. Lateral view in extension, showing correct joint line level and normal position of the patella.
c. Posterior drawer stress view, showing functioning PCL; posterior drawer is 5mm.

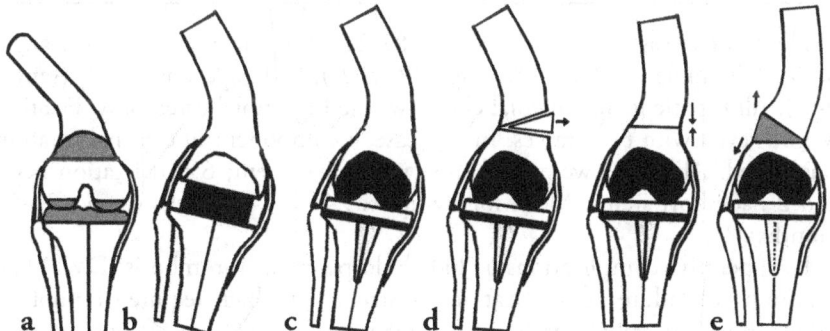

Fig. 8. – Femoral malunion.
a. Tibial cut and anterior/posterior femoral cuts are performed with the knee flexed.
b. Distal femoral cut is performed parallel to the tibial cut, with the knee extended.
c. Insertion of both components.
d. Medial closed-wedge osteotomy of the distal femur.
e. Lateral open-wedge osteotomy of the distal femur. Strong fixation is achieved with a plate in both cases.

needs correction. An osteotomy is performed to achieve an overall neutral axial alignment. It may be either an open-wedge or a closed-wedge osteotomy. However, with an open-wedge osteotomy, one seldom gets a stable osteofibrous hinge as in the tibia, and stiff, bulky fixation devices are necessary (screw plate or blade plate). Prior to inserting the fixation devices, radioscopy must be used to identify the center of the femoral head and check for correct alignment of the lower limb.

Results of TKA + osteotomy in severe genu valgum after failed osteotomy

There were 8 cases of overcorrected valgus tibial osteotomy. Mean age of the patients was 69 ± 7 years (range, 60 to 79 years). Mean delay between initial tibial osteotomy and TKA was 8.4 years (range, 11 months to 13 years). Results are presented in table I.

Table I – Preoperative and postoperative status: 8 cases of TKR + osteotomy.

8 cases	Preoperative	Postoperative
Age	69 ± 7 (60-79)	
IKS Knee Score	32 ± 4 (20-57)	83 ± 9 (66-96)
IKSK: gain		51 ± 11 (39-64)
IKS: function	52 ± 8 (45-65)	68 ± 34 (25-100)
IKSF: gain		24 ± 13 (10-40)
HSS Score	47 ± 11 (37-63)	90 + 5 (85-97)
HSS: gain		42 ± 8 (34-51)
Flexion	110 ± 13 (90-130)	115°± 10 (90-130)
HKA Angle	197 ± 9 (187-210)	179 ± 2° (175-181)
Gape	3 ± 2 (0-5)	0.2 ± 0.2° (0-1)
Bone Deformity	11.5 ± 4.7 (9-17)	
Position of Patella	0.7 ± 0.3 (0.3-1)	0.67 ± 0.3 (0,44-1)
Operation Time		135 ± 17min (110-160)
Blood Loss		1090 ± 350mL (620-1,650)

HKA angle was 197 ± 10 ° (range, 187-210°), F angle was 91 ± 3° (range, 88-97°), T angle was 99 ± 3° (range, 94-102°), and gape was 3 ± 2° (range, 0-5°). All 8 patients had medial closed-wedge high tibial osteotomy. Fixation was achieved with two staples. In one case, a component of external rotation was added. All TKRs were implanted without cement; 6 had fixation pegs, and 2 had short stems. Mean follow-up was 46 ± 24 months (range, 20-57 months).

Postoperative complications included: deep venous thrombosis (DVT) (1), beginning of failure of the fixation construct (1) which required immobilization in a resin splint for 6 weeks, and nonunion (1) which required surgical revision with bonegrafting at 6 months. Arthrolysis was performed in 1 case at removal of the fixation devices, which provided an increase in flexion from 80° to 110°.

Mean time to union was 5 months ± 4 (range, 4-13 months).

Mean HKA angle was 179 ± 2° (range, 175-181°); mean decrease in HKA angle between surgery and follow-up was 3 ± 3°.

Good results were achieved with an IKS knee score of 83 ± 9 points (range, 66-96 points) and an IKS fonction score of 72 ± 23 points (range, 25-100 points). Total IKS score increased by 79 ± 21 points on a 200-point scale. HSS score was 90 ± 5 points (range, 85-97 points) with an increase of 42 ± 8 points (range, 34-50 points). Flexion was 115° ± 10° (range, 90-130°).

Mean radiological anterior drawer was 6 ± 2mm (range, 4-8mm).

Mean radiological posterior drawer was 7 ± 4mm (range, 0-10mm).

What should be performed first: total knee arthroplasty or osteotomy?

As far as we are concerned, we think that TKA provides adequate soft tissue balance, stability of the prosthetic joint, and correct realignment of the leg. Performing the osteotomy prior to implanting the prosthesis would have the advantage of allowing the use of the dedicated instruments and cutting guides both on the tibia and the femur, thus eliminating a technical issue. On the other hand, this would mean anticipating the amount of correction necessary, whereas the correction provided by the prosthesis and the soft tissue balance are still unknown parameters.

Where should the osteotomy be performed?

Obviously, the osteotomy should be performed where the deformity is the greatest. Wolff (60) showed that the closer the osteotomy is from the apex of the deformity, the milder the correction; this could be a strong argument to perform the osteotomy at the apex of the deformity. However, in cases of diaphyseal malunion, two separate approaches would be necessary: one for the osteotomy, and another one for the prosthesis. Furthermore, it is a known fact that diaphyseal osteotomies take more time to unite than metaphyseal osteotomies. Therefore, the osteotomy must be performed in a well vascularized cancellous bone segment to promote healing, but far enough from the prosthesis to allow insertion of fixation devices. Based on this, we have selected to perform our osteotomies in the metaphyseal region, proximal to the femoral condyles or proximal to the tibial tuberosity (or even at the tibial tuberosity if it has been elevated).

Design of the tibial component

Many of the current designs have more or less long stems, others (particularly earlier designs) have pegs.

As previously mentioned, with pegged or short stem components, the osteotomy can be performed with the prosthesis *in situ*. Stem components make staple or plate fixation somewhat more difficult to perform; however, stems may assist in stabilizing osteotomies, especially long stems. Inserting a central stem into a deformed bone may be problematic, due to a possible anatomic mismatch between the center of the medullary canal and the center of the proximal tibia. In sequelae of overcorrected osteotomy, inserting the prosthesis first may result in cortical violation (Neyret *et al.* (44)).

In such cases, it is advisable to perform the osteotomy with the knee extended, using a spacer block to maintain soft-tissue tension, or with the trial components *in situ*, and take care to check the correction achieved, under fluoroscopy. Then, the final components can be inserted; fixation of the osteotomy is the last step.

In most cases, the realignment osteotomy brings the stem back into correct position. Some authors think that the stem is, indeed, effective in stabilizing the osteotomy. But only a very long stem can have this beneficial effect, and the axis of the stem is seldom aligned with that of the tibial shaft, unless under a combination of favourable circumstances not likely to be replicated. Uchinou (56) used this method to correct a severely overcorrected high tibial osteotomy (40° valgus), and we also used it in two knees. The use of offset stems has been proposed to address this technical issue.

What type of osteotomy should be performed?

In our series, open-wedge osteotomies combined with autografts united more rapidly and, more importantly, were much more stable. Actually, it is the method of choice for femoral osteotomies, particularly when there is shortening. However, we favour medial closed-wedge osteotomy in valgus deformity secondary to valgus tibial osteotomy, because open-wedge osteotomy would carry an excessive risk of peroneal nerve palsy.

What are the best fixation methods?

For tibial osteotomies, the ideal fixation method is staples: small size device, easy to insert, provides adequate stability during healing.

As we have seen, locking the osteotomy site with a long stem component could be a good solution to improve the stability of the construct, but we now think that it actually generates additional technical problems. Fixation of a femoral osteotomy is always challenging. The difficulty lies in the fact that a satisfactory trade-off must be found between the necessity to perform the osteotomy not too proximally to allow for proper healing, and the need to insert at least two screws for placement of a screw plate below the osteotomy in order to stabilize the construct.

Indications for combined osteotomy plus TKA

This treatment method which associates osteotomy and TKA is reserved for those rare cases where a major extra-articular deformity is combined with severe osteoarthritis. This indication is exceptional: during the period when

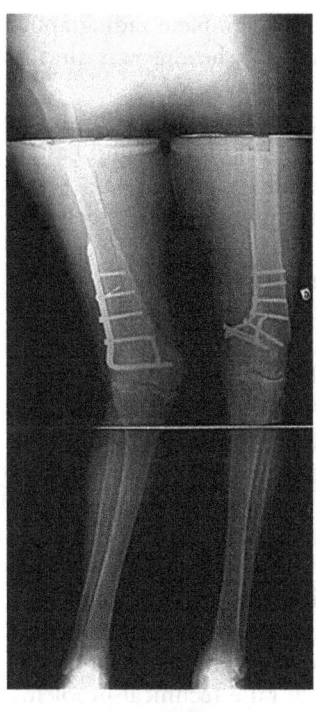

Fig. 9. – Femoral valgus malunion on the right side and varus malunion on the left side: a typical indication for TKR + supracondylar osteotomy.

these 19 procedures were performed, 985 non-constrained prostheses were implanted and 623 osteotomies were performed.

Main indications included sequelae of tibial or femoral osteotomy (fig. 9), post-traumatic malunion, and congenital deformity.

Preoperative planning may include Wolff's experimental calculations (60) as well as measurements taken from stress views (forced valgus and varus). The overall deformity results from a combination of wear, convex-side laxity, and extra-articular bone deformity. Laxity and wear are standard parameters in every preoperative planning for total knee replacement. Additionally, one must determine whether the bone deformity can be corrected by a prosthesis, and what size of tibial insert will best fit the joint space after the release procedures have been performed. This will allow identification of the worst cases in which, according to us, it is preferable to combine TKA and osteotomy rather than to try and correct everything with the prosthesis alone, due to poor stability and considering all the drawbacks previously mentioned.

Based on the degree of the extra-articular deformity in our series (mean valgus deviation of 11.5°, and mean varus deviation of 14.6°), it is easy to determine the threshold values that have been used to place our indications: below these threshold values, the deformity was managed with a cruciate-retaining prosthesis and soft tissue balancing. Indications will be fine-tuned later on, when a larger number of cases is available.

Discussion

The joint line level could be maintained in all the knees, thanks to retention of the PCL. For the same reason, position of the patella remained almost unchanged, which greatly facilitated restoration of flexion.

In our series, mean operation time was 135 minutes versus 152 minutes in a series of prostheses implanted by Krackow in knees with severe valgus deformities (31). In his series, mean blood loss was 1,386mL versus 1,091mL in our own series. It can be concluded that the combined osteotomy did not adversely affect the operation time and blood loss.

In our series, the healing process was quite slow. It is one of the reasons why some authors like Cameron (9) select to perform a two-stage procedure with osteotomy as the first stage. However, it should be pointed out that what we considered as a sound union was the evidence of complete radiographic healing, which explains this long healing time. Actually, healing was already achieved and the patients had resumed weight bearing.

Our results are consistent with those reported in the literature by Insall (23), Ranawat (47), Goodfellow (19), Cloutier (11), Dejour (12), and Laskin (32). Achieving 111° flexion is, indeed, a good result.

There are very few publications regarding implantations of TKRs for treatment of severe genu valgum.

Krackow's series (31) consisted of cruciate-retaining prostheses with a mean follow-up of 54 months. He defined three types of genu valgum: Type I and Type II were structural valgus deformities with more or less significant wear (LCL strech-out in Type II); Type III was the result of an overcorrected valgus proximal tibial osteotomy. His series consisted essentially of Type I and Type II deformities, whereas our series included eight Type III, and yet, our results were as good as his and even better as regards flexion. Furthermore, Krackow (31) had three peroneal nerve palsies; we never had this complication. In Stern's series (52) which consisted of posterior stabilized or constrained prostheses with 4.5-year follow-up, the inclusion criterion was anatomic valgus of more than 10°; 19 patients had an anatomic valgus greater than 25°. Making a comparison is very difficult because angular deviation, preoperative laxity, or the etiology of valgus deformity are often unknown; furthermore, this series includes very different cases which raise technical problems of varying complexity. As a matter of fact, posterior stabilized or hinge prostheses were implanted in cases where it seemed just impossible to balance the knee, and 3% of peroneal nerve palsy have been reported. Miyasaka's series (42) consisted of 60 total knee prostheses implanted in valgus knees (anatomic valgus superior to 10°) with a mean follow-up of 14 years. Results were rated as good, but surgical revisions had been excluded from the study as well as 10 constrained prostheses (total condylar III). Aglietti (1) with 51 TKRs implanted in knees with a preoperative anatomic valgus of 19.5°, and Lootwoet (39) in his series of knees with a mean HKA angle of 196°, achieved very good results (table II). The results of our small series of severe valgus knees are excellent and yet, our cases were much more challenging than those in the published series.

Comparison with the literature as regards sequelae of overcorrected osteotomy is most interesting. Many authors set out to analyse the results of total knee replacement after failed valgus tibial osteotomy. Most of these results are presented in table III. Very often, they were not as good as those of primary

Table II – Results reported in the literature regarding TKRs in valgus knees.

	IKS knee score	HSS score	Flexion
Krackow (1991)	87.6		103°
Stern (1991)		86	
Miyasaka (1997)	88.7		101°
Aglietti (1997)	91% excellent & good		
Lootvoet (1997)	93.6		
Lerat	89.5	89.9	115°

Table III – Results of TKA after failed osteotomy (review of the literature).

	Excellent & good	IKSK score	HSS score	Flexion
Staheli (1987)	89%			
Gill (1995)		87.3		109°
Toksvig-Larsen (1998)			85	104°
Amendola (1989)	88%		86	101°
Katz (1997)	81%			95°
Neyret (1992)			77	98°
Mont (1994)	64%			
Krackow (1990)	100%			95°
Lerat TKR + osteotomy	80%	77.8	83.5	114°

total knee replacements. Staehli (51), Gill (17), and Toksvig–Larsen (55) in their respective series, obtained similar results to those achieved in a comparative series of primary knees. Amendola (2) studied 42 TKAs performed for sequelae of osteotomy; the HSS score was identical to that in the control group, but the study group had 14° less flexion than the control group. In contrast, in several other studies (Katz (25), Windsor (59), Neyret (44), Laskin (33), Mont (43), and Cameron (9)), results were not as good as those of primary knees.

Katz (25) studied 21 TKRs: there were flexion contractures, and only 81% of good/excellent results versus 100% in the control group. Windsor (59) compared TKAs performed for sequelae of osteotomy, with revision total knee arthroplasties and not with primary knee arthroplasties. Laskin (33) analysed the results of a series in which a Coonse-Adams approach was used 23 times, together with a quadricepsplasty to improve exposure. Excluding failures and complications, the results were still lower than in primary total knee arthroplasties, with lesser range of motion. Cameron (9) reported a 27% incidence of complications at less than 6-year follow-up. The functional and anatomical results achieved in our series were consistent with those reported in the literature, but flexion was better. The few series in which results are as good as those obtained with primary knees do not include any severe valgus knees. Unfortunately, none of these studies analysed the results relative to the degree of preoperative deformity. In Gill's series (17), 10% of the patients had a valgus deformity greater than 10°, but the results have been analysed with no specific focus on this subgroup. Mont (43) emphasized some aggravating factors, such as history of algodystrophy and number of pevious operations, and industrial accidents, but he did not study the influence of preoperative deformity or nature of tibial malunion. Neyret (44) and Lerat (37) analysed the technical difficulties according to the type of malunion, but the results have not been specifically analysed in each group. Krackow (30) reported the results of 5 TKRs implanted in patients with failed osteotomy, 25° of valgus deformity, and medial ligament laxity. He actually used a special technique for tightening the posteromedial structures.

Mean operation time in our TKAs combined with osteotomies was similar to that in Krackow's series (30), except when he used his special tightening technique which increased the operation time by as much as 50 to 100%.

Therefore, our series of TKAs performed for sequelae of tibial osteotomy includes cases that are considered by all other authors as the most technically challenging. And yet, postoperatively, mean flexion was better than, and functional scores similar to those reported in large published series which do not differentiate the types of sequelae of osteotomy (major or minor). Loss of correction (2.4°) that we have noted at the osteotomy should be reduced in future, using a more efficient fixation system, and allowing a more gradual resumption of weight bearing.

Conclusion

In the majority of cases, treatment of osteoarthritis in valgus knees is not technically more challenging than in varus knees, and yields similar results.

Ligament balancing aims at maintaining the joint space in the healthy medial compartment. Realignment of the knee joint is achieved through standardized lateral soft tissue release procedures, allowing restoration of both the Q-angle and the patellofemoral joint balance. Up to 20° of deformity, a non-constrained cruciate-retaining prosthesis may be used.

Deformities greater than 20° are technically much more challenging, particularly when combined with extra-articular bone deformities (after over-corrected osteotomy or post-traumatic malunion).

The use of posterior stabilized implants with excision of cruciate ligaments and extensive concave-side release may correct severe deformities, as has been demonstrated in the literature. However, this suffers from numerous drawbacks, the major ones being: elevation of the joint line due to a thick tibial insert, lowering of the patella, increased tension on the extensor mechanism and neurovascular structures, and lengthening of the lower limb.

Alternatively, in these special cases, one may select to use a non-constrained prosthesis combined with an osteotomy (to correct bone deformity). We think it preferable to perform TKA and osteotomy at the same time rather than in two stages. Therefore, osteotomies did not adversely affect the results of TKAs which are actually better than those reported in the literature for similar indications.

References

1. Aglietti P , Buzzi R, Giron F et al. (1996) The Install-Burstein posterior stabilized total knee replacement in the valgus knee. The American Journal of Knee Surgery 9: 8-12
2. Amendola A, Rorabeck Ch, Bourne RB et al. (1989) Total knee arthroplasty following high tibial osteotomie for osteoarthridtis. Arthroplasty 4: 511-7
3. Arima J, Whiteside LA, Martin JW et al. (1998) Effect of partial release of the posterior cruciate ligament in TKA. Clin Orthop 353: 194-202
4. Arima J, Whiteside LA, Mccarthy DS et al. (1995) Femoral rotational alignment, based on the anterior posterior axis, in total knee arthroplasty in a valgus knee. A technical note. J Bone Joint Surg 77-A: 1331-4

5. Berger RA, Rubash HE, Seel MJ et al. (1993) Determining the rotational alignment of the femoral component in total knee arthroplasty using the epicondylar axis. Clin Orthop 286: 40-7

6. Boisrenoult P, Scemama P, Fallet L et al. (2001) La torsion épiphysaire distale du fémur dans le genou arthrosique. Étude tomodensitométrique de 75 genoux avec arthrose médiale. Rev Chir Orthop 87: 469-76.

7. Buechel FF (1990) A sequential three-step lateral release for correcting fixed valgus knee deformities during total knee arthroplasty. Clin Orthop 260: 170-5

8. Burdin P (1996) Équilibre ligamentaire du genou et prothèse du genou. Annales Orthop Ouest 28: 19-20

9. Cameron HU, Park US (1996) Total knee replacement following high tibial osteotomy and unicompartmental knee. Orthop Research 19: 807-8

10. Churghill DL, Incavo SJ, Johnson CC et al. (1998) The trans-epicondylar axis approximates the optimal flexion axis of the knee. Clin Orthop 356: 111-8

11. Cloutier JM (1983) Results of total knee arthroplasty with a non-constrained prothesis. J Bone Joint Surg 65-A: 906-19

12. Dejour H, Neyret P (1991) Les Gonarthroses. 7 Journées Lyonnaises de Chirurgie du Genou, Lyon, Monographie. p.412

13. Delfico AJ, Tria AJ (1996) Surgical techniques and the management of fixed deformities in total knee arthroplasty. The American Journal of Knee Surgery 9: 82-90

14. Elias SG, Freeman Mar, Gokcay EI (1998) A correlative study of the geometry and anatomy of the distal femur. Clin Orthop. 260: 88-103

15. Faris PM (1994) Soft tissue balancing and total knee arthroplasty. In Fu FH, Harner CD, Vince KG Knee surgery, William & Wilkins eds, Baltimore II, 73: 1385-89

16. Freeman MAR, Sulco T, Todd RC (1977) Replacement of the severely damaged arthritic knee by the ICLH (Freeman-Swanson) arthroplasty. J Bone Joint Surg 59 B: 64

17. Gill T, Schemitsch EH, Brick GW et al. (1995) Revision total knee arthroplasty after failed unicompartment arthroplasty or high tibial osteotomy. Clin Orthop 321: 10-18

18. Godenèche A (1998) Prothèses totales du genou et ostéotomies dans le même temps opératoire pour gonarthrose avec déviations axiales majeures (à propos de 11 cas). Thèse Médecine, Lyon

19. Goodfellow JW, O'Connor J (1986) Clinical results of the Oxford knee surface arthroplasty of the tibio-femoral joint with a meniscal bearing prosthesis. Clin Orthop 42: 205-21

20. Healy WL, Iorio R, Lemods DW (1998) Medial reconstruction during total knee arthroplasty for severe valgus deformity. Clin Orthop 356: 161-9

21. Hungerford DS, Lennox DW (1984) Fixed valgus deformity. In: Hungerford DS, Krackow KA and Kenna RV (eds). Total Knee Arthroplasty – A Comprehensive Approach. Baltimore, Williams & Wilkins p. 167-78

22. Hungerford DS, Insall JN (1997) Extra-articular deformity in TKA. 14th Annual Current Concepts in Joint Replacement. Cleveland, Session XVII. Paper 86 and 87

23. Insall JN (1984) Surgery of the knee. New York, Churchill Livingstone: 587-696

24. Insall JN, Scott WN, Keblish PA et al. (1994) Total knee arthroplasty exposures and soft tissue balancing. In: Insall JN, Scott WN (eds) Video Book of Knee Surgery. Philadelphia: JB Lippincott

25. Katz MM, Hungerford DS, Krackow KA et al. (1997) Results of total knee arthroplasty after failed proximal tibial osteotomy for osteoarthritis. J Bone Joint Surg 69-A: 225-32

26. Karachalios T, Sarangi PP, Newman JH (1994) Severe varus and valgus deformities treated by total knee arthroplasty. J Bone Joint Surg 76-B: 938-42

27. Keblish PA (1991) The lateral approach to the valgus knee: Surgical technique and analysis of 53 cases with over two-year follow-up evaluation. Clin Orthop 271: 52-62

28. Keblish PA (1995) Valgus deformity in TKR. The lateral retinacular approach. Orthop Trans: 9-28

29. Krackow KA (1984) Management of fixed deformity at total joint arthroplasty. In: Hungerford DS, Krackow KA, Kenna B (eds) Total knee arthroplasty: Baltimore, Aspen. 163-78

30. Krackow KA, Holtgrewe JL (1990) Experience with a new technique for managing seve-rely overcorrected valgus high tibial osteotomy at total knee arthroplasty. Clin Orthop 258: 213-4

31. Krackow KA, Jones MM, Teeny SM *et al.* (1991) Primary total knee arthroplasty in patients with fixed valgus deformity. Clin Orthop 273: 9-18

32. Laskin RS (ed) (1991) Total Knee Replacement. London, UK: Springer-Verlag: 41-74

33. Laskin RS (1993) Total knee replacement after high tibial osteotomy. In American Academy of Orthopaedic Surgeon 60th Annual Meeting, San Francisco: 18-23

34. Laskin RS (1995) Flexion space configuration in TKA. J Arthroplasty 10: 657-60

35. Lecuire F, Jaffar-Bandjee Z (1994) Luxation postérieure du tibia sur prothèse totale du genou: à propos de 6 cas. Rev Chir Orthop 80: 525-31

36. Lerat JL, Moyen B, Renouard D *et al.* (1990) Les échecs des ostéotomies de valgisation pour arthrose du genou, réopérés par prothèse avec conservation des deux ligaments croisés. SOFCOT 66 réunion annuelle: Symposium sur les échecs des ostéotomies tibiales: 115-8

37. Lerat JL (2000) Les ostéotomies dans la gonarthrose. Cahiers d'Enseignement de la SOFCOT Paris, Ed Elsevier: 165-201

38. Lerat JL, Godenèche A, Moyen B *et al.* (2001) Total knee arthroplasty associated with osteotomy for gonarthrosis with major extra-articular deformity (19 knees). ISAKOS congress, Montreux, Switzerland

39. Lootvoet L, Blouard E, Himmer O *et al.* (1997) Prohèse totale du genou sur grand genu valgum. Revue rétrospective de 90 genoux opérés par abord antéro-externe. Acta Orthopaedica Belgica 63, 4: 278-86

40. Mantas JP, Bloebaum RD, Skedos JG *et al.* (1992) Implication of reference axes used for rotational alignment of the femoral component in primary and revision knee arthroplasty. J Arthroplasty 7: 531-5

41. Merritt P, Conaty JP Dorr LD (1987) Effect of soft tissue release on results of total knee replacement. In: Rand JA and Dorr LD Proceedings of the Knee Society Rock Ville, Aspen Publishers 25-9

42. Miyasaka KC, Ranawat CS, Mullaji A (1997) Total knee arthroplasty in the valgus knee: intermediate term results and technique for ligament balancing. J Arthroplasty 12 (2): 220

43. Mont MA, Antonaides S, Krackow KA *et al.* (1994) Total knee arthroplasty after failed high tibial osteotomy: a comparaison with a matched group. Clin Orthop 299: 125-30

44. Neyret P, Dejour H, Deroche P *et al.* (1992) Prothèse totale du genou après ostéotomie tibiale de valgisation. Problèmes techniques. Rev Chir Orthop 78: 438-48

45. Pagnano MW, Hanssen AD, Lewallen DG *et al.* (1998) Flexion instability after primary posterior cruciate retaining total knee arthroplasty. Clin Orthop 356: 39-46

46. Poilvache PL, Insall JN, Scuderi GR *et al.* (1996) Rotational landmarks and sizing of the distal femur in total knee arthroplasty. Clin Orthop 331: 35-46

47. Ranawat CS, Rose HA, Rich DS (1984) Total condylar knee arthroplasty for valgus and combined valgus flexion deformity of the knee. In: Murray JA (Ed.) Intructional Course Lectures. St Louis, CV Masby: 412-6

48. Ritter MA, Faris PM, Keating EM (1988) Posterior cruciate ligament balancing during total knee arthroplasty. J Arthroplasty 3 (4): 323

49. Shoemaker SC, Markolf KL, Finerman GA (1982) *In vitro* stability of the implanted total condylar prosthesis. Effects of joint load and of sectioning the posterior cruciate ligament. J Bone Joint Surg 64-A: 1201-13

50. Scott WN (1994) The knee. St Louis: CV Mosby, Vol II

51. Staeheli JW, Cass JR, Morrey BF (1987) Condylar total knee arthroplasty after failed proximal tibial osteotomy. J Bone Joint Surg 69-A: 28-31

52. Stern SH, Moeckel BH, Insall JN (1991) Total knee arthroplasty in valgus knees. Clin Orthop 273: 5-8

53. Sthiel JB, Abbott BD (1995) Morphology of the transepicondylar axes and its application in primary and revision total knee arthroplasty. J Arthroplasty 10: 785-9

54. Teeny S, Krackow KA, Hungerford DS *et al.* (1991) Primary total knee arthroplasty in patients with severe varus deformity. Clin Orthop 273: 19-3

55. Toksvig-Larsen S, Magyar G, Onsten I *et al.* (1998) Fixation of the tibial component of total knee arthroplasty after high tibial osteotomy. A matched radiostereometric stydy. J Bone Joint Surg 80-B: 295-7
56. Uchinou S, Yano H, Shinizu K (1996) Case reports. A severly overcorrected high tibial osteotomy. Revision by osteotomy and a long stem component. Acta Orthop Scand 67(2): 193-4
57. Whiteside LA (1993) Correction of ligament and bone defects in total arthroplasty of the severely valgus knee. Clin Orthop 288: 234-45
58. Whiteside LA, Arima J (1995) The anteroposterior axes for femoral alignment in valgus total knee arthroplasty. Clin Orthop 321: 168-72
59. Windsor RE, Insall JN, Vince KG (1988) Technical considerations of total knee arthroplasty after proximal tibial osteotomy. J Bone Joint Surg 70-A: 547
60. Wolff AMN, Hungerford DS (1990) The effect of extra-articular varus and valgus deformity on total knee arthroplasty. Clin Orthop 271: 35-51
61. Yoshii I, Whiteside LA., White SE *et al.* (1991) Influence of prosthetic joint line position on knee kinematics patellar position. J Arthroplasty 6: 169

Total knee arthroplasty for the stiff knee

J.N. Argenson, H. Vinel, J.M. Aubaniac

Definition

A stiff knee can be defined as a knee with less than 50° range of motion, but there is a wide variation in presentation (1, 9).

An ankylosed knee can be defined as a knee with a fixed preoperative range of motion of 0° (2), resulting from the spontaneous evolution of various pathological knee conditions.

An arthrodesed knee is a knee with fixed preoperative range of motion of 0°, resulting from previous intentional surgical fusion of the knee.

Etiology

The most common causes are osteoarthritis and rheumatoid arthritis.

Ankylosis may also result from hemophilic arthropathy or psoriatic arthritis.

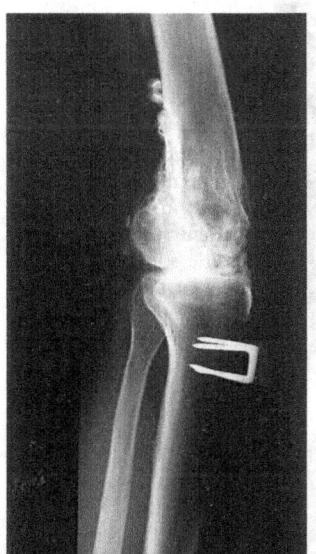

Previous infection of the knee or previous injury to the knee are also involved.

Some knee arthrodesis have been indicated for neuromuscular disorder or severe pain in young adults.

Previous surgery of the knee (fig. 1) is frequently found as a source of stiffness including: arthrotomy, osteotomy, or previously failed knee arthroplasty usually for infection (3, 11).

Indications

The underlying cause of stiffness of the knee must be carefully evaluated when considering the risks and benefits of the procedure, which

Fig. 1 – Lateral view of an ankylosed knee following recurrent infection in a multi-operated 46-year old patient.

is always difficult and a potential source of complications. Although there is always difficulty in determining which complications are related directly to an ankylosed or stiff knee, and which are related to the patient's underlying disease, some conditions should discourage the surgeon to perform the arthroplasty (7). This includes: reflex sympathetic dystrophy, poor neuromuscular conditions, inedequate bone quality, low-grade sepsis and painless successfully arthrodesed knee. It should be stated at this point that cases of primary knee fusion have not been found to present the same degree of long-term complications of back pain that are associated with successful hip fusion (3, 11). When all these contraindications are eliminated, total knee arthroplasty for a stiff or ankylosed knee may be considered to relief pain, improve range of motion and provide better walking and day-living ability.

Preoperative evaluation

The clinical evaluation must assess the preoperative range of motion, the knee may be ankylosed in extension or with a flexion contracture. Any previous scar incision must be recorded and located as well as the state of the extensor mechanism like fibrosis of the quadriceps muscle and shortening or thightness of the collateral ligaments.

The radiographic evaluation should include full weight bearing view of the two limbs (fig. 2) to assess mechanical axis and identify intra-or extra-articular deformity, fibrosis or bony blocks. The planing also include anteroposterior, lateral and when possible patellofemoral views. Stress X-rays, whenever

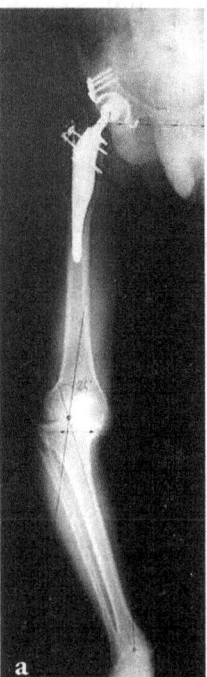
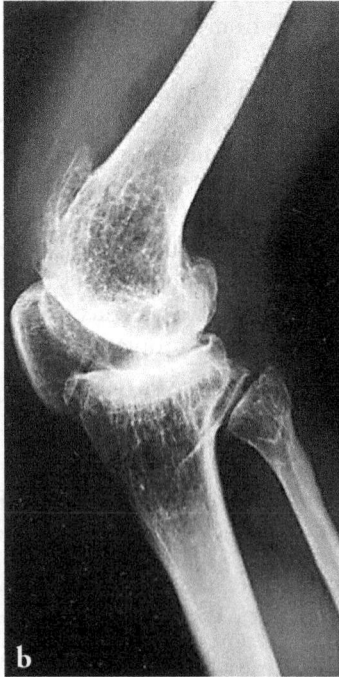

Fig. 2 – Full weight bearing view of the limbs (fig. 2a) showing an important varus deformity (24°) in a 66-year-old patient with an ostearthritic stiff knee, showed on a lateral view (fig. 2b), under a previous total hip arthroplasty following hip fusion.

possible, may be useful in case of asymetrical retractions and computed tomography may help to locate new bone formation. Finally any hardware present about the knee must be identified to obtain appropriate instrumentation for removal.

The choice of the prosthesis which need to be used rely on the surgeon options, but most of the time on the state of the ligaments. With severe deformity, the posterior cruciate ligament is usually abnormal and the prosthesis must substitute for it (9). It is also generally agreed that the soft-tissue release necessary to gain flexion for stiff knees require the sacrifice of both cruciate ligaments and the use of a posterior stabilized prosthesis (1, 2). Additionally because the flexion gap is quite often larger than the extension gap, a posterior stabilized prosthesis is also helpful to solve the discrepancy (1). After previous knee surgery and specially knee fusion or when extensive soft-tissue releases are required, the potential inadequacy of the collateral ligament structures may need the use of a more constrained prosthesis.

Surgical technique

The skin incision should be straight midline, incorporating as much as possible old incisions.

A medial parapatellar arthrotomy is then perfomed starting superiorily between the rectus and vastus medialis and finishing inferiorly 1cm medial to the tibial tuberosity. The medial aspect of the proximal tibia is released at this time and the subperiosteal dissection is extended posteriorly and distally in varus knees. Any adhesions between the quadriceps and the femur on either side of the patella are released and the lateral retinacular release is performed early in the procedure.

At that time of the procedure the main surgical technical difficulty is the eversion of the patella, with a high risk of avulsion of the patellar tendon. An external rotation of the tibia is helpful to take tension off the patellar tendon, as well as a release of the patellofemoral ligament and an inside/out or preferentially outside/in lateral retinacular release. Scar tissue at the joint line are excised, as well as cruciate ligaments and menisci. If the knee is ankylosed, an osteotomy using a power saw is performed at the joint line or after careful identification of the fusion site. If the knee cannot be flexed more than 40° at that time, several procedures are possible.

A quadriceps release as proposed by Ranawat and Flynn (9), by a controlled Z-lengthening (fig. 3) can be done at the level of the rectus femoris and the vastus intermedius muscles, using six to eight small incisions. With each Z, the flexion of the knee increases in a controlled fashion until 80° is reached.

A modified V-Y quadricepsplasty (fig. 4) is the second option in which the triangular, distally based flap including the patella, is "turned down" anterolaterally (1, 4).

A tibial tubercle osteotomy is the third option (fig. 5 and 6), with two requirements: a long distal osteotomy and the preservation of the medial edge of the tubercle. The osteotomy can be fixed by screws or wires (8, 12).

The release is then continued laterally including the lateral capsular structures, the lateral collateral ligament, the iliotibial band and the popliteus in some valgus knees. In case of flexion contracture, a complete posterior capsule release or a capsulotomy may be required.

The rest of the operation is then continued in the usual manner with tibial and femoral cuts. The flexion/extension gaps are checked using spacer blocks with the flexion gap, usually the greater of the two. A posterior stabilized insert will allow in many cases appropriate stability (fig. 7).

The closure of the arthrotomy is realized, after draining, at 15° of flexion to avoid excessive tension.

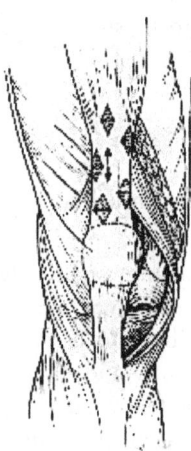

Fig. 3 – Anterior view of Z-lengthening, according to Ranawat and Flynn.

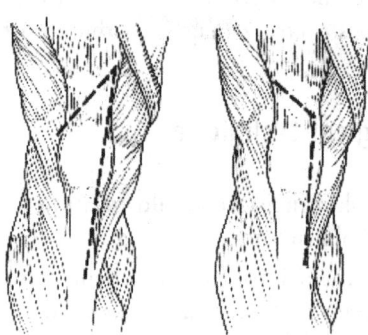

Fig. 4 – The inverted V-Y quadricepsplasty, with turndown of patellar mechanism, as modified by Insall.

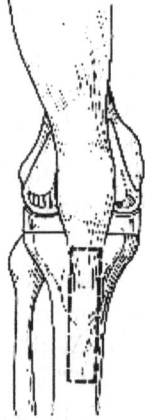

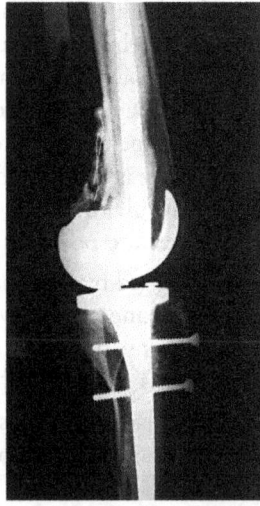

Fig. 6 – Lateral view of a tibial tubercle osteotomy (same patient as in fig. 1).

Fig. 5 – The tibial tubercle osteotomy, from Nordin.

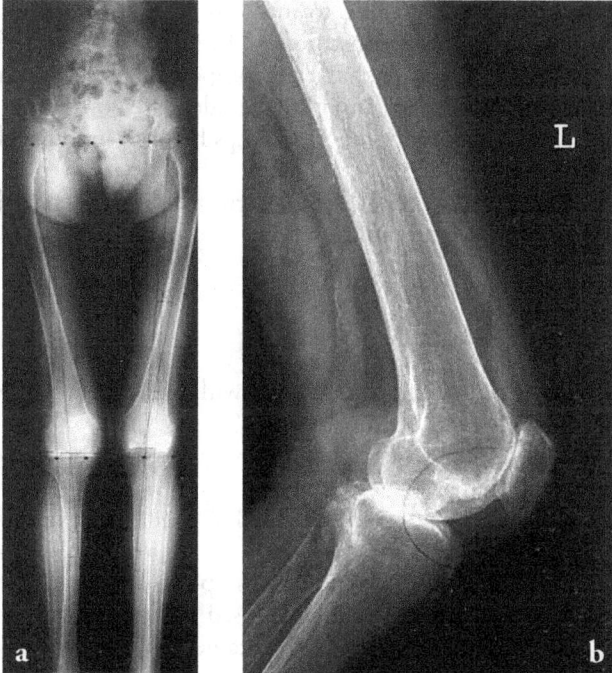

Fig. 7 – Anteroposterior (fig. 7a) and lateral view (fig. 7b) of a rheumatoïd stiff knee with valgus deformity and flexion contracture (15°) in a 74-year-old woman.

Postoperative management

The motion should be started as early as possible and epidural anesthesia may be useful permitting to be maintained postoperatively on continuous infusion.

A continuous passive motion machine can be set initially to 30° and increased as tolerated by about 10° per day (9).

A vigorous manual therapy protocol realized two hours daily by a physical therapist consisting in knee flexion exercices and straight leg raises has proven to increase significantly postoperative range of motion in previously ankylosed joints (6).

In case of preoperative flexion contracture the patient is kept in a knee immobilizer for night. In case of quadricepsplasty the range of motion exercices may be delayed.

Complications

Avulsion of the patellar tendon or tibial tubercle - subperiosteal mobilization, external rotation of the tibia, and one of the extensor mechanism: "eversion techniques" are useful to avoid this complication.

– Recurrent joint stiffness: this may require manipulation under anesthesia at 4 or 6 weeks, or surgical arthrolysis.

– Delayed wound healing: need to interrupt motion exercices and sometimes may require a flap for reconstruction. In knees with multiple incisions the use of soft-tissue expansion has been proposed before the knee arthroplasty. The skin expanders help to provide adequate soft-tissue for wound closure and the expander under the quadriceps helps to mobilise the extensor mechanism (5).

– Deep infection: may require long-term antibiotics, staged revisions, arthrodesis or above knee amputation.

Results

In 1983, Mullen (6) obtained in 13 knees with a preoperative flexion from 0° to 90°, a range of motion from 0° to 95°.

In 1987, Bradley et al. (2) obtained an average arc of motion of 64° in 9 previously ankylosed knees.

In 1988, Holden and Jackson (3) obtained 0° to 90° of flexion in 2 patients with previous arthrodesis.

In 1989, Aglietti et al. (1) obtained a postoperative average arc of motion of 68°, in 20 stiff knees, 6 of which ankylosed in flexion.

In 1990, Schurman and Wilde (10) obtained in 3 ankylosed knees respectively 65°, 85° and 115° of maximum postoperative flexion.

In 1996, Naranja et al. (7) retrospectively reviewed a large multicentric series of 35 knees without any preoperative knee motion. The range of motion after a mean follow-up of 90 months averaged 7° lack of extension and 62° flexion.

Discussion

All the reports in the literature indicate that the results are routinely lower than those obtained with routine primary total knee replacement. The morbidity is high, specially for previously ankylosed or arthrodesed knees, with a 57% overall complication rate in the larger group reported by Naranja et al. (7).

However, in stiff knees, a significant improvement in range of motion can be observed, due to correction of both flexion and quadriceps contractures (1). The surgeon must explain to patients with less than 50° of flexion before the arthroplasty, that a 80° of motion achieved at 8 to 10 months postoperatively should be considered as a successful outcome (9).

In ankylosed knees, the postoperative flexion is usually significantly lower than the one obtained for stiff knee in which a motion from 0° to 50° was still present before the arthroplasty.

In previously surgically arthrodesed knees, despite anecdotal successful reports (3, 5) our own experience with only one success without complications in five knees lead us to believe, like others (1, 7), that the risks and benefits of the procedure should be carefully considered before any indication of total knee arthroplasty in this situation.

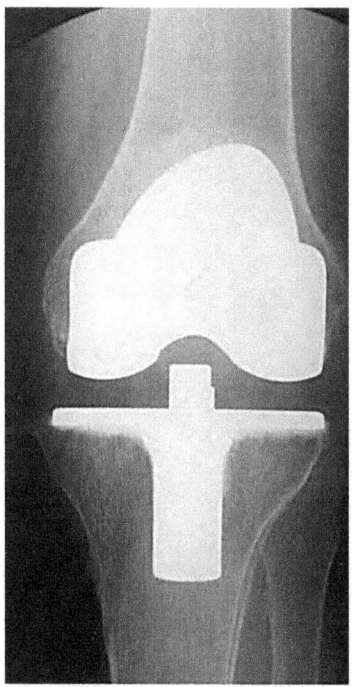
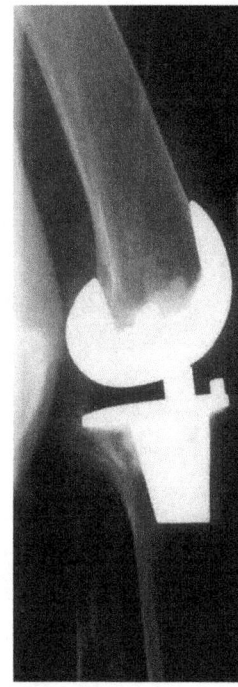

Fig. 8 – Postoperative anteroposterior (fig. 8a) and lateral view (fig. 8b) of the same patient (as in fig. 7) achieving 115° of knee flexion six months after posterior stabilized mobile knee arthroplasty.

a.   b.

References

1. Aglietti P, Windsor RE, Buzzi R *et al.* (1989) Arthroplasty for the stiff or ankylosed knee. J Arthroplasty 4: 1-5
2. Bradley GW, Freeman MAR, Albredktsson BEJ (1987) Total prosthetic replacement of ankylosed knees. J Arthroplasty 2: 179-83
3. Holden DL, Jackson DW (1988) Considerations in total knee arthroplasty following previous knee fusion. Clin Orthop 227: 223-8
4. Insall JN (1984) Surgical approaches to the knee. In: Insall JN (ed) Surgery of the knee. Churchill Livingstone, New York, p. 47
5. Mahomed N, Mc Kee N, Solomon P *et al.* (1994) Soft tissue expansion before total knee arthroplasty in arthrodesed joints. J Bone Joint Surg 76-B: 88-90
6. Mullen JO (1983) Range of motion following total knee arthroplasty in ankylosed joints. Clin Orthop 179: 200-3
7. Naranja RJ, Lotke PA, Pagnano MW *et al.* (1996) Total knee arthroplasty in a previously ankylosed or arthrodesed knee. Clin Orthop 331: 234-7
8. Nordin JY (1996) Les prothèses totales de genou difficiles de première intention. In: Duparc J (ed) Cahiers d'enseignement de la SOFCOT. Expansion Scientifique française, Paris, p. 47
9. Ranawat CS, Flynn WF (1995) The stiff knee. In: Lotke PA (ed) Knee Arthroplasty. Raven Press, New York, p. 141
10. Schurman J, Wilde A (1990) Total knee replacement after spontaneous osseous ankylosis. J Bone Joint Surg 72-A: 455-9
11. Stulberg SD (1982) Arthrodesis in failed total knee replacements. Orthop Clin North Am 13: 213-7
12. Whiteside L, Ohl M (1990) Tibial tubercle osteotomy for exposure of the difficult total knee arthroplasty. Clin Orthop 260: 6-9

Total knee arthroplasty after tibial valgus osteotomy

F. Gougeon

Introduction

High tibial osteotomy (HTO) produces four major changes to the periarticular area which will interfere with total knee replacement: skin incision, medial or lateral approach which will affect the collateral ligaments or their insertions, bone resection or bone augmentation which will modify the geometry and/or strength of the tibial epiphysis, and at last, insertion of fixation devices. Modification of bony and ligamentous structures will be a source of technical problems during later total knee arthroplasty. As a matter of fact, performing a total knee replacement (TKR) after a high tibial osteotomy (HTO) is a double challenge in terms of: technical difficulties due to prior osteotomy, and quality of results. The question is whether valgus osteotomy may compromise the outcome of subsequent TKR.

Skin incisions

Skin incisions may be difficult to deal with, depending on their number and location. One must differentiate between vertical and horizontal skin incisions.

Vertical incisions

When vertical surgical incision scars are located close to the midline skin incision, it is advisable to use them or extend them, even if subfascial dissection is necessary to perform the desired arthrotomy. One can generally use prior anterolateral incisions which just need to be extended proximally, whereas medial incisions are usually more posterior and can seldom be used. As a rule, skin flaps with reversed pedicles in which the isthmus opens downwards are never used, and narrow flaps or parallel incisions are not recommended. As far as we are concerned, we use the most anterior incision, and dissect the superficial fascia to perform a medial parapatellar arthrotomy.

Horizontal incisions

Medial or lateral horizontal surgical incision scars are less problematic. They allow any recommended approach for the selected implant. A midline anterior incision intersects the horizontal scar at 90°, thus creating a broad superior pedicle flap with good viability.

Removal of fixation devices

Fixation devices (if still present) may be removed as the first stage of a two-stage procedure with a few weeks' delay between removal and TKR, or at the same time as TKR (1). The two-stage procedure has one major drawback: it implies two anesthesias, two surgeries, two hospital stays. On the other hand, one advantage is that a bacteriological sample can be taken from the first operative site (11), and only limited dissection is needed if the approaches are different. The second advantage is that a limited approach is subsequently required for TKA, and there is no risk of hematoma at the removal site. A two-stage procedure is mandatory when there is suspicion of bacterial contamination. It is advisable in the following cases: If two different approaches (one for the osteotomy, one for the prosthesis) are necessary; if a very extensive approach is required; if the fixation devices are very bulky or difficult removal is anticipated. In cases where small-size devices have been used, the removal procedure is straightforward, slightly extending the approach or making a counterincision, and it can be combined with TKA (1).

Evaluation of technical difficulties

The main intraoperative difficulties during surgical revision for failed osteotomy arise from bone deformity produced by prior osteotomy, and patent or potential ligament imbalance resulting from correction of malunion. Although these two elements cannot be dissociated, bony problems will be addressed first.

Malunions

In the coronal plane, three situations can be encountered:

- valgus malunion due to overcorrection;
- increased valgus angulation due to progressive wear of the lateral compartment;
- recurrence of the varus deformity due to progression of medial wear.

In the sagittal plane, and particularly if a lateral closing-wedge valgus osteotomy has been performed, the epiphysis may have been translated posteriorly due to the inferior-posterior direction of the oblique osteotomy. On the other

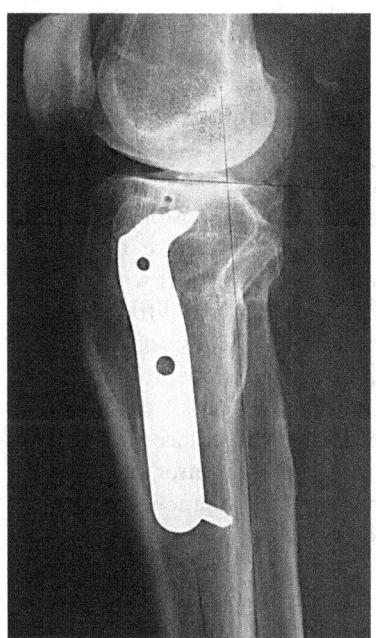

Fig. 1. – Increased tibial slope after tibial valgus osteotomy. Development of flexion contracture.

hand, a closing-wedge or opening-wedge osteotomy that is not symmetric anteriorly and posteriorly may result in flexion contracture or recurvatum (more rarely) (fig. 1).

In the horizontal plane, there may be a rotational malunion. This is commonly seen in closing-wedge osteotomy where the hinge is the medial cortex which is not in a true sagittal plane.

Evaluation of some of these deformities can be difficult.

Coronal plane deviation is quite easy to measure from a standing orthoroentgenogram in the absence of articular flexion contracture. Posterior displacement of the epiphysis is visible on a lateral view, although difficult to quantify.

Flexion contracture or recurvatum at the osteotomy site may be manifested by a clinical deformity of the knee or asymmetric range of motion (ROM). It can be assessed from a lateral view of the knee, but it cannot be quantified with accuracy because the proximal fragment is too small.

Evaluation of rotational malunion, although critical, is very difficult. It is due to the fact that anterior landmarks are altered. In particular, the anterior tibial tubercle cannot be used for rotational alignment of the tibial component. Severe anomalies can be detected, based on clinical analysis of the overall rotation of the tibia (foot axis with patella placed in the coronal plane), foot progression angle, range of external/internal rotation of the distal end of the lower extremity. A preoperative CT scan (provided that internal fixation devices have been removed) may help evaluate with accuracy this rotational disturbance.

Quantification of these anomalies allows the anticipation of intraoperative difficulties to restore correct alignment of the lower limb. The difficulty to achieve adequate correction depends on the severity of the deformity and its origin.

Axial deviation due to extra-articular malunion (resulting directly from the osteotomy) must be differentiated from axial deviation due to wear and intra-articular deformity within the ligamentous envelope.

Some extra-articular malunions cannot be corrected during TKA and require prior corrective osteotomy or combined TKA and osteotomy: either because the deformity is too severe, or because performing intra-articular correction of the deformity would produce an amount of laxity that could not be corrected by the type of prosthesis used.

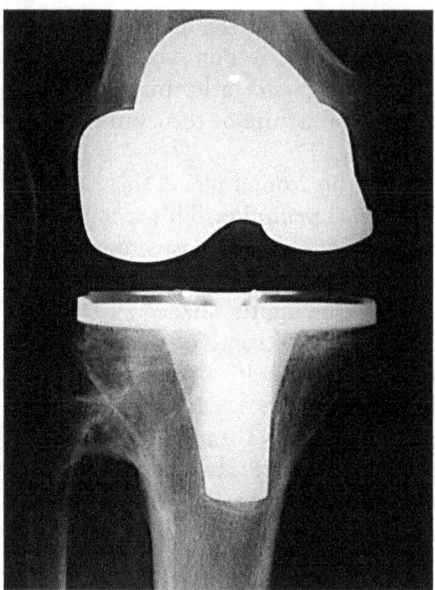

Fig. 2. – Impingement between tibial stem and medial cortex.

Rotational malunion cannot be corrected by a prosthesis. A fixed tibial bearing does not provide correction of the rotation induced by lateral closing-wedge osteotomy. As a matter of fact, if the metal tray is properly positioned on the resected tibial surface to achieve good cortical support without overhang, there is very little room for correction. The use of a rotating platform will allow proper positioning of the tibial tray on the resected tibial surface and realignment of the extensor mechanism, thus reducing rotational malunion. Nevertheless, correction is still limited to a few degrees, and any rotational malunion equal to or greater than 10° cannot be corrected by a prosthesis.

Translational malunion (anteriorly or posteriorly) cannot be corrected by a prosthesis either. Good preoperative planning based on AP and lateral views is critical. Templates are available to check for absence of impingement between the tibial keel and the cortices. One must be careful to differentiate between the cases where the tibial keel will be properly positioned and those where malunion is so severe that the tibial keel will inevitably impinge upon one of the cortices (fig. 2). In this situation, three options are available:

– use a thinner and longer stem;
– use an offset stem;
– if the previous options are not appropriate, perform a corrective osteotomy.

This corrective osteotomy may be performed as the first stage of a two-stage procedure, particularly if several planes are involved. However, in most cases, one single procedure is sufficient to perform both osteotomy and TKA, using a long stem component with distal locking, or adding a short fixation plate to control rotation.

Flexion or recurvatum malunion can generally be corrected with total knee arthroplasty. Correction is achieved by performing an asymmetric (anteriorly or posteriorly) tibial cut (more bone is removed posteriorly for correction of a recurvatum). However, intra-articular correction of an extra-articular deformity produces laxity in flexion. In this situation, Insall (11) insists on the necessity of linking the femoral and tibial cuts by increasing the thickness of the tibial component, and then recutting the distal femur in order to achieve good soft tissue balance both in flexion and extension. Therefore, we believe, like Insall (11), that it is preferable to use an implant that requires linked bone cuts, beginning with the tibial cut and then adjusting the distal femoral cut to achieve adequate soft tissue balance both in flexion and extension.

In the coronal plane, an overcorrected valgus high tibial osteotomy can be corrected by removing more bone from the medial tibial condyle. But this asymmetric resection produces medial laxity (fig. 3). On the other hand, a valgus deformity resulting from intra-articular wear can be corrected within the ligamentous envelope, using a thicker tibial component (fig. 4). A varus deformity due to progression of medial compartment wear can be corrected within the ligamentous envelope, using a thicker tibial component; however, this has the deleterious effect of recreating the excessive valgus produced by the osteotomy (fig. 5). Partial correction of medial compartment wear to restore correct axial alignment will result in residual medial laxity as that caused by resection.

Ligament balancing

Ligament balancing to achieve symmetric flexion and extension gaps is the most difficult part of total knee arthroplasty for failed osteotomy. Quality of the "ligamentous envelope" is always compromised by the initial surgery (1, 4, 8, 10). The ligament imbalance results from initial disturbances, iatrogenic injuries caused by the osteotomy, and lesions occurring secondarily to the osteotomy. Its analysis is rather complex.

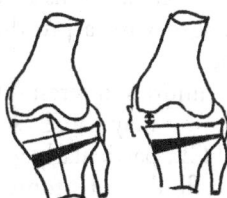

Fig. 3. – Severe resection of the medial tibial condyle.

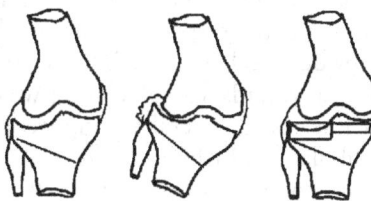

Fig. 4. – Correction within the ligamentous envelope of a valgus deformity due to wear.

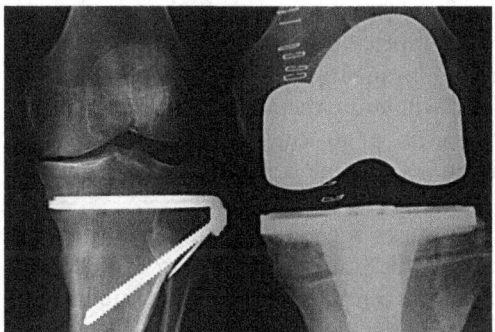

Fig. 5. – Correction of a varus deformity due to wear after tibial valgus osteotomy, within the ligamentous envelope. Thick tibial component.

Typical initial anomalies include overstretching on the convex side of the deformity (lateral side) and contracture on the concave side (medial ligaments). However, in our experience, contractures were an exceptional occurrence.

As regards iatrogenic injuries, one must differentiate between medial opening-wedge osteotomy and lateral closing-wedge osteotomy.

In medial opening-wedge osteotomy, injuries interest the superficial MCL. Depending on the surgical technique used, it is either sectioned close to its insertion to afford access to the medial aspect of the tibia, or released from its insertion with an attached bone block (fig. 6). In the former case, the open-wedge osteotomy is performed beneath MCL insertion; the MCL is not stretched, but its insertion area is reduced so that any attempt at lengthening is hazardous, even through decortication. In the latter case, the bone block is reattached at the osteotomy or proximal to the osteotomy, that is, above the normal insertion site of MCL; this results in relative lengthening of the ligament. Therefore, in case resection of the medial tibial plateau is performed to achieve correct alignment of the leg, the resulting laxity will be more severe in the second case than in the first one.

Furthermore, as quality of both the ligament and its insertion area is compromised by detachment and reattachment of the distal insertion, lengthening (if needed) through subperiosteal dissection or decortication is rather difficult. The distal insertion of the ligament is inevitably weakened. This weakness, particularly in recurrent varus deformity, may lead to rupture of the superficial MCL in case lengthening is required to achieve adequate stability of the implant. This rupture will destabilize the prosthesis, and in a non-constrained prosthesis this destabilization is unmanageable . This is why we think that these specific cases would be best managed with a prosthesis that provides mechanical stability in the coronal plane.

Now, as regards lateral closing-wedge osteotomy, injuries interest LCL and/or fascia lata. Lateral closing-wedge valgus osteotomy may cause ascent of the fibular head which results in slackening of the LCL, particularly when tibial osteotomy is not performed in conjunction with fibular osteotomy. At last, the lateral approach often results in loss of flexibility of the lateral soft tissues, particularly tensor fascia lata, which makes balancing even more difficult to achieve (3).

Any additional tibial resection performed for correction of a deformity will inevitably produce laxity on the side of the resection. According to Wolff *et al.* (12), intra-articular correction of 10° metaphyseal malunion produces – for a 10cm wide epiphysis 1.5cm asymmetry in bone resection. In the case of a lateral closing-wedge osteotomy, balancing the knee in extension will require lengthening of the MCL and will lead either to elevation of the joint line if the flexion gap is also asymmetric, or to lengthening of the femur if the flexion gap is correct. Both situations will entail significant consequences for the patellofemoral joint.

The amount of convex-side laxity varies according to the severity of the initial deformity. True joint laxity due to dislocation may also occur. It is generally concomitant with destruction of the central pivot and joint subluxation in the frontal plane. It then adds to the laxity caused by resection. Depending

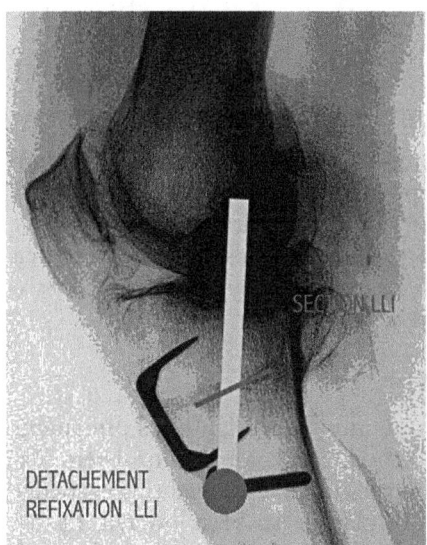

Fig. 6. – MCL released and reattached with a screw.

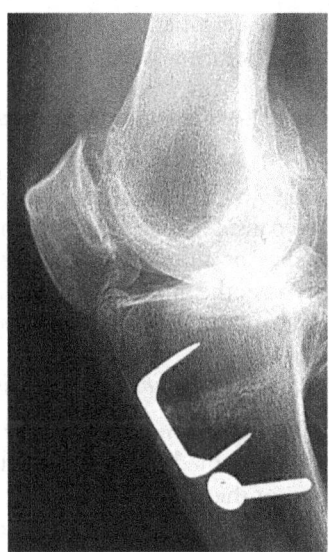

Fig. 7. – Patella baja after tibial valgus osteotomy.

on the degree of severity, it may require the use of a prosthesis that is highly constrained in the coronal plane.

Specific issues

Patella baja

Patients may have patella baja after a valgus osteotomy (fig. 7). In our experience, it was a rare occurrence with lateral closing-wedge osteotomy (2). Other authors reported a much higher incidence: 24% for Badet *et al.* (1) with closing-wedge tibial osteotomy, and even 80% for Windsor *et al.* (11).

If patella baja is not associated with joint stiffness, and flexion is still superior or equal to 90°, the prosthesis can generally be inserted, taking care to protect the distal insertion of the patellar tendon with a pin (to avoid avulsion). Otherwise, lengthening of the extensor mechanism is necessary.

Preoperative stiffness

In knees with significant preoperative stiffness, lengthening of the extensor mechanism may be performed either by elevating the anterior tibial tubercle or by lengthening the quadriceps tendon. Elevation of the tibial tuberosity facilitates exposure and protects the patellar tendon, but it is limited by the position of the tibial plateau. Furthermore, this procedure carries the risk of iatrogenic complications including: fracture of the tibial tubercle, nonunion, sepsis... Lengthening may be achieved either through a V-Y plasty or a rectus snip. Some authors (3, 7, 10) are quite happy with the results of V-Y plasty, but we personally experienced frequent extension lags, much more often than with the rectus snip.

Opening-wedge osteotomy plus bone substitute

As this technique is gaining popularity, the presence of an inert bone void filler which becomes more or less incorporated must be taken into account. We consider that in the absence of incorporation (confirmed by preoperative X-rays or noted intraoperatively), it is preferable to use a long stem that bypasses the grafted area, and replace this inert material by an autograft consisting of bone material removed during resections.

Thickness of the tibial cut and joint line level

When total knee arthroplasty is performed after failed high tibial osteotomy, the worn medial tibial condyle cannot be used as a landmark for determination of the appropriate bone resection. Furthermore, if a lateral closing-wedge osteotomy was performed, the lateral tibial plateau has been lowered (fig. 8); if a medial opening-wedge osteotomy was performed, wear of the medial compartment is more or less compensated by bone augmentation. During total knee arthroplasty, it is logical to correct the bone loss or bone augmentation resulting from osteotomy.

After a lateral closing-wedge osteotomy, one must determine the exact amount of bone to be removed, in order to minimize the medial laxity caused by bone resection; lowering of the lateral tibial plateau must be compensated for by a lateral reconstruction procedure.

After a medial opening-wedge osteotomy, one must remove the exact amount of bone that corresponds to the thickness of the component, without performing any ligament release.

Maintaining the joint line level is particularly important to avoid patella baja.

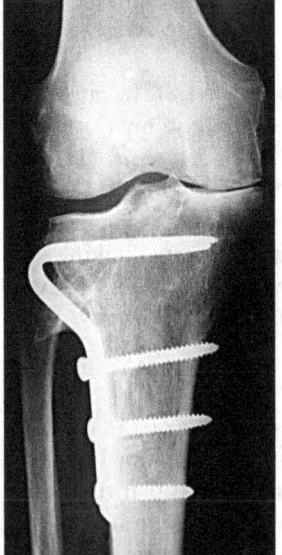

Fig. 8. – Lateral tibial condyle lowered after tibial valgus osteotomy.

Technical solutions

Moderate under- or overcorrection (inferior to 10°)

Lateral closing-wedge osteotomy

In the case of a moderate varus or valgus deformity, the technical difficulties are very similar to those in primary total knee arthroplasty.

In the case of moderate recurrence of the varus deformity, the lateral tibial plateau generally shows minimal to no wear; at the very most, there is some cartilage wear. Therefore, the lateral tibial plateau is a suitable landmark for determination of the level of resection, knowing that the thickness of the cut must be decreased by 1-2mm (maximum) to allow for the amount of wear. Less bone will be removed from the medial tibial condyle. In theory, medial release should be necessary in all the cases, but due to prior osteotomy, lateral ligaments have lost flexibility so that the lateral laxity caused by resection is very mild and ligament balancing is quite easy.

In moderately overcorrected valgus knees, axial realignment after tibial resection will often necessitate more extensive lateral release than in primary TKA, involving the tensor fascia lata, sometimes the popliteal tendon, rarely the LCL. This situation requires utmost care to maintain integrity of the medial portion of the ligamentous envelope. In the vast majority of cases, soft tissue balancing allows correction of this mild intra-articular deformity, and the epiphyseal deformity does not necessitate any special procedure.

Medial opening-wedge osteotomy

In the case of recurrence of the initial varus deformity, three main causes have been identified: undercorrection of the initial deformity, collapse of the graft, impaction of the bone substitute into the proximal fragment. In any event, the metaphyseal deformity is moderate. Bone resection will produce mild lateral laxity which will be easily balanced for by a limited medial release. As the risk of complete rupture of the MCL (as mentioned above) is low, but not zero, a highly constrained prosthesis can be necessary. The amount of resection is based on the lateral tibial condyle.

Determining the amount of tibial resection in an overcorrected valgus knee is much more difficult. The severe medial resection will produce medial laxity which will add to a possible iatrogenic laxity resulting from damage to the MCL during prior surgery (fig. 9). Therefore, extensive lateral release will be necessary to compensate for this medial laxity. If the deformity is moderate, performing the cut flush with the surface of the lateral tibial condyle does not usually produce an amount of laxity that is not correctable. In such cases, determination of the joint line level is critical, as simply filling the tibiofemoral space may lead to patella baja. On the other hand, using a prosthesis that imposes linked bone cuts and a tibial-cut-first approach, and fills the extension space by moving the distal femoral cut distally, increases tension on the extensor mechanism. Overtensioning may even lead to lateral subluxation of the patella or excessive stresses being placed on the patellar polyethylene bearing.

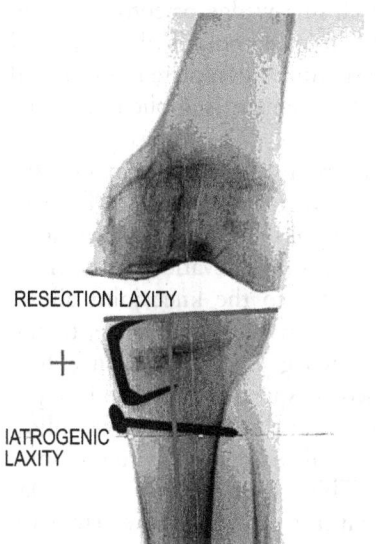

RESECTION LAXITY

+

IATROGENIC LAXITY

Fig. 9. – Medial laxity resulting from bone resection plus iatrogenic injury to MCL.

Valgus overcorrection (superior to 10°) under 70 years of age

The problem is correction of juxta-articular malunion, which is typically associated with deformity of the tibial metaphysis. Two management options are
available: prior correction of the deformity as a two-stage procedure or a one-
stage procedure (combined with TKA); intra-articular correction through tibial
resection, using augmentation (i.e. metal augments, bone grafts…) and performing release procedures. The indication for the appropriate treatment
method is based on the degree of severity of the deformity in the coronal
plane and any concomitant deformities. Osteotomy is the treatment of choice
for severe and/or multiplanar deformity (12). We personally think that it
should be combined with TKA whenever possible. Stability is provided by a
long press-fit stem which bypasses the osteotomy, and by fixation devices for
rotatory stability. We always perform the tibial cut first, and then the osteotomy. As other authors (1), we think that it may be advisable to elevate the
anterior tibial tubercle and position the osteotomy at some distance from the
tibial cut, in order to avoid weakening of the metaphysis or the potential risk
of metaphyseal necrosis. In cases where correction is needed only in the coronal
plane, one simple solution is to perform a curviplanar osteotomy, either just
above the tibial tuberosity or distal to the tibial tuberosity, after it has been
elevated. This avoids increasing bone loss. Osteotomy is initiated by making
multiple holes (postage stamp technique) with a compass point and then
connecting them using a bone chisel. Compression is applied to the osteotomy site by the peroneal splint during reduction. The osteotomy is bypassed
by the long stem of the component and a short screw plate may be added
for rotatory stability. If the tibial tuberosity has been elevated, it can be secured
with screws or cerclage wires.

In the other cases, we perform a medial closing-wedge osteotomy, again
after the tibial tuberosity has been elevated; the osteotomy is also bypassed
by the long stem of the component, and a short antirotation plate is also added
at the end of the procedure. Whenever possible, cement is applied proximal
to the osteotomy site.

In cases where intra-articular correction has been selected, the main difficulty, in a lateral closing-wedge osteotomy, lies with the presence of fibrosis,
contracture of the lateral structures, and epiphyseal deformity. In such cases,
the use of a lateral approach is mandatory, and routine elevation of the tibial
tuberosity can be most helpful. Lateral approach to the knee joint allows
release of the tensor fascia lata from its insertion on Gerdy's tubercle, taking
care to maintain continuity with the fascia of the leg. The lateral retinaculum
is routinely incised; this opening can be closed by spreading out the infrapatellar fat pad which is still pedicled to the vessels of the lateral synovial plica.
The popliteal muscle tendon must often be sacrificed as well as the femoral
insertion of the posterolateral corner capsule. This release procedure is similar
to that performed in primary TKA, except that it is generally more extensive,
due to loss of flexibility of the lateral structures.

Unless there is convex-side laxity (evidenced by medial lift-off), the amount
of bone removed from the medial condyle should correspond to the thick-

ness of the component. The lateral cut must be performed using a special cutting guide for stepped resection; the sagittal cut is critical and requires caution to avoid malrotation. The epiphyseal deformity can be corrected by an offset stem.

In cases of overcorrected medial opening-wedge osteotomy, malunion is usually less of a problem. The main issue is weakening of medial capsuloligamentous structures. Therefore, particularly in these severe deformities, one must be prepared to deal intraoperatively with incompetent capsuloligamentous structures and have a highly constrained TKR available for this purpose.

Severe valgus deformity over the age of 70

In this situation, we often use a highly constrained TKR. The tibial cut is done first, lateral capsuloligamentous structures are lengthened to accommodate a tibial component that will provide adequate stability of the medial compartment in flexion and extension. Adjustment of the ligament balance is provided by the spine/cam mechanism. As in the previous case, a stepped tibial cut may be performed, and the step filled with a metal block. Now, one may also perform a flat cut which will remove a greater amount of bone. We think that stem extensions are necessary with these highly constrained prostheses. Offset stems generally solve the problem of metaphyseal deformities. This solution is simple and effective in restoring axial alignment of the lower limb; furthermore, it eliminates the need for extensive soft tissue release, simplifies the procedure, and allows immediate resumption of weight bearing in all the cases.

Results

Actually, it is difficult to make a meaningful comparison between the published series reporting the results of total knee arthroplasty after failed osteotomy, because different scores are used and the groups of revised patients are also different and poorly documented.

Publications reflect two diverging opinions. Some of the early publications (8, 11) report significantly lower results for TKA after failed osteotomy. Other publications, often more recent, report similar or slightly lower results.

Authors of early publications emphasize the difficulties with approach and exposure, mainly due to patella baja. In Insall's series, osteotomies were stabilized using cast immobilization, which probably explains his poor results. Krackow's study (7) shows that the main predictors for a poor prognosis for TKA after failed osteotomy are algodystrophy, work accident, and persistent pain following osteotomy. A comparison was made between the patients treated with this method and two control groups; results in the TKR/osteotomy treatment group were significantly lower than in the control groups. However, it should be pointed out that Krackow (5) systematically uses a low-

constraint knee design and achieves stability by performing ligament procedures: retensioning of the posteromedial corner capsule, and distal anterior
transposition of the distal insertion of the superficial MCL. We personally
think that in aged patients, this type of ligamentoplasty may be a cause of
anatomic failure and/or persistent pain.

The second group of authors claims that results are similar or slightly lower
than those of primary knees. As early as 1987, Staeheli (9) reported identical
results in a group of patients who, however, had no significant deformity in
the frontal plane (only 2 overcorrections in 35 patients). Ritter (6) found no
difference in results between the TKR/osteotomy group and the primary TKR
group. Badet (1) reported a series with poorer results on pain control as compared to the overall HLS series, but almost identical results regarding other
evaluation criteria.

Restoration of mechanical axis

Although in these early series, no reference is made to the mechanical axis of
the lower limb, which makes analysis somewhat inaccurate, it seems that full
correction of the frontal deformity has often been achieved. Postoperative
tibiofemoral axis was 7° (range, 3-12°) in Insall's series (11), and 6.5° (range,
3-17°) in Merrill Ritter's series (6). In another series consisting of not previously operated valgus knees, Insall achieved a mean postoperative axis of
7°, that is, an overall mechanical axis close to 180°. This is consistent with
the results reported by Neyret (8) and Badet (1). Staeheli's series (9) also shows
good restoration of the mechanical axis.

Component fixation

No problems with component fixation have been reported in the literature
in series of TKAs after failed valgus osteotomy. Toksvig-Larsen (10) used RSA
(roentgen-stereophotogrammetric analysis) to compare a series of 40 primary
knee arthroplasties versus 40 TKAs after failed osteotomy, and confirmed these
data. There was no difference in migration or tendency to migration, and no
difference in component position or alignment between the two series.

Comparison with revision TKA after failed unicompartmental knee arthroplasty

Gill (3) compared the technical difficulties and results of total knee arthroplasty after failed UKA versus TKA after failed osteotomy, and concluded
that the revision procedure is technically more challenging after failed unicompartmental knee arthroplasty (more reconstruction required).
Furthermore, clinical results are not as good (IKS score: 87 after failed HTO
versus 78 after failed UKA). We also found that revision of a unicompartmental knee replacement to a total knee replacement is a more major procedure which involves more reconstruction and is potentially more difficult

in terms of ligament balancing. Indications are likely different: osteotomy remains an excellent indication in patients with a regular occupation or activity (e.g., DIY, gardening), whereas unicompartmental knee replacement is particularly well suited to females or patients engaged in a moderately active occupation.

Conclusion

Revision to total knee replacement, although technically demanding, provides a solution that is generally (but not always) mechanically and functionally satisfactory. Advanced age of patients, sequelae of prior surgeries, severity of the axial deformity at the time of surgery, presence of an epiphyseal malunion, are strong predictors of a poor prognosis. Highly constrained prostheses are a very simple solution to restore correct alignment and soft tissue balance in the elderly. In other patients, most situations can be addressed by: accurate preoperative planning including evaluation of anticipated difficulties, and sufficient inventory of components offering a variety of options for augmentation or control of laxity in case of ligament deficiency. In knees with very severe deformities, combined TKA and osteotomy (one-stage procedure) may be effective in restoring the anatomic conditions required for implantation of a total knee prosthesis. In this respect, our results are consistent with those reported in recent publications: total knee prostheses implanted after failed tibial valgus osteotomy yield as good results (or nearly as good) as primary knee prostheses, thus allowing to maintain the specific indications for HTO.

References

1. Badet R, Neyret P. Prothèse totale du genou après ostéotomie tibiale de valgisation 9ᵉ Journées Lyonnaises de chirurgie du genou et de l'épaule. p. 235-45
2. Dohin B, Migaud H, Gougeon F et al. (1993) Effets de l'ostéotomie de valgisation par soustraction externe sur la hauteur de la rotule et l'arthrose fémoro-patellaire. Acta orthop Belg 59, 1: 69-75
3. Gill T, Schemitsch E.H, Brick GW et al. (1995) Revision total knee arthroplasty after failing unicompartmental knee arthroplasty or high tibial osteotomy. Clin Orthop 321: 10-8
4. Katz MM, Hungerford D, Krackow KA et al. (1987) Results of total knee arthroplasty after failed proximal tibial osteotomy for osteoarthritis. J Bone Joint Surg 69-A, 2: 225-33
5. Krackow KA, Holtgrewe JL (1990) Experience with a new technique for managing severely overcorrected valgus high tibial osteotomy at total knee arthroplasty. Clin Orthop 258: 213-24
6. Meding JB, Keating EM, Ritter MA et al. (2000) Total knee arthroplasty after high tibial osteotomy. Clin Orthop 375: 175-84
7. Mont MA, Krackow KA, Hungerford DS (1994) Total knee arthroplasty after failed high tibial osteotomy. Clin Orthop 299: 125-30
8. Neyret P, Deroche P, Deschamp G et al. (1992) Prothèse totale de genou après ostéotomie tibiale de valgisation. Problèmes techniques. Rev Chir Orthop 77: 438-48

9. Staeheli JW, Cass JR, Morrey BF (1987) Condylar total knee arthroplasty after failed proximal tibial osteotomy. J Bone Joint Surg 69-A, 1: 28-31

10. Toksvig-Larsen S, Magyar G, Onsten I *et al.* (1998) Fixation of the tibial component of total knee arthroplasty after hight tibial osteotomy. J Bone Joint Surg 80-B, 2: 295-7

11. Windsor RE, Insall JN, Vince KG (1988) Technical considerations of total knee arthroplasty after proximal tibial osteotomy. J Bone Joint Surg 70-A, 4: 547-55

12. Wolff AM, Hungerford D, Pepe CL (1991) The effect of extra-articular varus and valgus deformity on total knee arthroplasty. Clin Orthop 271: 35-51

Total knee arthroplasty after failed unicompartmental knee arthroplasty

R. Verdonk, K.F. Almquist

Introduction

Unicompartmental knee arthroplasty revision is a rare complication in arthroplastic knee surgery. Indeed, the results obtained in primary cases (13) appear to be extremely satisfactory, regardless of whether fixed or mobile tibial plateau elements are used.

Complications occur when the proper indication was not established, or when the surgical technique was not perfect.

Moreover, lateral unicompartmental knee arthroplasty evolves differently from medial unicompartmental knee arthroplasty as the lateral compartment is subject to more ligament constraints and to potential extreme rotatory motion.

Apart from general considerations related to skin incision and potential complex problems in knee revision arthroplasty, the surgeon should remain very cautious regarding bone stock issues and implant fixation problems, which are essentially located at the tibial level.

Like total knee arthroplasty after preceding corrective tibial or femoral osteotomy, unicompartmental revision arthroplasty is encumbered with potential problems and thus should not be considered as simple straightforward surgery. Issues relating to revision of a unicompartmental knee prosthesis with a subsequent unicompartmental implant will not be discussed because they are beyond the scope of this chapter.

Indications and contraindications

Introduction

There has been a tendency to overlook both medial and lateral unicompartmental knee arthroplasty as an approach to solve unicompartmental degenerative arthrosis. Patients with progressive inflammatory diseases should obviously not be considered for this type of surgery (12).

Indications for unicompartmental arthroplasty

Age, malalignment, obesity, osteoporosis or a combination of these have been considered a contraindication for this type of surgery.

Age: in candidates for total knee arthroplasty, physical age and not calendar age should be taken into account. Moreover, cartilage degeneration in both compartments of the knee joint increases with increasing physical age thus compromising the contralateral compartment which is painfree at the time of surgery (7, 9, 16, 18, 20).

Malalignment is a major consideration when it gives rise to knee dysfunction. In the young and active population one should first look into possibilities for corrective varus or valgus osteotomy.

Since varus malalignment is more frequent than valgus malalignment, it progressively induces regression of the joint space. The surgeon will be confronted with this finding in potential realignment surgery and unicompartmental arthroplasty (fig. 1, 2).

Lootvoet (10) clearly illustrated that when more than half of the normal (contralateral) joint space has disappeared, good to excellent long-term results after corrective valgus osteotomy cannot be obtained, even though age can be of influence.

Morbid obesity and disease-induced osteoporosis will not be discussed, since proper therapeutic measures to treat the underlying disease are required.

Obesity as such does not prove to be a contraindication for unicompartmental arthroplasty if malalignment and age are given proper consideration.

Disuse osteoporosis will disappear after pain-relieving unicompartmental surgery and should not be considered a contraindication for weightbearing knee compartmental surgery.

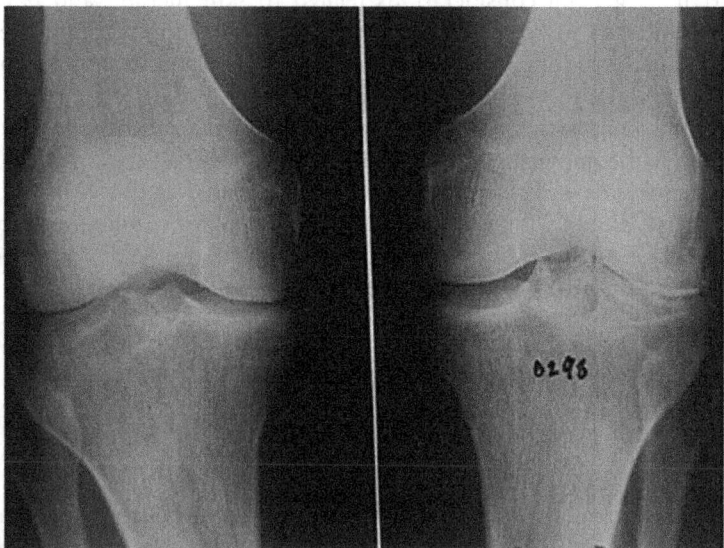

Fig. 1 – Progressive degenerative arthrosis develops in the lateral compartment of the left knee, as seen on Schuss X-ray showing narrowing of the joint line after lateral meniscectomy.

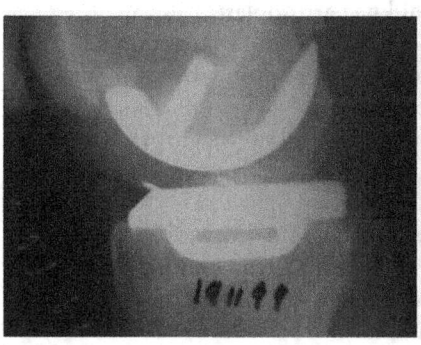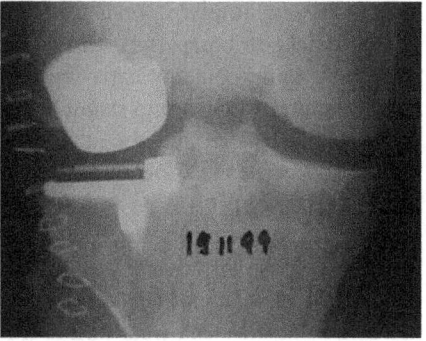

Fig. 2 – A lateral compartment arthroplasty is performed using an Oxford knee prosthesis with appropriate positioning of the implant.

Contraindications for unicompartmental arthroplasty

Goodfellow *et al.* (5) and Murray *et al.* (13, 14, 15, 19) have rightly retained **ligament instability** (most commonly ACL deficiency) of the knee joint as a contraindication for mobile medial plateau unicompartmental knee arthroplasty. The possibility of meniscal dislocation, obviously requiring reduction, is always present. But also in fixed medial plateau bearing, polyethylene erosion cannot be avoided (1).

Presently, unicompartmental lateral mobile knee arthroplasty appears to be ill-advised.

Whether or not **patellofemoral arthrosis** is to be considered a major contraindication for unicompartmental knee arthroplasty remains controversial.

Manifest patellofemoral trochleodysplasia (3, 4) would warrant total knee arthroplasty since in these cases neither patellofemoral arthroplasty nor unicompartmental knee arthroplasty would offer permanent pain relief considering potential tricompartmental degeneration.

Even though symptomatic **limited avascular necrosis** both of the femur (most often) and of the tibia is no limiting factor in unicompartmental knee arthroplasty, massive avascular necrosis, as best illustrated on MR in case of e.g., cortison-induced joint line discrepancy, requires total knee arthroplasty.

Indications for revision in failed unicompartmental arthroplasty

Although excellent results of unicompartmental arthroplasty, both using mobile and fixed plateau bearings of a recent design have been reported, all authors (1, 5, 6, 11, 17, 20) emphasize strict adherence to indications and surgical technique prerequisites.

Meniscal dislocation in case of a mobile insert should be reduced at once (fig. 3, 4). In lateral compartment arthroplasty it can be expected to be a recurrent event implying revision to total knee arthroplasty.

In medial compartment arthroplasty dislocation could be traumatic in origin. One should consider early reduction possibly requiring better medial collateral ligament tensioning using a larger implant.

Anyhow, the orthopaedic surgeon should not allow weightbearing before reduction in case of dislocation, so as to keep the metallic implants intact, and total replacement.

Iterative traumatic ligament (ACL) rupture might jeopardize future knee function, particularly with mobile bearing unicompartmental implants. With fixed tibial plateau elements this issue remains controversial but will lead to increased polyethylene wear and lamination.

Aseptic loosening might be caused by progressive avascular necrosis, more specifically in the femoral condyle.

Sepsis and septic loosening have no particular therapeutic considerations different from total knee arthroplasty, and will not be discussed further in this chapter (2).

Even though nowadays mostly obviated – because of appropriate implant sizes and matches – prosthesis conformity with special reference to the tibial plateau rim has been a potential clinical problem. As in total knee arthroplasty, one should consider proper tibial plateau covering in order to obtain cortical support and subchondral epiphyseal fixation.

Because of the variety of medial and lateral tibial contours it was not always possible in the past to obtain optimal tibial coverage, resulting in prosthesis irritation and bursitis, which could produce progressive dysfunction and necessitate revision.

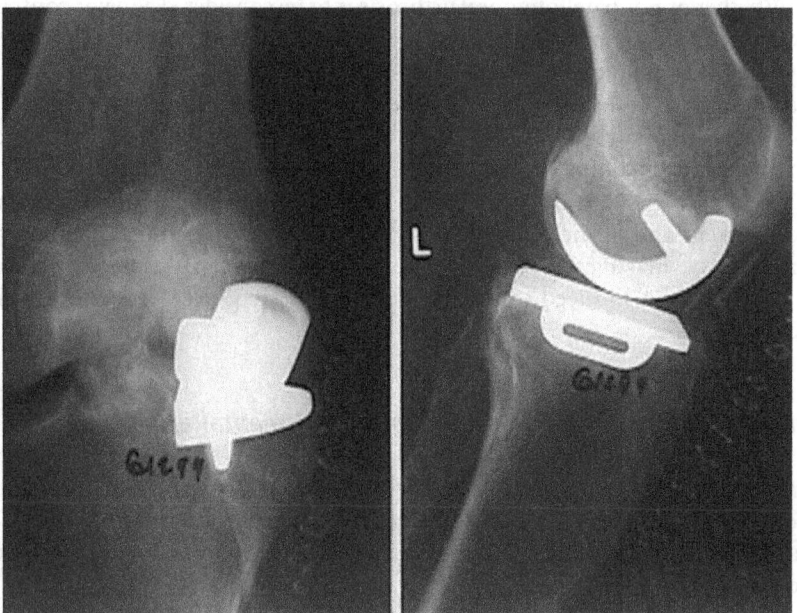

Fig. 3 – Displacement of the implant occurs, necessitating revision three weeks postinsertion.

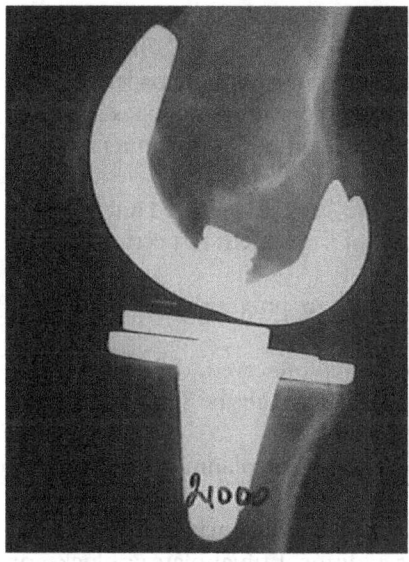

Fig. 4 – A posterior saving total knee arthroplasty is necessitated because of lateral compartment failure.
More than extensive bone resection has been performed on the tibial level.

Surgical technique

Introduction

Since revision arthroplasty in unicompartmental knee prosthesis can be fraught with unexpected surgical problems, one should consider a midline knee approach as a standard procedure.

Revision of a unicompartmental prosthesis with a similar implant will not be considered here, because it is beyond the scope of this chapter.

The initial clinical evaluation will have outlined the ligament balance and quality with special attention to the collateral structures. If collateral ligament stability appears to be completely insufficient, the orthopaedic surgeon should consider totally constrained devices for implantation.

Central pivot ligament quality is almost irrelevant as peroperatively it will be decided whether or not the posterior cruciate ligament will be saved.

However, ACL-retaining procedures in early stages of primary arthroplasty in inflammatory diseases do not represent a clinical or peroperative issue within the scope of this chapter.

Surgical technique

Medial compartment

The midline knee approach with a subvastus or transvastus muscle incision allows for full medial unicompartmental evaluation.

Appropriate respect for the patellar tendon is mandatory and will be possible in most cases, particularly if revision arthroplasty is performed after minimally invasive primary surgery.

For technical reasons, and after appropriate evaluation of all three compartments of the knee, it is preferable to approach the femoral condyle first. When confronted with a cemented component, small chisels and osteotomes are preferably used to remove the prosthesis, respecting the underlying bone as much as possible.

With a non-cemented component even more skill is required to remove the femoral prosthesis.

In case of pertinent loosening, the prosthesis is easily removed and the surgeon's attention is then drawn to the removal of the cement respecting the surrounding bone stock.

The same chisels and osteotomes are used to progressively remove the cemented or non-cemented tibial implant.

Even though femoral bone stock is usually well preserved, the design of the femoral implant device notwithstanding, one can easily be surprised by the amount of bone stock loss in tibial plateau revision.

It is this element that should be borne in mind when planning to revise unicompartmental prostheses.

In some rare instances medial tibial plateau bone stock loss is massive, necessitating (preferably) bone grafting or additional tibial plateau blocks, or even longer-stem tibial plateau implants.

Using appropriate revision ancillary instruments necessitates the use of half blocks in order to restore proper ligament balancing. From this moment, according to the surgeon's preference, ligament tension is evaluated in flexion and subsequently in extension, or the other way around, leading to proper total knee implantation.

Also according to the surgeon's preference and experience the patella will be approached in the most efficient way. This issue is not discussed in this chapter.

Lateral compartment

Using a midline skin incision the knee is opened laterally with a midline approach to the quadriceps tendon. Hoffa fat pad dissection and lateral reflection, as described by Keblish (8), are performed, allowing for medial patellar dislocation and easy access to the lateral compartmental implant.

The same surgical steps as described for the medial compartment will ensure proper removal and reimplantation.

Conclusion

One should not consider unicompartmental knee arthroplasty as an inbetween surgical step from knee joint degenerative arthrosis to total knee arthroplasty. Possible need for revision can be caused by infection and is beyond the scope of this chapter.

Progressive avascular necrosis with implant loosening, traumatic ligament disruption, recurrent dislocation of meniscal implants in case of mobile tibial plateau, and implant-related pain at the tibial rim can necessitate revision.

As the midline incision should be the rule, it will allow a proper medial or lateral approach to the knee joint and implant removal with due respect for bone stock. In case of a bone defect, bone grafts will be required or possibly a tibial block insert to equalize the joint line.

In any case, the surgeon should be aware of probable and possible pitfalls regarding unexpected loss of bone stock, and inform the patient accordingly in order to obtain good postrevision results.

References

1. Cartier P, Cheaib S (1987) Unicondylar knee arthroplasty. 2-10 years of follow-up evaluation J. Arthroplasty 2: 157-62
2. De Winter F, Van De Wiele C, Vogelaers D *et al.* (2001) Fluorine-18 fluorodeoxyglucose-positron emission tomography: a highly accurate imaging modality for the diagnosis of chronic musculoskeletal infections. J Bone Jt Surg, 83A 651-60
3. Dejour D, Rocatelli E (2001) Patellar instability in adults. Ed. Scientifiques et Médicales Elsevier SAS (Paris), Surgical Techniques in Orthopaedics and Traumatology, 55-520-A.10 p. 6
4. Dejour H, Walch G, Neyret P *et al.* (1990) La dysplasie de la trochlée fémorale. Rev Chir Orthop 76: 45-54
5. Goodfellow JW, O'Connor J (1986) Clinical results of the Oxford knee. Surface arthroplasty of the tibiofemoral joint with a meniscal bearing prosthesis. Clin Orthop 205: 21-42
6. Heck DA, Marmor L, Gibson A *et al.* (1993) Unicompartmental knee arthroplasty. A multicenter investigation with long-term follow-up evaluation. Clin Orthop 286: 154-9
7. Insall JX (193) Historical development, classification and characteristics of knee prosthesis. Surgery of the Knee, Livingstone, Philadelphia p. 677-717
8. Keblish PA (1991) The lateral approach to the valgus knee. Surgical technique and analysis of 53 cases with over two-year follow-up evaluation. Clin Orthop 271: 52-62
9. Lootvoet L, Burton P, Himmer O *et al.* (1997) A unicompartmental knee prosthesis: the effect of the positioning of the tibial plate on the functional results. Acta Orthop Belg 63: 94-101
10. Lootvoet L, Massinon A, Rossillon R *et al.* (1993) Upper tibial osteotomy for gonarthrosis in genu varum. Apropos of a series of 193 cases reviewed 6 to 10 years later. Rev Chir Orthop Réparatrice Appar Mot 79: 375-84
11. Mallory TII, Danyi J (1983) Unicompartmental total knee arthroplasty: a five- to nine-year follow-up study of 42 procedures. Clin Orthop 175: 135-8
12. McIntosh DL, Hunter GA (1972) The use of the hemiarthroplasty prosthesis for advanced osteoarthrosis and rheumatoid arthritis of the knee. J Bone Joint Surg 54B: 244-55
13. Murray DW, Goodfellow JW, O'Connor JJ (1998) The Oxford medial unicompartmental arthroplasty: a ten-year survival study. J Bone Joint Surg 80B: 983-9
14. Murray DW (2000) Unicompartmental knee replacement: now or never? Orthopaedics 23: 979-80
15. Psychoyois V, Crawford RW, O'Connor JJ *et al.* (1998) Wear of congruent meniscal bearings in unicompartmental knee arthroplasty: a retrieval study of 16 specimens. J Bone Joint Surg 80B: 976-82
16. Puddu G (2000) Osteotomies about the athletic knee. Operative techniques in sports medicine 8: 1
17. Romagnoli S *et al.* (1998) La protesi mono nel compartimento esterno. Atti del Convegno Internazionale. The Uni Prosthesis of the Knee, Milano 27/28 marzo 1998 – Libreria Cortina Milano 75-9
18. Stern SH, Becker MW, Insall JN (1993) Unicondylar knee arthroplasty: an evaluation of selection criteria. Clin Orthop 286: 143-8
19. Weale AE, Murray DW, Crawford R *et al.* (1999) Does arthritis progress in the retained compartments after "Oxford" medial unicompartmental arthroplasty? A clinical and radiological study with a minimum ten-year follow-up. J Bone Joint Surg 81B: 783-9
20. Witvoet J, Peyrache MD, Nizard R (1993) Prothèses unicompartimentaires du genou type Lotus dans le traitement des gonarthroses latéralisées : résultats de 135 cas avec un recul moyen de 4,6 ans. Rev Chir Orthop 79: 565-76

Soft tissue balancing in total knee arthroplasty

G. Deschamps

Soft tissue balancing in total knee arthroplasty (TKA) includes:
– analysis of the various types of laxity that are encountered in TKA, and their respective causes and consequences;
– technical procedures which can be performed to correct a ligament imbalance, particularly in the coronal plane.

We will consider these two aspects, based on our own experience and published data.

Concept of soft tissue balancing in TKA

This mainly interests sliding prostheses since hinged knee systems do not use the same implantation principles.

Goal

TKA has two absolute requirements:
– restoration of axial alignment which is critical to the long-term success of the arthroplasty (in terms of wear and loosening);
– soft tissue balancing which is also critical because any significant imbalance may adversely affect the short-term outcome (instability due to laxity, or stiffness resulting from a persistent contracture). Even a moderate imbalance may lead to wear or loosening in the long run.

In the past, the reasonable clinical lifespan for a Total Knee Replacement (TKR) was 10 years, which means that only the severe laxities that are responsible for immediate failures were to be feared (i.e., medial laxity in the valgus knee which is responsible for instability with walking; anterior/posterior instability in flexion which may cause dislocation – particularly posterior dislocation – in some posterior stabilized knee designs).

The improved service life and level of performance offered by current knee designers imposes more accuracy in soft tissue balancing and more caution in the analysis of results. Thus, a "yawning" in the coronal plane, particularly if it is asymmetrical, or the presence of anterior/posterior laxity due to a slack PCL (retained and yet non-functional), must now be considered as objectionable imperfections in implants which are expected to last for a minimum of 20 years (1, 2).

Then, we think it necessary to analyse the various types of laxity that may be encountered in TKA, their causes, and how to avoid them.

Types of laxity

Both the coronal plane, in extension and flexion, and the sagittal plane must be considered. This leads us to differentiate between true laxity due to stretched ligaments on the one hand, and what is considered as a ligament imbalance resulting from the bone cuts that are performed to restore axial alignment, on the other hand (3).

Coronal laxity in extension

The difference between laxity due to stretch-out and laxity resulting from bone cuts is best appreciated in the coronal plane.

Laxity due to stretched ligaments

This type of laxity is very uncommon in the varus knee.

In contrast, it is frequently seen in the valgus knee. The main problem with this type of deformity is that laxity will mainly show within the first 20 to 30° of flexion, not when the knee is fully extended. This is clearly demonstrated by the analysis of plain radiographs of knees with lateral tibiofemoral osteoarthritis. Actually, X-rays taken in full extension may not show any deformity or wear. Only schuss views will reveal a tight lateral compartment, sometimes associated with an open medial compartment (fig. 1 **a.** and **b.**).

When performing a TKA, we routinely test the knee in extension. With the hand placed on the anterior aspect of the thigh, we force the knee in extension to check whether proper balance has been achieved. The subsequent control x-rays will often reveal the persistence of a space medially due to a few degrees of flexion, which may not have any functional consequences.

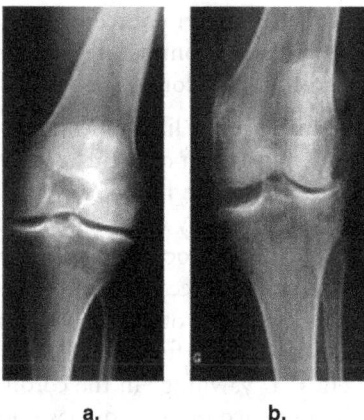

a.   **b.**

Fig. 1. – Lateral compartment osteoarthritis.
a. Normal extension gap;
b. Stress view that reveals a tight space and medial laxity.

However, one should differentiate between a knee that is unlocked, slightly flexed, and gapes, and whose appearance can be improved by the recovery of full extension, and a knee in which lateral releases have been insufficient. In the latter case, the "yawning" will persist, and excessive pressure on the lateral compartment will be generated, that will cause accelerated wear of the polyethylene (PE) (fig. 2).

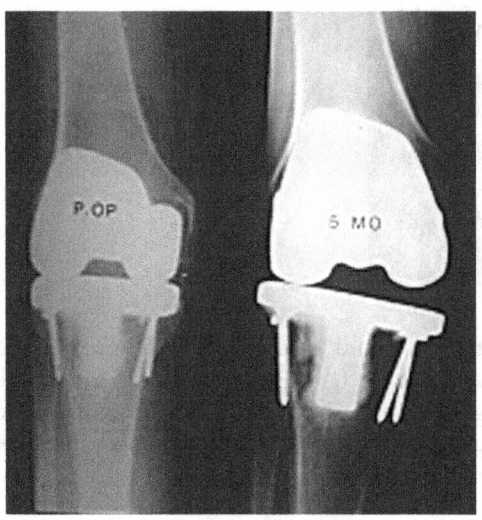

Fig. 2. – TKR in a genu valgum. No postoperative laxity in extension. The X-ray taken in mild flexion shows recurrent medial laxity.

Laxity resulting from bone cuts

Both the causes and effects of this type of laxity are radically different. It is due to bone deformity and will exist independent of any ligament stretch-out.

This type of laxity results from bone cuts. As a matter of fact, in knees with a metaphyseal/diaphyseal deformity, asymmetrical resections are necessary to restore a neutral mechanical axis.

For instance, in a genu varum with a proximal tibial deformity (tibia vara) (fig. 3), the tibial joint line slopes medially by 7, 8 or even 10° relative to the mechanical axis of the tibia. In order to restore a joint line that is perpendicular to the mechanical axis, one must remove approximately 7 to 10mm more bone from the lateral tibial condyle than from the medial tibial condyle. This creates a trapezoidal tibiofemoral space with a large lateral side which results in lateral laxity.

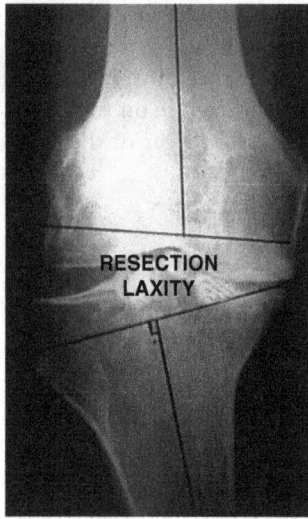

Fig. 3. – Laxity resulting from bone cuts in a tibia vara.

A similar situation is found in the genu valgum, but there, the femoral resection is generally at fault (genu valgum due to a femoral deficiency). In this case, resecting more bone from the medial femoral condyle in order to restore a joint line that is perpendicular to the mechanical axis of the femur will create a trapezoidal space with a large medial side (fig. 4) which will result in medial laxity.

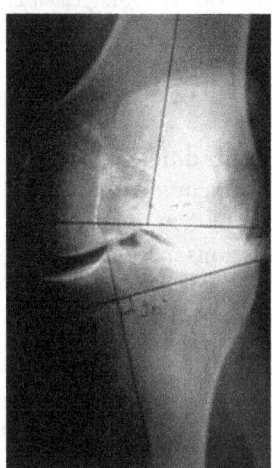

Fig. 4. – Laxity resulting from bone cuts in a valgus knee (femur being predominantly involved).

Thus, the laxity resulting from bone cuts is always:
– lateral in a genu varum;
– medial in a genu valgum.

It is important to note that the laxity involved by bone cuts will always add to the laxity (if any) caused by stretched ligaments.

It is often underestimated during the preoperative planning. However, it is critically important because it may have a pernicious influence on soft tissue balancing, particularly when the PCL is retained. As a matter of fact, it potentiates any axial malalignment that may persist after insertion of the prosthetic components. It is all the more prejudicial because experience shows that the mildest imperfection will always tend to replicate the initial deformity: residual varus in a genu varum, residual valgus in a genu valgum. Although the laxity is often very mild and does not affect the immediate outcome, it adversely affects the long-term outcome and should not be neglected.

Coronal laxity in flexion

The causes are the same as those of laxity in extension, particularly for laxity due to stretch-out.

In contrast, for laxity resulting from bone cuts, rotation of the femoral component should be taken into account.

For instance, if the tibial cut is made perpendicular to the mechanical axis of the tibia and the posterior femoral cut parallel to the posterior condyle line, the flexion gap is often asymmetrical:

– larger laterally in a tibia vara;
– larger medially in a valgus deformity.

Should one strive to create a strictly rectangular flexion space? The answer is not unequivocal. As a matter of fact, from a physiological point of view, there is always more laxity laterally than medially; the medial compartment is the one that provides stability. However, we feel it important to differentiate, particularly in the genu varum, between asymmetrical flexion gaps with tight medial compartments which may cause joint stiffness and PE wear, and asymmetrical flexion gaps merely resulting from a physiological lateral laxity, without any medial tightness, that is, with proper ligament balance.

Asymmetrical resections performed with an external rotation have the advantages of consistently creating a perfectly rectangular flexion space (fig. 5).

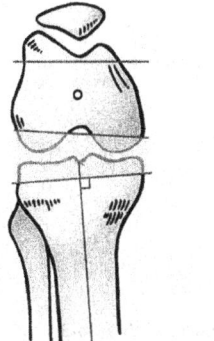 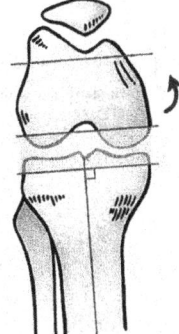

Fig. 5. – Externally rotated posterior femoral cut creating a rectangular flexion space.

Although they do palliate any excessive medial tightness that may result from the 90° tibial cut, and provide recentring of the patella on the femoral canopy, it must be reminded that femoral external rotation generates varus stresses in the lower limb. We shall revert to the potential consequences of this technical trick on ligament balancing in the coronal plane. As a matter of fact, it may result in asymmetrical flexion/extension gaps if a release is performed secondarily on the concave side of the deformity, in extension, to balance the soft tissue. Then, the rectangular flexion space (created by the resection of the femur in external rotation) becomes trapezoidal due to the secondary release of the medial soft tissues, finally resulting in medial laxity in flexion (fig. 6).

One basic notion can be derived from this debate about coronal laxity. From a conceptual point of view, ligament balancing in TKA includes two aspects which have very different consequences on the outcome:

– *Laxity* is always found on the convex side of the deformity. Ligament stretch-out has the most deleterious effect because it may adversely affect the immediate functional result. A typical example is medial laxity in the genu valgum. Laxity resulting from bone cuts has only recently been acknowledged. It may seem negligible, and yet it may have very serious consequences in the medium run; as a matter of fact, because it builds up with the slightest axial malalignment, it may cause wear and loosening;

– *Contractures* are found on the concave side of the deformity. Failure to sufficiently release a contracture not only perpetuates the gape on the lax side, but it may also result in accelerated wear of the PE component due to excessive stresses. The difficulty is to evaluate as accurately as possible the amount of release that is both sufficient to correct the contracture and necessary to balance the ligaments. This is particularly critical in cases where the PCL is retained, as will be shown further on. As a matter of fact, when the PCL is present, it is not possible to correct a laxity on the convex side by releasing the concave side to an amount that exceeds the normal length of the PCL ligament.

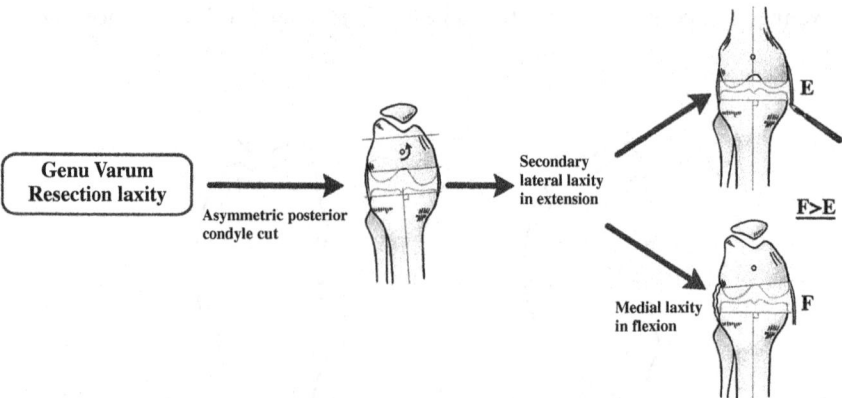

Fig. 6. – Varus deformity of the proximal tibia: the externally rotated cut creates a rectangular flexion space. But, in extension, the lateral laxity resulting from bone cuts imposes a medial release which, secondarily, produces medial laxity in flexion.

Sagittal laxity

Here again, one must first review the different types of laxity: laxity due to ligament stretch-out – either pre-existing or secondary to osteoarthritis – and laxity resulting from bone cuts, and then the methods available to correct this laxity.

Laxity due to ligament stretch-out

Posterior laxity is rare. The only problem with posterior laxity is that it is a contraindication to the use of cruciate retaining TKRs.

Anterior laxity is much more frequent. Osteoarthritis secondary to a chronic ACL rupture has been described by Dejour *et al.* (4). It is easy to identify on standing lateral X-rays which show anterior subluxation of the tibia under the femur, and wear (most often medially) with posterior bone loss. It is always associated with a PCL deficiency (at least histologically) (5). It is also associated with significant stretching of the posteromedial capsuloligamentous structures. Therefore, cruciate retaining TKRs should reasonably be contraindicated in such a situation. As a matter of fact, the lack of constraint of the tibial bearing and the posterior slope of the tibial cut which is recommended by many PCR total knee designers, may promote early redislocation due to anterior subluxation of the tibial component (6).

Laxity resulting from bone cuts

This type of laxity results from a complex combination of factors in relation with the type of deformity and the order of bone cuts that is dictated by each instrument system.

Three main factors may contribute to this type of sagittal laxity:

– *Performing the posterior femoral cut in external rotation.* Some instrument systems will impose a resection in 3° of external rotation in order to palliate the asymmetry of the flexion gap resulting from the 90° tibial cut. This is based on Moreland's study (7) which states that an individual with neutral axial alignment has 3° of mechanical tibial varus. As a result, performing a tibial resection at 90° in the coronal plane and a femoral resection parallel to the femoral condyles will inevitably result in a knee that is tight medially. This can be compensated by performing a 3° externally rotated posterior femoral cut which removes more bone medially than laterally and thus increases the space medially. Besides the fact that Moreland's statement is questionable, it should be pointed out that if the varus deformity is associated with a medial contracture, and there is a significant proximal tibial deformity, the space created by the distal femoral cut (which must be perpendicular to the mechanical axis of the femur) will necessarily be trapezoidal with a large lateral side. This means that a medial release will be mandatory to achieve a perfect balance in extension. But, secondarily, this may produce medial laxity in flexion, which will be detrimental if an externally rotated femoral cut is routinely performed (removing more bone from the medial condyle) (fig. 6).

In a genu valgum with medial laxity due to overstretching, the situation is different. In this case, even though an externally rotated femoral cut is advisable, it must remove less bone from the lateral posterior condyle and not more bone from the medial posterior condyle. Externally rotating the femoral component contributes to the ligament balance in flexion since the lateral release that is necessary to achieve adequate balance will increase the flexion gap laterally. In these cases, frequently associated with lateral subluxation of the patella and contracture of the lateral retinaculum, external rotation of the femoral component is, indeed, effective in improving patella kinematics.

– *Correcting laxity in extension by lowering the distal femoral cut.* This option which is offered with some instrument systems, has the advantage (as we shall see further on) of avoiding elevation of the joint line and lowering of the patella, contrary to the correction that is achieved by increasing the thickness of the tibial component. However, this option authorizes the use of a thinner PE component in extension which may prove insufficient to provide adequate stability in the sagittal plane in flexion. Then, the use of a posterior stabilized implant will be necessary.

– *Sectioning the PCL intraoperatively.* Some recent knee systems include ultra-congruent component options. Being initially reserved for cruciate-substituting rotating knees, they were later on proposed by some designers for use with cruciate-retaining knees, adding anterior-posterior sliding to rotation. Anterior-posterior sliding allows the femur to move posteriorly on the tibial component during flexion. Besides the fact that this often results in a paradoxical motion which is the very opposite of what is wanted (fig. 7) and which has been described by Matsuda and Whiteside (8), some authors recommend that the PCL be secondarily sacrificed if it does not function properly during trialing. Their argument is that the conforming design of the tibial component provides the necessary stability even if the PCL is eventually sacrificed. However, we think it important to point out that sectioning the PCL results in 4 to 5mm (on average) widening of the flexion gap only. Then, there is a high risk of having a knee that is stable in extension and loose in flexion (4mm represents the increment between two PE component thicknesses). Therefore, if the surgeon does not opt for a thicker PE component, there is a high risk of dislocation in flexion after the PCL has been sectioned, and if it does, there is a risk of flexion contracture.

Obviously, the causes and consequences of ligament imbalance are numerous and complex. We thought these had to be analysed before tackling the difficult problem of correction of laxity.

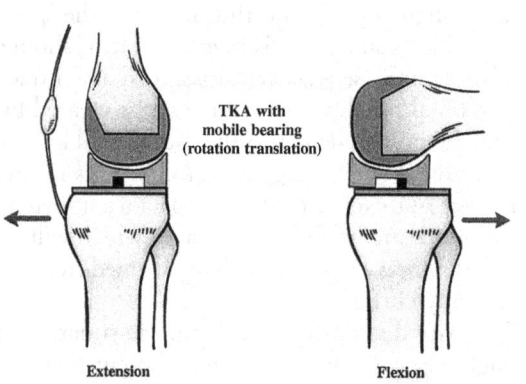

TKA with
mobile bearing
(rotation translation)

Extension

Flexion

Fig. 7. – Anterior-posterior sliding: reverse paradoxical movement.

Correction of laxity in TKA

There are two types of problems and associated consequences:
  – Should the PCL be retained or sacrificed?
  – From a technical point of view, is it more appropriate to increase the thickness of the PE tibial component or change the position of the femoral component?

Retention/sacrifice of the PCL

First of all, it must be pointed out that the resections that are necessary for insertion of a TKR create a gap between the femur and the tibia. Because of the flexion-extension range of motion, there are (schematically) two gaps: an extension gap and a flexion gap. These two gaps are delimited by ligamentous structures.

In the absence of laxity, the gap created by the bone cuts is filled with prosthetic material. The components are intended to replace exactly the amount of bone that has been resected (fig. 8 **a.**).

In contrast, where there is some laxity, any soft tissue release will artificially increase the tibiofemoral space (height L representing the amount of laxity) (fig. 8 **b.** and **c.**). In this case, the prosthetic components will not only have to compensate the resection, but they will also have to fill the additional space resulting from the soft tissue release. This correction can be achieved either by moving the femoral component to a more distal position or by selecting a thicker PE component. Each of these options has specific consequences on the joint line level and ligament tensioning both in extension and flexion. Ideally, one should achieve equal and symmetrical spaces with balanced ligaments both in extension and flexion.

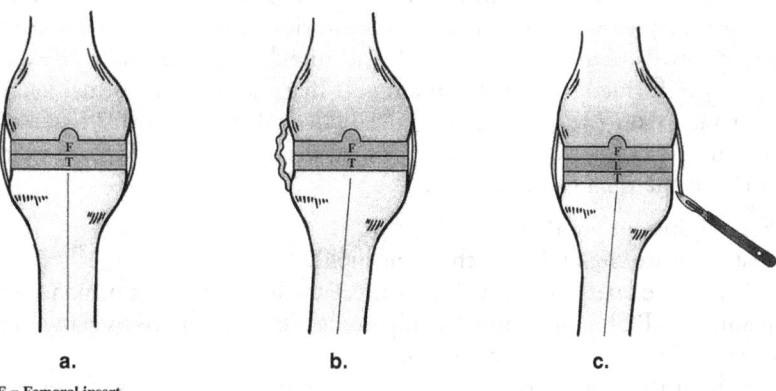

a.   **b.**   **c.**

F = Femoral insert
T = Tibial insert

Fig. 8. – a. In the absence of a laxity, the prosthetic components will fill the space created by the bone cuts.
b. In the presence of a laxity, filling the space with prosthetic material is not sufficient to correct the laxity.

Three situations must be avoided:
– coronal laxity in extension which produces instability;
– excessive tightness of one compartment in flexion which may result in
stiffness;
– anterior/posterior laxity in flexion (risk of dislocation).

Regarding the flexion gap, we think it is essential to achieve at least medial
compartment stability. In the case of an asymmetrical flexion gap (imbalance
between the lateral and medial ligamentous structures), the procedure will
depend on the ligament tensioning status in extension:
– either the extension gap also is asymmetrical: soft tissue balancing should
be resumed;
– or the extension gap is symmetrical, that is, there is no laxity in extension:
a mild laxity in flexion can be ignored as long as the medial compartment is
stable, with no excessive tightness.

PCL sacrifice

In this case, the rules of ligament balancing are very simple: lengthening of the
ligaments on the concave side until they are equal both in length and tension
to those on the convex side.

These procedures have identical and symmetrical effects on the flexion and
extension gaps. Only the way of correcting the laxity will affect the level of the
joint line and the amount of tension on the peripheral ligaments in extension
and flexion. But, we shall revert to this further on.

A typical example is the genu valgum with medial laxity (fig. 9 **a.** and **b.**).

PCL retention

The PCL is the third element that comes into play in ligament balancing and
makes it more tricky. In this situation, any excessive release on the concave
side is faced with the problem of the limited length of the PCL. It is not possible, contrary to what was done in the previous case, to simply release the
tight concave side to balance it with the stretched convex side. If excessive
release is performed, that is, to an amount that exceeds the normal length of
the ligaments on the concave side, the PCL will become overstretched and
stiff, acting as a "presser foot" (fig. 9 **c.** and **d.**) which will cause anterior dislocation of the tibia (no LCA) (6).

Several options are then available :
– also release the PCL, which seems highly hazardous;
– ignore the laxity, which will also affect the long-term performance of the
implant. The PCL alone cannot compensate a coronal laxity, as shown in the
history of chronic anterior laxity (4);
– tighten the ligaments on the convex side (fig. 9 **e.**). We shall review the
limitations of these techniques in a next section.

However, it should be pointed out that in the presence of a laxity on the
convex side of the deformity, independent of its cause (overstretching and/or
bone cuts), retention of the PCL leads to technical imperfections or uncertain

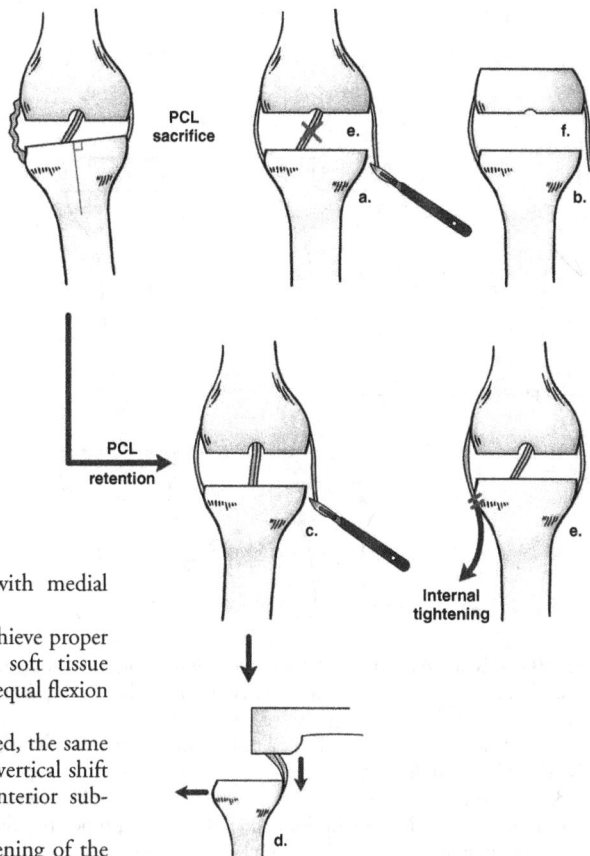

Fig. 9. – Genu valgum with medial laxity.
a. & **b.** PCL sacrificed to achieve proper balance of the peripheral soft tissue through lateral release, with equal flexion and extension gaps.
c. & **d.** If the PCL is retained, the same lateral release will induce a vertical shift of the PCL resulting in anterior sub-luxation of the tibia.
e. The only option is tightening of the medial structures.

options. This is the reason why, in this situation at least, we routinely sacrifice the PCL as advocated in many publications (1, 8, 10-12).

Correction of a laxity

– Thicker PE component (fig. 10 **c.** and **c.'**)

It is the most common method of correction of a laxity: it is simple, and a thicker PE component has the advantage of affecting both the flexion and extension gaps.

Unfortunately, where there is severe laxity, particularly in the valgus knee, this method induces elevation of the joint line relative to the tibial attachments of the ligaments. Furthermore, bone distraction results in lowering of the patella via the patellar tendon. Elevation of the joint line combined with traction on the patellar tendon may eventually result in a patella baja which generates postoperative pain (9), all the more as correction of a laxity is always associated with leg lengthening which stretches the extensor mechanism.

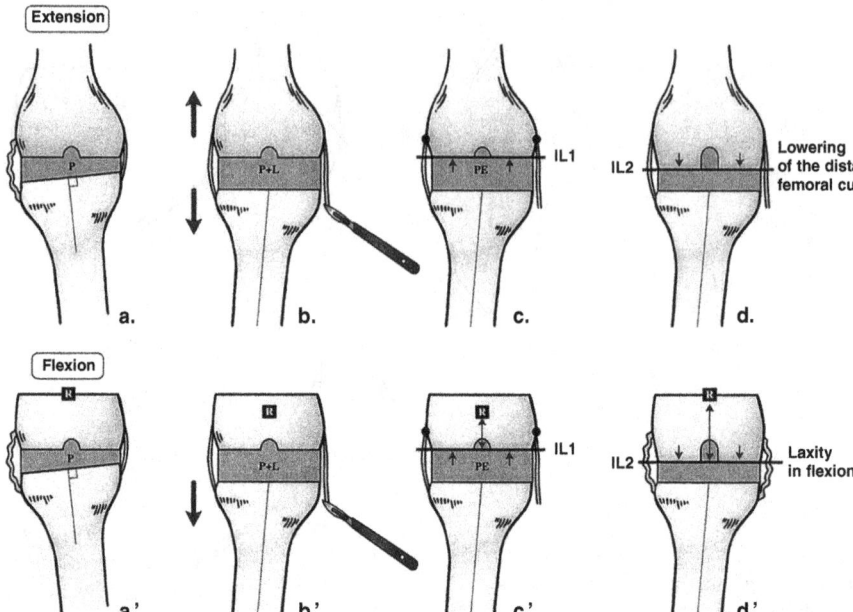

Fig. 10 – a. & a.': Asymmetrical space resulting from ligament stretching-contracture and bone cuts.
b. & b.': Increased flexion and extension gaps, due to ligament release performed on the concave side of the deformity.
c. & c.': Space filled with a thicker tibial component, which results in elevation of the joint line (IL1) and patella baja.
d. & d.': Proper balance achieved in extension through lowering of the distal femoral cut. This allows restoration of the joint line (IL2) and proper patella level. However, some residual laxity may persist in flexion, which will require the use of a posterior stabilized prosthesis.

– Moving the femoral component to a more distal position (Fig. 10 **d.** and **d.'**)

This has always been our favourite method with the HLS® total knee prosthesis (TORNIER, Saint-Ismier, France).

It consists in performing the distal femoral cut at a late stage of the procedure, after ligament balancing. Correction of a laxity is achieved by lowering the distal femoral cut level instead of increasing the thickness of the PE component. The main advantage of this method is that, in the presence of a laxity, the joint line and the patella are equally lowered, which eliminates the risk of inducing or worsening a patella baja.

But this method has no effect on the flexion gap. Where there is severe laxity, the PE component may not be thick enough in flexion, which will require the use of a posterior stabilized implant. Therefore, when performing extensive release in extension, it is recommended to always check again the flexion gap afterwards, using spacers. This way, any significant increase in the flexion gap resulting from the releases performed in extension will not be overlooked. Therefore, the distal cut level will be set according to the PE thickness that is required to stabilize the knee in flexion. This will ensure symmetrical flexion and extension gaps, in all cases.

Now, one must admit that in the presence of a laxity, no TKR will restore a perfect joint line, except a highly constrained prosthesis which can contour the problem of ligament balance.

– Retention of the PCL is the worst solution because it implies some "trade-offs" which affect the durability of the implant, and this is incompatible with today's requirements.

– Sacrifice of the PCL using a regular posterior stabilized device is a wiser, simple option. But it means increasing the amount of prosthetic material to compensate both the laxity and bone resections, which results in leg lengthening (by an average of 4mm).

– Increasing the thickness of the PE component may induce or worsen a patella baja. The resulting detrimental effect cumulates with stretching of the extensor mechanism due to leg lengthening.

– Moving the femoral component to a more distal position avoids lowering of the patella. But the flexion gap needs to be carefully checked again after the soft tissue releases so as to avoid a laxity in flexion (which will not be fully controlled with posterior stabilization).

Ligament balancing procedures

General considerations

Two types of procedures can be performed.

Soft tissue release

This interests the ligaments located on the concave side of the deformity. It has been extensively discussed in the English literature and the word "release" is now commonly used in French publications.

Soft tissue releases include capsular-periosteal detachments as is performed on the tibia in the varus knee, and transections as is the case for the popliteal tendon or LCL in the valgus knee, or the posterior capsule in a flexion contracture. Capsular-periosteal detachments have a more progressive and controlled relaxing effect than transections which may have more severe effects than what was expected. This is the reason why a detailed description of the sequential release procedure is necessary. Furthermore, this will be different whether the contracture is on the medial or lateral side, and whether it is performed on the femur or the tibia. Whereas medial release procedures seem to be routinely standardized, lateral release procedures are not, as will be shown.

Retensioning procedure

Actually, a few lateral tensioning procedures were described in the early days of modern TKRs, but none of them showed long-term efficacy.

Only medial tensioning procedures which specifically address residual laxity after correction of a genu valgum are still described in the literature (15).

Although some authors state that these procedures lose their efficacy in the long run because they are performed on weakened tissue, we think that they should be considered on condition that precise technical rules are defined and adhered to. In particular, one should be careful to perform a perfect release on the concave side of the deformity, because excessive tightness will promote recurrence of the laxity.

At last, whether a release or tensioning procedure is performed, restoration of axial alignment is a prerequisite to ensure long-term success of the arthroplasty.

Two situations must be avoided:
– try to palliate a residual laxity or protect a ligament reconstruction by overcorrecting a deformity as is done in an osteotomy;
– compensate a ligament contracture by undercorrecting the alignment during frontal bone cuts.

Soft tissue balancing in the genu varum

Contrary to the genu valgum, medial releases are standardized (type and sequence). They are always performed on the tibial side (anteromedial aspect of the tibia). The releases are performed in an anterior-posterior direction as follows:

1) anterior capsule;
2) deep MCL and meniscal attachments;
3) semimembranosus;
4) medial posterior capsule.

Release of the superficial MCL or pes anserinus is very rare. This is, indeed, a major release. Because it affects much more the flexion gap than the extension gap, it may cause laxity in flexion and thus compromise the stability of the implant in flexion (16). Only severe deformities may require release of the MCL from its tibial attachment; should the case occur, it will be performed in the first place, prior to any other medial release, and only if there is a severe contracture in flexion (17).

Due to the risk of instability that is associated with excessive release of the medial structures, it is advisable to determine and plan – as much as possible – the amount of release that will be necessary to achieve adequate soft tissue balance. Johnson et al. (18) noted that where a deformity greater than 10° in extension could be corrected in flexion, no release was necessary. Instead, they propose a test called the "CLEFT" test (Collateral Ligament Flexion Extension Test) which assists in evaluating the need for a release.

This theoretical analysis shows that medial contracture and true lateral laxity are most infrequent in the genu varum. Most ligament asymmetries occurring in this type of deformity are associated with bone deformities (tibia vara). 90° tibial cuts create an asymmetrical trapezoidal space because more bone is removed from the lateral than the medial tibial condyle. This results in a pseudo lateral laxity (due to bone cuts), and a pseudo medial contracture that may be worsened in case of severe downward tibial slope. In such cases, if the tibial cut has been measured in the midportion of the lateral tibial condyle, it may be insufficient to allow the insertion of the smallest tibial trial (fig. 11).

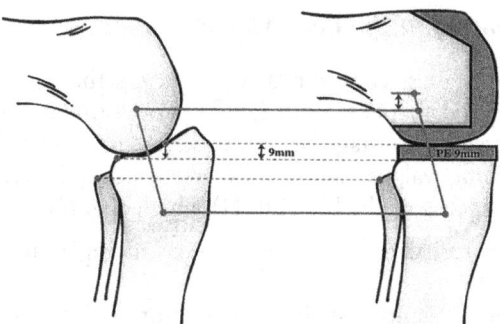

Fig. 11. – Significant posterior slope that will induce insufficient tibial resection if the tibial cut is measured in the midportion of the tibial plateau.

In this situation, a medial release will result in excessive lengthening of the medial ligamentous structures, elevation of the joint line and lowering of the patella. Furthermore, in cases where the PCL has been retained, the PCL will shift toward a vertical position, inducing anterior subluxation of the tibial plateau (Fig. 9 **c.** and **d.**).

As far as we are concerned, determination and planning of medial releases in the genu varum are based on the preoperative X-rays.

The standing AP and lateral full-length X-rays show the mechanical axis of the tibia and the tibial slope. If the measurements reveal a severe deformity and the tibial cut has been measured in the midportion of the tibial plateau, a thicker resection will be necessary (e.g., 10 or 11mm for a templated 9mm tibial component). In the case of a moderate deformity (mechanical axis superior to 85°, slope inferior to 5°), a more conservative resection should be performed (inferior to 9mm for a templated 9mm tibial component).

These X-rays may be completed with stress views (forced valgus) to better appreciate the reducibility of the deformity.

– If the deformity can be reduced and the tibial cut does not permit the insertion of the smallest spacer block, the first thing to do prior to any soft tissue procedure, is to recut the proximal tibia.

– If the deformity cannot be reduced, one must check for any ligament imbalance in extension. Should the lateral compartment gape in extension, a medial release will have to be performed, incrementally and carefully, until proper balance is achieved in extension. Then, either the spacer block can be inserted in flexion without any excessive tension on the medial ligaments, and proper balance is achieved, or the smallest spacer block still does not go into the space, and the proximal tibia needs to be recut by a few millimetres.

At this stage of the discussion, it is necessary to define the amount of tibial deformity that can be corrected and balanced by a simple balancing procedure. According to some surgeons, any coronal tibial deformity in excess of 10° should be managed with a high valgus tibial osteotomy in association with the total knee arthroplasty (19,20).

Soft tissue balancing in the genu valgum

The genu valgum is a less common deformity than the genu varum. As it is much better tolerated, patients with lateral compartment osteoarthritis will often present quite late, at a stage where the disease is associated with ligament overstretching. Some valgus deformities are associated with an ipsilateral developmental dysplasia of the hip (DDH) which aggravates the stretching.

The worst case scenario where ligament balancing is really challenging, combines :

– dysplasia predominantly involving the femur, with hypoplasia of the lateral condyle both posteriorly and distally;

– medial ligament stretching which reveals itself in the early stages of flexion, and is characterized in combined hip/knee cases by the tibia in flexion-external rotation;

– lateral ligament contracture often occurring after a few years.

This allows to understand the technical goals of ligament balancing in this particular case.

– In terms of bone reconstruction, restoration of the joint line mainly involves the femur. It can be achieved by : moving the femoral component to a more distal position to correct the laxity resulting from bone cuts, in extension, and externally rotating the femoral component to compensate the hypoplasia of the posterior lateral condyle. It is important to emphasize that external rotation of the femoral component should be achieved by resecting less bone from the lateral posterior condyle and not by resecting more bone from the medial posterior condyle, which would increase the medial laxity in flexion. There is no risk of generating excessive pressure since a lateral release is systematically performed.

– As regards ligament balancing procedures, and more particularly correction of medial laxity, it should be reminded that stretching will best reveal itself in the early stages of flexion. This is frequently observed a few months postoperatively, which explains the recurrence of medial "yawnings" in knees which initially seemed to be perfectly balanced (fig. 2). Therefore, achieving stability in full extension should not be considered sufficient in severe valgus deformities. A perfect balance should be achieved both in extension and in 20° of flexion; in this position, "yawning" is not permissible. A knee that spontaneously gapes in 20° of flexion indicates that lateral release has been insufficient; if this occurs only on forced valgus, it means that the medial ligamentous structures are somewhat slack, and a tightening procedure may be considered.

Lateral release procedures

There is no real consensus regarding these procedures.

Hereunder are suggested procedures:

– release of the lateral collateral ligament (LCL) and popliteal tendon from their attachments to the femoral condyle;

– release of the tensor fascia lata from its attachment to the Gerdy tubercle;

– sectioning of the lateral posterior capsule;

– release of the biceps femoris has been given up by many authors.

As far as we are concerned, we have tried several methods and have found that the most reliable procedure is that recommended by Whiteside (17) :

– in cases where there is a contracture both in flexion and extension, release the popliteal tendon and LCL from their femoral attachments;

– if there is a residual contracture in extension, release the tensor fascia lata from its tibial attachment, and then section the lateral posterior capsule using scissors or a scalpel.

In our experience, the use of a distractor in extension has proved most helpful to perform a step-by-step balancing. The instrument that we are currently using (HLS® TORNIER) allows to determine the thickness of the distal femoral cut only after proper balance in flexion and extension has been achieved, which meets the requirements of femoral bone reconstruction, as previously discussed.

It is important to point out that the medial release must be limited to the amount that is necessary to expose and dislocate the knee joint in an antero-medial approach. This is why some authors advocate the anterolateral approach (Keblish approach). Its main advantage is that it does not compromise the medial compartment, but exposure is more difficult and often requires elevation of the tibial tubercle. Furthermore, it does not permit any medial tightening procedure.

Medial tightening procedures

Medial tightening procedures have recently been redefined by Munjal and Krackow (16). However, these procedures raise very little enthusiasm because of some reported failures. As a matter of fact:

– efficacy and reliability of medial tightening is very much dependent on whether sufficient lateral release has been performed;

– medial tightening should be performed on strong soft tissue, preferably the anterior portion of the medial capsuloligamentous structures, to be effective in the early stages of flexion;

– medial tightening should not restrict the range of motion and cause stiffening of the knee joint.

This is why we think that proximal tightening (femoral) is associated with the risk of stiffening due to the development of medial condylar adhesions.

Only distal tightening (tibia) seems acceptable to us. However, to be efficient, it must stabilize the knee in the position where laxity usually occurs, that is, in 20 to 30° of flexion, not in full extension. But, in this position, it is the most anterior fibers of the capsule and MCL that come into play and stabilize the medial compartment, not the MCL itself.

Two years ago, we started to perform medial tightening procedures in knees which are stable in full extension, but will gape in mild flexion. With the knee positioned in 20° of flexion and varus-internal rotation, we tighten the anterior lip of the capsule inferiorly and anteriorly and fix it with one or two staples (fig. 12). Since we have been doing this, we have not observed any spontaneous gape as may be seen on postoperative standing X-rays taken in slight flexion-external rotation, which is a typical posture in patients with a long-standing fixed valgus deformity (fig. 12).

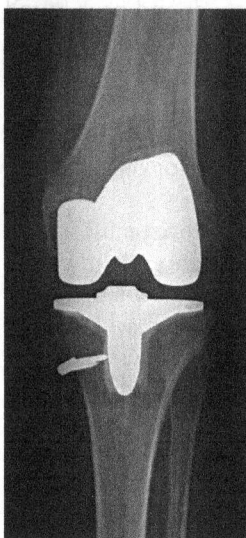

Fig. 12. – Anteromedial capsular tightening.

Soft tissue balancing in the presence of a flexion contracture

Flexion contracture can have several causes:

– Intra-articular mechanical causes such as a wedge-shaped bone block due to osteoarthritis or sequelae of an articular fracture. Bone resections and joint debridement which are performed in TKA will readily eliminate the flexion contracture;

– Extra-articular mechanical causes such as malunion in the sagittal plane. When the extra-articular flexion contracture is greater than 10°, a deflexion osteotomy should be considered. However, where an osteotomy is associated with the arthroplasty, one must carefully select the implant to be used and the intramedullary fixation method, particularly for femoral osteotomies;

– Contracture of the posterior capsule, which is predominantly seen in inflammatory rheumatism, is the third cause. In the absence of a predominant intra- or extra-articular mechanical cause of a severe flexion contracture, it may be interesting to try and reduce the deformity preoperatively using physical therapy.

In addition to the osteotomy that may be required to correct a malunion, some specific release procedures may be necessary. But these can only be considered after posterior debridement has been performed. These include transection or release of the capsule from its attachment to the femoral condyle.

One should always bear in mind that the vessels in the popliteal fossa are very close by and that this release should be performed on a flexed knee. One will seldom recut the femur to correct a flexion contracture; this should be performed as a last resort, after all the posterior releases are completed.

But it is also true that postoperative rehabilitation alone cannot possibly correct a residual flexion contracture.

Conclusion

Soft tissue balancing in total knee arthroplasty is a rather complex subject which includes both conceptual and technical data. We thought it was important to analyse these two aspects because this surgical step is, indeed, critical to the clinical success of a total knee replacement.

Also, we think it is indispensable to understand that the goals and effects of the procedures performed may vary according to the knee prosthesis that is selected. As a matter of fact, knowing this may help select the implant design that will best address the specific needs of a patient.

References

1. Pagnano MW, Hanssen AD, Lewallen DG et al. (1998) Flexion instability after primary posterior cruciate retaining Total Knee Arthroplasty. Clin Orthop 356: 39-46
2. Matsuda S, Miura H, Nagamine R et al. (1999) Knee stability in posterior cruciate ligament retaining Total Knee Arthroplasty. Clin Orthop 366: 169-73
3. Neyret Ph, Dejour H (1991) Axes, Équilibrage ligamentaire. 7ᵉ Journées Lyonnaises de Chirurgie du Genou. Lyon 290-8
4. Dejour H, Deschamps G, Walch G et al. (1987) Arthrose du genou sur laxité chronique antérieure. Rev Chir Orthop 73: 157-70
5. Caton J, Boulahia A, Patricot LM (1999) Histoire naturelle du ligament croisé postérieur dans les gonarthroses. In: Chambat P, Neyret Ph, Deschamps G (eds) Chirugie prothétique du genou. Montpellier: Sauramps médical 305-8
6. Julliard R (1991) Communications particulières, 65ᵉ réunion annuelle de la SOFCOT. Paris Rev Chir Orthop 77 (suppl 1): 161
7. Moreland JR, Bassett LW, Hanker GJ (1987) Radiographic analysis of the axial alignment of the lower extremity. J Bone Joint Surg 69 (A): 745-9
8. Matsuda S, Whiteside LA, White SE et al. (1999) Knee stability in meniscal bearing Total Knee Arthroplasty. J Arthroplasty 14: 82-90
9. Deschamps G (2001) L'interligne prothétique lors du changement. Ph Burdin, D Huten. Les Reprises de Prothèses Totales de Genou. Symposium. Rev Chir Orthop 87 suppl 5 IS: 186-91
10. Stiehl JB, Komistek RD, Dennis DA et al. (1995) Fluoroscopic analysis of kinematics after posterior cruciate retaining knee arthroplasty. J Bone Joint Surg 77B: 884-9
11. Dennis DA, Komistek RD, Hoff WA (1996) In vivo knee kinematics derived using an inverse perspective technique. Clin Orthop 331: 107-17
12. Wilson SA, Mc Cann PD, Gotlin RS et al. (1996) Comprehensive gait analysis in posterior stabilized knee arthroplasty. J Arthroplasty 11: 359-67
13. Laskin RS (1996) The Insall Award. Total Knee Replacement with Posterior Cruciate Ligament Retention in Patients with a Fixed Varus Deformity. Clin Orthop 331: 29-34
14. Dennis DA, Komistek RD, Colwell CE Jr et al. (1998) In vivo anteroposterior femorotibial translation of total knee arthroplasty: a multicenter analysis. Clin Orthop 356: 47-57

15. Munjal S, Krackow KA (2000) Surgery of the medial collateral ligament in patients under-going Total Knee Replacement. Medscape Orthopaedics and Sports Medicine 4
16. Mihalko NW, Miller C, Krackow KA (2000) Total Knee Arthroplasty ligament balancing and gap kinematics with Posterior Cruciate ligament sacrifice and preservation. Am J Orthop 29 (8): 610-6
17. Krackow KA, Mihalko WM (1999) The effect of medial release on flexion and extension gaps in cadaveric knees: implications for soft tissue balancing in Total Knee Arthroplasty. Am J Knee Surg 12(4): 222-8
18. Johnson R, Barry K, Elloy MA (1994) The Collateral Ligament Flexion Extension Test (CLEFT) in Total Knee Replacement. J R Coll Surg Edinb 39: 127-30
19. Neyret Ph, Zanone X, Ait Si Selmi T (1999) Prothèse totale du genou et ostéotomie tibiale simultanées pour genu varum excessif. In: Chambat P, Neyret Ph, Deschamps G (eds) Chirugie prothétique du genou. Montpellier: Sauramps médical 259-66
20. Franceschina MJ, Swienckowski JJ (1999) Correction of varus deformity with tibial flip autograft technique in Total Knee Arthroplasty. J Arthroplasty 14: 172-4
21. Wihteside LA (1999) Selective ligament release in Total Knee Arthroplasty of the knee in valgus. Clin Orthop 367: 130-40

Extensor mechanism related complications in total knee arthroplasty
Diagnosis – Treatment – Prevention

P. Beaufils

For many reasons, management of patella in total knee arthroplasty is an important issue:

– The natural or prosthetic patellofemoral joint is subjected to tremendous compressive or shear forces, up to 8 times the body weight, and these forces may exceed the strength of polyethylene (61);

– Contact areas between the patellar component and the trochlear groove are always smaller than in the normal patellofemoral joint; this is true for all patellar designs (21% according to Rand) (55);

– Kinematics of a prosthetic patellofemoral joint during flexion does not reproduce the kinematics of a normal knee. One of the differences is the medial contact that occurs in the prosthetic joint (63, 64);

– Patellofemoral joint is an integral part of the knee joint and cannot be isolated. There are inseparable interactions between the tibiofemoral joint and the patellofemoral joint: any tibiofemoral malpositioning may adversely affect the patellofemoral kinematics;

– At last, no patellar component design is able to address the anatomic spectrum of the trochlear groove and patella (25).

Because currently available designs are unable to meet all the above requirements, a trade-off is inevitable, which partly explains the frequency of patellofemoral complications after total knee arthroplasty: instability, polyethylene wear, loosening, osteolysis, tendon rupture, or patella fracture.
Patellofemoral complications, or insufficient results due to the patellofemoral joint, are a very common cause of surgical revision (1, 5, 10, 15, 19, 33, 55). Actually, this etiology is the second most important cause of revision, just after loosening and before instability or stiffness (18%) (10, 20). In spite of favorable factors including: improvements made in knee replacement designs (21, 46, 52, 62), decrease in the need for lateral retinacular release (contributor to devascularization) (57), better understanding of the relationship between position of the femoral and tibial components and patellar complications (2, 11), the rate of patellofemoral complications is still high; in our prospective evaluation performed between September 1999 and June 2000, they were still responsible for 15% of TKR revisions (10, 20).

Patella resurfacing versus non-resurfacing

In view of these complications, many authors (7, 16, 17, 24, 26, 35, 42) suggested to leave the patella unresurfaced. However, this continues to be controversial as it means using a femoral component with a "patella-friendly" design.

Non-resurfacing is usually accompanied by peripheral denervation through circumferential sectioning of the synovium, and some surgeons also perform a spongialization procedure.

Results remain a subject of controversy. Some surgeons are convinced that resurfacing yields a better outcome (16, 24), whereas others consider that similar results (7, 26, 35) or even better results are achieved with non-resurfacing (17). In 1988, Lindstrand (43) presented the results from the Swedish Register for Osteoarthritis (table I). The number of surgical revisions is the same whether the patella has been resurfaced or not. Of course, complications are different: pain (7) and instability in the non-resurfaced group; instability, loosening, pain, and fracture in the resurfaced group.

It can be concluded that:

– patella resurfacing is mandatory in patients with inflammatory arthritis;
– patella resurfacing is desirable in arthritic patients with a severely worn or lateralized patella;
– in all other cases, the natural patella may be retained provided that a "patella-friendly" femoral component design is used (1).

Table I – Revision of TKR: data from the Swedish Register (Lindstrand [43]).

	Number non-resurfaced	Number Resurfaced
Total	10,928	5,139
Surgical revision	168	82
Revision for patellar problem	99	36
Patellar pain	78	4
Patellar instability	21	–
Component dislocation	–	14
Component loosening	–	11
Component failure	–	5
Patellar fracture	–	2
Type of procedure		
Secondary implantation	91	–
Realignment	8	10
Revision of patellar component	–	15
Removal of patellar component	–	11

Patellofemoral complications and treatement

Patellofemoral complications include:

- functional instability;
- pain;
- rupture of the extensor mechanism: patella fracture or tendon rupture.

Functional instability almost always manifests itself by dislocation, whether permanent or occasional.

Patella-related anterior knee pain may occur:

- in knees with a non-resurfaced patella;
- in patients with a well-fixed patellar component;
- in patients with confirmed patellar loosening.

At last, ruptures of the extensor mechanism, whether acute (from trauma) or progressive, can be divided into patella fractures and ruptures of the patellar tendon or quadriceps tendon.

Excluding the latter which are a specific problem, patellofemoral complications can be managed either with a special extensor mechanism procedure or with replacement of the femoral and tibial components. Preoperative planning requires, in addition to standard X-rays, a CT scan assessment (in all the cases) to evaluate any malrotation of the femoral and/or tibial component.

Dislocations

They are easy to identify since there is a permanent, occasional, or habitual dislocation of the patella (fig. 1).

Radiological assessment allows evaluation of the degree of anatomic involvement. In the series presented during the SOFCOT Meeting (10), the average tilt was 26° and the lateral shift 30mm.

Isolated extensor mechanism procedures include medial displacement of the tibial tuberosity which may be combined with a proximal soft tissue procedure (38, 45, 63) or an isolated soft tissue procedure; exceptionally, patellectomy will be performed if it is impossible to reposition the patella.

Evidence of rotational malpositioning of the femoral and/or tibial component requires replacement of the prosthesis.

Clinical results are rather modest (30% relief of pain). Patellar tracking is restored in only 50% of the cases: Where components are replaced, or where a combined tibial tuberosity and soft tissue procedure is performed. An isolated procedure involving either the tibial tuberosity or the soft tissues usually does not restore patellar tracking.

Furthermore, there is a high risk of complications (about 25%) which mainly involve the extensor mechanism.

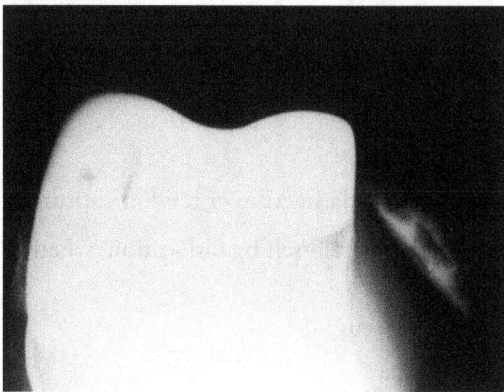

Fig. 1 – Patellar dislocation after TKA.

Pain

Non-resurfaced patella

According to Barrack (7), 10% of non-resurfaced patellae require secondary resurfacing due to residual anterior knee pain or secondary joint space narrowing (fig. 2). Surgical treatment usually consists in implantation of a new cemented all-poly patellar component, which generally gives good clinical results. It is in this group of patients that results of surgical revision are the best, with a low complication rate.

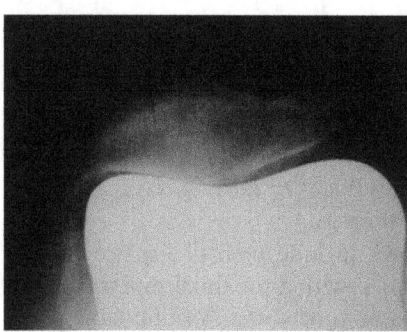

Fig. 2 – Non-resurfaced patella in TKA. Note secondary joint space narrowing.

Patients with a well-fixed patellar component

In these patients, it is very difficult to identify the patella as the source of anterior knee pain, because the anomalies are not always clearly significant. It is generally diagnosed as a lateral impingement (fig. 3a) between the uncovered lateral aspect of the patella and the lateral side of the trochlear groove, even in the absence of tilt or subluxation.

Treatment is partial patellectomy (lateral portion of the patella) and sectioning of the lateral retinaculum in order to eliminate the cause of lateral impingement (fig. 3b). In case of malpositioning of the femoral and/or tibial component, it is recommended to replace them both. In this situation, medial displacement of the tibial tuberosity is not justified.

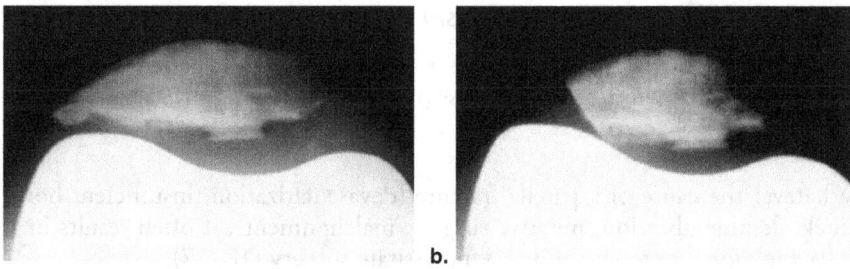

Fig. 3 – a. Impingement between the uncovered lateral aspect of the patella and the trochlear groove of the femoral component.
b. Partial vertical patellectomy of the lateral portion of the patella.

Unfortunately, this gives poor functional results. Actually, the worst results of the patellofemoral series are found in this group of patients, which brings to question the very concept of lateral impingement.

Isolated patellar loosening

Isolated patellar loosening is more frequently seen in metal-backed components (fig. 4) (15% in our series) (8, 10, 39, 44) than in all-poly patellar components (10, 28) (4% in our series [10]).

Complete revision of the prosthesis is often required, particularly if the primary patellar component is metal-backed. This owes to the fact that the trochlear groove of the femoral component is damaged by the metal baseplate of the patellar component.

Patellar procedures (with or without replacement of the femoral and tibial components) are generally limited to replacement of the patellar component whenever sufficient bone stock is available; sometimes, simple removal of the patellar component is performed, alone or combined with a spongialization procedure.

Only fair results are achieved, and the rate of late complications and surgical revision is dramatically high (35%), particularly if isolated patellar procedures are performed.

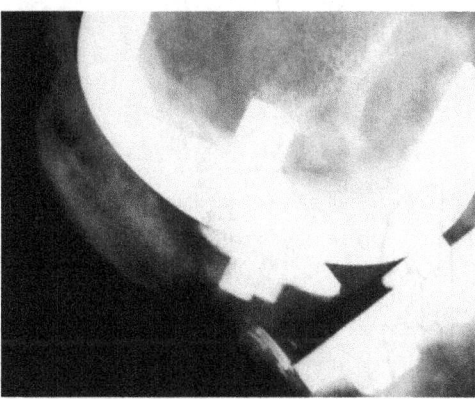

Fig. 4 – Loosening of a metal-backed patellar component.

Rupture of the extensor mechanism

It may be an acute or chronic rupture. In the latter case, the patient will report anterior knee pain and/or gradual loss of active extension.

Patella fracture

Whatever the cause of a patella fracture (devascularization, insufficient bone stock, demineralization, iterative surgery, malalignment), it often results in a poor functional outcome and may necessitate surgery (18, 27).

To evaluate the situation, one must check for continuity of the extensor mechanism and status of the patellar component (well-fixed or loose). These two factors will determine the appropriate treatment option. The Goldberg classification (30) is rather complex and inconsistent with this approach. The classification (40) which is based on evaluation of the continuity of the extensor mechanism is much more appropriate (fig. 5).

Considering that the surgical management of this type of fracture is rather challenging, in patients with satisfactory function and continuity of the extensor mechanism (full active extension), preference should be given to non-oper-

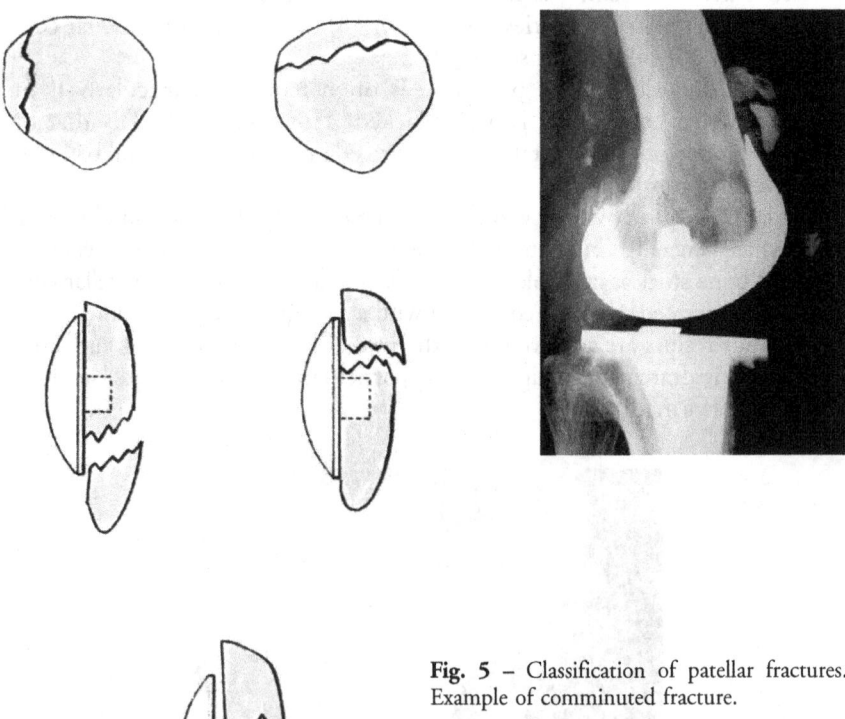

Fig. 5 – Classification of patellar fractures. Example of comminuted fracture.

ative treatment with splinting and full weight bearing until bone union or at least stiff non-union is achieved.

Surgery is indicated in patients with loss of continuity of the extensor mechanism and loss of complete active extension, or in case of locking or pain due to an unstable patellar component. Several surgical treatment options are available:

– partial or complete patellectomy with removal of the patellar component;
– simple removal of the patellar component;
– removal of the patellar component and fixation of the fracture;
– insertion of a new patellar component (exceptionally possible).

In our experience, the lower results achieved with internal fixation compared to simple removal of the patellar component or patellectomy are due to the fact that this technique was used only in patients with true rupture of the extensor mechanism.

Thus, iterative cement fixation of the patellar component never seemed possible in this type of fracture. The treatment of choice is removal of the patellar component, alone or combined with patellectomy (partial or complete) in multifragmentary stellate fractures (40). Internal fixation should be reserved for fractures with complete loss of continuity, knowing that this will likely yield poor results.

In any event, in view of the poor quality of results, one must be very careful when placing the surgical indications. Non-operative treatment should be preferred whenever there is satisfactory knee function and continuity of the extensor mechanism.

Tendon rupture

Rupture of the patellar ligament or quadriceps tendon: this complication tends to occur in multiply operated knees (2nd or 3rd revision). The main reason for consultation is functional instability with active extension lag.

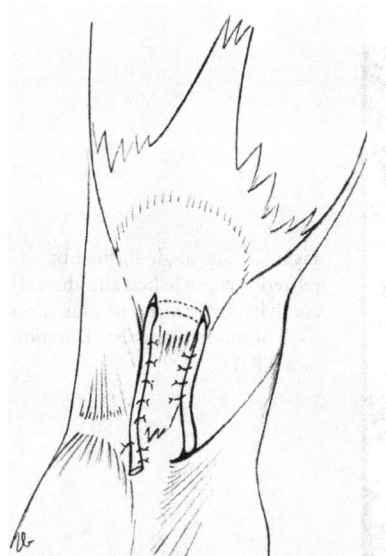

Fig. 6 – Technique of reconstruction of the patellar tendon using hamstring tendons.

Rupture of the patellar ligament which manifests radiographically with patella alta should be managed with sutures reinforced with a tendon graft (medial hamstring tendons in most cases). The tendons remain attached to the tibia and are passed transversely through the patella to provide a supportive frame (19) (fig. 6). Aracil suggested the use of a synthetic ligament (3), Nazarian (49) and Kulkarni (36) the use of extensor mechanism allografts.

Ruptures of the quadriceps tendon are managed with sutures and reinforcement graft, either using the hamstring tendons, or turning over the quadriceps tendon as performed by Bosworth for repair of the Achilles tendon.

In our experience, these procedures have been shown to significantly increase active extension (from -18° to -9°, on average). However, no significant change has been noted in the position of the patella (which is used for evaluation of the stability of the repair).

Conclusion

Excluding rupture of the extensor mechanism, the analysis of patellofemoral complications and subsequent treatment led us to the following conclusions.

Best treatment option: revision total knee arthroplasty or isolated extensor mechanism procedure ?

Any problem involving the extensor mechanism after total knee replacement requires a CT scan to evaluate rotation of the femoral component (fig. 7) and tibial component (Berger (11)). A severe anomaly will require revision of the femoral and/or tibial component.

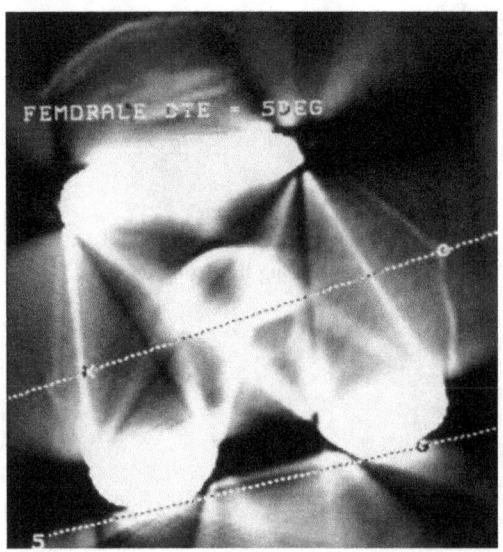

Fig. 7 – The angle formed by the posterior condyle line and the epicondylar axis can be measured on a CT scan, even after implantation of a TKR.

Frequency of complications

Secondary complications after surgical revision for extensor mechanism problems are frequent (about 1 out of 3 cases). The rate of occurrence is the same whether or not the prosthetic components have been replaced, but the distribution depends on the type of complication: in cases where an isolated patellar procedure is performed, the risk of secondary extensor mechanism complications (fracture, tendon rupture, malalignment, loosening) is 25% versus 8% when components are replaced.

Fair clinical results

The best clinical results are achieved with placement of a patellar component in an initially non-resurfaced patella. The poorest results are obtained in patients with well-fixed patellar components: these bad results which are similar to those reported after revision TKA for "unexplained pain" raise the question of the real source of pain (15). The so-called "lateral impingement" should probably be questioned.

Dislocation

Combined procedures (tibial tuberosity + soft tissues), or revision TKA for a confirmed rotational problem, give better results than isolated procedures involving the tibial tuberosity.

Patellar loosening

Patellar loosening is typically associated with a high rate of complication and revision. These are much more frequent when an isolated patellar procedure has been performed. Isolated patellar loosening is a rare entity. Patellar loosening should always prompt a surgeon to investigate for gross loosening of the prosthesis in which patellar loosening would only be an indicator, or to check for patella malpositioning. Anyway, in both situations, revision total knee arthroplasty should be contemplated.

Prerequisite for optimal patelloplasty

The decision to insert a patellar component implies taking into consideration patella non-related factors and pure patella-related factors. Insertion of a patellar component is not a simple and straightforward procedure that is performed at the end of the surgery. Each step of the arthroplasty may influence the success of the patellar resurfacing.

Extrinsic factors include: design of the trochlear groove, rotation of both femoral and tibial components and position of the tibiofemoral joint line.

Patellar factors include type of patellar component (inlay or onlay), component design, positioning on the patellar bone, balance of patellar retinaculi as well as patellar and femoral component sagittal profile.

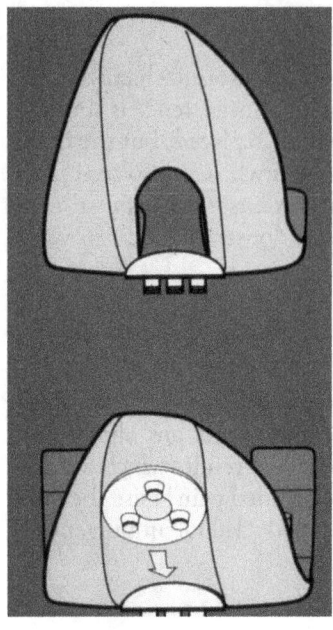

Fig. 8 – Design of the trochlear groove with proximal and lateral obliquity.

Extrinsic factors

Design of the trochlear groove should be as close to anatomy as possible (fig. 8): deepened trochlear groove, particularly at the junction between the trochlea and the condyles, 7° superior-lateral obliquity, prominent lateral flange.

Rotational alignment of the femoral component is a critical step which is meant to:

– balance the flexion gap;

– lateralize the proximal patellar track. It is the trochlear groove that must capture the patella rather than the patella shifting laterally to engage the patellar groove. The importance of external rotation is very controversial. It can be achieved using a special instrument set to a fixed external rotation of 3° or 5° (depending on the instrument system used), or based on balanced collateral ligaments. Personally, we prefer to adjust rotation according to the skeleton morphology in order to position the femoral component parallel to the epicondylar axis. We have shown in a CT scan study the high variability (between 0° and 9°) of the angle formed by the epicondylar axis and the posterior condyle line (13) (fig. 9a). Therefore, it is an illusion to think that correct external rotation can be achieved with preset instruments. It can also be adjusted intraoperatively, based on the epicondylar axis which, however, is difficult to identify. One can also use the anteroposterior axis as described by Whiteside (passing through the deepest part of the patellar groove) which is supposed to be perpendicular to the epicondylar axis. There is one last option which may be preferable: preoperatively measure this angle on a CT scan image (fig. 9b) and then position the femoral component accordingly. In a near future, computer assisted surgery will allow accurate determination of femoral component rotation (CT scan image);

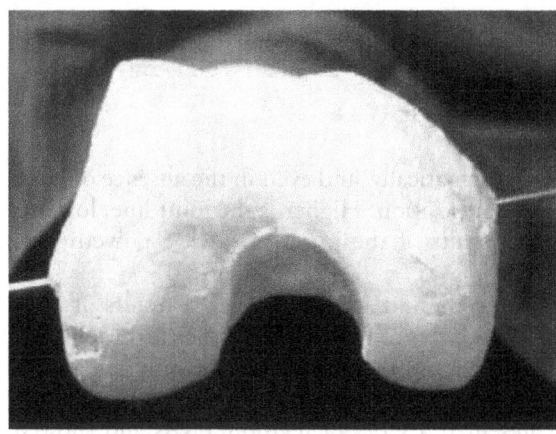

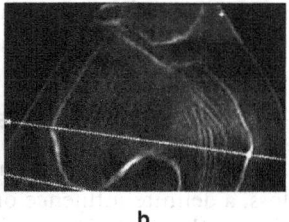

b.

Fig. 9 – a. Anatomic view of the angle formed by the epicondylar axis and the posterior condyle line.
b. CT scan image.

a.

– an externally rotated femoral component should be moved laterally, again, to "capture the patella".

Rotation of the tibial component is equally important (fig. 10). Internal rotation of the tibial tray (which is easier when a medial approach is used) automatically results in lateral shift of the tibial tuberosity, which causes patellar instability. Conversely, excessive external rotation results in medial shift of the tibial tuberosity and provides smooth patellar tracking, but it places the foot in internal rotation. In practice, the midportion of the baseplate is usually aligned with the medial margin of the tibial tubercle. Then, patellofemoral tracking is tested in flexion; increase in baseplate external rotation should be contemplated only if instability persists.

Berger (11) showed how component malrotation can affect patellar stability. Based on a comparison between a TKR group with postoperative patellar

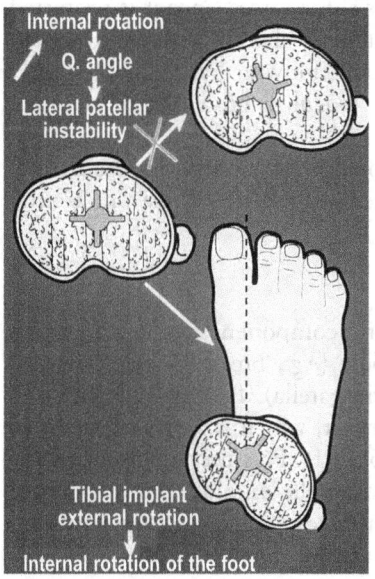

Fig. 10 – Rotation of the tibial component.

symptoms and a symptom-free TKR group, he showed that patellar problems are all the more severe as combined component internal rotation is significant.

Influence of joint line level

Prosthetic joint line level has, mathematically, and even in the absence of bone loss, a definite influence on patellar position. Higher is the joint line, lower is the patella (23). This generally results of the use of a thicker polyethylene insert to correct laxity.

There is no consensus regarding the impact on functional results of knee arthroplasty. Partington (51), in his series of revision total knee arthroplasties, noted that a joint line elevation of more than 8mm significantly affects the functional outcome. During the SOFCOT meeting headed by P. Burdin and D. Huten, Deschamps (23) presented a series of revision TKAs and showed that the joint line level influences the functional outcome through lowering of the patella, particularly in knees with patella baja. He concluded that:

– elevation of the joint line causes or aggravates patella baja, and adversely affects the functional outcome;

– patella baja is extremely difficult to treat with simple adjustment of the joint line level;

– maybe specific extensor mechanism procedures should be considered to treat severe patella baja (such as elevation of the tibial tubercle).

Intrinsic factors

Type and design of patellar component

As yet, no study has demonstrated the superiority of the inlay design over the onlay design (29).

The inset patella theoretically sustains less shear forces since it is protected by a natural bony rim. Its main disadvantage is that it requires a certain amount of bone stock. Furthermore, it cannot be fully medialized. At last, part of the patellar bone makes contact with the trochlear groove of the femoral component.

The resurfacing or onlay patella allows for free positioning on the natural patella. However, it sustains high shear forces and needs not just one central fixation peg, but three pegs.

Symmetric versus asymmetric patellar component

Biomechanically (29, 32, 61), an asymmetric component that is congruent with the trochlear groove is more appropriate (*e.g.*, Freeman saddle-shaped patella, sombrero-shaped patella, asymmetric patella). Its chief advantage is that it provides increased patellofemoral contact, which is a crucial factor in wear performance of polyethylene (29, 48, 55, 61). Pressures are dramatically decreased, but shear forces are high: due to patellofemoral congruity, these forces can only apply to the bone-implant interface. This stress concentration will be aggravated by patellar malposition and tilt.

In contrast, the symmetric dome-shaped design as described by Insall (34) and used by many authors (1), maintains a linear contact with the trochlear groove, which produces extremely high "normal" stresses. However, as it is a non-conforming component, shear forces are borne by the joint, sparing the bone-implant interface. At last, persistent tilt will be better tolerated because the symmetric design ensures an even distribution of loads, whatever the amount of tilt.

Patellar component positioning on patellar bone

Malpositioning of a patellar component that results in tilt or lateral shift of the component may have clinical consequences: Trousdale (1998 AAOS meeting) showed that in a series of TKRs with patellar tilt, 52% of the patients underwent revision surgery or complained of anterior knee pain. Malpositioning may also lead to premature wear, particularly in metal-backed components (fig. 4) (39, 59).

Positioning the patellar component as accurately as possible is critical. Implantation of the patellar component requires the same care as femoral and tibial components (6).

The goal is to achieve, after proper balancing of the patellar retinaculi:

– a patellar component that is aligned with the trochlear groove;

– good patellar tracking with the patellar component well centred in the trochlear groove.

On a patellofemoral view:

– Patellar tilt is defined as the angle formed between the proximal patellar track and the resection plane of the patella;

– Patellar shift represents the distance from the middle of the trochlear groove to the middle of the patellar component; direction of the patellar shift, where present, is usually lateral;

– Subluxation is defined as a combination of the previous motions. Isolated tilt is not subluxation, since congruity is maintained;

– M/L patella position of the patellar component relative to the bony patella is defined by the distance between the anatomic center of the bony patella and the center of the patellar component (fig. 11). When the component is centralized, this distance is zero (0). A component is said to be medialized when it rests on the medial aspect of the patella. It is seldom lateralized.

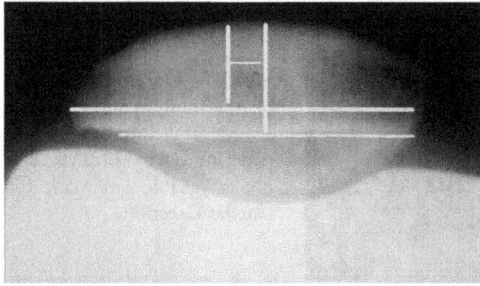

Fig. 11 – Definitions:
M/L patella position: distance between the center of the patellar component and the center of the resected patellar surface. It refers to the position of the component on the patellar bone.

Balanced patellar retinaculi

Sectioning of the lateral retinaculum has long been proposed to palliate mal-positioning of the patellar component. In certain series, more than 30% of the lateral retinacula have been sectioned (55). This was mainly due to the lack of consideration paid to:

– design of the trochlear groove (symmetric or flat);
– rotation of both femoral and tibial components.

Yet, sectioning may be highly detrimental: devascularization of the patella, which may cause fracture or necrosis; medial tilt of the patellar component (57). Early in our experience, we sectioned the lateral retinaculum in 15% of our cases: in this group, the rate of medial tilt greater than 5° was 8.6% versus 2% in the group with intact retinaculum.

Patellar cut

Bindelglass (12), Gomes (31), Ranawat (54), and Rand (55) reported a high rate of residual tilt or shift. Gomes (31) stressed the importance of using accurate instruments to avoid residual tilt. Free-hand cuts resulted in residual tilt of 8.35°. Referencing the cut off the anterior aspect of the patella, which is supposed to be parallel to the proximal patellar track, reduced the tilt to an average of 1.82°.

Actually, the anterior aspect of the patella is not a reliable anatomic landmark (fig. 12). In case of patellar dysplasia – even if there is no tilt – the anterior aspect of the patella may face anterolaterally; using it as a reference would inevitably result in an oblique patellar resection.

Actually, the trochlear plane is the only reliable landmark. Still based on the idea that it is the trochlear groove which "captures" the patellar component rather than the component shifting laterally to engage the patellar groove, it seemed logical to reference the patellar resection off the trochlear groove. In practice, this can be done using a special instrument assembled to the trial femoral component. This instrument provides two fundamental landmarks (fig. 13):

– proximal trochlear plane (guide pins for patellar resection are placed parallel to this plane);
– midline of the prosthetic trochlear groove to correctly position the patellar component relative to the center of the trochlear groove and not to the center of the natural patella.

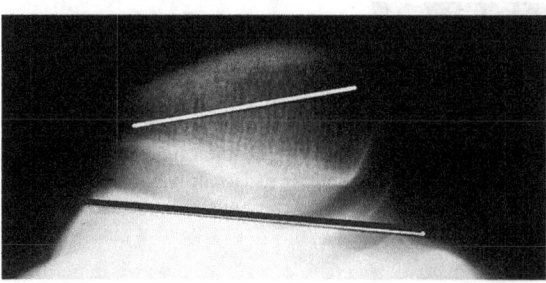

Fig. 12 – The anterior surface of the bony patella is not always parallel to the proximal patellar groove. Therefore, it is not a reliable landmark for patellar resection.

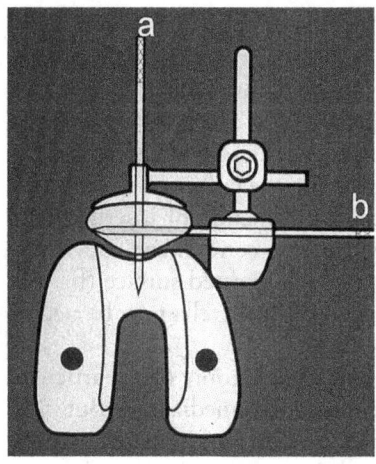

Fig. 13 – The two fundamental landmarks are: **a.** center of the trochlear groove; **b.** plane of the trochlea.

It goes without saying that, as for the tibiofemoral joint, patellar resection must be performed after proper balance of the patellar retinaculi and correct component rotation have been achieved.

The sequence of surgical steps is as follows:

– femoral component insertion (external rotation and lateral positioning);

– tibial component insertion (midportion of the baseplate is aligned with the medial margin of the tibial tubercle);

– resection of patellar osteophytes;

– repositioning of the patellar component on the trial tibial/femoral components, and evaluation of patellofemoral kinematics in flexion. If a tendency to subluxation is noted, one begins by adjusting tibial component rotation. Should subluxation persist, the lateral retinaculum is sectioned. At last, exceptionally, medialization of the tibial tubercle may be necessary.

Once proper balance of the patellar retinaculi and proper component rotation have been achieved, the patellar cut is performed. With the patella well centred in the trochlear groove, a first pin is drilled through the patella into the center of the femoral groove (reference point for central placement of the patellar component), then another two pins are inserted into the patella, parallel to the femoral groove, to mark the patellar resection plane. The thickness of the cut depends on the initial amount of wear.

We used this method (9, 41) and analysed 532 X-rays at 3 months postoperatively: the patellar component was perfectly centred in the trochlear groove in 97.2% of the cases. The average tilt was 0.25° (SD = 2.3°); in 87% of the knees, tilt ranged from -2° to +2°. Interestingly, the postoperative position of the patella was not influenced by the preoperative tilt (if any). As a matter of fact, there was no significant difference in postoperative position between preoperatively centralized, tilted or subluxated patellae, which confirms that this resection system works independently.

M/L position of the patellar component on patellar bone

Insall (34) and Whiteside (63, 64) stressed the necessity to place the component on the medial aspect of the patella. Whiteside demonstrated in a cadaver study that this improves patellar kinematics.

The use of an asymmetric design should theoretically provide better coverage of the resected patellar surface while medializing the center of the component, but we previously pointed out the technical difficulty of inserting this type of component. Medialization of a symmetric component inevitably results in lack of coverage of the lateral aspect of the resected surface (fig. 3). Partial vertical patellectomy of the lateral portion of the patella may be necessary if the uncovered area is too large.

In fact, medial placement is meant to replicate the anatomy of the articular surface of the patella since the patellar crest is most often medialized. But, this is not always the case: in knees with a symmetric kneecap, the patellar component must be centralized and not medialized. In our experience, using the above described instrument, two-thirds of our components were medialized and one-third were centralized.

Patellar component positioning and surgical approach

Which is the best surgical approach in patients with severe preoperative patellar subluxation: medial or lateral approach? The lateral approach described by Keblish or the lateral approach with elevation of the tibial tubercle (but generally without medialization), essentially used in genu valgum, is a good option to get a balanced patella, whether or not there is a valgus deformity.

The medial approach usually requires extensive sectioning of the lateral retinaculum, which ends in almost complete devascularization of the patella (medial arthrotomy + lateral sectioning).

The lateral approach preserves integrity of the medial retinaculum, allows subperiosteal partial patellectomy (lateral portion of the patella) and reattachment of the lateral retinaculum to the patellar periosteum. We have compared two groups of TKRs in patients with severe patellar subluxation (65). Both groups were matched for etiology and preoperative tibiofemoral axis. There was no significant difference in residual shift, but there was a statistically significant difference in tilt in favour of the lateral approach. Considering the low morbidity rate associated with the lateral approach, we have selected to use it in preference to the medial approach.

Prosthetic volume in the sagittal plane

Both thickness of the patellar component (22, 57) and combined A/P dimensions of the femoral and patellar components in the sagittal plane are involved (58).

Patellar thickness

Daluga (22) showed that there is a strong correlation between increased patellar thickness, increased rate of postoperative knee manipulation (under general anesthesia) and decreased flexion ROM.

As a matter of fact, a thicker patella causes excessive tensioning of the retinacula, which results in decreased range of motion and increased contact pressures.

Boisrenoult (14), Oishi (50), and Starr (60) showed in cadaver studies that a 5mm increase in patellar thickness results in 30% increase in the compressive force from 40° of flexion.

Therefore, one must not yield to the temptation of performing a minimal resection just to preserve as much patellar bone as possible. When there is little or no wear, thickness of the resection must be equal to the thickness of the patellar component (this avoids the risk of thickness buildup). Most instruments are designed to provide controlled resection.

It is only in severely worn patellae (less than 12mm thick) where resection would dramatically weaken the bone that a minimal resection is justified: the aim is to restore initial patellar thickness (before wear).

Prosthetic volume in the sagittal plane

Both thickness of the patellar component and anterior-posterior dimension of the femoral component are involved.

Due to the increase in dimensions of femoral components in the sagittal plane, any incorrect size selection may lead to a purely femoral component-related error of several millimetres. Using the anterior surface of the femur or the posterior condyles to determine the size of the femoral component does not change this fact. Influence on range of motion and stresses is the same as that of increased patellar thickness. Combination of these two factors is of course highly deleterious (14, 58).

Conclusion

Patella resurfacing in total knee arthroplasty necessarily implies a trade-off that precludes restoration of normal patellofemoral kinematics. This is the reason why many authors advocate non-resurfacing, either systematically (at least in osteoarthritis) or in specific cases. Both techniques seem to give similar results. Although the rates of insufficient results are almost identical, these insufficient results are different in nature.

The better results achieved with patella resurfacing are attributable to the insertion technique rather than the design of the component: no difference has been noted between inset and onlay patellar components, between symmetric and asymmetric designs, and between constrained and unconstrained designs.

Success of patelloplasty depends on two main factors:

– consideration paid to the close relationship between the patellofemoral joint and the tibiofemoral joint. The knee joint forms a whole. Fixation of the patellar component is only the final step of a global surgical protocol which includes: selection of a femoral component with a suitable trochlear groove; correct external rotation and lateralization of the femoral component; appropriate AP dimension of the femoral component; correct external rotation of the tibial tray; restoration of the joint line level. There is no clear evidence that mobile-bearing designs provided a significant improvement;

– care used in positioning the patellar component: proper balance of patellar retinaculi and bone cut accuracy are as critical as in the previous tibiofemoral steps. In this respect, patellar instruments should not only allow maintenance of patellar thickness, but also perfect centring of the component in the trochlear groove, and correct resection parallel to the proximal patellar track.

Proper application of these principles should help decrease the rate of patella-related complications.

References

1. Aglietti P, Baldini A, Buzzi R et al. (2001) Patella resurfacing in TKR; functional evaluation and complications. Knee Surg, Sports Traumatol, Arthrosc 9, suppl 1: 27-33
2. Akagi M, Matsusue Y, Mata T et al. (1999) Effect of rotational alignment on patellar tracking in total knee arthroplasty. Clin Orthop 366: 155-63
3. Aracil J, Salom M, Aroca JE et al. (1999) Extensor apparatus reconstruction with Leeds Keio ligament in total knee arthroplasty. J Arthroplasty 14: 204-8
4. Aubriot JH (1993) Problèmes rotuliens des prothèses totales de genou semi-contraintes. Conf d'Enseignement de la SOFCOT, J Duparc ed, Exp Scient Fr, Paris 45: 1-11
5. Bartlett DH, Franzen J (1993) Accurate Preparation of the Patella During Total Knee Arthroplasty. J Arthropl 8: 75-82
6. Barrack RL, Wolfe MW, Waldman DA et al. (1997) Resurfacing of the Patella in Total Knee Arthroplasty. A prospective randomized double blind study. J Bone Joint Surg 79A, 1121-31
7. Bayley JC, Scott RD, Ewald FC et al. (1988) Failure of the metal backed patellar component after total knee replacement. J Bone Joint Surg 70A: 668
8. Beaufils P, Hossenbaccus M, Bouraly JP et al. (1995) Positionnement de l'implant rotulien dans la prothèse de genou à partir de la trochlée prothétique. Rev Chir Orthop 81, suppl II: 178
9. Beaufils P (2001) Complications sur l'Appareil Extenseur. Symposium SOFCOT. Les reprises de prothèse totale de genou. Directeurs Ph Burdin, D Huten. Rev Chir Orthop 87, suppl. 1 à paraître
10. Berger RA, Crossett LS, Jacobs JJ et al. (1998) Malrotation causing patellofemoral complications after total knee arthroplasty. Clin Orthop, 1998, 356, 144-53
11. Bindelglass DF, Cohen JL, Dorr LD (1993) Patellar tilt and subluxation in total knee arthroplasty. Clin Orthop 286: 103-9
12. Boisrenoult Ph, Scemama P, Fallet L et al. Groupe diomed (2001) Étude tomodensitométrique de la torsion fémorale distale sur genou arthrosique, Rev Chir Orthop 87
13. Boisrenoult Ph, Beaufils P, Diop A et al. Groupe Diomed (1997) Étude expérimentale de l'effet des variations de l'encombrement antéro-postérieur sur l'effort fémoro-patellaire dans la prothèse tri-compartimentale. Rev Chir Orthop 83, suppl 2: 30
14. Bonnin M, Deschamps G, Neyret Ph (2000) Les Changements des Prothèses Totales de Genou non Infectées. Analyse des résultats d'une série continue de 69 cas. Rev Chir Orthop 86: 694-706
15. Boyd AD, Ewald FC, Thomas WH et al. (1993) Long-term Complications after Total Knee Arthroplasty with or without Resurfacing of the Patella. J Bone Joint Surg 75A: 674-81
16. Bourne RB, Rorabeck CH, Vaz M et al. (1995) Resurfacing versus not resurfacing the patella during Total Knee Replacement. Clin Orthop 321: 156-61

17. Bourne RB (1999) Fracture of the patella after total knee replacement. Orthop Clin North Am 30, 287-91
18. Burdin Ph (1999) L'articulation fémoro-patellaire et prothèses tricompartimentales du genou. In Pathologie Fémoro-patellaire D Goutallier ed, Cahiers d'enseignement de la SOFCOT, Exp Scient Fr, Paris 71: 161-74
19. Burdin Ph, Huten D (2001) Les Reprises de Prothèses Totales de Genou, symposium SOF-COT 2000, Rev Chir Orthop 87, suppl I, à paraître
20. Chew JT, Stewart NJ, Hanssen AD et al. (1997) Differences in patellar tracking and knee kinematics among three different total knee designs. Clin Orthop 345: 87-98
21. Daluga D, Lombardi AV, Mallory TH et al. (1991) Knee manipulation following total knee arthroplasty. Analysis of prognostic variables. J Arthropl 6: 119-28
22. Deschamps G, Bonnin M, Ait si Selmi T et al. (2001) L'interligne prothétique dans les reprises. In: Les Reprises de Prothèses Totales de Genou SOFCOT 2000 Directeurs: Ph Burdin, D Huten. Rev Chir Orthop 87, suppl I sous presse
23. Enis JE, Gardner R, Robledo MA et al. (1990) Comparison of Patellar Resurfacing versus Non-resurfacing in Bilateral Total Knee Arthroplasty. Clin Orthop 260: 38-42
24. Feinstein W, Noble P, Kamaric E et al. (1996) Anatomic Alignment of the Patellar Groove. Clin Orthop 331, 64-73
25. Feller JA, Bartlett RJ, Lang DM (1996) Patellar resurfacing versus retention in Total Knee Arthroplasty. J Bone Joint Surg 78B: 226-8
26. Figgie HE, Goldberg VM, Figgie MP et al. (1989)The effect of alignment of the implant on fractures of the patella after condylar total knee arthroplasty. J Bone Joint Surg 71 A: 1031-9
27. Francke EI, Lachiewicz PF (2000) Failure of a cemented all-polyethylene patellar component of a Pres Fit condylar Total Knee Arthroplasty. J Arthroplasty 15: 234-7
28. Freeman MAR, Samuelson KM, Elias SG et al. (1989) The Patellofemoral Joint in Total Knee Prostheses. Design Considerations. J Arthropl 4, suppl S: 69-74
29. Goldberg VM, Figgie HE, Inglis AE et al. (1988) Patellar fracture type and prognosis in total condylar total knee arthroplasty. Clin Orthop 236: 115-22
30. Gomes LS, Bechtold JE, Gustilo RB (1988) Patellar prosthesis positioning in Total Knee Arthroplasty. A roentgenographic study. Clin orthop, 236, 72-81
31. Hsu HP, Walker PS (1989) Wear and deformation of patellar components in total knee arthroplasty. Clin Orthop 246: 260-6
32. Huten D (2001) Revision surgery in failed total knee arthroplasty arthroplasty. European Instructional Course Lectures. Thorngren, Soucacos, Hran, Scott ed, Br Ed Soc of Bone Joint Surg, London, 207-15.
33. Insall J (2001) The patella in total knee arthroplasty: does it matter? Knee Surg, Sports traumat, Arthroscopy 9, suppl 1: 2
34. Keblish PA, Varma A, Greenwald AS (1994) Patellar Resurfacing or Retention in Total Knee Arthroplasty. A prospective study of patients with bilateral replacements. J Bone Joint Surg 76B: 930-7
35. Kulkarni S, Sawant M, Ireland J (1999) Allograft reconstruction of the extensor mechanism for progressive extensor leg after total knee arthroplasty and previous patellectomy: a 3-year follow-up. J Arthroplasty 14: 892-4
36. Kurk P, Rorabeck CH, Bourne RB et al. (1992) Management of recurrent dislocation of the patella following total knee arthroplasty. J Arthroplasty 7: 229-33
37. Laskin R, Bucknell A (1990) The Use of Metal-Backed Patellar Prostheses in Total Knee Arthroplasty. Clin Orthop, 260: 52-5
38. Le AX, Cameron HU, Otsuka NY et al. (1999) Fracture of the patella following total knee arthroplasty. Orthopaedics 22, 395-8
39. Levai JP, Peronne E, Groupe Diomed (1999) Prothèse totale de genou cimentée dans la gonarthrose: revue à 5 ans de recul d'une série de 225 cas. Rev Chir Orthop, 85, suppl 3: 86
40. Levitsky KA, Harris WJ, Mc Manus J et al. (1993) Total Knee Arthroplasty without patellar resurfacing. Clin Orthop 286: 116-21
41. Lindstrand A, Robertson O, Lewold S et al. (2001) The patella in total knee arthroplasty

resurfacing or non resurfacing of the patella. Knee Surg, Sports Traumatol, Arthrosc 9, suppl 1, 21-3

42. Lombardi AV, Engh GA, Volz RG *et al.* (1988) Fracture dissociation of the polyethylene in metal-backed patellar components in total knee arthroplasty. J Bone Joint Surg 70: 675-9

43. Merkow RL, Soudry M, Insall JN (1985) Patellar dislocation following total knee replacement. J Bone Joint Surg 67A 1321-7

44. Mont MA, Yoon TR, Krackow KA *et al.* (1999) Eliminating patellofemoral complications in total knee arthroplasty: clinical and radiographic results of 121 consecutive cases using Duracon system. J Arthroplasty 14: 446-55

45. Munzinger U, Pettrich J, Boldt JG (2001) Patella resurfacing in total knee arthroplasty using metalbacked rotating bearing components: a 2 to 10 year follow-up evaluation. Knee Surg, Sports Trauma, Arthrosc 9, suppl 1: 34-42

46. Nazarian DG, Booth RE (1999) Extensor mechanism allografts in total knee arthroplasty. Clin Orthop 367: 123-9

47. Oishi CS, Kaufman KR, Irby SE *et al.* (1996) Effects of Patellar Thickness on Compression and Shear Forces in Total Knee Arthroplasty. Clin Orthop 331 283-90

48. Partington P, Sawhney J, Rorabeck C (1999) Joint Line Restoration after Revision Total Knee Arthroplasty. Clin Orthop, 367: 165-71

49. Petersilge WJ, Oishi CS, Kaufman KR *et al.* (1994) The effect of trochlear design on patellofemoral shear and compressive forces in trochlear design. Clin Orthop 309: 124-30

50. Ranawat CS (1996) The patellofemoral joint in total condylar knee arthroplasty. Clin Orthop 205: 93-9

51. Rand JA (1994) The patellofemoral joint in total knee arthroplasty. J Bone Joint Surg 76A: 612-20

52. Ritter MA, Pierce MJ, Zhou H *et al.* (1999) Patellar complications (total knee arthroplasty). Effect of lateral release and thickness. Clin Orthop 367: 149-57

53. Rouvillain JL, Kanor M, Favuto M *et al.* (1999) Modifications sagittales induites par l'arthroplastie du genou: étude radiologique. Rev Chir Orthop 85: 450-7

54. Stulberg SD, Stulberg BN, Hamati Y *et al.* (1989) Failure mechanisms of metal-backed patellar components. Clin Orthop 249: 79-96

55. Star MJ, Kaufman KR, Irby SE *et al.* (1996) The effects of patellar thickness on patellar forces after resurfacing. Clin Orthop, 322: 279-85

56. Takeuchi T, Lathi V, Khan A *et al.* (1995) Patellofemoral contact pressures exceed the compressive yield strength of UHMWPE in Total Knee Arthroplasties. J Arthropl 10: 363

57. Theiss SM, Kitziger KJ, Lotke PS *et al.* (1996) Component design affecting patellofemoral complications after total knee arthroplasty. Clin Orthop 326: 183-7

58. Whiteside LA (1997) Distal realignment of the patellar tendon to correct abnormal patellar tracking. Clin Orthop 344: 284-9

59. Yoshii I, Whiteside LA, Anouchi YS (1992) The effect of patellar button placement and femoral component design on patellar tracking in total knee arthroplasty. Clin Orthop 275: 211-19

60. Zniber B, Beaufils P (2001) Influence de la voie d'abord sur le positionnement rotulien dans les prothèses totales de genou sur gonarthrose avec grande subluxation externe de rotule. Rev Chir Orthop 87, suppl, à paraître

Femoral rotation in totak knee arthroplasty

J.G. Boldt, U. Munzinger

Femoral rotation positioning is critical for successful TKA. Three different methods of referencing are generally accepted. These include the transepicondylar axis (TEA), as advocated by Insall, arbitrary external rotation from the posterior condyles, and the so-called Whiteside line. Another less well recognized method, which has been used for over twenty years is referencing femoral component rotation perpendicular to the tibial shaft axis via a balanced flexion tension gap. Placing the femoral component parallel to the TEA leads to a biomechanically sound knee motion in full flexion and extension. However, this method has potential errors including any anatomical deviations of the distal femur, which may occur in cases with severe varus or valgus angle deformity, condylar dysplasia, or other rotational pathology of the lower extremity.

Clinical outcomes after TKA are dependent upon multifactorial issues; one of which is femoral component rotational alignment. Prosthetic design and implantation of femoro-tibial components vary with different total knee systems. The surgeon must evaluate and address variables that include varus-valgus alignment, extra-articular deformities, soft tissue contractions, exaggerated Q angle, patella position, size and shape as well as femoro-tibial rotation. Intraoperative variables include surgical approach, femoro-tibial stability, soft tissue management, extensor mechanism and patella treatment, prosthetic selection and positioning. Femoral component rotational alignment has gained more attention in the recent literature, since component mal-positioning "negatively" influences knee kinematics, including patello-femoral tracking and range of motion.

The TEA is the most commonly referenced anatomic landmark for rotational positioning of the femoral component in TKA. It is reported as being more predictable than Whiteside's line or the posterior condyle. However, the TEA depends on estimated landmarks and may be altered in both varus and valgus knees and/or other pathological variations that may change lower limb rotational axes. Tibial rotation position, an important consideration in fixed bearing designs, is also a factor that affects gap balance and the patello-femoral joint. Tibial rotational positioning is of lesser concern in mobile-bearing TKA because of the ability (of the bearing) to adapt to tibio-femoral rotation in flexion and extension.

Rotational malpositioning creates a trapezoidal rather than rectangular flexion gap with an altered patello-femoral articulation and unbalanced femoro-tibial kinematics. Instability in flexion with a tighter medial and laxer lateral compartment occurs when the femoral component is internally malrotated. This is frequently combined with lateral patello-femoral subluxation and instability (lift-off) of the lateral compartment in flexion. In most TKA systems, for a given amount of tibial resection, there is an appropriate amount of posterior condylar resection required to create a symmetric flexion gap. Different opinions of surgical approach exist regarding soft tissue releases, tibia first or femoral first bone cuts, as well as the femoral rotation resection. The most common method of tibial resection is perpendicular to the mechanical axis with some posterior inclination.

The three established methods of determining femoral rotational positioning in TKA consist of: the transepicondylar axis as advocated by Insall (fig. 1) Whiteside's line, or a line perpendicular to the antero-posterior femoral axis (fig. 2), referencing 3 to 4° external rotation from the posterior condyles (fig. 3). The posterior condylar reference as described by Hungerford (fig. 4) is seldom utilized since it results in consistent femoral internal rotational positioning, often excessive. The LCS method is based on the tibial shaft axis and balanced flexion gap and has been utilized since 1977 with mobile bearing TKA (fig. 5). Potential advantages and errors of each method will be discussed.

Olcott and Scott have recently reported that these three widely accepted methods were consistent in yielding a symmetric, balanced flexion gap within 3°. However, significant variable and inconsistencies were noted. The transepicondylar axis failed to yield flexion gap symmetry in 10% of neutral

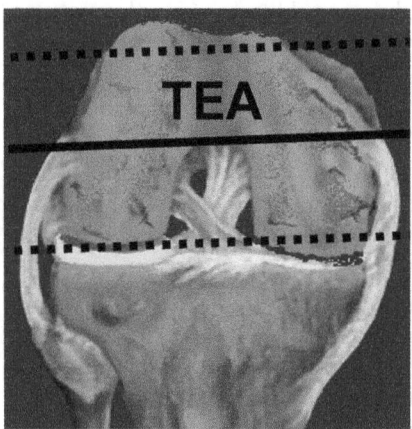

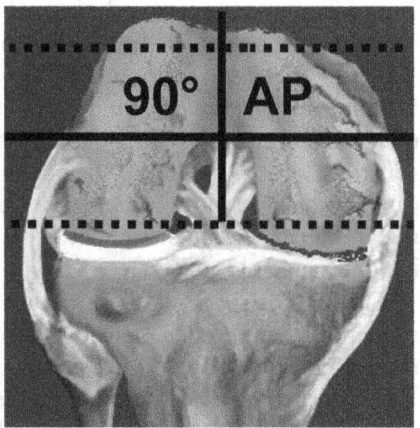

Fig. 1 – The transepicondylar axis (Insall) is identified after intraoperative identification of both lateral and medial femoral epicondyles. Potential errors are landmark inconsistencies, previous trauma, femoral rotation, and ability to digitally identify both medial and lateral epicondyles.

Fig. 2 – The antero-posterior femoral axis method (Whitesides's line) references femoral rotation perpendicular to that line, which places the component approximately parallel to the transepicondylar line. Potential errors are femoral rotation variables, previous trauma, or patello-femoral diseases that may hinder anatomical identification.

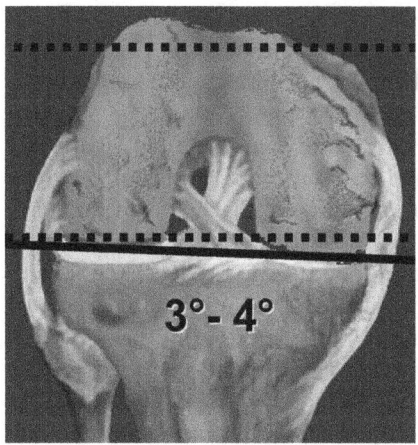

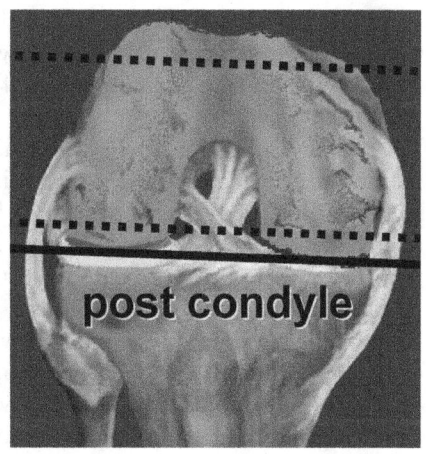

Fig. 3 – Referencing femoral rotation in 3-4° external rotation to the posterior condylar line leads to a component positioning that approximates to the transepicondylar line, but has a large angular range. This method is arbitrary, based on estimates with variable reference lines in possibly distorted condyles, particularly in valgus or varus deformities.

Fig. 4 – Referencing femoral rotation from the posterior condylar line leads to an internally malrotated component positioning with an average of 4-5° to the transepicondylar axis, which requires varus tibial resection and increased valgus femoral resection to achieve a balanced rectangular flexion tension gap. Internal rotation will also have negative impact to the patello-femoral articulation.

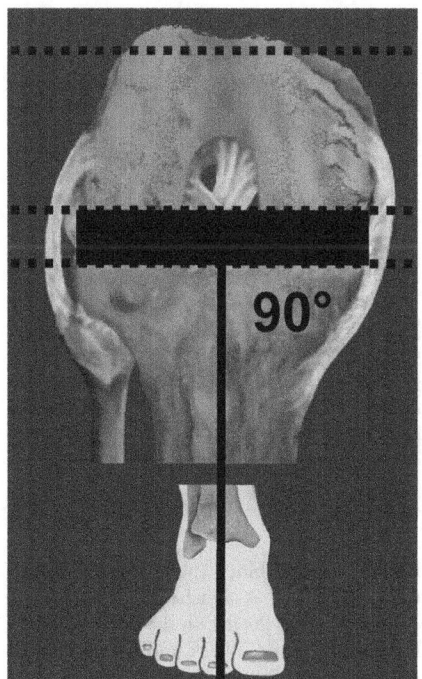

Fig. 5 – Referencing femoral rotation perpendicular to the tibial shaft axis and a balanced flexion tension gap (LCS method) leads to prospectively predictable alignment parallel to the transepicondylar axis (mean 0.3°).

varus TKA and 14% valgus TKA, with discrepancies varying from 9° too little to 6° too much external rotation, which is less than desirable. The authors recommended using a combination of these methods to avoid potential malresections.

Clinical studies by Stiehl and Cherveny compared the tibial shaft axis method to other methods for determining femoral rotation in four different fixed bearing knee systems utilizing a femoral first approach. With the postcondylar method, 72% required lateral release with 7% of patella fractures reported. When 4 to 5° of external rotation method was used, 28% of lateral release were reported. When the tibial shaft axis method was utilized, femoral component placement was reported within 1° of external rotation compared to the TEA. There were decreased number of lateral releases required and no patella complications. Katz *et al.* showed in a cadaver study of eight knees (a three surgeon evaluation) that determination of femoral component rotational positioning was more reliable using a balanced flexion gap and the anteroposterior axis. A similar study performed by Jerosch *et al.* emphasized that the inaccuracy of anatomically identifying the TEA of the femur by eight surgeon in three knee cadavers was 23°. Intraoperative evaluation of the femoral epicondyles and the TEA is less predictable and accurate than previously established methods. The method used to define femoral rotation with the LCS system is referenced on a tibial cut perpendicular to the tibial shaft axis and a symmetrical (rectangular) flexion gap. This method automatically defines the position of the free moveable femoral resection guide (fig. 6), avoiding the need of identifying anatomical landmarks. A rectangular spacer block is then applied to the rotationally unconstrained femoral component and sits flat on

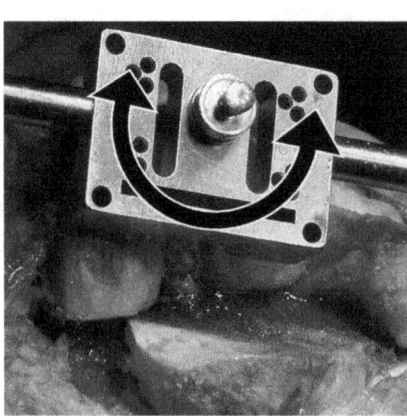
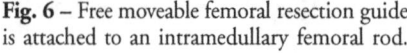
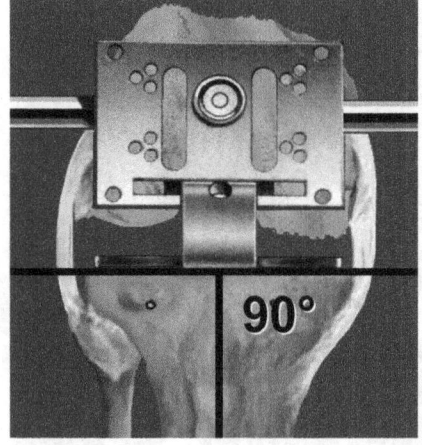

Fig. 6 – Free moveable femoral resection guide is attached to an intramedullary femoral rod.

Fig. 7 – Spacer block (perpendicular to the tibial shaft axis) is attached to the femoral component and sits flat on the tibial resection for flexion balance check and determination of femoral rotational alignment.

the tibial resection. The flexion tension is set and checked for proper balance (fig. 7, 8). The extension gap is balanced to the flexion gap with a distal femoral resection, establishing the mechanical axis. (fig. 9, 10).

Comparison of this tibial axis method with the TEA methods adds to our understanding of this most important technique step in TKA. CT scan eval-

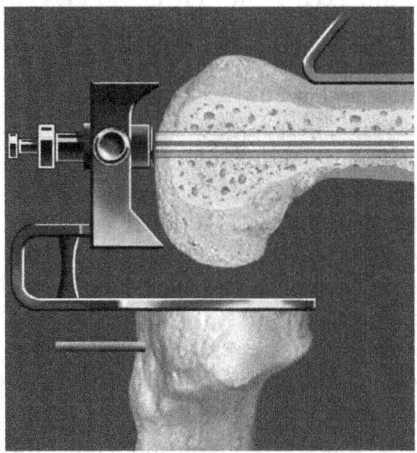

Fig. 8 – Tibial resection is perpendicular to the tibial shaft axis and femoral resection block parallel to the tibial resection.

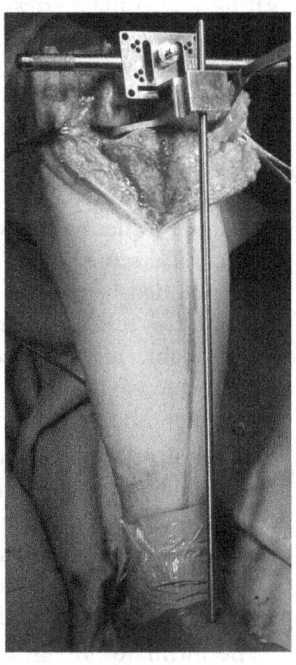

Fig. 9 – Spacer block determines rotational alignment of the femoral resection block with a balanced rectangular flexion tension gap setting the guide parallel to the tibial shaft axis.

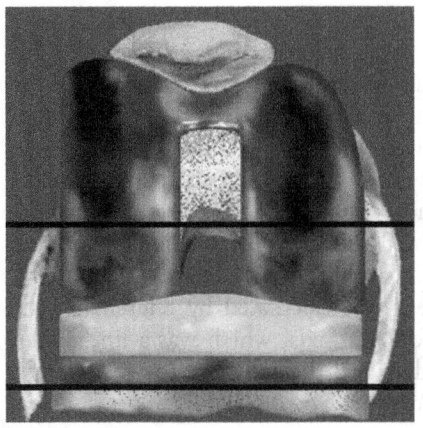

Fig. 10 – Femoral component alignment parallel to transepicondylar axis ensures optimum patello-femoral tracking.

uation is the most accurate method to objectively assessing femoral component rotational placement compared to a known anatomic landmark post TKA. In order to clinically investigate the accuracy of the LCS method with regard to femoral component rotational positioning, we performed a study in which helical CT scan investigation was used referencing the femoral prosthetic placement to the transepicondylar axis. From a cohort of 3,058 mobile bearing low contact stress (LCS, Depuy Int, Leeds, UK) TKAS, 40 (1.3%) clinically well functioning knees were randomly selected for evaluation of femoral component rotational alignment. All patients with TKA in this center underwent routine clinical examination and follow-up radiographs at 1 week, 6 weeks, 1 year, 5 years, or when complications occurred. Mean age in this cohort was 67 years (range 54 to 77). Inclusion criteria for this subset was range of motion (ROM) over 100°, lack of pre- or postoperative complications, and excellent or good clinical results according to a modified HSS 100-point clinical score with a mean of 91.2 points (81 to 100). One patient had to be excluded because of inability to identify appropriate anatomical landmarks on CT scans, and another patient refused CT investigation. Of the 38 cases available for this study, the patella was left unresurfaced in 36 (95%) cases, one was previously patellectomized, another patella was resurfaced using a metal-backed rotating patella component.

Follow-ups at regular intervals included a clinical evaluation and X-ray protocol. Radiographic analysis was focused on patella tracking, congruency, and patella tilt with comparable pre- and postoperative skyline radiographs. Patella tracking was based on alignment of the femoral trochlear sulcus and the crown of the patella and measured in millimeters of lateral deviation on comparable pre- and postoperative skyline views.

The ultimate 38 cases were randomly selected from patients who were scheduled by a computerized system for 1-, 5-, or 10-year routine follow-up. These patients were invited to participate in the study until the appropriate number was obtained. Of the two cases eliminated one patient refused to participate, another was eliminated for technical reason as noted. Of this group all patients had excellent or good clinical results and no patient refused participation. The local university ethics committee approved the study.

All cases were investigated by one of two consultant musculoskeletal radiologists with CT experience of more than fifteen years. Before the start of the examination they examined a few patients not included into the investigation in order to use the same criteria, which were identical to those used for everyday examinations. The radiologists were not aware of the patients' knee status (single blinded). They were instructed not to talk with the patients about the status of their knees but about technical CT aspects only. All data for femoral component rotational positioning were analyzed using a helical CT scanner. Femoral component rotational alignment was calculated by referencing the two posterior condyles to the transepicondylar axis, which was a line drawn between the spike of the lateral epicondyle and the sulcus of the medial epicondyle as recently recommended by Yoshino et al. (fig.11). One case was excluded because of inability to identify the medial sulcus despite 2mm cuts. Angles were calculated utilizing sophisticated helical CT-implemented software.

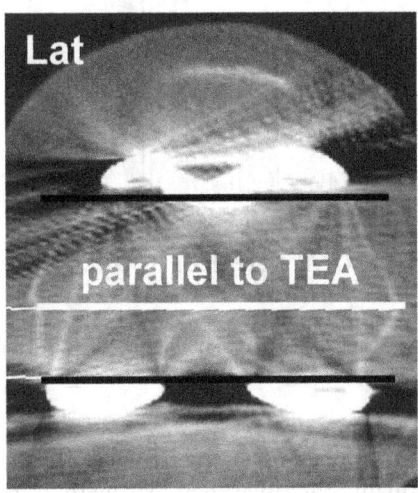

Fig. 11 – Transversal CT scans are a practical method for accurate determination of femoral component rotational positioning in TKA best referenced to the transepicondylar axis. Example of a well-aligned femoral component parallel to the TEA.

An independent statistician analyzed all data. The distribution of angles in each group was analyzed using the one-sample Kolmogorov-Smirnov test which indicates whether the number of cases is sufficient and a normal "bell-curve" distribution is demonstrated. A positive Kolmogorov-Smirnov test validates further parametric statistical analyses.

The subset of 38 cases (follow-up: 12 to 120 months) studied in this series had clinical results comparable to a larger cohort group of over 3,000 TKAS. All cases were well functioning knees with good or excellent clinical results. The mean ROM was 115° (range 100 to 135). Preoperatively, 3 of 38 cases had documented patella subluxation and tilt of more than 6°. Postoperatively all 3 achieved perfect patello-femoral tracking. Decreased height and sclerosis of the lateral patella facet was seen in two case without clinical symptoms. There were no fixation failures, no patella failures and no reoperations for any reason in this group.

Mean femoral alignment was near parallel (0.3° internal rotation) to the TEA with a range of 6° internal to 4° external rotation.

Standard deviation was 2.2 and standard error 0.4. All angles were normally distributed using one-sample Kolmogorov-Smirnov test, which validates a statistical mean value and outliers. Four cases fell outside of the predicted mean value (more than 3° internal or external rotation). Three had internal rotation and one case had external rotation. All four cases with maximum internal and external rotation showed perfect patello-femoral tracking on skyline views (fig.12).

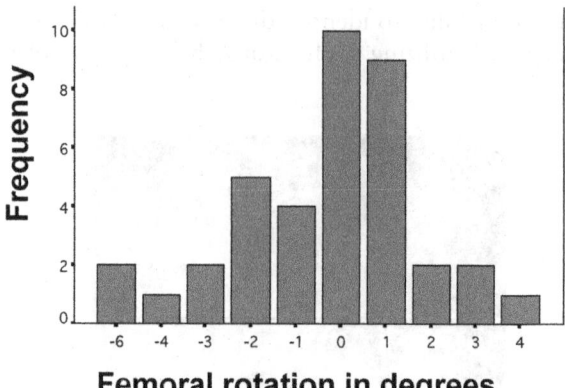

Femoral rotation in degrees

Fig. 12 – Graph showing normal distribution of femoral component rotational alignment in the subset group. Mean rotation of the femoral component was parallel (0.3°) to the trans-epicondylar axis, ranging from 6° internal to 5° external rotation.

The data of our study emphasizes that correct femoral component rotational positioning, utilizing the tibial shaft axis method, results in a high level of consistency for accurate patello-femoral alignment and predictable clinical outcome.

In summary, femoral rotational alignment based on the tibial axis and balanced flexion tension is an instrumented technique that:

1) avoids relationship to arbitrary landmarks;

2) establish a precise flexion gap which allows for a stable relationship to the corrected biomechanical axis;

3) is patient-specific regarding bone and soft tissue variations;

4) is reproducible (especially in severe deformities such as the valgus knee);

5) results in predictable patella outcomes in reported series. Femoral component rotational alignment is technique- and instrument-dependent and influences patella tracking, gap balance, and soft tissue kinematics. Deviation into internal rotation results in less than ideal patello-femoral tracking and clinical outcomes. Potential complications, such as the painful and/or stiff TKA (arthrofibrosis), have been shown to correlate with significant internal rotation of the femoral component. The tibial shaft axis method as used with the LCS system provides perfect rotational alignment without anatomical landmark identification, and is, therefore, felt to be as or more predictable than all other currently practiced methods.

Acknowledgement:

J. Hodler MD and M. Zanetti MD for helical CT data (Zurich, Switzerland)
T. Drobny MD for clinical support (Zurich, Switzerland)
P. Keblish MD for critical manuscript review

References

1. Akagi M, Matsusue Y, Mata T et al. (1999) Effect of rotational alignment on patellar tracking in total knee arthroplasty. Clin Orthop 1999 Sep (366): 155-63
2. Arima J, Whiteside LA, McCarthy DS et al. (1995) Femoral rotational alignment, based on the anteroposterior axis, in total knee arthroplasty in a valgus knee. A technical note. J Bone Joint Surg Am 77(9): 1331-4
3. Berger RA, Crossett LS, Jacobs JJ et al. (1998) Rotation causing patellofemoral complications after total knee arthroplasty. Clin Orthop (356): 144-53
4. Berger RA, Rubash HE, Seel MJ et al. (1993) Determining the rotational alignment of the femoral component in total knee arthroplasty using the epicondylar axis. Clin Orthop 1993 Jan (286): 40-7
5. Buechel FF (1982) A simplified evaluation system for the rating of the knee function. Orthop Rev 11(9): 97-101
6. Churchill DL, Incavo SJ, Johnson CC et al. (1998) The transepicondylar axis approximates the optimal flexion axis of the knee. Clin Orthop (356): 111-8
7. Dennis DA, Komistek RD, Walker SA et al. (2001) Femoral condylar lift-off in vivo in total knee arthroplasty. J Bone Joint Surg Br 83(1): 33-9
8. Eckhoff DG, Piatt BE, Gnadinger CA et al. (1995) Assessing rotational alignment in total knee arthroplasty. Clin Orthop 1995 Sep (318): 176-81
9. Engh GA (2000) Orienting the femoral component at total knee arthroplasty. Am J Knee Surg 13(3): 162-5
10. Fehring TK (2000) Rotational malalignment of the femoral component in total knee arthroplasty. Clin Orthop 380: 72-9
11. Fehring TK (2000) Rotational malalignment of the femoral component in total knee arthroplasty. Clin Orthop Nov (380): 72-9
12. Griffin FM, Insall JN, Scuderi GR (2000) Accuracy of soft tissue balancing in total knee arthroplasty. J Arthroplasty 2000 Dec 15(8): 970-3
13. Griffin FM, Insall JN, Scuderi GR (1998) The posterior condylar angle in osteoarthritic knees. J Arthroplasty 13(7): 812-5
14. Hungerford DS (1995) Alignment in total knee replacement. Instr Course Lect 44: 455-68
15. Katz MA, Beck TD, Silber JS et al. (2001) Determining femoral rotational alignment in total knee arthroplasty: Reliability of techniques. J Arthroplasty 16(3): 301-5
16. Lonner JH, Siliski JM, Scott RD (1999) Prodromes of failure in total knee arthroplasty. J Arthroplasty 14(4): 488-92
17. Mantas JP, Bloebaum RD, Skedros JG et al. (1992) Implications of reference axes used for rotational alignment of the femoral component in primary and revision knee arthroplasty. J Arthroplasty 7(4): 531-5
18. Nagamine R, Miura H, Bravo CV et al. (2000) Anatomic variations should be considered in total knee arthroplasty. J Orthop Sci 5(3): 232-7
19. Nagamine R, Miura H, Inoue Y et al. (1998) Reliability of the anteroposterior axis and the posterior condylar axis for determining rotational alignment of the femoral component in total knee arthroplasty. J Orthop Sci 3(4): 194-8
20. Olcott CW, Scott RD (2000) A comparison of 4 intraoperative methods to determine femoral component rotation during total knee arthroplasty. J Arthroplasty 15(1): 22-6
21. Olcott CW, Scott RD (1999) The Ranawat Award. Femoral component rotation during total knee arthroplasty. Clin Orthop (367): 39-42
22. Poilvache PL, Insall JN, Scuderi GR et al. (1996) Rotational landmarks and sizing of the distal femur in total knee arthroplasty. Clin Orthop (331): 35-46
23. Scuderi GR, Insall JN, Scott NW (1994) Patellofemoral Pain After Total Knee Arthroplasty. J Am Acad Orthop Surg 1994 Oct 2(5): 239-46
24. Stiehl JB, Abbott BD (1995) Morphology of the transepicondylar axis and its application in primary and revision total knee arthroplasty. J Arthroplasty 10(6): 785-9
25. Stiehl JB, Cherveny PM (1996) Femoral rotational alignment using the tibial shaft axis in total knee arthroplasty. Clin Orthop (331): 47-55

26. Stiehl JB, Dennis DA, Komistek RD *et al.* (1999) *In vivo* determination of condylar lift-off and screw-home in a mobile-bearing total knee. J Arthroplasty 14(3): 293-9
27. Stiehl JB, Dennis DA, Komistek RD *et al.* (1997) *In vivo* kinematic analysis of a mobile bearing total knee prosthesis. Clin Orthop (345): 60-6
28. Whiteside LA, Arima J (1995) The anteroposterior axis for femoral rotational alignment in valgus total knee arthroplasty. Clin Orthop 1995 Dec (321): 168-72
29. Yamada K, Imaizumi T (2000) Assessment of relative rotational alignment in total knee arthroplasty: usefulness of the modified Eckhoff method. J Orthop Sci 5(2): 100-3
30. Yoshino N, Takai S, Ohtsuki Y *et al.* (2001) Computed tomography measurement of the surgical and clinical transepicondylar axis of the distal femur in osteoarthritic knees. J Arthroplasty 16(4): 493-7

Bone loss with total knee replacement

P. Burdin, S. Lautman, J. Brilhault

Introduction

Implanting a knee prosthesis while respecting the tension of the capsulo-ligamentous envelope implies that the amount of bone resected is adapted to the implant and shared evenly between the femur and the tibia so that the prosthetic joint line can be maintained in its anatomic position.

Destruction of the bone surrounding the prosthesis can occur in different circumstances. These osseous destructions appearing after the bone resections necessary during the first surgery are usually named bone loss (BL).

There are several causes of the BL, witch can be associated:

– Loosening of a prosthetic component will act as a grater, gnawing the bone on which it is laid. The prosthesis usually sinks into the bone creating asymmetric BL;

– Periprosthetic osteolysis. Infiltration of particles between the prosthesis and the bone (wearing debris of polyethylene, cement particles in loosening, metallic particles if the wearing leads to a metal-metal contact), gives birth to a granuloma, determined by a mechanism that is now well known (5), that fragilize bone structure and can originate loosening;

– Osteopenia by constraint stealing (stress shielding). Its preferred site is the femur, posterior to the prosthetic trochlea. The bone does not completely disappear but becomes so fragile that the removal of the femoral component can sometimes create a real BL;

– Bone Loss can be due to the surgeon:

• During surgery: If a mistake is made in a bone cut (too important or wrongly orientated) its correction at revision surgery will make the BL apparent;

• While removing the prosthesis (and more so if a component is not loose) and even if great caution is taken in the matter, a part of the bone attached to the components can be ripped off in the process.

When it becomes necessary to change the prosthesis the BL must be managed:

– To restore a solid support for the new prosthesis;
– To conserve or restore a normal mechanical axis for the limb;
– To conserve or restore a prosthetic joint line in its anatomical position;

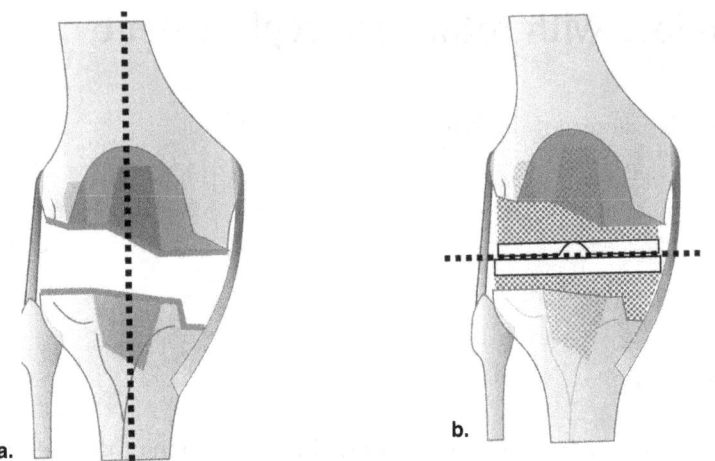

Fig. 1 – a. The mechanical axis of the lower limb is restored. The ligaments are in tension. BLs are observed.
b. A standard size prosthesis restores the height of the articular space, and differentiates the BLs concerning the femur from that of the tibia.

– To conserve a correct tension in the capsulo-ligamantous envelope in all positions of knee flexion.

One is therefore naturally brought to provide a definition of BL: It is, after removal of the prosthesis, the bone defects between the remaining bone and a new prosthesis of normal volume and ideally positioned (fig. 1-a et 1-b).

Different methods can be employed to treat these BL in revision surgery, but none have yet proven itself the best (probably none can apply itself to all situations).

To evaluate the results of these different techniques and establish their indications, some authors tried to describe the situations in which they were employed thus proposing a classification of BL.

Dorr (2), in 1989, classified them in central and peripheric, without defining their importance or localization.

Rand (6), in 1991, established a BL classification from peroperatory observations. There are four types by combination of the height and volumes of the defects. They are also described as central or peripheric.

Bargar et Gross (1), in 1992, differentiate segmentary or cavitary BL, and describe their volume on preop X-rays, with reference to anatomic landmarks (bi-epicondylary line for the femur, and top of the tibial tuberosity and fibula head for the tibia). They introduced a score by adding up points.

Engh (3, 4) accused Bargar et Gross's classification of being too complex (because it mounts up to individualizing too many situations) and also established on only preop radiographs (often difficult to read), and proposed a new classification, AORI (because developed at Anderson Orthopedic Research Institute).

This classification has great qualities:

– It uses the same terminology for the femur and the tibia;

– Information comes from perop observations and preop radiographs, as well as the type of reconstruction that was necessary;

– BL are described in both the tibial and femoral metaphysis, and limited by the same landmarks as those chosen by Bargar and Gross (bi-epicondylary line for the femur, and top of the tibial tuberosity for the tibia). There are three types: Type I when the metaphyseal region is moderately altered and the stability of the new prosthesis is not compromised; type II when a reconstruction will be or was necessary because of the importance of the metaphyseal damage (in the type II-A the BL is unilateral, in the type II-B the BL concern both tibial plateaus or femoral condyles); type III when the BL destroyed most of one or two condyles or one or two tibial plateau (reaching the limit of the metaphyseal zone, implying possible loss of the insertion of a collateral ligament or patellar tendon).

But we feel it has certain flaws:

– The terms central and peripheric, or continent and non-continent disappear (the authors arguing the in that metaphyseal zone there is no cortical bone);

– The type II (the most frequent because of the size of the metaphyseal zone) includes very different situations. The author finds this advantageous because of the possibility of statistical analysis. We feel that it induces a lack of precision.

Because we think that there are flaws in these classifications, during the November 2000 SOFCOT symposium on TKA, we proposed a new classification that intended to synthesize the existing ones, largely inspired by Engh's principles.

The goals of a classification

The goals of a classification are:

– To describe as precisely as possible the morphology of the bone (femur or tibia) receiving the new prosthesis and the possible elements of augmentation (cement, wedge, graft…);

– To describe the importance of the BL to be treated, but also the quality of the receiving bone and possible elements of augmentation. This in order to compare the different types of reconstruction available. For the moment we are still far from having established a consensus on this subject and the list of problems is long: When should one use a centro-medullary stem? What should be its length and diameter? Should it be cemented? Should a cavitary BL be filled with cement or bone graft? Should one use allograft, autograft, or bone substitutes? Should a segmentary BL be filled with bone or a metallic wedge? …)

A classification should allow retrospective usage by analysis of operator protocols and radiographs in order of avoid losing an experience that is becoming important.

It should allow statistical analysis of the results, thus coherent groupments of population or, on the contrary, division of certain groups, in order to analyze the influence of certain parameters, should be possible secondarily.

General principles

– Tibial and femoral BL are evaluated separately;
– It is not based on preop radiographs (since these often underestimate the importance of the BL) but on perop observations and the analysis of postop radiographs;
– The perop evaluations of BL are done after removal of the prosthesis (that sometimes increases them) and after possible "cleaning" bone cuts;
– It is precise and therefore implies many undergroups, but when it is necessary for result analysis, it can be simplified by creating coherent groups in regard to the projected analysis.

Classification of tibial BL

The upper extremity of the tibia is divided into three zones (A, B, and C) by two planes perpendicular to its mechanical axis. The superior plane is tangent to the upper extremity of the fibula, the inferior one is two centimeters lower (fig. 2).

The superior surface of the tibia is divided into three sectors: medial, central and lateral (fig. 2).

Three types of BL are individualized (fig. 3): central (cavitary), peripheric (cavitary) and segmentary.

The tibial grade is defined by the highest zone on which the new prosthesis, with its possible added elements, sits on the remaining tibia (possibly after "cleaning" cuts).

Therefore there are three tibial grades: A, B and C (fig. 4).

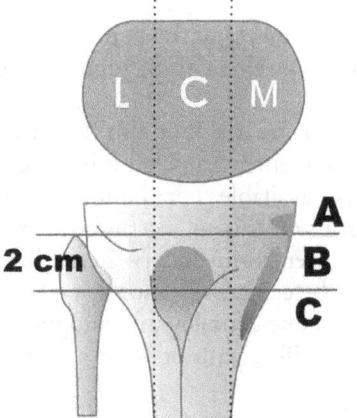

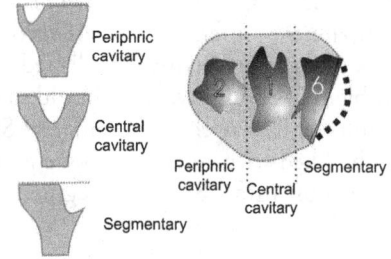

Fig. 2 – The three zones and sectors of the tibia.

Fig. 3 – The three types of BSLs.

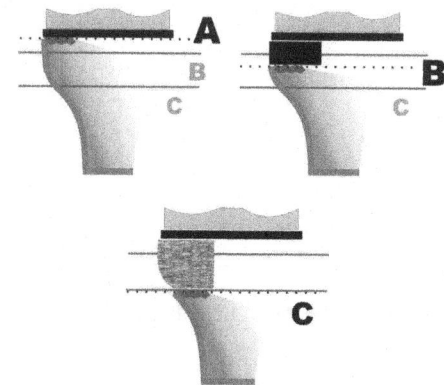

Fig. 4 – The three tibial grades.

Each grade can be followed by an index that defines whether the sitting zone is medial (index [M]) or lateral (index [L]) or bilateral (index [ML]).

The state of the bone surface receiving the new prosthesis is defined by a "surface score" resulting from an addition of points: 1 point for a central BL, 2 points for a peripheric BL, and 6 points for a segmentary BL (peripheric cortical defect) (fig. 3). The number of points for each BL was not defined in order to quantify the gravity of each but in order to obtain a score (addition of points) that could be the result of an only situation. A fast lecture is possible: An odd score implies a central BL, a score superior or equal to 6 implies the presence of a segmentary BL.

Within the same grade, the classification can quantify the importance (the depth) of a possible segmentary BL, by a last "depth" index:

– If a segmentary BL remains in the same tibial zone as that of the grade, the index is the same as the grade (a) for a grade A, (b) far a grade B and (c) for a grade C;

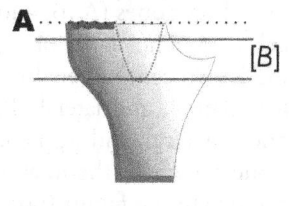

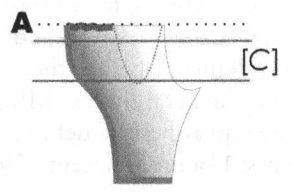

– If the segmentary BL is in a deeper zone than that of the grade, the index is defined by this zone: (b) or (c) for a grade A, (c) for a grade B and (d) for a grade C (implying an extension to the diaphyse) (fig. 5).

Therefore the code for the tibia has the following structure:

Grade (side index) Surface score (depth index)

Here are some examples (fig. 6).

B (L) 8 [c] wich means and can only mean that:

– The "cleanness" cut was made in the B zone;

Fig. 5 – The depth index.

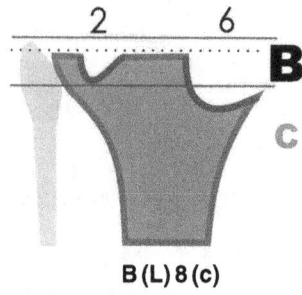

B (L) 8 (c)

Fig. 6 – Two examples of tibial BSLs.

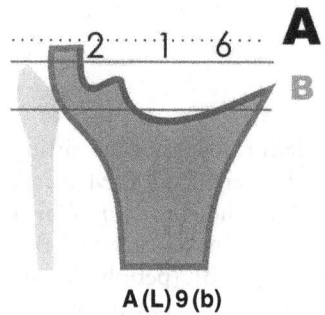

A (L) 9 (b)

– On the lateral side;
– On the medial side there is a segmentary BL reaching the C zone;
– On the lateral side after the bone cuts there remained a peripheric BL;
– The surface score is even (there are no Central defects).
A (L) 9 [b] wich means and can only mean that:
– The "cleanness" cut was made in the A zone;
– On the lateral side;
– On the medial side there is a segmentary BL reaching the B zone;
– On the lateral side after the bone cuts there remained a peripheric BL;
– The surface score is odd (there is a central defect).

Classification of femoral BL

The principles are the same as for the tibia (fig. 7).

The lower extremity of the femur is divided into three zones (A, B, and C) by two planes perpendicular to its mechanical axis. The superior plane includes the bi-epicondylar line, the inferior plane is two centimeters lower.

The femur is divided into three sectors: medial, central, and lateral. Three types of BL are defined: central (cavitary), peripheric (cavitary), and segmentary.

The femoral grade is defined by the deepest zone on which the new prosthesis sits (with its possible added elements) on the remaining femur (possibly after "cleaning cuts"). Therefore there are three femoral grades A, B and C.

Each grade can be followed by an index that defines whether the sitting zone is medial (index [M]) or lateral (index [L]) or bilateral (index [ML]).

The state of the bone surface receiving the new prosthesis is defined by a "surface score" resulting from an addition of points: 1 point for a central (cavi-

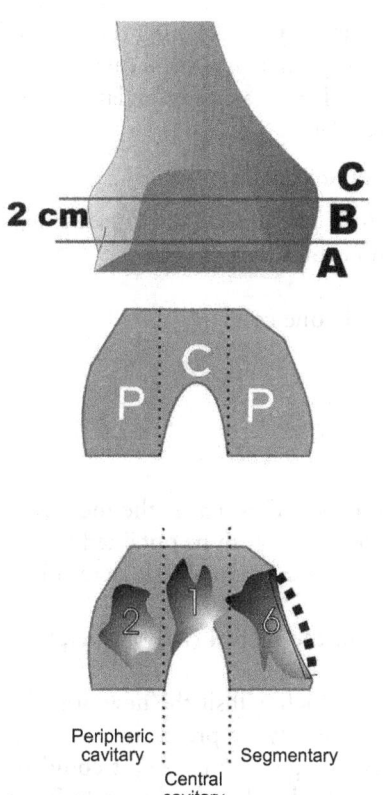

cavitary

Central
cavitary

Segmentary

Fig. 7 – Distal femoral BSLs.

tary) BL, 2 points for a peripheric (cavitary) BL, and 6 points for a segmentary BL (fig. 7).

Within the same grade, the classification can quantify the importance (the depth) of a possible segmentary BL, by a last "depth" index. If the segmentary BL remains in the same femoral zone as that of the grade, the index is the same as the grade (a) for a grade A, (b) far a grade B and (c) for a grade C. If the segmentary BSL is in a deeper femoral zone than that of the grade, the index is defined by this zone (b or c) for a grade A, (c) for a grade B and (d) for a grade C, implying an extension to the diaphyse.

The only difference with the tibia is that it is possible to signify the existence of segmentary BL in the posterior condyles, by giving a last "posterior condyle score" for each of both condyles (fig. 8): 0 point if there are no BL, 1 point for a posterior condyle segmentary BL without distal segmentary BL on the same side, 2 points for a posterior condyle segmentary BL associated with a distal segmentary BSL on the same side.

Therefore the code for the femur has the following structure:
Grade (side index) Surface score (depth index) (posterior condyle index)
Here are some examples.
A (M) 7(b) (3) which means and can only mean that:
– The distal "cleanness cut" was in zone A on the medial side;

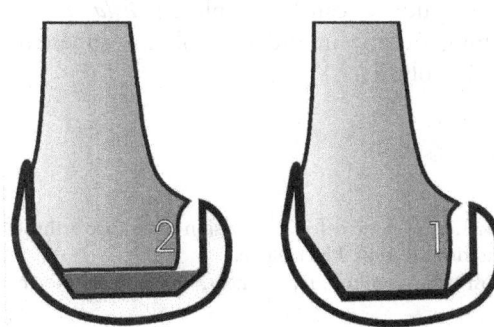

Fig. 8 – The "posterior condyle" score.

– On the lateral side there was a distal Segmentary BL reaching the B zone;

– The depth score is odd therefore in the center there is a distal cavitary BL;

– There is a posterior segmentary medial BL and a posterior lateral segmentary BL (as well as the distal segmentary BL).

A (ML) 4 (a) (1) which means and can only mean that:

– The distal "cleanness cut" was in zone A on the medial and lateral side;

– There are two lateral cavitary BL and no central BL;

– There are no distal segmentary BL;

– There is a posterior segmentary BL of only one condyle.

How should one proceed?

For the femur as well as the tibia:

– Determine the zone in which the "cleanness cut" is made (the most economical, if a step-off cut was made). This information can be obtained by the perop observations and/or the immediate postop radiographs. It determines the A, B, or C grade;

– Indicate whether the grade was defined in the medial (M) or lateral (L) or both (ML) compartments;

– Describe the state of the bone surface on which will sit the new prosthesis. This information can be obtained peroperatively by presenting the new prosthesis without the augmentation devises (wedges, graft...) that could be necessary, sitting on the "cleanness cut". It can also be obtained by analysis the immediate postop radiographs by drawing the line perpendicular to the mechanical axis of the bone, tangent to the "cleanness cut". The surface score is then obtained by adding the different points;

– Determine in which zone is a possible cortical defect on the opposite side to the one defining the grade. This information comes from perop observations and/or analysis of immediate postop radiographs;

– For the femur, indicate the posterior condyle score. This information comes from perop observations.

This classification that can describe all situations seems at first too complex.

In fact, with a little experience, with a single lecture one can visualize the situation to which the surgeon was confronted.

Mostly following the goals of the study, it can be simplified *"a la carte"*, neglecting certain items or grouping others, in order to obtain coherent groups in regard to the problem to be solved.

References

1. Bargar WL, Gross TP (1992) A classification of bone defects in revision total knee arthroplasty. Presented at the Knee Society Interim Meeting, Philadelphia
2. Dorr LD (1989) Bone graft for bone lost with total knee replacement. Orthop Clin North Am 20(2): 179-87

3. Engh GA, Ammeen DJ (1998) Management of bone loss during revision hip or knee replacement. Classification and preoperative radiographic evaluation: knee. Orthop Clin North Am 29(2): 205-17
4. Engh GA (1997) Bone defect classification. In: Engh GA, Rorabeck CH (eds) Revision total knee arthroplasty. Williams & Wilkins, Baltimore, p. 63
5. Harris WH (2001) The osteolysis phenomena in total hip and total knee replacement surgery. In: Rieker Cl, Oberholzer S, Wyss U (eds) World tribology forum in arthroplasty, Hans Huber, Bern, p. 17
6. Rand JA (1991) Bone deficiency in total knee arthroplasty. Use of metal wedge augmentation. Clin Orthop 271: 63-71

Revision total knee arthroplasty for aseptic failure

M. Bonnin

Revision total knee arthroplasty is a difficult procedure. The functional outcome is less satisfactory than that of primary implants and there is a high rate of complications and failures. The results are also less good than those of total knee replacements after failure of unicompartmental prostheses or tibial valgus osteotomies (table I). Because of these mediocre results, meticulous preoperative analysis is even more imperative in order to discover the cause of failure (loosening, instability, stiffness...) and the contributory factors. These may be surgeon-related (malpositioning, poor soft tissue balance) or patient-related (activity, excess weight, associated lesions), or may arise from the implant itself (design, polyethylene).

Implant replacement raises several problems:

1. Technical difficulties related to replacement itself (surgical approach, retrieval of the material, stages of reconstruction);

2. Specific difficulties depending on cause of failure (restoration of bony defects, soft tissue balance);

3. Correction of factors leading to failure (initial faulty soft tissue balance, incorrect component size and position);

4. Patient-related difficulties which may have contributed to failure (rheumatoid arthritis, previous knee surgery, associated joint disease).

These must all be identified and analyzed before surgery and preoperative planning is of crucial importance, more than in any other procedure. Here we will only address certain technical aspects of total knee revision, the specific pro-

Table I – Result of primary total knee arthroplasty (TKA), after failure of unicompartmental knee arthroplasty (UKA), osteotomy (HTO) or total knee arthroplasty (TKA) (1, 3, 8).

Indication for TKA	Follow-up	Global IKS Score/200
Failure of UKA (n = 54)	4 years (1-12)	147
Failure of HTO (n = 90)	6.5 years (2-12)	145
Failure of TKA (n = 69)	3 years (1-9)	131

blems of analysis of bone loss and how it should be filled. Choice of constraint and failure related to the patellofemoral joint are dealt with elsewhere.

Preoperative planning

Goniometry, comparative anteroposterior and lateral views of the weight bearing knee and axial views of the patellas are required to plan the procedure. These images make it possible to assess instability, to anticipate the amount of bone loss and the deformity to be corrected. Templates are routinely used to judge the optimal size of the implant in relation to local anatomy. This size serves as a basis for reconstruction but will be modified depending on constraints related to soft tissue balance.

Positioning of the components is planned using templates based on anatomic landmarks: the femoral medullary canal, the tibial medullary canal and the anterior femoral cortex. At this stage, the use of offset stems can be anticipated. This expedient may avoid misdirection through cortical bone and to a lesser extent impingement of the stem on cortical bone, which leads to residual pain.

The optimal joint line level can now be evaluated using comparative views obtained with the same (known) magnification coefficient. This is a crucial factor which has an impact on patellofemoral and tibiofemoral kinematics and partially conditions the functional result. Partington (30) obtained better results if the joint line was elevated by less than 8mm. Deschamps (10) did not confirm these results but in his multicentre series the joint line position had altered less than in the series of Partington. In various series of the literature, the joint line was lowered by 1.72mm (3) and elevated by 12mm (30).

If there is no ligament distension, placing the joint line in relation to fixed anatomic landmarks gives an optimal level. The head of the fibula can be used if preoperative comparative images are available. The epicondyles can be used as landmarks during surgery. Griffin (21) (fig. 1) established a fixed relationship between the transepicondylar diameter (TED) of the knee and the distance from the epicondyles to the joint line (DEJ): medially, DEJ = TED 0.36 in women or 0.35 in men; laterally, DEJ = TED 0.32 in women or 0.31 in men.

If the ligaments are distended, stability in extension is obtained at the cost of joint "lengthening" and the notion of a joint line becomes a complex one (fig. 2):

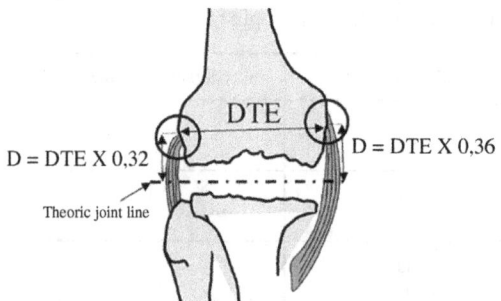

DTE

D = DTE X 0,32

D = DTE X 0,36

Theoric joint line

Fig. 1 – Determination of the position of the joint line using the epicondyles, using Griffin's measurements (21).

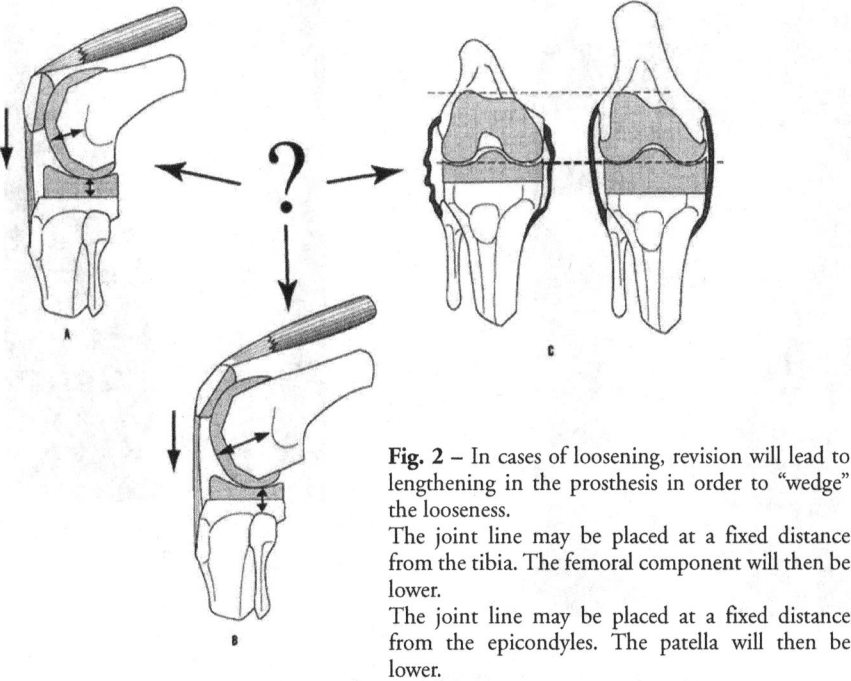

Fig. 2 – In cases of loosening, revision will lead to lengthening in the prosthesis in order to "wedge" the looseness.

The joint line may be placed at a fixed distance from the tibia. The femoral component will then be lower.

The joint line may be placed at a fixed distance from the epicondyles. The patella will then be lower.

The joint line may be placed halfway from the insertions of the peripheral ligaments. The patella will then be lower.

1. If we place the emphasis on the patellofemoral joint, patellar height must be used as a basis. As the patella remains at a fixed distance from the tibia (subject to retraction or distension of the patellar tendon or to anterior tibial tubercle osteotomy), the ideal landmark is the tibia or the fibula if we do not wish to alter the relationship between the joint line and the patella. However this leads us to "wedge" the laxity by distal reconstruction of the femur, resulting in stiffness and considerable patellofemoral strain.

2. If we place the emphasis on tibiofemoral kinematics, the ideal position is halfway between the tibial and femoral insertions of the collateral ligaments. However, this results in a relative drop of the patella in relation to the new joint line (subject to anterior tibial tubercle osteotomy) and the patella will be too low.

3. The third possibility is to determine the joint line level in relation to the epicondyles. This means that laxity is corrected by the thickness of the tibial polyethylene alone, which can lead to a low patella.

In practice, there is no ideal solution which automatically positions the joint line. It is important to use several anatomic landmarks during surgery and to check the position of the patella in relation to the final joint line at the end of the procedure. The joint line level is determined by referring to preoperative radiographs and using templates: An area of the prosthesis which is considered to be in a satisfactory position from the standpoint of the joint line is identified. This "ideal" point is then located during the procedu-

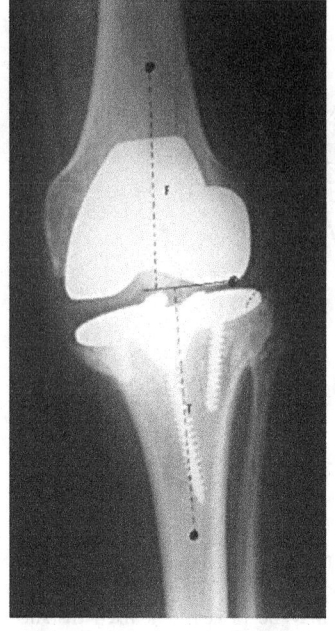

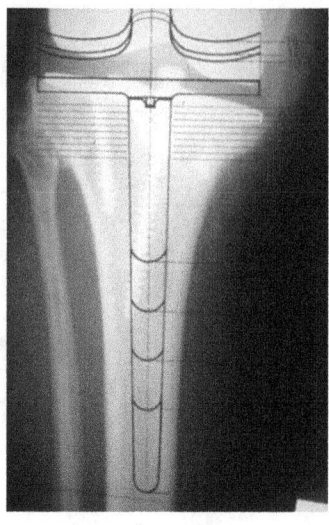

b.

c.

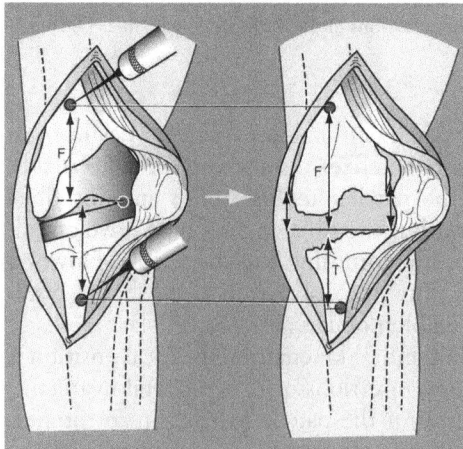

Fig. 3 – Locating the height of the joint line (from [4] with permission).
a. A point on the tibial component which is judged to be in a correct position is identified on preoperative radiographs: It represents the desired position of the joint line.
b. Use of templates on the radiographs help to identify the "ideal" joint line.
c. During the procedure, a landmark (drill hole or pin) is marked on the tibia and the femur at a known distance (distance T and F) from this reference point. When the prosthetic components have been removed, using the tibial and femoral marks the desired level of the joint line can be found.

re, before the implant is removed. A landmark (pin or drill hole) is then indicated on the tibia and the femur at a measured distance from this "ideal" point. After the components have been removed, even if there is considerable bone loss, the reference point in relation to which the joint line should be placed can be identified (fig. 3). This reference level can be modified later if necessary according to soft tissue balance in flexion and in extension (see below).

The course of the procedure

Skin and pre-existing incisions

If numerous cutaneous incisions are made, a few simple rules must be followed in order to reduce the risk of cutaneous necrosis. In difficult cases, it is preferable to obtain the opinion of a plastic surgeon on the utility of preventive techniques and to anticipate rapid secondary surgery if necrosis does occur.

Articular approach

This consists of two successive stages: subluxation of the patella and tibiofemoral subluxation. These must be carried out with prudence and with patience as on them depends the remaining course of the procedure.

Patellar subluxation

No attempt at removing the prosthetic components can be made before the patella has been subluxated. This is made easier by good preparation with a wide approach and incision carried high on the quadricipital tendon, release of the suprapatellar bursa and patellar adhesions, as well as progressive release of attachments between the patella tendon and the anterior border of the tibial plateau. The assistant can then detach the patella with a retractor and gently attempt to evert it. Detachment from the patellar tendon of adhesions, in particular at the external angle of the tibial plateau (for an internal approach) then resection of the external flange from the tibia to the vastus lateralis muscle and external vertical patellectomy can help to subluxate the patella (fig. 4). It is often distal rather than proximal release which enables mobilisation of the patella. The patellar tendon insertion can be protected by placing a pin in the anterior tibial tubercle (ATT).

If it is impossible to subluxate the patella, technical expedients can be used.

– Elevation of the ATT must follow strict rules. It must be anticipated from the start when planning the procedure in at-risk cases: low patella, previous

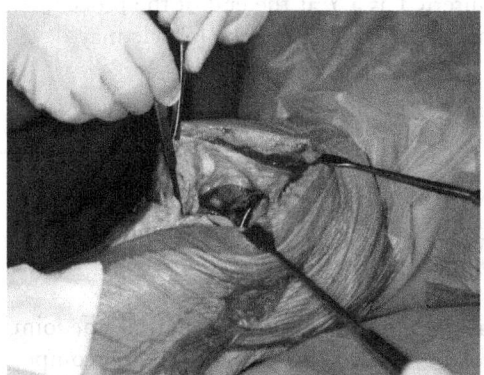

Fig. 4 – Progressive release of the patella.

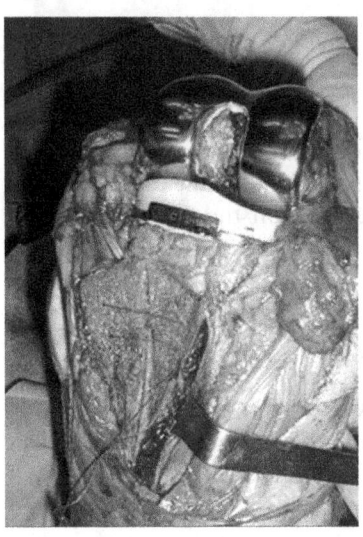

Fig. 5 – Elevation of the anterior tibial tubercle.

surgery on the knee, history of ATT osteotomy, of high tibial osteotomy or knee stiffness. In principle, it should then be done at the beginning of the procedure. In other cases, the decision must be made quickly and not after repeated, fruitless attempts at an articular approach. The portion of bone must be long (6cm) and thick (1cm). The internal cortical bone is detached with a stryker saw, as is the distal extremity. The external cortical bone is detached with an osteotome and the portion of bone must retain an external pedicle on the anterior tibial muscle. If the approach was external, it retains an internal pedicle on the periosteum. Fixation is done at the end of the procedure by three bicortical screws, though some operators prefer metal wire (fig. 5). This technique has the advantage of simplicity; it does not damage the quadriceps and allows early rehabilitation. Its drawback is the risk of pseudarthrosis, fracture of the ATT or even the tibia, and the increased risk of cutaneous necrosis if the preliminary incisions intersect at this level. However these complications are rare (4, 39) and this technique can be widely applied.

– Oblique incision of the quadricipital tendon, or quadriceps snip (18), consists of incising the tendon obliquely in the proximal part of the incision, in a distal to proximal direction and medially to laterally up to the fibres of the vastus lateralis muscle. This technique allows a wide approach and easy subluxation of the patella without putting bone or skin at risk. It is particularly useful in cases where the skin is of poor quality or if many incisions intersect on the ATT. Closure of the tendon must however be meticulous and of good quality in order to avoid residual active flexion contracture.

– Complete elevation of the quadricipital tendon after V-incision has been described in difficult cases. It is reinserted as a Y at the end of the procedure. This technique puts the extensor apparatus at risk and the muscle may develop residual weakness (35).

Tibiofemoral subluxation

After patellar subluxation and flexing of the knee, tibiofemoral subluxation should be obtained with caution as the patellar tendon is still vulnerable. In difficult cases, it is obtained progressively as the first components of the implant are removed.

In the first stage, when the tibial polyethylene has been removed, the joint can be freed and the posterior condyles exposed (fig. 6). The femoral compo-

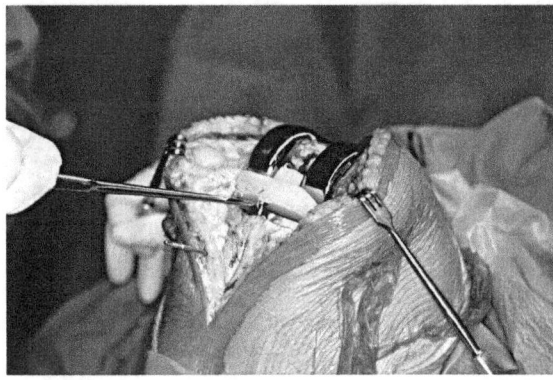

Fig. 6 – The tibial poly-ethylene is removed first in order to free the posterior condyles.

nent can then gradually be removed and tibiofemoral subluxation is rarely impossible at this stage. Forcible manoeuvres must be avoided such as using a retractor pressing into the intercondylar notch, which would increase loss of bone stock. It is rarely necessary to resort to the expedient of Engh (15) who carried out osteotomy of the medial epicondyle, raising *en bloc* the internal lateral ligament and the medial epicondyle, which is then reinserted at the end of the procedure. This is in fact an approach technique but it may be used for internal release if there is marked varus.

Component removal

Components must be removed very gradually to avoid further loss of bone stock. This may be very easy with a loosened prosthesis but very difficult in other cases, in particular if the prosthesis is cementless. Tibial polyethylene is removed first, then the femoral component and lastly the metal tibial base-plate.

The femoral component must be progressively mobilized by sliding small osteotomes between the prosthetic trochlea and the femur (fig. 7) or an alternating saw, avoiding any movement of leverage on the bone. A Gigli saw is conventionally used. After mobilisation of the entire femoral compo-nent, extraction is completed using a bone collector. If there is a long intra-

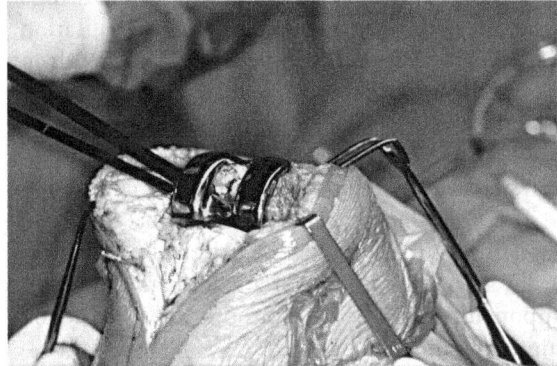

Fig. 7 –The femoral com-ponent is gradually removed using fine osteotomes. The tibia can then be subluxated anteriorly before passing on to the next stage.

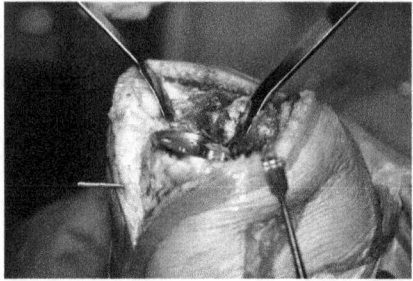
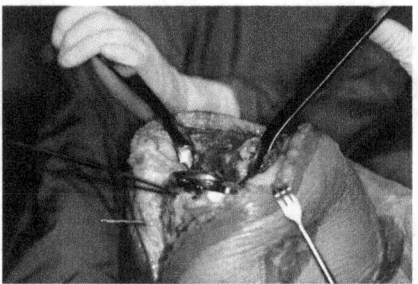

Fig. 8 – a. After removal of the femoral component, the tibia can be dislocated. **b.** The tibial component is mobilised little by little using fine osteotomes.

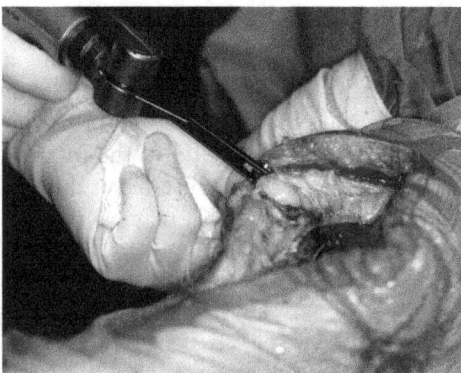

Fig. 9 – Removal of the patellar component.

medullary stem, anterior corticotomy can be carried out at varying heights on the femur, or an anterior femoral window. The remaining cement is then removed using the same instruments as in revision total hip arthroplasty. The window or corticotomy is closed at the end of the procedure using cerclage wires.

The metal tibial baseplate can only be removed after complete tibiofemoral subluxation (fig. 8). The same rules apply (no levering movement) and the same instruments are used. When the metal tray has been detached from the central plot, removal can be done in two stages. Usually, detachment of the tibial tray and its mobilisation make it possible to remove the whole using a bone collector. If fixation of the central medullary stem prevents mobilisation, and if the baseplate can be removed, the stem is progressively detached from the top using small osteotomes. If this is not possible, a tibial window must be created, either anterior and internal, or from the elevation of the ATT, which is a comfortable approach.

The patellar button is not systematically removed. The patellar component must be changed only in the case of loosening, faulty resection or metal-backed patella. When the patella is firmly fixed, it may be extremely difficult to remove and can fracture. Ideally, an oscillating saw or an alternating saw slipped under the prosthetic component should be used but this requires adequate bone stock and may be limited by metallic pegs (fig. 9).

Evaluation of bone stock deficiencies

When the components have been removed, the bony extremities must be carefully curetted, with removal of cement debris, curettage of lytic defects, synovectomy and abundant lavage. The material removed must be sent for bacteriological analysis (fig. 10).

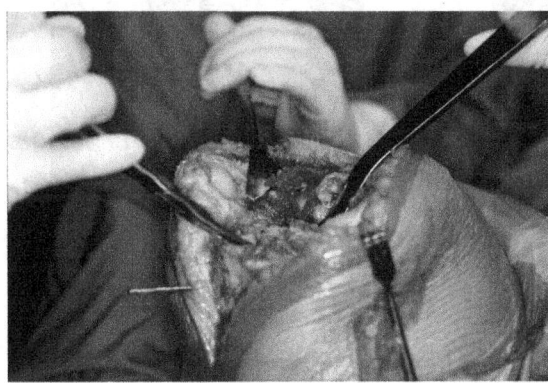

Fig. 10 – Curettage and removal of cement debris and membranous residue on the bony extremities.

At this stage loss of bone stock can be evaluated and reconstruction considered. Minimal resection to cleanse the bony surface can be done. It must always be minimal but is necessary if there was a resection error on the primary prosthesis or if the revision prosthesis requires a different slope. In any case, this resection should not go beyond zone B (fig. 2 – chapter 34). In the femur resection is rare, unless there was a manifest initial error with insufficient resection.

Reconstruction of bony defects

Filling of the bony defect depends on its size, its site and whether it is cavitary or segmental. Its aim is to restore the normal alignment of the knee, with good strain distribution and maximal preservation of bone stock.

Considerable resection of the tibia is to be excluded as the mechanical resistance of spongy bone decreases very quickly and a smaller tibial diameter would require the use of small trays, increasing the mechanical strains and limiting *ipso facto* the size which can be used on the femur. In another respect, cortical support is often a limiting factor in reconstruction and it is preferable to keep a cavitary defect and graft it rather than to resect to obtain homogeneous but more distal support. Cases with resection in zone C (fig 2 – chapter 34) of the tibia had less good results (26). Some authors advise translating the tibial component in order to avoid bearing on the loss of substance, so that support is given by healthy bone. However this technique necessitates the use of small-sized components and can only correct small-sized defects (25).

Filling of a bony defect always requires the use of long intramedullary stems (13, 22, 28, 34, 38, 40). These prevent tilting of the implants and give better

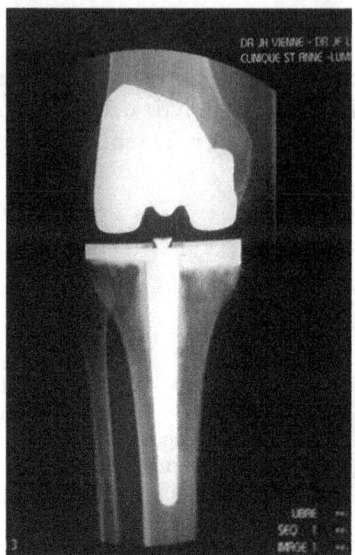 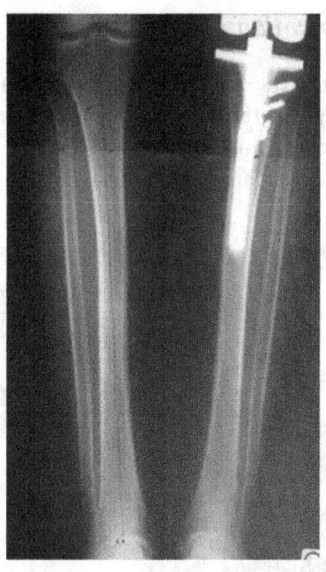

Fig. 11 – Reconstruction from the epiphysis: Risk of misdirection and the stem must be cemented.

Fig. 12 – Reconstruction from the diaphysis. A system offsetting the stem in relation to the plateau is required.

distribution of mechanical stresses. There are two types of stem, corresponding to two different techniques of reconstruction.

– *Reconstruction from the epiphysis*: the tibial component, with its wedges if any, is adapted to the configuration of the epiphysis and correction is determined using extramedullary or fine intramedullary guidewires. In the last stage, a long intramedullary prosthetic stem is inserted. This stem is small in size: It must not take up the entire medullary canal because of the risks of misdirection, of tilting after impaction or of impingement of the extremity of the stem on cortical bone. With this technique the stem must be fully cemented, which may lead to technical problems if later revision is required.

– *Reconstruction from the diaphysis*: after reaming, a "press-fit" intramedullary stem is inserted into the medullary canal. It thus fits perfectly into the medullary canal of the upper part of the tibial diaphysis. Reconstruction is then carried out on this stem. Here the stem is large, because it is adapted to the medullary canal, there is no risk of tilting after impaction, risk of misdirection is minimal and the stem is not cemented. On the other hand, because of frequent misalignment between the medullary canal and the epiphysis with this option it is necessary to be able to alter the alignment of the tibial tray relative to the stem (fig. 12) (23).

Several techniques may be used to fill a bony defect. If it is minimal (< 5mm) filling with cement with or without fixation screws seems mechanically reliable and has been supported by certain authors. At the present time this type of filling is reserved only for circumscribed irregularities on the tibia or small cavitary defects of the condyles. A central cavitary lytic defect may be filled by morselised grafts of spongy bone (auto- or allograft). Bone stock is thus restored without making the cortex more fragile.

With a tibial defect extending to the cortex (segmental deficiency), filling may be done in several ways. Cement is not sufficient in such cases, even if reinforced by screws (6). Horizontal or oblique metal wedges give a base in healthy bone and good stability of the implant with satisfactory stress distribution (29). The wedges may be modular, which provides more versatility, or monobloc in relation to the metal baseplate, which gives more rigidity to the system. Brooks has shown that modular wedges are equivalent to custom-made components regarding rigidity (6). Oblique wedges make it possible to limit bone excision, but they must not be too oblique. Support on horizontal wedges leads to greater bone excision but essentially at the expense of spongy bone, and horizontal support is preferable from a mechanical viewpoint. Fehring, in an *in vitro* study observed slightly less strain with horizontal wedges, but the difference was minimal and the author recommends adapting the type of reconstruction to the shape of the defect in order to sacrifice as little bone as possible (17). Chen in an *in vitro* study observed greater rigidity when horizontal wedges were used for peripheral defects from 20° to 35° (9)

Massive bone grafts (auto- or allografts) can be used to reconstruct large segmental bone deficiencies or to fill a massive central cavity. There is however a risk of secondary rupture after four to five years (12, 19, 33, 36).

Morselized grafts, whether auto- or allografts, seem to have better potential for incorporation (31). Some authors observed a high failure rate (25). Impacted morselized graft techniques similar to the technique described by Gie (20) in the hip have their supporters (5, 41). Cavitary defects were first filled by forced impaction of morselized grafts. Impaction is then applied using a phantom and the long-stemmed prosthetic component is forcibly inserted in the bed of compacted grafts. The segmental defect is then filled by grafts impacted into the residual space between the prosthesis and the remaining cortical bone. Unlike the hip, this technique is used with cementless implants, as Bradley observed more failures when cement was used (5).

At the condyles, a small circumscribed defect can also be filled with spongy bone grafts but this is a rare situation and in general the defect involves the entire thickness of the condyle and metal wedges must be used, depending on the size and placement chosen for the femoral component during soft tissue balance. Here again filling can be done by morselized graft impaction with cementless implants (5).

Reconstruction and soft tissue balance

Reconstruction and soft tissue balance should be carried out progressively with the aim of using minimal constraint, that is a conventional posterior stabilised prosthesis. This type of prosthesis can in fact be used in the majority of reconstructions. Only if it is not possible to stabilise the knee with a prosthesis of this type should we consider passing on to a constrained prosthesis, either a constrained posterior stabilized prosthesis of constrained condylar knee (CCK) type or a rotational hinged prosthesis (RH). This choice can thus be made only at the end of the procedure, after having carried out trials with a standard posterior stabilised plateau. Use of a constrained prosthesis does not dispense with the need to follow the rules of balance and reconstruction. Constraint must not be a "cover-up" and a poorly positioned constrained prosthesis will lead to early failure.

If constraint must be used, a rotational hinged prosthesis should be preferred in the rare cases with persistent laxity in extension and a constrained posterior stabilized prosthesis should be chosen if there is good stability in extension but persistent laxity in flexion (table II) (24).

Table II – Choice of constraint according to residual laxity at the end of the procedure.

Stability in flexion	Stability in extension	Choice of constraint
+	+	PS
±	+	PS
−	+	CCK
−	−	RH

The principle of soft tissue balance is to analyse flexion and extension separately (table III).

Flexion space is governed by:
1. the thickness of the tibial polyethylene;
2. the size of the femoral prosthetic component (the larger its size, the greater its anteroposterior diameter and the smaller the flexion space);
3. by the use of an offset femoral stem (offset in a forward direction increases the flexion space, offset in a backward direction decreases the flexion space).

Table III – Factors influencing flexion and extension spaces in revision total knee arthroplasty.

	Flexion gap	Extension gap
Polyethylene	+	+
Size of femoral component	+	−
Position of femoral component	−	+
Posterior offset of femoral component	+	−

Extension space is governed by:
1. the thickness of the tibial polyethylene;
2. and by the positioning of the femoral component (the more distal it is, the more restricted the extension space).

Phase 1: Tibial reconstruction

This is the initial phase which, whatever the mode of reconstruction chosen (metal wedges, cement, grafts) should make it possible to find a reference basis for the following stages (14, 16, 27, 37). The frontal and sagittal axis is maintained by a long intramedullary stem in the medullary canal. The initial position of the joint line has already been determined during preoperative planning.

The position in rotation must now be carefully analysed by identifying the ATT, the posterior plane of the tibial plateaus and the axis of the foot.

The trial tibial component is then positioned with a polyethylene plateau located at the reference level established from comparative preoperative radiographs and identified before the components were removed.

Phase 2: Soft tissue balance in flexion

When the trial tibial component is in place, the femoral stage can begin (fig. 13). A trial femoral component on an intramedullary stem is inserted. Its initial size is determined by:

1. preoperative radiographic analysis using templates, and possibly radiographs of the opposite knee;

2. the size of the tibial component selected during the previous phase. The relationship between tibial size and femoral size varies according to the prosthetic system used and the type of constraint chosen. The possible size differences are greater with standard posterior stabilised prostheses than with constrained posterior stabilised prostheses. Certain systems which impose "same size" conformity make it impossible to regulate soft tissue balance in flexion by resection of the femoral component. When choosing a prosthetic system, it is important to take into consideration this possibility of using different sized femoral and tibial components.

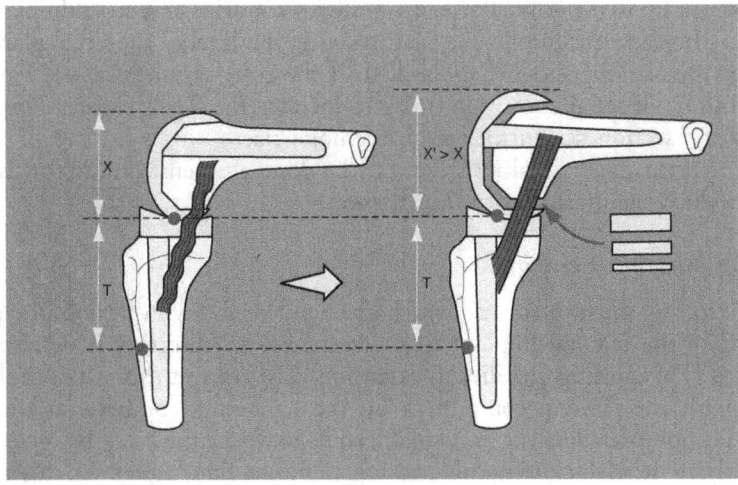

Fig. 13 – Soft tissue balance in flexion. After placing the tibial component according to the preoperative plan (height T in relation to the initial landmark) laxity in flexion is corrected by increasing the size of the femoral component. The posterior loss of substance is then compensated by posterior condylar metal wedges.

Rotational positioning is crucial at this stage as the reference posterior bicondylar plane has disappeared and bone loss makes the remaining condyles and the trochlea totally unreliable. Only the transepicondylar axis can thus be used as a landmark (2, 11, 32). Any rotational malalignment of the primary prosthesis must be corrected, and posterior condylar wedges may be necessary on one side or the other.

Soft tissue balance is then established by adjusting the size of the femoral component, which must be chosen to allow good stability in flexion without excessive lateral and medial overhang. The posterior bone defect appearing between the residual posterior condyle and the prosthesis is filled by metal wedges.

Several situations may arise:

1. The initial size gives good stability in flexion (we can move on to extension);

2. Laxity in flexion;

2.1 – The initial size is too small. We then successively try increasing sizes until we find the size which gives good stability in flexion. If this size is compatible with femoral shape (no lateral overhang) and with the size of the tibial component, we can move on to extension. If this is not the case, we try the following expedients until good stability is obtained;

2.2 – If (2.1) fails, we can offset the femoral stem posteriorly, which offsets the femoral component in the same direction;

2.3 – If (2.2) fails or is not possible (no offset stems), the thickness of the tibial polyethylene is increased but in a controlled manner to avoid excessive modification of the joint line;

2.4 – If (2.3) fails, we move on to a constrained system.

3. Stiffness restricting flexion.

3.1 – The initial size gives too limited a flexion space: use a smaller femoral component up to the limit allowed by posterior condylar support and tibial size;

3.2 – In case of failure in the first instance, the level of the tibial platform and the tibial slope should be checked. If these are satisfactory, the femoral stem can be offset anteriorly in order to increase the flexion space. Posterior condylar resection can further reduce femoral size;

3.3 – If this fails, tibial resection can be done after ensuring that this will not produce significant laxity in extension.

Phase 3: Balancing in extension

After selecting the implant size which gives good stability in flexion, the positioning of the femoral implant in a proximal/distal direction is determined (fig. 14). This governs stability in extension. The error at this stage would be to support the femoral component on the remaining condyles, as there is generally bone deficiency. This would lead us to wedge the laxity by increasing the polyethylene thickness, this making the joint line higher. At this stage, positioning must be guided by stability alone and three situations may arise:

1. The positioning spontaneously gives good stability in extension. We then ensure the whole of the mobile sector is stable and can consider fixing the permanent components;

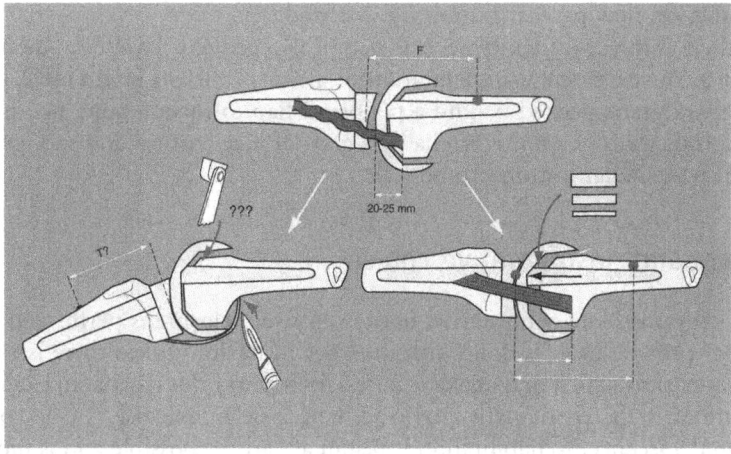

Fig. 14 – Soft tissue balance in extension. Laxity in extension is corrected by distally translating the femoral component. Distal condylar loss of substance is then compensated by metal wedges. Stiffness is corrected (1) by soft tissue release, (2) minimal femoral resection and (3) tibial resection.

2. Laxity in extension;

2.1 – Symmetric laxity in extension. The femoral component must be offset distally until good stability is obtained. The distal femoral defect thus created is filled by metal wedges giving good condylar support;

2.2 – Asymmetric laxity in extension. The taut side is released and we are now in the previous situation;

2.3 – If stabilisation is impossible even after maximal displacement of the femoral component (limits related to the distal femoral wedges), the thickness of the tibial polyethylene must be increased. This however will have the effect of restricting the flexion space, and this must be compensated by decreasing the size of the femoral component;

2.4 – If stability is insufficient in spite of maximum polyethylene thickness, a constrained system must be used.

3. Stiffness in extension.

3.1 – Extension is impossible even though the femoral component is in contact with the bony condyles. The first thing to do is posterior release involving the capsule and any remains of the posterior cruciate ligament;

3.2 – Extension is impossible in spite of posterior arthrolysis. Economical distal condylar resection can be envisaged, checking the position of the joint line in relation to the epicondyles;

3.3 – Extension is impossible in spite of distal resection. Consider tibial resection. However, this will affect the flexion space, which must be compensated by increased resection of the femoral component.

Phase 4: Patellar reconstruction

Patellar reconstruction is difficult if there is little residual bone stock. It may be necessary to leave the bony patella in its original state but results appear to be better if a new patellar button can be fixed (7).

If there is major difficulty, several technical expedients have been described: use of biconvex patellas, implantation of a neo-patella in Hydrocel®, use of morselized grafts packed behind a periosteal flap to form a bony neo-patella, or reconstitution of a bony patella by a graft of iliac cortical and spongy bone in which a patellar button can be sealed.

Closure and postoperative course

Once the prosthetic components have been fixed, closure is performed as for primary prostheses. It is done with the knee in flexion unless there is excessive skin tension which may make it necessary to carry out closure in extension. Closure must be particularly meticulous because of the risks of necrosis or wound dehiscence. Rehabilitation is begun as early as possible and is modulated depending on the state of the skin and the associated procedures carried out on the extensor apparatus.

References

1. Badet R, Aït Si Selmi T, Neyret Ph (1999) Prothèse totale du genou après ostéotomie tibiale de valgisation. In: La chirurgie prothétique du genou. Chambat, Neyret, Deschamps. Sauramps, Montpellier, p. 241-58
2. Berger RA, Rubash HE, Steel MJ et al. (1993) Determining the rotational alignment of the femoral component in total knee arthroplasty, using the trans-epicondylar axis. Clin Orthop 286:40-47.
3. Bonnin M, Deroche P, Palazzolo P (1999) Les reprises de prothèses totales du genou. In: La chirurgie prothétique du genou. Chambat P, Neyret Ph, Deschamps G. Sauramps, Montpellier, p. 177-202
4. Bonnin M, Deschamps G, Neyret Ph et al. (2000) Les changements de prothèses totales du genou non infecté. Rev Chir Orthop 86: 694-706
5. Bradley GW (2000) Revision total knee arthroplasty by impaction bone grafting. Clin Orthop 371: 113-8
6. Brooks J, Walker PS, Scott RD (1984) Tibial component fixation in deficient tibial bone stock. Clin Orthop 184: 304-8.
7. Caton J, Reynaud P, Marabet Z (2001) La rotule lors des changements de prothèses totales du genou. Rev Chir Orthop 87 (suppl. 15): 195-6
8. Chatain F, Richard A, Deschamps G (1999) Reprise de prothèse unicompartimentales par prothèse totale du genou. In: La chirurgie prothétique du genou. Chambat P, Neyret Ph, Deschamps G. Sauramps, Montpellier, p. 159-68
9. Chen F, Krackow KA (1994) Management of tibial defects in total knee arthroplasty A biomechanical study. Clin Orthop 305: 249-57
10. Deschamps G, Bonnin M, Aït Si Selmi T et al. (2001) L'interligne prothétique dans les reprises de prothèses totales du genou. Rev Chir Orthop 87 (suppl. 15): 186-91
11. Eckhoff DG, Metzger RG, Vandewalle MV (1995) Malrotation associated with implant alignment technique in total knee arthroplasty. Clin Orthop 321: 28-31
12. Engh GA, Herswurm PJ, Parks NL (1997) Treatment of major defects of bone with bulk allografts and stemmed components during total knee arthroplasty. J Bone Joint Surg Am 79: 1030-9
13. Engh GA, Parks NL, Ammeen DJ (1994) Tibial osteolysis in cementless total knee arthroplasty. A review of 25 cases treated with and without tibial component revision. Clin Orthop 309: 33-43

14. Engh GA, Mc Auley JP (1997) Joint line restoration and flexion-extension balance with revision total knee arthroplasty. In: Revision total knee arthroplasty. Engh GA, Williams Wilkins, Baltimore p. 235-51
15. Engh GA (1999) AAOS Annaheim Fev. 1999
16. Fehring TK, Valadie AL (1994) Knee instability after total knee arthroplasty. Clin Orthop 299: 157-62
17. Fehring TK, Peindl RD, Humble RS et al. (1996) Modular tibial augmentations in total knee arthroplasty. Clin Orthop. 327: 207-17
18. Garvin KL, Scuderi GR, Insall JN (1995) Evolution of the quadriceps snip. Clin Orthop 321: 131-7
19. Ghazavi MT, Stockley I, Yee G et al. (1997) Reconstruction of massive bone defects with allograft in revision total knee arthroplasty. J Bone Joint Surg Am 79: 17-25
20. Gie IA, Linder L, Ling RSM (1993) Impacted cancellous allograft and cement for revision total hip arthroplasty. J Bone Joint Surg 75B: 14-21
21. Griffin FM, Mark K, Suderi GR et al. (2000) Anatomy of the epicondyles of the distal femur. MRI analysis of normal knees. J Arthroplasty 15:354-9
22. Haas SB, Insall IN, Montgomery W et al. (1995) Revision total knee arthroplasty with use of modular components with stems inserted without cement. J Bone Joint Surg Am 77: 1700-7
23. Hicks CA, Noble P, Tullos H (1995) The anatomy of the tibial intramedullary canal. Clin Orthop 321: 111-6
24. Huten D, Vandevelde D, Angotti P et al. (2001) Le choix de la contrainte prothétique lors des changements de prothèses totales du genou. Rev Chir Orthop 87(suppl. 1S): 182-6
25. Laskin RS (1989) Total knee arthroplasty in the presence of large bony defects of the tibia and marked knee instability. Clin Orthop 248: 66-70
26. Mathieu M, Rizk S (2001) Les reprises de prothèses totales du genou pour descellement: facteurs de pronostic. Rev Chir Orthop 87(suppl. 1S): 178
27. Mont MA, Delanois R, Hungerford DS (1989) Balancing and alignment. Surgical techniques on how to achieve soft tissue balancing. In: Revision total knee arthroplasty. P Lotke, J Garino, Lippincott-Raven Philadelphia p. 173-86
28. Murray PB, Rand JA, Hanssen AD (1994) Cemented long-stem revision total knee arthroplasty. Clin Orthop 309: 116-23
29. Pagnano MW, Trousdale RT, Rand JA (1995) Tibial wedge augmentation for bone deficiency in total knee arthroplasty follow-up study. Clin Orthop 321: 151-5
30. Partington PF, Sawhney J, Rorabeck C et al. (1999) Joint line restoration after revision total knee arthroplasty. Clin Orthop 367: 165-71
31. Scuderi GR, Insall JN, Haas S et al.(1989) Inlay antogenic bone grafting of tibial defects in primary total knee arthroplasty. Clin Orthop 248: 93-7
32. Stiehl JB, Abbott BD (1995) Morphology of the transepicondylar axis and its application in primary and revision total knee arthroplasty. J Arthroplasty 10:785-789
33. Stockley I, Mc Aulmey JP, Gross AE (1992) Allograft reconstruction in total knee arthroplasty. J Bone Joint Surg 74B: 393-7
34. Takayashi Y, Gustilo RB (1994) Non constrained implants in revision total knee arthroplasty. Clin Orthop 309:1 56-62
35. Trousdale RT, Hansen AD, Rand JA et al. (1993) V-Y quadriceps plasty in total knee arthroplasty. Clin Orthop 286: 48-55
36. Tsahakis PJ, Beaver WB, Brick GW (1994) Technique and results of allograft reconstruction in revision total knee arthroplasty. Clin Orthop 303: 86-94
37. Vince KJ (1998) Constraint in revision knee arthroplasty AAOS – Instructional course. New Orleans. March 1998
38. Vince KG, Long W (1995) Revision total knee arthroplasty: The limits of press medullary fixation. Clin Orthop 317: 172-7
39. Whiteside LA (1995) Exposure in difficult total knee arthroplasty using tibial tubercule osteotomy. Clin Orthop 321: 32-5
40. Widel JD (1994) Non-cemented revision total knee arthroplasty. Clin Orthop 309: 110-5
41. Whiteside LA (1998) Morselized allografting in revision total knee arthroplasty. Orthopedics 21: 1041-3

Management of bone defects in revision total knee arthroplasty

D. Huten

Some degree of bone loss is typically encountered in all cases of revision total knee arthroplasty, particularly revisions for loosening.

Causes of bone loss include (37, 77):

– initial osteoarticular destruction;

– bone resections performed during prior knee replacement(s);

– bone wear caused by motion of loose components;

– osteolysis instigated by the macrophage reaction to particulate wear debris;

– sometimes, periprosthetic fracture, infection, and even osteonecrosis resulting from surgical devascularization (37, 67);

– components that are difficult to remove, particularly well-fixed components or ingrown uncemented components.

Additionally, decrease (of varying severity) in distal femoral bone mineral density (BMD) is observed, which promotes fractures and makes revision surgery even more challenging (40, 42, 47, 56, 69). Decrease in BMD was evaluated using plain radiographs (47), or measured with DEXA (40) or quantitative computed tomography (QCT) (69). At the distal femur, and particularly at the anterior aspect of the epiphysis, bone loss occurs within the first postoperative year and does not progress further (47). At the tibia, measurements showed that bone loss ranged from 0.4 to 3.6% per month, with no further progression after the first year (69). Cemented central tibial stems, even short ones, have been shown to promote bone resorption (42). Decrease in BMD is even more significant in rheumatoid patients, and after prolonged unloading.

Bone loss mainly affects the epiphyseal region, but it may extend to the metaphysis and even the diaphysis if the revised components had stem extensions. It is often underestimated during preoperative planning, particularly at the distal femur, because on X-rays it is concealed by the femoral component (9, 11, 14).

Several classifications of bone loss in revision TKA are available (12, 14, 20, 28, 57, 67, 68). All of them distinguish between contained defects with cancellous bone loss and no cortical loss, and non-contained defects without peripheral bony rim. However, there is no consensus regarding grading of the severity of the defect which determines the complexity and the outcome of a revision procedure. As a matter of fact, there is a world of difference between an epiphyseal bone loss limited to the distal 10-15 mm of the distal femur, just above the joint line, and a bone defect that involves the metaphysis and even the diaphysis.

Bone resections minimize or even eliminate bone defects, but they also remove healthy bone. A minimal resection provides a large but discontinuous surface area for the component and a weak support due to the bone loss, but it preserves integrity of the healthy bone (9, 46, 57).

Reconstruction of bone defects is meant to:
– provide the best possible support to the new prosthesis;
– allow even transfer of loads to bone;
– correct any malpositioning resulting, for example, from a varus tibial cut or femoral malrotation;
– restore the joint line and, consequently, normal patella position.

Reconstruction techniques vary according to the site and the severity of bone loss:
– cement, reinforced or not with screws;
– modular or custom prosthesis;
– autografts, or, more often, morsellized or structural allografts.

Classification of bone defects

A classification of bone defects is indispensable to a surgeon to make a prognosis, plan the procedure, and compare the results achieved with the different techniques.

The severity of bone loss is often underestimated during the preoperative planning because on X-rays it is concealed by the metal components; furthermore, bone loss is increased by removal of the old components. Evaluation of bone loss is more difficult on the femoral side: on the AP view, the epiphysis is almost completely concealed by the metal component; on the lateral view, both condyles are superimposed, so that osteolysis of one condyle may be hidden from view by the intact contralateral condyle. It is best appreciated by examining the superior aspect of posterior condyles where the cancellous bone is exposed and fixation often weaker. This explains why axial migration of the femoral component is detectable only by comparing a sequence of roentgenograms.

We compared the results of the preoperative radiographic evaluation with the intraoperative findings described in the operation report: tibial bone loss was radiographically underestimated in more than 50% of the cases, and femoral bone loss in more than 60% (9). Therefore, intraoperative findings are most valuable, as well as immediate postoperative X-rays which clearly show the resection levels and the quality of the reconstruction. Because of this radio-anatomic discrepancy, it is important to use a revision total knee system which offers a wide range of options to address any bone loss.

In 1986, Dorr proposed a classification of tibial bone defects based on their localization: central cavitary or peripheral (12). This classification can be used both for primary and revision total knee arthroplasty (TKA). He advocated bone grafting of defects involving more than 50% of the resected tibial condyle and more than 5mm deep.

Rand based his classification on the following: symmetry/asymmetry of the defect, site and severity (57). A bone defect can by symmetric (component migration occurred in both femoral condyles or both tibial condyles) or asymmetric (unilateral migration of the component with varus or valgus deviation in the frontal plane), central or peripheral, and at the femur: distal, posterior, or both.

After all bone cuts have been completed, bone loss is graded according to the degree of severity:

– Type I (minimal) involves less than 50% of a tibial or femoral condyle; less than 5mm deep;

  – Type II (moderate) between 50% and 70%; 5-10mm deep;

  – Type III (extensive) between 70% and 90%; depth $\geq$ 10mm;

  – Type IV (massive, cavitary) > 90%, with two subcategories:

  • intact peripheral bony rim;

  • discontinuous peripheral bony rim.

Gross classified bone defects as contained (with a peripheral bony rim) and non-contained. Uncontained defects are divided into circumferential and non-circumferential, and the latter are subdivided into defects greater than or smaller than 3 cm. A tibial bone defect smaller than 3cm can be filled with a modular metal wedge; when greater than 3cm, it can only be managed with an allograft or a custom prosthesis (20).

Engh defined three types of tibial metaphyseal bone defects (T1, T2, T3) and three types of femoral metaphyseal bone defects (F1, F2, F3), based on preoperative X-rays, operative findings, and retrospectively, on the procedures performed during revision arthroplasty (14):

– Type I (intact metaphysis): no component migration, minimal bone loss (< 1cm^3), strong cancellous bone. A stemless component can be used.

– Type II (metaphysis involved): component migration, bone loss > 1cm^3, cancellous bone damaged. Small metaphyseal bone cysts may be present proximal to the tibial tuberosity or distal to the epicondyles. Bone loss may affect one tibial condyle (T2 A) or both tibial condyles (T2 B), one femoral condyle (F2 A) or both femoral condyles (F2 B). Filling with cement, modular augment, or bone graft is necessary to restore the joint line. A stemmed revision component is required;

– Type III (metaphysis partly destroyed): bone loss involves most of one or both tibial or femoral condyles; it may extend further and cause detachment of the collateral ligament or patellar ligament. This requires the use of structural bone grafts or custom components, stemmed components, and sometimes a hinge prosthesis.

The recent Rubash classification of femoral defects based on intraoperative findings also takes into consideration the position of the defect relative to the epicondyles (28). Distinction is made between minor bone defects smaller than 1cm^3 and located distal to the epicondyles, and defects greater than 1cm^3 or located proximal to the epicondyles; each type is subclassified as contained bone defect involving only the cancellous bone, and non-contained bone defect without peripheral bony rim.

The HSS (Hospital for Special Surgery) classification includes bone defects which involve the diaphysis, and takes into consideration the bone loss process (67, 68):

– cystic bone defects (bone cysts which were filled with cement during prior knee arthroplasty, focal osteolysis, fixation pegs);
– wedge-shaped bone defects: wedge shape results from asymmetric migration of components. May be contained or non-contained;
– central cavitary defects: seen during revision of stemmed components;
– defects resulting from bone perforation or fracture;
– segmental defects: destruction of most of one or both femoral or tibial condyles. May cause detachment of ligaments.

Most of these classifications rely on the condition of bone ends after the old components have been removed. We think, as many other authors (46, 57), that it is much more logical to evaluate the bone stock after all bone cuts have been performed. This classification (9) uses three parameters:

– resection level. Three zones (A, B, C) have been defined for the femur and the tibia to grade bone defects. Insertions of the collateral ligaments are located in upper zone B on the femur and in zone C on the tibia. Insertion of the popliteal ligament is located in lower zone B on the lateral femoral condyle, and is therefore the most susceptible to be damaged during femoral resection (fig. 1);
– symmetry / asymmetry of bone cuts on the medial and lateral sides. An index has been defined: 1 for symmetric medial and lateral cuts, 2 for an oblique or stepped femoral resection. Should resection involve two zones, the zone to be considered is that which is the most distant from the joint line;
– condition of bone surface: no bone loss, cavitary defect, segmental defect. In this classification, non-contained defects are described as "segmental" defects, whereas North American classification systems use this term for defects involving most of a femoral or tibial condyle (67, 68).

Three areas have been defined for femoral and tibial defects. A score is allocated according to the area involved: 1 point for a central cavitary defect, 2 points for a medial or lateral cavitary defect, 6 points for a medial or lateral segmental defect. Altogether, six grades (from A1 to C2) and a 17-point scale are used for each epiphysis. For the femur, a special posterior score denotes the position (A or B) of the posterior condylar resection; condition of bone surface after the resection is not taken into consideration. For each condyle, 1 point is allocated for resection in zone A, and 3 points for resection in zone B.

Intra- and inter-investigator reproducibility of the above classification sys-

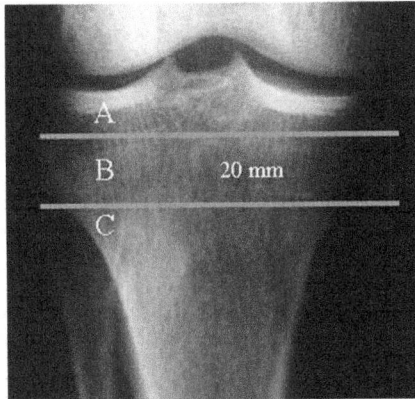
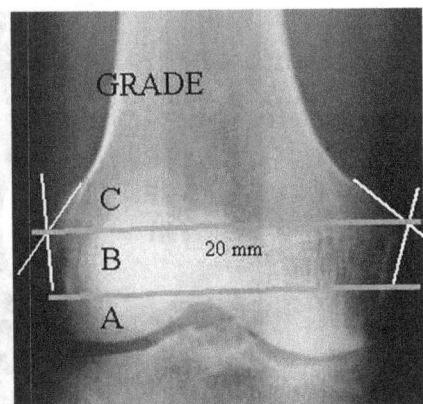
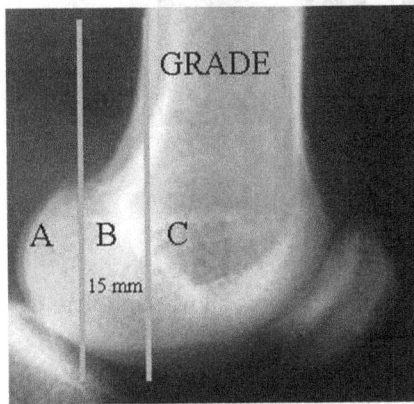

Fig. 1 – Definition of the three grades of bone defects, based on resection level.
A. Tibia.
B. Distal femur.
C. Posterior condyles.

tems has not been assessed. A longer follow-up and prospective studies will be necessary to assess their value.

Femoral and tibial bone defects

Elimination of the defect

During revision arthroplasty, bone resections are performed to provide flat surfaces for placement of the new components and remove all necrotic bone. They also reduce bone defects, if any. To completely eliminate a bone defect, one can remove a greater amount of bone and / or slightly translate the component. This technical trick is mostly used in the tibia, as a wide array of tibial component sizes is available (width and thickness; components more than 20mm thick) as well as a large load-bearing area (fig. 2). In contrast, few knee systems offer very thick femoral components. Furthermore, the femur does not offer a large uninterrupted load-bearing area, and translation is very limited. At last, translation implies that a smaller femoral component is used (smaller M-L and A-P dimensions), and this presents a potential risk of instability during flexion and notching of the anterior femoral cortex.

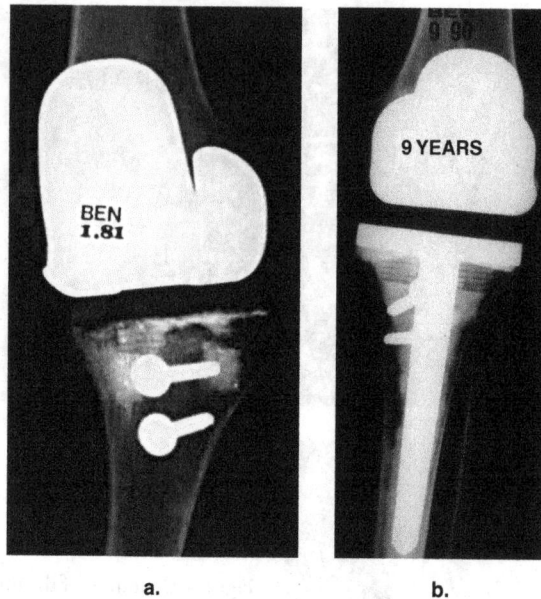

Fig. 2 – Grade C tibial bone defect (A) managed with bone resection (B).

Resecting the proximal tibia at the base of the defect allows complete elimination of the bone loss, but there are several drawbacks:

– the tibial component will rest on weakened bone. As a matter of fact, in the metaphyseal region, cancellous bone strength rapidly decreases with distance from the surface (26, 30, 70). Bone strength at 35mm distal to the joint line is only one-third of that measured at 5mm. Nevertheless, the greatest decrease is observed within 0 to 5mm of the joint line (26, 30, 70). According to Rand (57), the proximal tibial resection should not exceed 10mm (starting from the joint line), whereas Lotke thinks that a tibial resection of up to 20mm is acceptable (43);

– cancellous bone density is lower, and therefore, fixation is less reliable;

– as width of the resected surface is smaller, the tibial component must be downsized and may not have adequate cortical support;

– at last, the geometry of the cut is altered; its rounded-off contours may induce component malrotation.

According to Ritter, there is no evidence that a thick proximal tibial cut can potentially cause loosening; bone may even remodel and strengthen with loading. Therefore, thickness of the tibial cut is limited more by ligament insertions than by bone strength (21).

Translation of the tibial component has several advantages: it provides a larger area of healthy bone to support the component, and it leaves the defect outside the load-bearing area and thus eliminates the need for reconstruction (83). This technique has mainly been used in primary TKA. However, it has been shown that tibial tray translations of more than 4mm increase the incidence of radiolucency and loosening (38), particularly in cementless components (34). Therefore, translation should not exceed 4mm. Lotke used this technique for primary replacements in knees with a tibial defect involving less than 50% of either tibial plateau and deeper than 20mm (44). In addition, he increased the thickness of the tibial cut and used a cement wedge. At 5-11 year follow-up, non-progressive radiolucent lines were observed in 83% of the knees. Using this technique, the tibial tray is moved to the weaker side, there is a risk of patella maltracking in case of medialization, and it may be necessary to downsize the tibial tray.

Its specific drawbacks include:

– reduced contact area, less cortical support: excessive pressure is exerted upon the cancellous bone of the proximal tibia. Bourne's experiments showed that loss of tibial component-cortex contact results in 33% reduction (laterally) and 60% reduction (medially) of the loads sustained by the cortices (6). As a result, cancellous bone is overloaded, which may lead to debonding at the bone-cement interface or collapse of the cancellous bone, particularly where proximal tibial resection exceeds 10mm (starting from the joint line) (6);

– the tibial component may be too small to be associated with the appropriate size femoral component which would provide stability in flexion;

– if the femoral component is not translated by the same amount, there is a potential risk of subluxation.

In primary TKA, these techniques are reserved for bone defects involving less than 50% of either tibial plateau and less than 20mm deep (44, 57), and are preferably used in the elderly.

Their role in revision TKA is difficult to establish. Influence of the resection level has been evaluated in a series of 329 revision TKAs and the results were presented during the 2000 SOFCOT meeting. Tibial iterative loosening rate tended to increase with the thickness of the cut, particularly for cuts located in zone C (below the horizontal line, 20mm distal to the line passing through the top of the fibular head). Nevertheless, resection in zone B to completely eliminate the bone loss was preferable to resection in zone A (above the horizontal line passing through the top of the fibular head), allowing for persistence of a residual bone loss (23).

As regards femur, Nakabayashi showed that bone strength decreases over the distal 12mm of the femur and more particularly over the distal 6mm, and that at a depth ≤ 6mm, the lateral condyle is weaker than the medial condyle (51). Furthermore, bone strength is higher in femur than in tibia, both at the surface and in depth (26, 51). This is not consistent with Hvid's conclusions which state that femoral bone strength increases with increasing depth, and is lower than tibial bone strength (30). Results of the series presented during the 2000 SOFCOT meeting did not demonstrate a clear influence of the femoral resection on the iterative loosening rate (23), which is consistent with experimental data.

Cementing of bone defects

General points

Cement offers the advantage of ease of fit into a bone defect; furthermore, it is the least expensive filler material. But, it is not a biological material that can promote healing or union with the host bone. It fills a void but does not actually repair the defect. At last, cement cannot be efficiently pressurized into large bone defects or non-contained defects, so that its indications are rather limited. It has poor mechanical properties: its compressive strength is higher than its shear strength and tensile strength. This has been confirmed by Chen who showed that significantly better mechanical results were achieved in quadrangular defects (vertical and horizontal surfaces) than in triangular defects (oblique shaped defects), that quality of results increased with angulation of the defect (there is a highly significant difference in results between a 20° and a 35° defect), and eventually, that an interposition membrane develops at the bone-cement interface (10). However, converting a triangular defect into a quadrangular defect requires additional bone removal; as a result, cement will rest on cancellous bone which unfortunately becomes weaker and weaker as distance to the joint line increases. This is why the mechanical strength of a quadrangular filling decreases as thickness increases (10).

Cementing technique

– Bone preparation should meet modern cementing technique requirements: interposition tissue is carefully removed to fully expose the healthy bone;

– An uneven surface must be created to promote cement fixation in the smooth condensed bone (drill 2-3mm diameter holes, make sawcuts);

– Use pressure lavage to remove all blood and debris from the bone surface;

– If necessary, cement may be reinforced with titanium screws (21) or CoCr screws (18), depending on baseplate material. Ritter recommends that screw heads are countersunk. As a matter of fact, cement pressurization and therefore, cement penetration into the trabecular bone cannot occur if the tibial component is in contact with a screw head. Nevertheless, screw heads may help stabilize a component during trialing and cementing; in this case, insertion depth of the screws must be adjusted so as to avoid component tilt (65). The number of screws to be used depends on the size of the defect. Screws should be placed as close to one another as possible. Screw length typically ranges from 25 to 40mm for 6.5mm diameter (21) (fig. 3);

– Cement may be injected into the bone defect using a cement gun, and then pressurized into bone interstices by direct finger pressure. It is easier to inject cement under pressure into contained bone defects and femoral bone defects;

– In non-contained bone defects, one uses a finger to contain the defect while pressing the cement with the other hand. Cement adheres to screws, which facilitates the maneuver. One must be careful not to insert the component too early as it must not rest directly on screw heads. It is recommended to apply cement to the screw heads and the inner surface of the component, wait until a sticky dough is obtained, and insert the component. This technique should seem to avoid radiolucent lines at the bone-cement interface (21);

– In contained bone defects, cement pressurization is much easier: prepare the bone surface, insert screws, insert the trial components and adjust screw insertion depth, as described above. After cement has been injected and pressurized, the final components can be inserted (21).

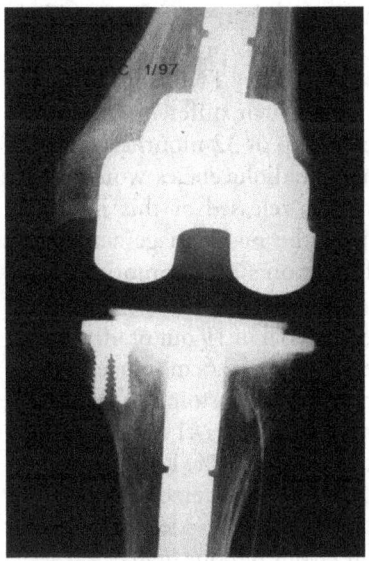

Fig. 3 – Bone defect filled with cement + screws.

Results

Very few publications are available:

– Bertin and Freeman reported the results of 45 revision TKAs with cementless stemmed prostheses and reconstruction of bone defects with cement. The average follow-up was only 18 months (range, 6 to 48 months). Radiolucent lines, most often incomplete, were seen at the bone-cement interface in 76% of the femoral components and 79% of the tibial components, and around 65 of the 74 stems. According to the author, cement fills the defect and transfers compressive loads to bone. Intrusion of cement into bone interstices improves only the rotatory stability (5).

– Ritter reported the results of 57 primary TKAs where peripheral bone defects were reconstructed with cement and screws. At 3 years postoperatively, there were 15 bone-cement radiolucencies around the defects, but no bone-cement radiolucencies around central stems or screws. These incomplete lucent lines less than 1mm thick were seen at 2 months postoperatively and did not progress thereafter (61). At 4-year follow-up, 10 of the 57 knee replacements showed radiolucencies. 47 knees were reviewed at an average follow-up of 6 years (range, 3 to 13 years) and did not show any radiographic changes

(62). He used the same technique in a series of 232 primary TKAs and 78 revision TKAs (30 tibial bone defects, 32 femoral bone defects, and 6 combined tibial / femoral bone defects) with equally good results (follow-up unknown); only 7 prostheses failed (due to infection, aseptic loosening, or other reasons) and were revised (21). According to Ritter, bone-cement radiolucent lines do not adversely affect the outcome as long as they are less than 2mm thick. They simply result from poor penetration of cement into condensed bone and likely develop immediately. Achieving good cement penetration is the best way to prevent radiolucencies. Adverse effects of heat necrosis and cement shrinkage, which are more severe in massive bone defects, are likely outweighed by the advantages provided by cement pressurization (21). Freeman also used this technique in a series of 18 primary TKRs, but his interpretation of bone-cement radiolucencies is very much different. He noted radiolucent lines in 17 knees at an average follow-up of 32 months, but none around screws. According to him, bone-cement radiolucencies would result from a macrophage reaction to cement particles released at this interface. Widening of lucent lines due to stimulation of the macrophage activity by substances released by dying cells in cases of component micromotions, bacteria, wear debris, may result in component loosening (18).

– Elia and Lotke used cement as a bone filler material in 19 out of 40 revision cases with medium size bone defects with a mean depth of 2.6cm (range, 1 to 14 cm) (13). In the other cases, they used bone grafts (12) or custom prostheses (9). All the components had stem extensions. Mean follow-up was 41 months (range, 2 to 9 years). Complication rate was 30%, and failure rate 10%. Results achieved with the three techniques were similar, with 52.5% of bone-cement lucent lines of more than 1mm being predominantly seen at the medial undersurface of the tibial tray. Nevertheless, cement was given up in favour of bone grafts.

– Murray also evaluated the reconstruction of bone defects with cement in a series of 40 revision TKAs (50). He used 25 cemented long stem tibial components and 38 cemented long stem femoral components due to poor quality of bone stock. Average follow-up was 58 months (range, 24 to 111 months). Immediate postoperative radiographs showed tibial bone-cement radiolucencies (undersurface of the tibial tray) in 5 knees (but none of them had progressed at the latest follow-up), and femoral bone-cement radiolucencies in 2 knees, one of which had progressed due to asymptomatic loosening. Incomplete radiolucencies of less than 1mm developed in 5 additional tibial components and 3 additional femoral components. The total incidence of tibial radiolucencies in this study was 32%. The authors did not report any adverse effects in cemented long stem components, in particular, no proximal osteoporosis or secondary fracture.

Discussion

In vitro studies show that cement, whether used alone or with screws, has poor performance. A cement wedge will deform under loads more than a metal wedge of the same size (8). Repeated deformations may lead to debonding at the cement-wedge interface and subsequent tilt of the tibial tray (10).

Other disadvantages of cement include:

– heat necrosis, all the more as a large amount of cement is used;
– shrinkage of approximately 2% during polymerization; influence of this phenomenon on cement-bone and cement-component interfaces is still unknown. Modern cementing techniques use high pressurization. Cement shrinkage has potential adverse consequences;
– capacity to spread in layers (lamination). When cement is reinforced with screws, there is a potential risk of corrosion: in case of contact between screws (fretting corrosion), or in case of association of two different metals (galvanic corrosion which takes place between two different metals joined together in the presence of an electrolyte). All screws are exposed to corrosion when placed in a physiologic environment; once buried in cement, they are protected. Titanium screws coated with an oxide film are more corrosion-resistant than stainless steel screws. Therefore, the best is to use a titanium tibial tray with titanium screws (21).

At last, should iterative loosening occur, loads will be transferred to bone through the cement (and screws, if any), through a long lever arm, thus aggravating the initial bone deficiency.

Indication

This technique is less and less used, likely due to the high rate of radiolucencies, and also because of the increasing tendency to use bone grafts for reconstruction of bone defects. It should be reserved for small contained bone defects (35), or peripheral defects less than 5mm deep and involving only 10% of a tibial plateau (57).

Modular prostheses and custom prostheses

Modular prostheses

All current revision knee systems offer tibial and femoral augments.
There are different tibial augments: blocks (quadrangular), and half or full wedges (triangular), each of them being offered in two or three sizes (31).
Femoral augments are all blocks (quadrangular): distal and / or posterior augments, each of them being offered in two or three thicknesses (depending on the knee system).
They provide easy and accurate filling of small defects which have previously been shaped with appropriate instruments. Both tibial and femoral augments provide adequate stability for the components and transfer the loads to the underlying bone. Posterior femoral blocks are often necessary to allow insertion of the appropriate size femoral component that will provide adequate stability in flexion; distal femoral blocks help restore the joint line. To increase external rotation of the femoral component, one will place a lateral posterior femoral augment and perform a posteromedial resection.

Most augments are made of metal and are secured to the components with screws (or snapped into place) or cement, which may cause fretting corrosion or cement fragmentation (fig. 4). Some knee systems offer cement augments which are fixed to the components with cement, so that it becomes impossible to distinguish the augment from the cement (fig. 5).

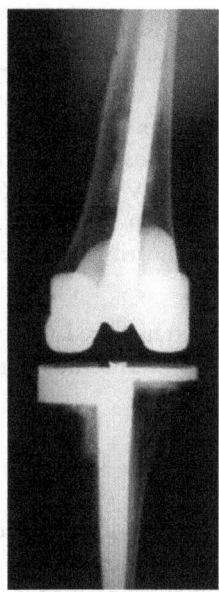

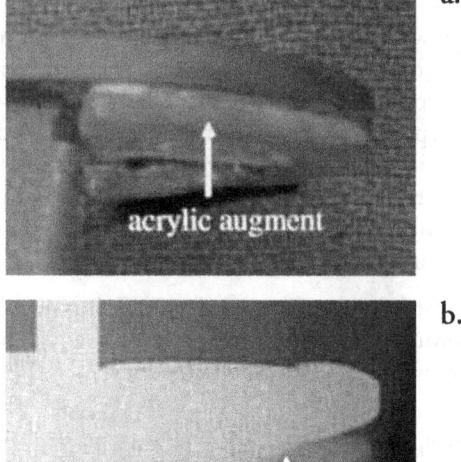

Fig. 4 – Bone defect filled with a metal block.

Fig. 5 – Cement augment fixed to the tibial component with cement.
a. Cement augment before implantation.
b. Cement augment after implantation.

In vitro *studies*

Brooks compared the mechanical behaviour of five filling options for a wedge-shaped bone defect in the medial tibial condyle: cement, cement and screws (to support the baseplate), custom prosthesis, metal wedge fixed to the baseplate with cement, Plexiglas® wedge (composition of Plexiglas® is very close to that of PMMA). Testing was performed under axial and varus loading conditions (8). Considering that deformation of the filler was 100% when cement alone was used, under axial loading conditions, it was 70% when screws were added, 32% when a Plexiglas® wedge was used, 17% with a metal wedge, and 9% with a custom prosthesis. Under varus loading conditions, it was 72%, 44%, 31%, and 17% respectively. Therefore, it can be concluded that cement alone is not appropriate for reconstruction of massive bone defects, and addition of screws provides only a slight improvement. Custom prosthesis is the best option, then comes metal wedge, and at last cement augment.

Chen compared the quality of the reconstruction achieved in a 20° oblique defect and in the same defect converted into a stepped pattern (quadrangular defect), using cement and metal augments (10). The poorest results were achieved with cement filling of a triangular defect, because of shear forces at the bone-cement interface and lower stiffness of cement. Metal blocks performed better than did step shaped cement constructs, which, in turn, performed better than did metal wedges (although differences were minimal, maybe due to imperfections in testing).

Fehring evaluated *in vitro* the transfer of loads to the proximal tibia through an IB II stemmed tibial baseplate, alone or augmented with a metal wedge or block, under axial and torsional load conditions (17). There were no significant differences between the three methods. Therefore, one can say that selection of the appropriate option is essentially based on the shape of the defect, although metal wedges are preferable in that they best preserve bone stock. Nevertheless, a metal block offers several advantages: owing to its higher resistance to torsional forces, it is a better option when a constrained prosthesis is used; bone preparation is easier; slightly lower loads are transferred to the medial side of the proximal tibia.

Technique points

Absolute accuracy of bone resection is mandatory.

This is why the first implantations were somewhat challenging (57): After the bone defect had been measured and the tibial resection completed, the wedge was affixed to the undersurface of the baseplate using wax, and dyed with methylene blue to visualize the point of contact with the resected bone. Then, the wedge was secured to the baseplate with cement at the desired place. A final check was recommended during cement setting.

Modern instruments ensure quick, accurate resections, so that this technique is gaining popularity. Resections are influenced by component rotation. Furthermore, stem extensions are used in such cases, and this influences the position of the tibial tray or the femoral component. Therefore, wedge cuts must be performed with the trial stem in place and after component rotation has been determined.

In cases where the metal wedge is in contact with sclerotic bone, it is recommended to drill a few holes to enhance cement penetration.

Results

Actually, very few studies have been performed regarding augments, and most of them concern primary knee replacements. Short-term results are satisfactory but no long-term results are available yet. Brand reported the results achieved in a series of 22 tibial metal wedges secured to the baseplate with cement, 5 of which were used in unicompartmental knee revisions (2) and in total knee revisions (3) (7). A 75mm stem was used in 3 knees. At a mean follow-up of 37 months, no loosening had occurred and no revision had been necessary. A non-progressive bone-cement radiolucency less than 1mm thick was present at the wedge in 27% of the knees and in 2 of the 3 total knee revisions.

Rand (57) used the same technique to insert 5 or 10mm augments in a series of 28 knees including only one total knee revision. At a mean follow-up of 2.3 years (range, 2 to 3.5 years), no complication had occurred. A non-progressive bone-cement radiolucency less than 1mm thick was present at the wedge in 46% of the knees, and was attributed to a faulty cementing technique. A radiolucency of less than 1mm was also noted at the baseplate-wedge interface.

Results in this series have been updated by Pagnano. 24 of the 28 knees were radiographically evaluated at a mean follow-up of 4.8 years. A bone-cement radiolucency was present at the wedge in 13 cases (54%): less than 1mm thick in 11 cases, and 1-3mm thick in the other 2 cases (52).

Scott (65) advocated the combination of augments and stem extensions in revision arthroplasty, but only three series have been reported so far.

Rand analysed at a mean follow-up of 3.1 years (range, 2 to 5.5 years) the results of 41 revision arthroplasties where tibial augments (6 medial and 4 lateral) and femoral augments (16 posterior, 2 distal, 12 distal / posterior) had been used (59, 60). Functional results were judged very satisfactory in 97% of the cases. Incomplete bone-cement radiolucency was noted in 61% of the knees. No revision was necessary.

Takahashi studied a series of 39 knees implanted with the same prosthetic design. Mean follow-up was only 20 months (74). The rate of early complications (i.e. hematoma, infection…) was rather high (20.5%), but these complications were unrelated to augments. Partial bone-cement radiolucent lines of at least 1mm were present in 72% of the knees, more often under the tibial tray than around the femoral component.

Haas' series included 67 revision arthroplasties with a mean follow-up of three and a half years (range, 2 to 9 years) (24). Tibial wedges were used in 25 knees, and femoral blocks (distal, posterior, or both) in 23 knees. Survivorship at 8 years was 83%. Main causes of failure were infection (4%) and aseptic loosening (3%); none of them seemed to be related to augments. The radiographic follow-up of augments has not been detailed in this series.

Therefore, radiolucencies although incomplete are frequently seen, particularly at the tibia where they are more readily visible than at the femur. Even though Rand considers that their high rate of occurrence owes to a meticulous radiographic technique (59), this rate is quite similar to that of cement fill with or without screws.

Discussion

The array of augmentation options varies according to knee systems, and no system offers anterior femoral blocks. Thickness is often limited, which precludes their use in massive bone defects. Several distal femoral blocks may be stacked and fixed to one another with cement (67, 68), but of course, this increases the number of interfaces. Maximum augmentation has not been clearly determined. Rand, in 1991, said that they should be reserved for peripheral bone defects of between 3 and 10mm (after resection) and advised against using them in defects more than 10mm deep (57). Brand thought they could be used to fill defects of 20-25mm depth before a resection that would remove 8 to 10mm of bone, leaving a residual bone defect of 10-17mm depth

(7). More recently, Gross advocated their use in tibial defects up to 3cm deep and in femoral defects 1cm deep (20), and Mason in tibial defects up to 2cm deep and in femoral defects up to 16mm deep (there is a knee system that includes a 16mm distal femoral block) (46). There is no consensus whatsoever.

Thick augments have several drawbacks which restrict their use:

– on the tibial side: they may cause pain due to impingement upon soft tissues inferiorly, and particularly inferomedially;

– on the femoral side: they do not leave much room for bone, particularly in small size femoral components;

– contrary to bone grafts, they do not facilitate re-revision;

– there is a potential risk of disassociation which, however, has not been reported so far. No fixation method outperforms the others, whether it be cement, screws, or snap-lock system. Studies of retrieved components are scarce. Rand evaluated the holding strength of a metal wedge that had been fixed with cement to the undersurface of a tibial tray, and was retrieved after 6.5 years: the force necessary to separate the wedge from the baseplate was 77% of the initial force (58);

– at last, there is a potential risk of particles of cement or metal being released, depending on the fixation method.

Longer follow-up will be necessary to evaluate their reliability. Meanwhile, it is cautious to reserve their use for small size bone defects, preferably in the aged.

Some knee systems include components with built-in augments (14) which offer exactly the same advantages as custom prostheses (greater stiffness, no risk of component disassociation and generation of wear particles), plus increased flexibility and reduced cost. However, this means that a significant inventory of components is required (large number of size and design combination options, right and left). Furthermore, this alternative offers less intraoperative flexibility than independent components and augments. Meticulous preoperative planning is mandatory. On the femoral side, it requires removal of a significant amount of bone from the less affected condyle since both prosthetic condyles have equal thickness.

Custom prostheses

Their mechanical characteristics are far superior to any other filling option (8). However, careful CT scan evaluation is required to determine the exact dimensions of the components, they take several weeks to manufacture, and they are costly.

Moreover, it is difficult to evaluate the exact shape and size of a bone defect preoperatively (defect is often larger than shown on preoperative images), so that the prosthesis may eventually not fit. This is why this alternative is not very popular and published series (13) are scarce.

Custom prostheses have been superseded by modular designs which accommodate intraoperative contingencies. As a matter of fact, current revision knee systems offer a wide selection of femoral and tibial augments, as well as stem extensions of various sizes, straight or offset, which allow for intraoperative customization of the prosthesis to the patient.

Therefore, custom prostheses now have very limited indications: diaphyseal offset that cannot be possibly managed with offset stems, severe epiphyseal destruction in the elderly where insertion of a custom-made tumor prosthesis has the advantage of reducing operation time. Modern hinge prostheses offer a certain degree of modularity which allows extemporaneous customization of components to meet patient needs.

Bone grafts

Bone grafts are used for reconstruction or filling of bone defects. Thus, they are the method of choice in young patients exposed to wear, osteolysis and loosening which require revision surgery. After healing, they are able to sustain loads: immediately for structural bone grafts, after incorporation and bone remodeling for cancellous bone grafts. They also allow for a uniform cement mantle.

Autografts

General considerations (19, 45)

Autografts have two major advantages:

– Actually, autografts are the ideal biological material. They include living osteoblasts which stimulate osteogenesis. Furthermore, they are both osteoconductive and osteoinductive so that they heal and incorporate more rapidly than allografts. In cancellous autografts, osteoblasts lay down new bone on necrotic trabecular bone as it is being resorbed by osteoclasts. Trabecular bone can be completely replaced with living bone. In cortical autografts, osteogenesis begins only after necrotic lamellar bone has been resorbed, which means that there is a long period during which bone is very weak. They never become fully ingrown;

– Of course, there is no risk of transmission of viruses.

But, autogenous grafts have two main drawbacks:

– Only a limited amount of bone is available for bone grafting in revision cases. Tibial and femoral resections are minimal and provide very little bone material which is often of poor quality. An additional amount of bone is provided by notch preparation when a cruciate-retaining TKR is revised, or if posterior resection of the lateral condyle is performed to increase external rotation of the femoral component. Some more bone can be taken from the iliac crest, but this lengthens the procedure, increases blood loss, and carries a potential risk of complications at the donor site (hematoma, infection, damage to the lateral femoral cutaneous nerve, postoperative pain);

– They often do not match the shape of the defect.

Bone grafting technique

A rigorous technique is mandatory. The recipient site must be carefully prepared. After removal of cement and interposition membranes, all sclerotic bone must be resected except at the periphery of the defect to avoid weakening of the rim. Multiple holes are drilled down to healthy bone.

It is easier to fill a bone defect with a geometric configuration. Giving a peripheral defect a triangular shape involves minimal bone removal, but the graft is subjected to shear forces; giving the defect a quadrangular shape involves more bone removal, but the graft is subjected to compressive loads. The Insall technique for reconstruction of central tibial defects consists in creating a trapezoid shape by resecting the peripheral rim before inserting a bone graft taken from the femoral notch (83).

The bone graft is temporarily fixed with pins and then cut flush with the resected tibial surface; if necessary, it can be secured with screws, taking care to countersink the screw heads which must not protrude above the resected surface and make contact with the undersurface of the metal baseplate.

One to three 3-4mm holes are drilled into the graft to facilitate cement penetration. One must be careful not to drill right through and reach the recipient bone-graft interface.

In case snug fit is not achieved, gaps may be filled with tightly packed morsellized grafts or a thin layer of cement to prevent intrusion of cement into the recipient bone-graft interface during cementing of the component.

A technique associating the use of wire mesh fixed with screws in the cortex adjacent to the bone defect, with impacted morsellized autografts has been described (71). It is very much similar to the technique described by Sloof for the acetabulum.

Resumption of weight bearing may be delayed or gradual to relieve the graft site from physiological loads until healing is achieved.

Results

Autografts have essentially been used in the tibia in primary cases where bone fragments from resections are available. Most of the time, functional and radiological results have been satisfactory (1, 3, 66). RSA (Roentgen-Stereophotogrammetric Analysis) demonstrated the quality of these reconstructions which is difficult to evaluate on plain radiographs (41). However, Laskin reported only 67% successful results at 5-year follow-up in a series of 26 knees (33). Underresection of sclerotic bone might explain this difference in results (17).

Autografts have been much less used in revision cases. Dorr reported 2 failures in 14 revisions, using 13 autografts and 1 allograft, in the tibia (12). The autogenous grafts had been collected during resections (9 cases) or harvested from the iliac crest (4 cases). They were not protected by a stem extension.

No published study is available for the femur.

Discussion

In revision arthroplasty, only small amounts of autogenous graft material are available, and grafts do not fit well. They are mostly used to fill small contained bone defects or at the junction between an allograft and the recipient bone. In some cases, they may be used to reconstruct small non-contained defects, but there is a risk of non-union which is all the higher as bone is sclerotic and poorly vascularized. It is recommended to use them in combination with stem extensions for graft protection, but one must keep in mind that a graft that is not sufficiently stressed will absorb.

Allografts

General considerations (19, 45)

Allograft is a biological material that is able to unite to the host bone, but allograft is "dead bone" which only has osteoconductive properties. Healing and incorporation process of allografts and autografts is similar, except that incorporation of cancellous bone and healing of cortical bone take more time. Weakening of cortical allografts due to resorption is slower than in autografts, which is an advantage in the short run. However, once union with the host bone has been achieved, allografts show very little remodeling and are therefore prone to fracture.

Massive allografts which include cortical and subchondral bone have the same mechanical properties as the missing bone fragment. Their strength is highly dependent on loading conditions; they tend to exhibit higher resistance to compressive forces. Femoral heads harvested during hip arthroplasties for osteoarthritis provide strong cancellous and subchondral bone. Morsellized allografts are unable to sustain loads immediately after implantation; they first need to heal and remodel.

Fresh frozen preservation is the best choice; it reduces enzymatic degradation and hardly affects torsional and bending strength. Bone grafts can be safely stored for 5 years at -70° C, and only 6 months at -20° C. Fresh-frozen femoral heads keep their cancellous structure and 70-85% of their initial strength (55). Freeze-drying has very little influence on compressive strength, but it decreases torsional and bending strength by as much as 90%. Two chief problems with allografts are supply and cost (although they are not as expensive as custom prostheses).

Advantages of allografts include:
– unlimited supply and possibility of cutting to the desired shape. As a matter of fact, allografts may be trimmed as needed and, if necessary, one can even use the same bone as the host bone for reconstruction. This intraoperative flexibility is a definite advantage over custom prostheses which cannot be shaped;
– they enhance component fixation by allowing easy intrusion of cement into cancellous bone.

However, allografts are also associated with a certain number of risks:
– potential risk (less than one in a million) of transmitting viral diseases (*e.g.* HIV, hepatitis, prions) (27, 72). This risk is higher with bulk grafts than with femoral heads which are double-checked after a quarantine period. This

risk can be further decreased by exposure to low-dose radiation (2.5mrads) which has little effect on breaking strength (55);

– due to the potential risk of non-union, fatigue fracture, fracture due to revascularization, resorption, allografts must be used under the best possible biomechanical conditions;

– infection. High infection rates have been reported in some series (72);

– immunologic reaction: due to the antigenicity of allografts, the presence of antibodies has been detected in recipients of allografts (2, 39). However, such reaction is variable and mild; it does not adversely affect the clinical outcome and has no influence on healing and histological findings (2). Nevertheless, it is advisable to remove as much bone marrow as possible by using pressure lavage and irrigation, and to check rhesus compatibility if the patient is a woman of child-bearing age.

Recipient site preparation is the same as for autografts. Necrotic or sclerotic bone is removed. One must be careful to preserve as much healthy bone as possible, particularly the peripheral bony rim of the defect which receives ligament insertions. The allograft is thawed in saline solution (60 minutes) which may be added with betadin. Bacteriological samples are taken. Soft tissues are removed. Lavage is used to remove as much bone marrow as possible. Morsellized or structural allografts may be used.

Morsellized allografts

Morsellized allografts are used in combination with long stem components that provide adequate stability. As a matter of fact, morsellized allografts are

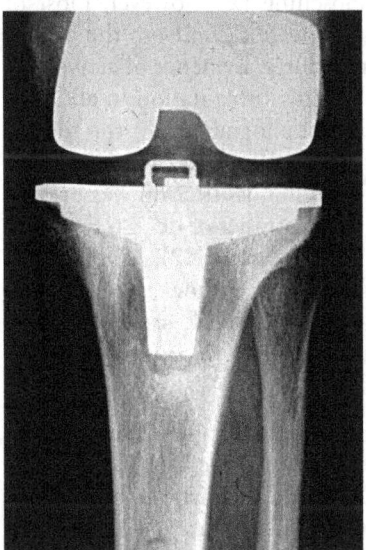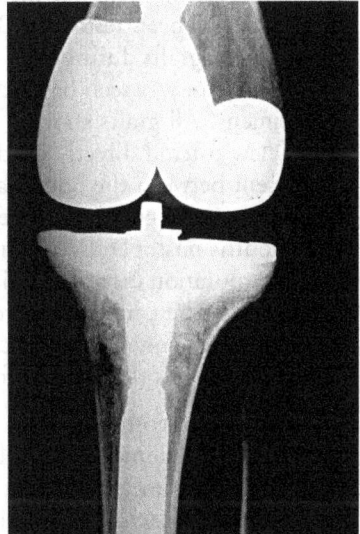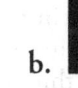

Fig. 6 – Central metaphyseal bone defect filled (**a.**) with morzellized bone grafts (**b.**).

not mechanically strong and are unable to support prosthetic components (fig. 6).

The first published series included only cementless prostheses.

The very first published series was that of Samuelson; it consisted of 22 Freeman-Samuelson revision knees (64). There were only contained bone defects filled with allografts: morsellized bone chips or 5-8mm bone fragments, and even bone blocks; the proportion of each type of graft material is unknown. Mean follow-up was only 15 months (range, 6 months to 2 years). 16 tibial grafts had incorporated, 5 were modified, 1 was unchanged. 14 femoral grafts had incorporated, 6 were modified, 2 were unchanged.

The Whiteside's series included 56 cases (80, 81), mostly non-contained large defects which did not involve more than 25% of the peripheral rim. Each cancellous allograft consisted of 1cm bone fragments that had been copiously lavaged; the allograft was compacted into the defect. Screws were used to secure 28 tibial components and 21 femoral components on the peripheral rim. A 15cm smooth long stem was systematically used in the tibia; in the femur, it was only used in cases where epiphyseal support was insufficient (39 cases). All stems were smooth uncemented stems that did not provide axial load transfer but offered high resistance to tilt. At 2-year follow-up, no failure had occurred. Bone mineral density of allografts had gradually increased (although femoral allografted areas were less visible than tibial ones). One femoral component had shifted into varus, and 26 of the 39 femoral stems showed radiolucencies. One tibial component had shifted into varus (with no worsening being noted thereafter), and 52 of the 56 tibial stems showed radiolucencies. When this series reached 63 cases, 14 had to be revised at between 3 weeks and 37 months postoperatively for various reasons: dehiscence (1), hematoma (2), painful cerclage (4), patellar ligament avulsion (2), patellar instability (1), tibiofemoral instability (2), loosening (2) (however, most of bone stock had been restored). Biopsy specimens were taken from the central portion of allografts during the 14 revision procedures. Evidence of active new bone formation was seen beyond 3 weeks following implantation in all biopsy specimens. All grafts showed (even deep in the allograft mass) the formation of new osteoid directly on dead allograft trabeculae, and vascular stroma was present between the bone fragments. Enchondral ossification was present at 6 months postoperatively together with a large number of dead trabeculae; at 18 months postoperatively, lamellar bone could be seen (82). All this indicates incorporation (at least partial) of the grafts. Other authors agree that this is actually the best method to restore bone stock. Rorabeck used it in large contained tibial bone defects (9 cases) and femoral bone defects (6 cases), with good results at less than 4-year follow-up (63).

Cementing of components in impacted morsellized allografts was recently reported (76). Technique is similar to that described for the hip (Exeter technique), using an intramedullary instrument to guide the distal impactor and the proximal impactor. A rotating hinge prosthesis was used. Clinical and radiographic results of the first three cases are encouraging but of course, follow-up is rather limited (18, 21, 28 months).

Structural allografts

The allograft is shaped to match the inside contour of the defect, with the trabeculae oriented in the line of weight bearing forces. Cancellous portions of the allograft should be placed next to the host bone. Junction between the recipient bone and the allograft must be as stable as possible: step, embedding (cylinder, segment of a sphere). It is recommended to avoid screw holes which promote on the one hand early revascularization followed by resorption and eventually collapse of the graft, and on the other hand secondary fractures (11, 15, 27, 72). It is much preferable to use an intramedullary stem (uncemented, if possible) that is firmly anchored in cortices. However, it may be necessary to use internal fixation with screws or plate, in spite of its drawbacks. If a cemented stem is used, care must be taken to avoid intrusion of cement into the host bone-graft interface. Adding autologous morsellized bone grafts to the junction promotes healing. As bone ingrowth into the porous surface of a metal component can only occur at the host bone-component interface, cement should be applied to the graft, not to the recipient bone.

Several techniques have been proposed, depending on whether the bone defect is on the femoral or tibial side, and on the severity and the shape of the defect.

The reconstruction techniques described for autografts also apply to allografts, but in most cases, allografts are preferably used in larger bone defects.

Engh suggested a technique that uses a femoral head from a bone bank (45). The cavity is reamed with a male reamer to a concentric hemisphere, in the line of weight bearing forces, until cancellous living bone is exposed. Then, the prepared femoral head (with a female reamer) is inserted into the cavity. The diameter of the male reamer is 2mm smaller than that of the female reamer. The graft is fixed with K-wires, but these must not interfere with bone preparation and particularly preparation of the housing for the stem extension. Then, bone resections are performed using dedicated instruments. If necessary, autografts or allografts may be used at the host bone-femoral head interface (68).

An allograft that fits the defect is best suited for reconstruction of a femoral or tibial condyle, or the entire epiphysis.

To reconstruct a femoral or tibial bone loss, the recipient bone is shaped to match the contour of the allograft (fragment of a bulk epiphyseal bone graft or femoral head) so as to achieve a stable junction. In spite of their disadvantages, screws remain the best fixation method (11, 20). Screws must not interfere with the stem (fig. 7).

In cases where both femoral or tibial condyles are affected, bone grafting of the entire epiphysis is necessary. Using a bone graft that is smaller than the epiphysis of the recipient allows embedding of the graft. A femoral bone graft with attached collateral ligaments or a tibial bone graft with attached patellar ligament may be required.

Once the appropriate allograft length (that allows full extension without recurvatum) has been determined, stability is achieved with impaction of the donor graft into the medullary canal of the recipient bone or by creating a step, taking rotation into account. One must bear in mind that excessive shaping of bone grafts tends to weaken them and will promote revascularization if the cancellous bone next to soft tissues is perforated or exposed. Should this occur, these areas must be cemented (27).

There is a tendency to move the joint line to the distal end for femoral grafts and to the proximal end for tibial grafts (11). Distance from the joint line to the fibular head is determined by using the contralateral knee as a reference. Where not possible, the joint line is set 1.5cm above the tip of the fibular head and 2.5cm below the medial epicondyle, level with the meniscal scar (if it can be identified).

Although not recommended, the use of stabilizing devices may be necessary (*i.e.* screws, plate, cerclage wires). Hemicylindric cortical allografts with cerclage wires can favourably replace screw plates, except in the tibia where cortical allografts and plates should be avoided because they make wound closure more difficult (11).

Selection of the appropriate component size is dictated by the dimensions of the recipient's epiphysis (measured on the contralateral knee), not by the size of the bone graft. Care must be taken to avoid bulky prostheses which may impinge upon adjacent soft tissues, particularly during the second stage of revisions for infection. Difficulties in wound closure may require patellectomy (27).

Both the component and the stem are fixed to the allograft with cement to prevent bone ingrowth (27). Insertion of a stem with or preferably without cement into the bone shaft results in compressive forces being exerted onto the junction (11, 15, 20, 27, 49, 75). Long stems are required (15). Harris recommends the use of 80mm cemented stems in the elderly, or uncemented stems with the distal end extending beyond the isthmus (27). No cement should be allowed into the host bone-graft interface (11, 15, 20, 27).

The junction should be bone grafted with autogenous grafts or a mixture of autogenous and allogeneic graft material (11, 20, 27, 75).

The remaining bone fragments with their attached ligament insertions (collateral ligaments, patellar ligament) are fixed to the bone graft (15, 20, 27, 49).

Postoperatively, a dynamic ROM knee orthosis allows early controlled motion. Weight bearing is gradually resumed after 4 to 6 weeks. Full weight bearing is allowed when the junction is soundly united, that is, approximately 3 months after implantation for the majority of patients.

Several series have been published (table I). However, comparison of results is very difficult because of a lack of consistency in: number of cases, etiology (some series include fresh or old fractures, others include primary knee replacements), revision rate for infection, type of bone deficiency (some series include only non-contained bone defects, others include both contained and non-contained bone defects), severity of bone loss (bone defect involving part or most of the epiphysis), type of bone graft used (bulk graft or femoral head), method of preservation (deep freezing or deep freezing plus irradiation), type of junction (embedding, transverse osteotomy or step osteotomy), method of fixation of the graft (stem extension, stem plus plate or screws), length of the stem

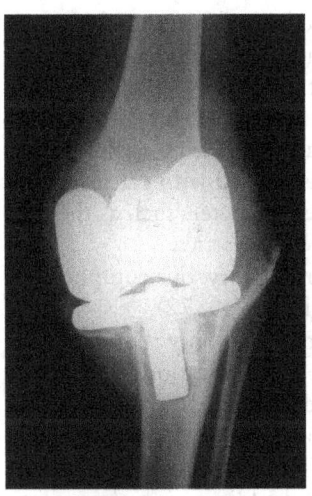

Fig. 7 – Bone loss managed with resection of the lateral tibial condyle and bone grafting of the medial tibial condyle.
a. Preoperative X-ray.
b. Bone reconstruction with screws.
c. Intraoperative view with the prosthesis *in situ*.
d. Postoperative X-ray.

a.

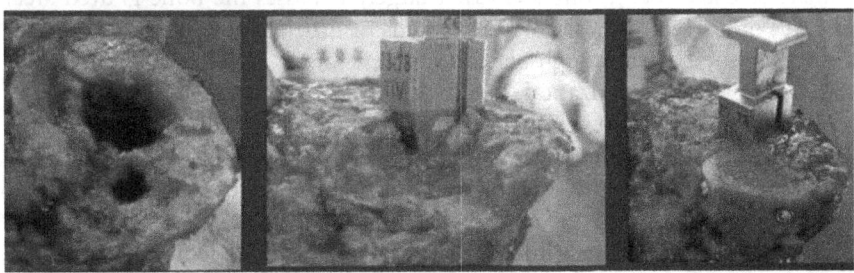

b.

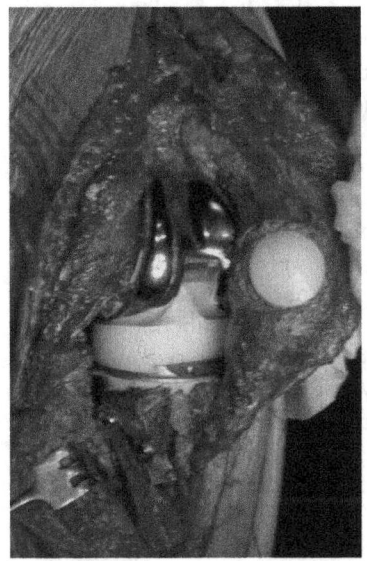

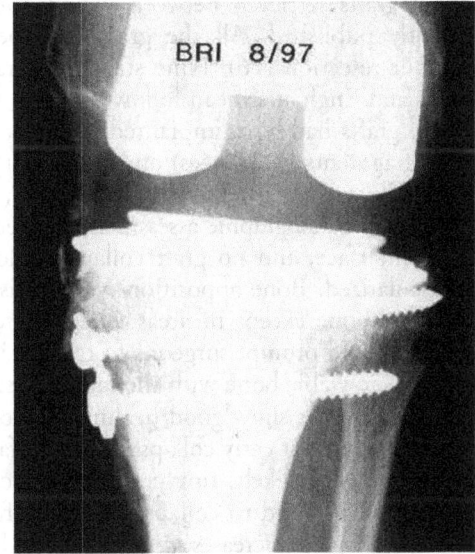

c.   d.

(largely bypassing or not the bone grafted area), method of fixation of the stem (cemented, uncemented, cemented to the graft but not to the shaft), presence or absence of bone graft at the recipient bone-graft junction, level of constraint of the prosthetic component (PS, varus / valgus constraint, hinge prosthesis either rotating or not), and follow-up. Some series also include morsellized bone grafts (63, 72), or hemicylindrical cortical allografts secured with cerclage wires where there is distal cortical perforation (72). Some parameters such as the type of prosthesis (72) may be highly variable within the same series.

Short-term and mid-term results are globally satisfactory, but complication rate varies a great deal and is sometimes quite high (20, 49, 72).

A summary is provided in Table I; we have considered only the cases with known results, structural bone grafts, and major complications (infection, non-union, fracture, loosening, laxity). Not all data were available in some series. It is very difficult to draw sound conclusions from series which are so dissimilar and sometimes inhomogeneous. However, some favourable factors have been identified: stable junction (step or embedding in preference to transverse osteotomy), long stem that largely bypasses the bone-grafted area, absence of hinge prosthesis. Where there is insufficient stability, internal fixation is required, even though plates and screws are known to weaken the graft and promote revascularization.

Infection is the most serious complication with a very uncertain outcome. Infection may have many causes: patient's general condition, numerous prior surgeries (sometimes with infection complication), length and complexity of the procedure, infection remote to the surgical site, massive epiphyseal allograft which carries a higher infectious risk than embedded femoral head (from bone bank). Having another team prepare the allograft shortens the operating time and therefore, may reduce the infectious risk (27, 75).

Histological studies are enlightening. A very interesting series of 73 massive allografts retrieved between 2 and 156 months after implantation was recently published. All the grafts had been used for reconstruction after tumour resection (16). Nine structural grafts were studied histologically by Parks and Engh at a mean follow-up of 41 months (range, 20 to 62 months). These grafts had been implanted in revision cases (1 distal femur, 6 femoral head fragments in 3 knees) and in primary cases (2 autografts in 1 patient) (54). All were retrieved grafts (5 allografts, 2 autografts) or biopsied grafts (2 allografts). Radiographic assessment showed no radiolucencies at the cement-bone interface, and no graft collapse. Allografts were intact. They had not revascularized. Bone apposition was consistently noted at the junction with the host bone except in areas where there was residual subchondral bone, which should prompt surgeons to remove it completely. The two autogenous grafts were viable bone with the same density as recipient bone.

These studies show good healing of allografts with slow revascularization, which means that early collapse is due to fatigue fracture rather than revascularization. Most likely, tiny cracks which cannot heal extend and propagate, and eventually lead to collapse of the graft. Therefore, using a long stem to protect the graft increases graft durability because the load is shared by graft bone, stem extension, and host bone (54).

Table I – Results achieved with bone allografts (this table includes only structural bone grafts).

Author and year	Nb of knees	Type of allograft	Preservation method	Type of junction	Internal fixation (other than stem)	Bone grafting of the junction	Hinge prosthesis	Type of intramedullary stem	Follow-up (in months)	Healing rate	Complications
Mnaymneh (1990)	10	massive, femur (6-16cm) massive, tibia (3-11cm) 7	deep freezing	embedding: 12 transverse osteotomy: 2	plate(s) and/or screws	+ if embedding	2	cemented to the bone graft	40 26 to 69	12/14 tibia: 100% femur:70%	1 infection 1 femoral bone loss 2 tibial loosen. 1 disloc.
Wilde (1990)	12	cancellous bone block: 5 massive, tibia: 7	deep freezing	embedding	plate and/or screws: in 5 of the 7 massive bone grafts	–	0	short, cemented	32 25 to 51	11/12	1 tibial bone loss
Krayy (1992)	7	massive, femur	?	?	none	+	3	long, cemented	44 32-57 (3 deaths)	complete:1 partial: 1 2: uncertain (3 deaths)	1 tibial loosening 1 dislocation 2 laxities
Stockley (1992)	20	massive, femur: 7 massive, tibia: 9 metaph./diaph bone graft: 7	deep freezing + 2.5mrads	embedding step	screws, sometimes	–	7	? (5 types of prostheses)	50 24 to 76	100%	3 infections 2 fractures
Tsahakis (1994)	15	massive, femur: 6 massive, tibia: 4 femoral head: 9	deep freezing	embedding step transverse osteotomy	screws, sometimes	+	0	stem cemented to the bone graft (16) or stem fully cemented (4)	25 12 to 48	100%	0

Table I –

Author and year	Nb of knees	Type of allograft	Preservation method	Type of junction	Internal fixation (other than stem)	Bone grafting of the junction	Hinge prosthesis	Type of intramedullary stem	Follow-up (in months)	Healing rate	Complications
Harris (1995)	14	massive, femur: 8 massive, tibia: 6	deep freezing	embedding (tibia) transverse osteotomy: 13	plates: 7	+	0	11 cases: stem cemented to the bone graft (5) or stem fully cemented (6), no stem or short stem: 3	43 29 to 63	13/14	1 infection 1 non-union 1 dislocation
Mow (1996)	13	massive, femur: 3 massive, tibia: 9 femoral head: 7	deep freezing or freeze-drying		none	+	0	long, uncemented (stem cemented to the bone graft: 7)	47 30 to 101	100%	1 tibial fx 1 tibial component fx 1 tibial loosen. (+ laxity)
Engh (1997)	30	massive, femur: 5 massive, tibia: 1 femoral head: 29	heads: deep freezing massive bone grafts: deep freezing + gamma radiation	embedding step	none	–	0	stem cemented proximally: 16 uncemented stem: 4	50 24 to 120	20/30	2 migrations (uncemented stems)
Ghazavi (1997)	30	massive bone graft	deep freezing + 2.5mrads	step for massive bone graft	screws or cerclage	+	5	long stem, uncemented	50 24 to 132	33/34	3 infections 1 femoral fx 1 femoral non-union 2 tibial loosen.
Rorabeck (1998)	10	massive, femur: 2 condyle: 1 massive, tibia: 2 medial plateau: 4	?	?	?	?	?	long stem, uncemented	< 4 years	1/10	1 infection 1 femoral non-union
Clatworthy (2001)	52	massive bone graft	deep freezing + 2.5mrads	step	screws, cerclage or plate	+	6	long stem, uncemented	97 60 to 180	64/66	4 infections 1 femoral fx 3 femoral loosen. 2 tibial loosen. 2 laxities

It is all very different in morsellized allografts. They are unable to sustain high loads during the immediate postoperative period, but bone ingrowth (at least partial) occurs as well as remodeling, so that restoration of strong bone stock can be expected. Structural allografts provide immediate strong support and can heal at the junction with the host bone, but no bone ingrowth or remodeling occurs with loading. This is why they are thought to have a limited future. Longer-term studies are necessary.

Conclusion

Selection of the appropriate treatment method for bone deficiency is based on:
– type of bone defect: contained or non-contained;
– severity (size and depth);
– quality of bone stock;
– patient's age and activity level.

Two important decisions must be made:
– Thickness of the resection: resection must remove all necrotic or weak bone to provide strong support for the prosthetic component and preserve as much of the healthy bone as possible. Resection should minimize and even eliminate the bone defect, and provide better peripheral support. Let's remind that in the series presented during the 2000 SOFCOT meeting, very distal tibial cuts (zone C) were unfavourable, and that resections in zone B which eliminate the defect seemed preferable to resections in zone A which allow persistence of a residual bone loss (23);
– Filling options:

• Contained bone defects are less of a concern because the peripheral rim remains intact and provides adequate support for the prosthetic component. Cement may be used in minor bone defects less than 5mm deep which may also be filled with impacted morsellized bone grafts (autografts, or more often, allografts). In all other cases, options include impacted morsellized bone grafts and structural allografts (generally a femoral head, or an epiphyseal allograft in a worst case scenario). The use of a structural bone graft seems perfectly justified in severe bone loss where the bone graft has a mechanical role to play. Nevertheless, some authors have obtained satisfactory results with impacted morsellized grafts (81). This technique implies that stable fixation of the prosthetic component is achieved pending bone ingrowth. It provides real incorporation and remodeling of the grafts (82);

• In non-contained bone defects, there is no peripheral bony rim:
Cement, with or without screws, has a poor mechanical behaviour (8) and is not recommended. Nevertheless, it can still be used in very small defects less than 5mm deep which involve less than 10% of a tibial or femoral condyle (57).

Metal wedges and blocks provide immediate filling of moderate bone defects, with satisfactory short-term results. However, radiolucencies are frequent, and the potential for disassociation and generation of cement or metal particles is difficult to evaluate. Very thick augments are available, but the size of the defects amenable to this technique has not yet been specified. Due to these uncertainties, surgeons are more inclined to use bone grafts in young active patients, at least in bone defects more than 10mm deep. In smaller defects, augments seem preferable because they do not carry the potential risk of non-union that is associated with small-size bone grafts inserted between the component and the host bone. This risk is higher in the femur where bone surface areas are smaller.

Other bone deficiencies require the use of allografts. At present, it is difficult to clearly establish the respective indications for morsellized allografts and structural allografts. Structural allografts are able to sustain and transfer loads, unite to host bone, and they provide sufficient cancellous bone surface area for cement fixation. But, they do not remodel and seem to be prone to mechanical complications in the medium term. Morsellized allografts do not provide immediate strong support, but bone ingrowth and remodeling occur. However, bone loss should not involve more than one-fourth of the peripheral rim. In larger bone defects, and where a tibial or a femoral condyle is almost completely destroyed, they seem indispensable. Nevertheless, in very aged patients, it may be preferable to opt for a tumour hinge prosthesis; it is a time-saving procedure with none of the complications associated with massive bone grafts. But, hinge prostheses have a limited lifetime due to mechanical complications (*i.e.* loosening, failure of the junction between the two components).

Custom prostheses have been supplanted by modular designs and now have very little place in reconstruction of bone defects.

A diaphyseal perforation (67, 68) is managed with a long stem component. A diaphyseal fracture may require the associated use of internal fixation. In both cases, the bone defect is filled with an autograft or an allograft, and hemicylindrical cortical allografts with cerclage wires may be added, provided that they do not hinder closure of soft tissues.

The long-term success of revision arthroplasty does not depend only on the technique of reconstruction of bone defects. Other critical factors are involved, which include:

– proper positioning of the prosthetic components in the frontal plane (correct alignment: between 2° of varus and 3° of valgus), in the sagittal plane, and in the horizontal plane (for tibiofemoral congruity and smooth patellar tracking);

– soft-tissue balance both in flexion and extension to avoid joint laxity.

– prosthetic constraint as low as possible to minimize stresses on fixation areas. Patients with deficient ligaments require the use of varus / valgus constrained prostheses or hinge prostheses even though they are known to be associated with mechanical complications (11, 15, 29, 78, 79).

– use of stem extensions to unload the proximal bone-grafted area; testings have demonstrated their efficiency (6, 8). Brooks showed that a 70mm cemented stem takes 30% of the load away from the metaphysis (6). The best choice is a stem that is long enough to largely bypass the bone-grafted area, and that is securely fixed (without cement, if possible); it will apply compression forces to the host bone-allograft junction (if any), avoid significant deviation of forces, and facilitate surgical revision (if necessary).

These essential aspects of revision surgery will be discussed further on in this book.

Patella

In case of patellar loosening, or after difficult extraction of a well-fixed patellar component, peg holes become enlarged, and the patellar bone is more or less thinned or even fractured. Implantation of a new component, although desirable, is sometimes impossible.

Several solutions have been proposed:

– biconvex patella with one single central peg (22) to fill a central defect. Laskin reported satisfactory results in a series of 85 cases, at 7-year follow-up, with one single secondary fracture (36);

– patellar component with peripheral pegs if the loose component had one central peg and conversely, filling old peg holes with morsellized bone grafts;

– reimplantation after reconstruction of the defect with an autograft fixed with screws. This interesting technique is seldom used and requires harvesting of an iliac crest graft (73);

– retention of patellar remnants: it is the only solution when the patella is too thin. The patella is shaped to fit the contours of the trochlear groove (patelloplasty). This technique yields lower functional scores than reimplantation. Furthermore, it is associated with persistent pain, difficulties to walk up and down stairs, and often with secondary fragmentation of the patella (4, 53).

In case of patellar fracture:

– any necrotic fragments are excised and other fragments are shaped (partial patellectomy). Care should be taken to preserve the bone fragment that receives the insertion of the patellar ligament because of the risk of secondary rupture (36);

– it may be necessary to repair the extensor mechanism, if torn. If this is combined with removal of all remaining bone fragments, it is a complete patellectomy;

– Hanssen recently proposed a new bone grafting technique (25) which consists in: retaining the periphery of the periprosthetic fibrous layer; filling the defect with impacted 5-8mm diameter cancellous bone grafts taken from the bone fragment resected during preparation of the femoral notch or from a bone-bank femoral head; taking a fibrous tissue flap from the suprapatellar or peripatellar region or the fascia lata (at some distance from the patella); suturing the flap to the patellar meniscus and patellar rim; at last, inserting a few additional bone grafts into this fibrous tissue pouch through an opening before closing it. Once closed, the pouch must be perfectly tight so that the bone grafts cannot migrate. The patellar retinaculum is temporarily closed and the knee is mobilized to fashion the bone grafts. After reconstruction, the patella should be at least 20mm thick. Satisfactory functional and radiological results have been reported in a small series of 9 cases. Fibrocartilaginous meta-plasia of the fibrous tissue developed in one patient who had been reoperated on for another reason. If need be, one may think of cementing a new patellar component in a reconstructed patella.

Simple cementing of a new standard patellar component is possible only where there is little bone stock, and a biconvex design would be more suitable (36). Component fixation after bone grafting is more uncertain. Patelloplasty which is sometimes performed in conjunction with reconstruction of the extensor mechanism, is often necessary in cases where the patella is too thin or fractured. Bone grafting of the residual patella is an interesting alternative and seems preferable to retaining patellar remnants, but it requires highly experienced hands.

The technique used is at least as important as rotation of the femoral and tibial components (which is critical to patellar tracking) and joint line level for the success of the arthroplasty.

Conclusion

Reconstruction of bone defects remains an important issue with many unans-wered questions. Augments are used in preference to cement. Bone grafting is desirable in young active patients, but a longer follow-up will be necessary to clarify the indications and appropriate techniques for use of morsellized and structural bone grafts.

Whatever solution is selected, the durability of the outcome depends on additional parameters which are critical to the success of the revision arthro-plasty: component positioning, soft tissue tensioning, level of constraint, use of stem extensions, joint line level. Absolute requirements include: correct ali-gnment (which contributes to even distribution of loads), absence of laxity, low constraint which minimizes stresses on fixation areas and use of stem extensions which help transfer part of the loads to the diaphysis.

References

1. Aglietti P, Buzzi R, Scrobe F (1991) Autologous bone grafting for medial defects in total knee arthroplasty. J Arthroplasty, 6, 4: 287-94
2. Aho AJ, Eskola J, Ekfors T et al. (1997) Immune response and clinical outcome of massi-ve human osteoarticular allografts. Clin Orthop 346: 196-206
3. Altchek D, Sculco TP, Rawlins B (1989) Autogenous bone grafting for severe angular defor-mity in total knee arthroplasty. J Arthroplasty 4, 2: 151-5
4. Barrack RL, Matzkin E, Ingraham R et al. (1998) Revision knee arthroplasty with patella replacement versus bony shell. Clin Orthop 356: 139-43
5. Bertin KC, Freeman MAR, Samuelson KM et al. (1985) Stemmed revision arthroplasty for aseptic loosening of total knee replacement. J Bone Joint Surg 1985, 67B, 2: 242-8
6. Bourne RB, Finlay JB (1986) The influence tibial component intramedullary stems and implant-cortex contact on the strain distribution of the proximal tibia folllowing total knee arthroplasty. Clin Orthop 208 : 95-9
7. Brand MG, Daley RJ, Ewald FC, Scott RD (1989) Tibial tray augmentation with modu-lar metal wedges for tibial bone stock deficiency. Clin Orthop 248: 71-9

8. Brooks PJ, Walker PS, Scott RD (1984) Tibial component fixation in deficient tibial bone stock. Clin Orthop 184l 302-08
9. Burdin Ph, Lautman S (2001) Classification des pertes de substance osseuse. In: Symposium de la SOFCOT 2000 sur les reprises de prothèses totales du genou. Rev Chir Orthop 87, 5: S172-S5.
10. Chen F, Krackow KA (1994) Management of tibial defects in total knee arthroplasty. A biomechanical study. Clin Orthop 305: 249-57
11. Clatworthy MG, Ballance J, Brick GW et al. (2001) The use of structural allograft for uncontained defects in revision total knee arthroplasty. A minimum five years review. J Bone Joint Surg 83 A, 3: 404-11
12. Dorr LD, Ranawatt CS, Sculco TA et al. (1986) Bone grafting for tibial defects in total knee arthroplasty. Clin Orthop 205: 153-65
13. Elia EA, Lotke PA (1991) Results of revision total knee arthroplasty associated with significant bone loss. Clin Orthop 271: 114-21
14. Engh GA, Ammeen DJ (1998) Classification and preoperative radiographic evaluation: knee. Orthop Clin North Am 29, 2: 205-217
15. Engh GA, Herzwurm PJ, Parks NL (1997) Treatment of major defects of bone with bulk allografts and stemmed components during total knee arthroplasty. J Bone Joint Surg 79A: 1030-39
16. Enneking WF, Campanacci D (2001) Retrieved human allografts: a clinicopathological study. J Bone Joint Surg 83 A: 971-86
17. Fehring TK, Peindl RD, Humble RS (1996) Modular tibial augmentations in total knee arthroplasty. Clin Orthop 327: 207-17
18. Freeman MAR, Bradley GW, Revell PA (1982) Observations upon the interface between bone and polymethylmethacrylate cement. J Bone Joint Surg 64 B, 4: 489-93
19. Garbuz DS, Masri BA, Czitrom AA (1998) Biology of allografting. Orthop. Clin. North Am 29, 2: 199-204
20. Ghazavi MT, Stockley I, Gilbert Y et al. (1997) Reconstruction of massive bone defects with allograft in revision total knee arthrplasty. J Bone Joint Surg 79A, 1: 17-25
21. Ginther JR, Ritter MA (1999) Management of severe bone loss. Methylmethacrylate as a fill. In: Revision Total Knee Arthroplasty. Lotke PA and Garino JP. edit., Lippincott-Raven edit., Philadelphie, p. 217-25
22. Gomes LSM, Bechtold JE, Gustilo RB (1988) Patellar prosthesis positioning in total knee arthroplasty. A roentgenographic study. Clin Orthop 236: p 72-80
23. Gougeon F, Tirveillot F, Migaud H (2001) Les recoupes osseuses. In: Symposium de la SOFCOT 2000 sur les reprises de prothèses totales du genou. Rev Chir Orthop 87, 5: S180-S1
24. Haas S, Insall JN, Montgomery W, Windsor R et al. (1995) Revision total knee arthroplasty with use of modular components with stems inserted without cement. J Bone Joint Surg 77A: 1700-7.
25. Hanssen AD (2001) Bone-grafting for severe patellar bone loss during revision knee arthroplasty, J Bone Joint Surg 83 A, 2: 171-6
26. Harada Y, Wevers HW, Cooke TDV (1988) Distribution of bone strength in the proximal tibia. J Arthroplasty 3, 2: 167-75
27. Harris AJ, Poddar S, Gitelis S et al. (1995) Arthroplasty with a composite of an allograft and a prosthesis for knees with severe deficiency of bone. J Bone Joint Surg 77A, 3: 373-86
28. Hoeffel DP, Rubash HE (2001) Revision total knee arthroplasty. Clin Orthop 380, 116-32
29. Huten D, Van De Velde D (2001) La contrainte prothétique lors du changement. Symposium de la SOFCOT 2000 sur les reprises de prothèses totales du genou. Rev Chir Orthop 87, 5: S182-S6
30. Hvid I, Hansen SL (1988) Trabecular bone strengh patterns at the knee. Clin Orthop 227: 210-21
31. Kirk PG (1997) Selecting an implant: a comparison of revision implant systems. In: Revision total knee arthroplasty. Engh GA., Rorabeck CH. edit., Williams and Wilkins edit., Baltimore Ch 7, p. 137-66
32. Kraay MJ, Goldberg VM, Figgie MP et al. (1992) Distal femoral replacement with allograft / prosthetic reconstruction for treatment of supracondylar fractures in patients with total kne arthroplasty. J Arhtroplasty 7, 1: 7-16

33. Laskin RS (1989) Total knee arthroplasty in the presence of large bony defects of the tibia and marked insability. Clin Orthop 248: 66-70

34. Laskin RS (1988) Tricon-M uncemented total knee arthroplasty. A review of 96 knees followed for longer than two years. J Arthroplasty 3: 27-38

35. Laskin RS, Saddler SC (1994) Bone defects in total knee arthroplasty. In: Knee surgery. Fu FH, Harner CD, Vince KG édit., Williams and Wilkins édit., Baltimore Vol II, 1399-405

36. Laskin RS (1998) Management of the patella during revision total knee replacement arthroplasty. Orthop Clin North Am 29: 355-60

37. Lewis PL, Brewster NT, Graves SE (1998) The pathogenesis of bone loss following total knee arthroplasty. Orthop Clin North Am 29, 2: 187-97

38. Lee JG, Keating M, Ritter MA (1990) Review of all polyethylene tibial component in total knee arthroplasty. A minimum seven-year follow-up period. Clin Orthop 260: 87-92

39. Lee MY, Finn HA, Lazda VA et al. Bone allografts are immunogenic and may preclude subsequent organ transplants

40. Levitz CI, Lotke PA, Karp JS (1995) Long-term changes in bone mineral density following total knee replacement. Clin Orthop 321: 68-72

41. Lindstrand A, Hansson U, Toksviig-Larsen S et al. (1999) Major bone transplantation in total knee arthroplasty: a 2 to 9 year radiostereometric analysis of tibial implant stability. J Arthroplasty 14, 2: 144-8

42. Lonner JH, Klotz M, Levitz C et al. (2001) Changes in bone density after cemented total knee arthroplasty: influence of stem design. J Arthroplasty 16, 1: 107-11

43. Lotke PA (1985) Tibial component translation for bone defects. Orthop Trans 9: 425

44. Lotke PA, Wong RY, Ecker ML (1991) The use of methylmethacrymate in primary total knee replacements with large tibial defects. Clin Orthop 20: 288-94

45. Mac Auley JP, Engh GA (1997) Allografts in revision total knee arthroplasty. In Revision total knee arthroplasty, Engh GA. and Rorabeck CH. edit., Williams and Wilkins edit., Baltimore, Chap. 14, 252-74

46. Mason JB, Scott RD (1999) Management of severe bone loss. Prosthetic modularity and custom implants. In: Revision Total Knee Arthroplasty Lotke PA and Garino JP edit., Lippincott-Raven edit., Philadelphie, 207-16

47. Mintzer CM, Robertson DD, Rackeman S et al. (1990) Bone loss in the distal anterior femur after total knee arthroplasty. Clin Orthop 260: 135-43

48. Mow CS, Wiedel JD (1996) Revision total knee arthroplasty using the porous coated anatomic revision prosthesis: six to twelve years results. J Arthroplasty 11, 3: 235-41

49. Mnaymneh W, Emerson RH, Borja F et al. (1990) Massive allografts in salvage revisions of failed total knee replacements. Clin Orthop 260: 144-50

50. Murray PB, Rand JA, Hanssen AD (1994) Cemented long stem revision total knee arthroplasty. Clin Orthop 309: 116-23

51. Nakabayashi Y, Wevers HW, Cooke TD et al. (1994) Bone strength and histomorphometry of the distal femur. J Arthroplasty 9: 307-15

52. Pagnano MW, Trousdale RT, Rand JA (1995) Tibial wedge augmentation for bone deficiency in total knee arthroplasty. Clin Orthop 321: 151-5

53. Pagnano MW, Scuderi GR, Insall JN (1998) Patellar component resection in revision and reimplantation total knee arthroplasty. Clin Orthop 356: 134-8

54. Parks NL, Engh GA (1997) Histology of nine structural bone grafts used in total knee arthroplasty. Clin Orthop 345: 17-23

55. Pelker RR, Friedlander GE (1987) Biomechanical properties of bone autografts and allografts. Orthop Clin North Am 18: 235

56. Petersen MM, Laurizten JB, Pedersen JG et al. (1996) Decreased bone density of the distal femur after uncemented knee arthroplasty. A 1-year follow-up of 29 cases. Acta Orthop Scand 1996, 67, 4, 339-44

57. Rand JA (1991) Bone deficiency in total knee arthroplasty. Use of metal wedge augmentation. Clin Orthop 271: 63-71

58. Rand JA (1995) Augmentation of a total knee arthroplasty with a modular metal wedge. A case report. J Bone Joint Surg 77A: 266-68

59. Rand JA (1996) Modularity in total knee arthroplasty. Acta Orthop Belg 62, Suppl. I: 181-6

60. Rand JA (1998) Modular augments in revision total knee arthroplasty. Orthop Clin North Am 29, 2: 347-53
61. Ritter M (1986) Screw and cement fixation of large defects in total knee arthroplasty. J Arthroplasty, 1, 2: 125-9
62. Ritter M, Keating M, Farris P (1993) Screw and cement fixation of large tibial defects in total knee arthroplasty. A sequel. J Arthroplasty 8: 63-5
63. Rorabeck CH, Smith PN (1998) Results of revision total knee arthroplasty in the face of significant bone deficiency. Orhop Clin North Am 29, 2: 361-71
64. Samuelson KM (1988) Bone grafting and non-cemented revision arthroplasty of the knee. Clin Orthop 226: 93-101
65. Scott RD (1988) Revision total knee arthroplasty. Clin Orthop 226: 65-77
66. Scuderi G, Insall JN, Haas SB et al. (1989) Inlay autogenic bone grafting of tibial defects in primary total knee artropolasty. Clin Orthop 248: 93-7
67. Sculco TP, Choi JC (1998) The role and results of bone grafting in revision total knee replacement. Orthop Clin North Am 29, 2: 339-46
68. Sculco TP, Choi JC (1999) Management of severe bone loss. The role and results of bone grafting in revision total knee replacement. In Revision Total Knee Arthroplasty, Lotke PA and Garino JP. edit., Lippincott-Raven edit., Philadelphie: 197-206
69. Seitz P, Ruegsegger P, Gschwend N (1987) Changes in local bone density after total knee arthroplasty. The use of quantative computed tomography. J Bone Joint Surg 69 B: 407-11
70. Sneppen D, Christensen P, Larsen H et al. (1981) Mechanical testing of trabecular bone in total knee arthroplasty . Development of an osteopenetrometer. Int Orthop 5: p 251-6
71. Springorum HW, De Nicola WL (1991) A new technique of defect filling in cementless total knee arthroplasty. In: Total knee replacement. Laskin RS édit., Springer Verlag édit., 232-4
72. Stockley I, Mc Auley JP, Gross AE (1992) Allograft reconstruction in total knee arthroplasty. J Bone Joint Surg 74B, 3: 393-7
73. Tabutin J (1998) Reconstruction osseuse de la patella par autogreffe vissée au cours des reprises des prothèses de genou. Rev Chir Orthop 84: 363-7
74. Takahashi Y, Gustilo RB (1994) Nonconstrained implants in revision total knee arthroplasty. Clin Orthop 309: 156-62
75. Tsahakis PJ, Beafer WB, Brick GW (1994) Technique and results of allograft reconstruction in revision total knee arthroplaty. Clin Orthop 303: 86-94
76. Ullmark G, Hovelius L (1996) Impacted morcellized allograft and cement for revision total knee arthroplasty. Acta Orthop Scand, 67, 1: 10-2
77. Van Loon CJ, de Waal Malefijt MC, Buma P et al. (1999) Femoral bone loss in total knee arthroplasty. Acta Ortop Belg 65, 2: 154-63
78. Vince KG (1996) Prosthetic selection in total knee arthroplasty. Am J Knee Surg 9: 76-82
79. Vince KG (1995) Revision knee arthroplasty. The limits of press fit medullary fixation. Clin Orthop 317: 172-7
80. Whiteside LA (1989) Cementless reconstruction of massive tibial bone loss in revision total knee arthroplasty. Clin Orthop 248: p 80-6
81. Whiteside LA (1993) Cementless revision total knee arthroplasty, Clin Orthop 286, 160-7
82. Whiteside LA (1998) Radiologic and histologic analysis of morselized allograft in revision total knee replacement. Clin Orthop 357: 149-56
83. Windsor RE, Insall JN, Sculco TP (1986) Bone grafting of tibial defects in primary and revision total knee arthroplasty. Clin Orthop 205: 132-7
84. Wilde AH, Schickendantz MS, Stulberg BN, Go RT (1990)The incorporation of tibial allografts in total knee arthroplasty. J Bone Joint Surg 72 A, 6: 815-24

Choice of constraint in revision total knee arthroplasty

K.G. Vince, M. Malo

General

Personal bias/statement

Constrained knee prostheses should be avoided when alternatives exist. When constraint is necessary, non-linked constrained devices are heavily favored over hinges and can be expected to solve virtually any stability problems when used appropriately. No constrained device, however, can provide a permanent solution when deforming forces, such as malalignment, persist in the knee. Linked constrained devices are misguided designs that ultimately make bad situations worse.

Introduction: the constrained prosthesis

Surgeons sometimes have an unfortunate and poorly considered reflex to a badly failed knee arthroplasty: "I need a constrained implant." Successful revision surgery will require far greater specificity and insight in planning, especially in the selection of a prosthesis. The final decision may not be possible until a later stage of the surgery itself. If constraint is indeed appropriate in a revision knee arthroplasty, it will not be due to bone loss or to correct deformity, but rather to compensate the instability that has resulted from soft tissue failure. Constraint should be regarded as a mechanical substitute for ligaments that have suffered plastic failure, or worse, have ruptured completely. Not all instability requires a constrained prosthesis. Knees can exhibit gross instability as a result of component loosening and bone loss. This will be solved not with constraint but with reconstitution of bone using implants and / or bone graft to restore tension to ligaments that have been intact but slack.

"Constrained", when used to describe a knee prosthesis, does not necessarily mean a hinge-linked device. Two major categories exist: linked and non-linked. The linked devices enclose two subgroups, the fixed-hinge and the rotating-hinge. While hinged devices date from the middle of this century, the first non-linked constrained device, the Total Condylar III prosthesis was introduced at the Hospital for Special Surgery in New York in about 1978. It followed the development of the Total Condylar I arthroplasty by Insall,

Walker and Ranawat at that institution in 1973. The Total Condylar I was designed to be implanted after sacrifice of the posterior cruciate ligament and included resurfacing of the patellofemoral joint. Stability came from an articular geometry with curved femoral condyles that sat in wells or dished surfaces on the tibial plateau, combined with a surgical technique that balanced flexion and extension gaps.

The difference between conformity and constraint

Comparison of the Total Condylar prostheses I and III highlights an important distinction between the concepts of "conformity" and "constraint". Conformity describes the degree to which the femoral and tibial articular surfaces match each other and accordingly the extent to which loads in the joint are disseminated across the bearing surface. Conforming articulations minimize contact stress by maximizing the surface area. In a hip arthroplasty for example, the radii of curvature of the acetabular and femoral surfaces are identical, with virtually one hundred percent of the hemispheric articular surface in contact with the femoral head. By contrast, early non-cemented, cruciate retaining knee arthroplasties had very flat tibial surfaces. The contoured femoral component made contact over a relatively small area of the tibia. These were highly non-conforming articulations that have been largely abandoned because of poor durability records.

Conformity is not necessarily constraint. Even though the conventional ball and socket of a hip arthroplasty may be completely conforming, it is not a constrained device. While conformity and constraint are separate concepts, increasing conformity eventually confers some constraint to an articulation. To make a hip arthroplasty constrained (and this is done only very rarely), a retaining ring must be added that locks the femoral head inside the socket.

Some degree of conformity has been regarded as important, if not essential, in the design of knee arthroplasty. In fact, conformity should probably be maximized in the design of knee replacements up to the point where it begins to impair knee kinematics, specifically the relationship between stability and mobility. The implant that is too conforming will tend to bind and limit motion.

Conformity then contributes to joint stability and reduces material wear, while constraint is a mechanical means to substitute for missing or damaged soft tissue structures and leads to higher loosening rates.

The development of constrained knee prostheses

The Total Condylar I prosthesis was conforming but not constrained. It represented a significant advance in knee arthroplasty design. During the early years of its implantation, the importance of alignment was recognized and the techniques for soft tissue releases to correct deformity were developed. In effect, surgeons learned how to resurface the articular cartilage, using the patients' own ligaments for stability.

Still, some difficult knee reconstructions required mechanical constraint.

The Total Condylar II was an ill-fated constrained device that suffered a high rate of loosening (18). It was abandoned before ever reaching significant production. The Total Condylar III ensued, featuring a prominent rectangular polyethylene spine on the tibial component that sat in a central box on the femoral component between the two femoral condyles (10). This construct was constrained though non-linked (fig. 1). The articulation of the two components provided stability to varus and valgus stresses as well as restraint to posterior tibial dislocation.

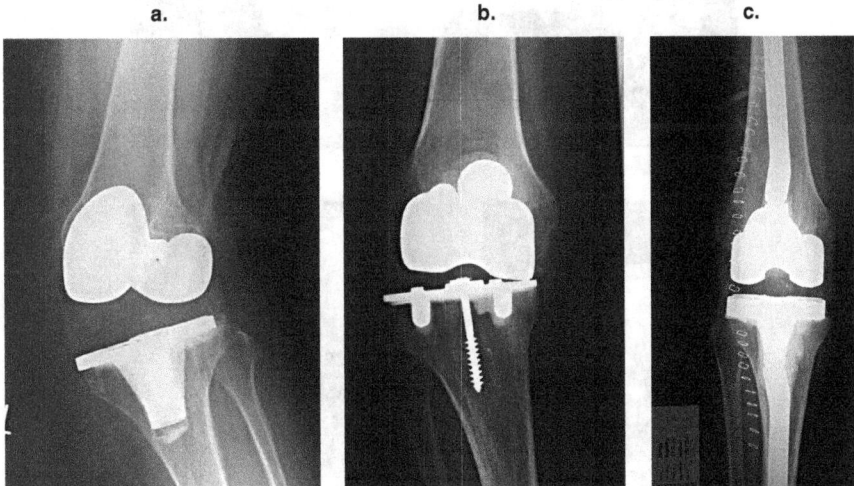

Fig. 1 – Unstable knee arthroplasties.
a. Valgus instability in primary knee arthroplasty due to failure of the medial collateral ligament. Many of these cases start with valgus deformity and a compromised medial collateral ligament. There is a high probability that this case will require a constrained prosthesis.
b. Varus instability in Porous Coated Anatomic (PCA) prosthesis that is the result of catastrophic polyethylene wear. The medial collateral ligament has not been stressed by this deformity and constraint should not be required.
c. Revision of the unstable primary arthroplasty in B. A (non-constrained) posterior stabilized articulation has been used. (Note there is no central eminence on the tibial component providing constraint.) Stem extensions have been used to enhance fixation.

Fixed-hinge designs were amongst the first prostheses to be introduced for knee replacement surgery (fig. 2) beginning in 1951 with the Walldius (45). Though a bold innovation at the time, the concept of a linked articulation was flawed. Many years passed before durable alternatives to hinged implants were perfected and about thirty years until one of the last fixed hinges, the European Guepar, was virtually abandoned. Numerous iterations of hinged knee arthroplasties had appeared and the linked constrained device has not died completely. There are even now misguided claims that rotating hinges can solve the problems of instability without high loosening rates. Hinges are to be avoided.

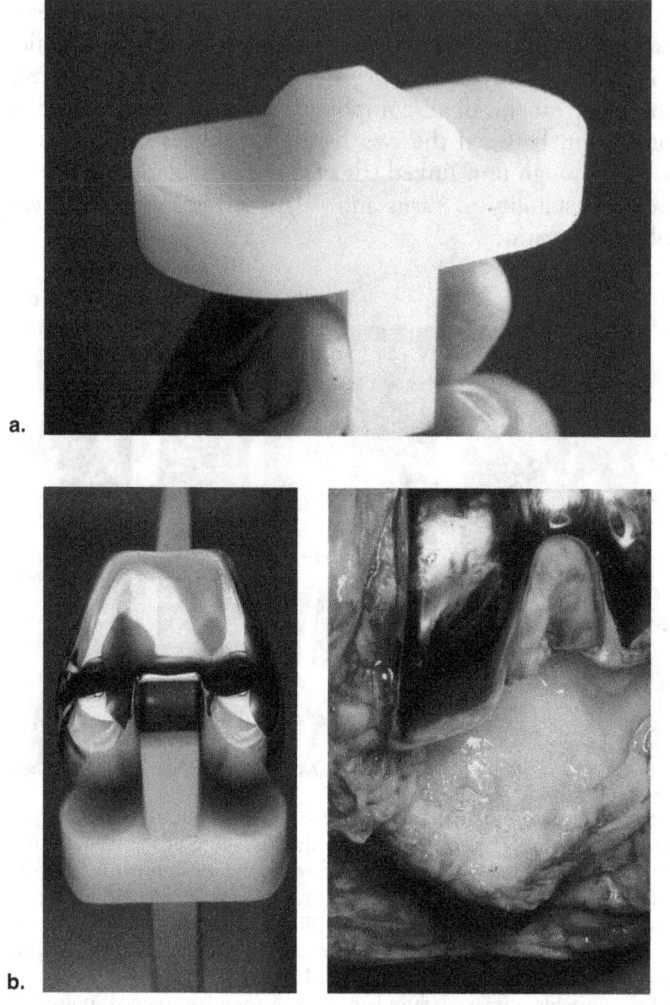

Fig. 2 – Conformity versus constraint.
a. All polyethylene tibias component from a Total Condylar cruciate sacrificing knee prosthesis. The "wells" on each tibial hemi-condyle provide stability and they also distribute load in the polyethylene.
b. The original Total Condylar III, with non-modular stems, substituted for collateral ligament function with a prominent central spine on the tibial, that was contained between the femoral condyles.
c. Lack of conformity, with flat polyethylene leads to rapid polyethylene wear. This is an extreme example of a "non-conforming articulation".

The relationship between stems and constraint

The rush to use a constrained device is sometimes predicated on the need for medullary fixation. The two concepts, constraint to compensate for ligamentous deficiency and medullary stems to augment fixation, should themselves be "unlinked". Stems can be used with or without constraint. They may be used to augment fixation when bone quality is poor, or when reconstruction with graft and'or augments is necessary. They may be employed with several different strategies:

1. modular press fit stems;
2. fixed or modular narrow diameter fully cemented stems;
3. fixed or modular narrow uncemented stems that gain three point fixation;
4. offset or curved uncemented stems that better match the internal shape and size of the canal (fig. 3).

a.   **b.**

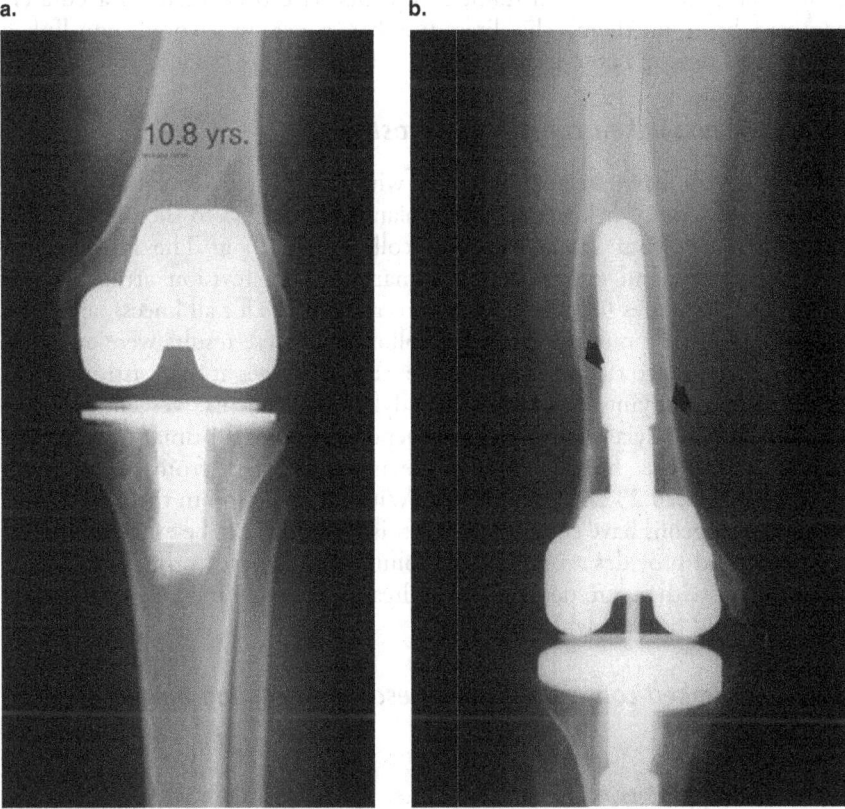

Fig. 3 – Constraint and loosening.
a. The Insall Burstein II, posterior stabilized knee prosthesis at over 10 years. This prosthesis depends on the patient's collateral ligaments for varus and valgus stability.
b. Failed constrained Condylar Knee Prosthesis. The combination of constraint, uncemented stem extension, malalignment and poor quality bone results in loosening and in this case femur fracture (arrows).

Constrained devices, when necessary because of instability from soft tissue compromise, should be implanted with intramedullary stem extensions to enhance fixation and to provide load sharing. While constrained devices will always use stems, non-constrained implants will require them only occasionally.

The hinge: Why is it so bad?

Are non-linked and linked constrained devices so very different from each other in terms of breakage and loosening rates? Isn't mechanical stabilization stressful to the interface whether or not the two components are linked together? There is currently, interest in rotating type-hinged arthroplasties, of which rotational freedom theoretically diminishes the high stresses on the articulation and at the bone-cement interface. This originated with the Kinematic Rotating Hinge(19), which has seemed some clinical use in the past two decades (5, 14, 27, 33, 36, 44). While it is difficult, because of the variety of clinical situations where constrained implants have been used, to accurately compare bpth of them, the literature has generally favored non-linked constrained device. Later, let's ask why.

Results of non-linked constrained prosthesis

Clinical series have been published with the Total Condylar III and Constrained Condylar knee (CCK) implants, from 1988 to the present. The first originated from Donaldson and colleagues (10) at The Hospital for Special Surgery, and described 17 primary and 14 revision arthroplasties. There were 5 failures (35.7% for revisions and 16.1% for all knees), all in the revision group at a mean of 3.8 years follow-up. These results were encouraging and superior to the previous experience with hinges at that institution. In other series studying the Total Condylar III and its descendant, the Constrained Condylar, no failures were reported amongst primary knee replacements and the failure rate in revisions ranged from 0 to 33% (8,11,13,15,16,20,23,24,26,30,32,43). Without exception in these published series, the surgeons have concluded that this prosthesis can be expected to perform well and provides an acceptable solution in complex primary and revision surgery with severe deformity and ligament instability. Less constrained devices should be used when possible.

Results of linked constrained prostheses and rotating hinges

Favor hinges

There are supporters of hinged implants, the most ardent of whom can be found amongst our European colleagues, who centime to use the largest numbers of hinges. Some, like Nieder and colleagues in Hamburg, Germany, prefer to decrease reliance on hinged prostheses, but leave them available for certain difficult cases (25). Others are more enthusiastic, in particular about rotating hinge designs. Blauth, in Kiel, Germany, has described with his colleagues excellent result of a rotating hinge design that bears his name. A total of 497 implants have been studied from 1 to 15 years with aseptic loosening complicating only in 1.2% of them. Deep infection complicated 3% of these (6). Other authors have advocated its use (7).

Rotating hinges have supporters. Smilowicz described a failure rate of 33% with non-rotating hinges compared with no failures amongst 15 rotating hinges followed during an average of 7 years and 11 months (35). Proponents of the Endo rotating hinge acknowledge problems with fixed-hinges but report a remarkable 10-year 94% of survivorship with the rotating version (12). These were largely primary knee arthroplasties and the results contrasted favorably with a much higher failure rate amongst non-constrained St. Georg Sled implants.

Oppose hinges

Vaczi and colleagues in Budapest, Hungary, have adopted a more North American view of the hinge (37). After reviewing their experience over 18 years with a variety of designs, they found in 59 revisions with hinges a complication rate of 17.8% and have reserved the hinges to very select cases. Hanssen and colleagues at the Mayo Clinic took a dim view of hinges when used for reimplantation after infection. They noted a generally poorer prognosis when a hinge was used and found that 3 of 4 limbs that required an above knee amputation had been reconstructed with hinges (14). Inglis, an American surgeon working in the United Kingdom, and Walker, a biomechanical design engineer, reported very poor results of first and second revisions with a fixed-axis hinge (Stanmore), concluding that revision of a fixed-hinge arthroplasty with another of the same design is unlikely to be successful 17). In Dundee, Scotland, Rickhuss and associates reported a 31% failure rate at 5-10 years with a Sheehan hinge, concluding that the device was obsolete (28).

Rotating hinges

The Kinematic rotating hinge has enjoyed some support amongst American surgeons. This prosthetic device was developed by a group of experienced engineers and surgeons acutely aware of the limitations and the high failure rate associated with fixed-hinge devices. Despite initial encouraging results (notably, a series of 38 knees reported by Shaw from Hershey, Pennsylvania with a minimum 25-month follow-up that yield a high percentage of satisfactory clinical results[33]), the long-term results continued to be disappointing. Rand and associates at the Mayo Clinic[27] reported on 38 rotating hinge knees at 50 months follow-up. There was a 22% rate of patellar instability, a 6% rate of component breakage, and a 16% rate of sepsis. They concluded that the prosthesis gave no better results than the previous non-rotating hinges.

The Noiles hinge has enjoyed mixed reviews in the past. The developers of the device published an enthusiastic review early on (1, 2). The device was met with considerable disappointment by other users. Shindell and associates (34) denounced the design and the claims of prior published reports in 1986. Serious flaws in the design were noted by Kester and colleagues who evaluated the mechanical failure modes in 12 retrieved devices (21).

Mechanical problems leading to breakage have been reported in other designs in the Lacey rotating hinge (31) and the Rotaflex Hinge (9, 47).

One of the difficulties in evaluating hinged arthroplasty designs is the relative dearth of clinical reviews with research methods and details that we have come to expect in arthroplasty surgery. As failures from breakage, wear, loosening and instability have been noted in the last decade with very promising non-constrained designs, one becomes skeptical about extrapolating early results from hinged designs to the long term. It would seem at times that the optimistic reports for hinges have been published in ignorance of the forty-year history of these devices (38).

Despite further design improvement in the more recent rotating hinge implants (3), their use should be reserved to oncologic procedures for tumors about the knee, and to salvage procedures in revision total knee arthroplasty (4, 5, 29, 36, 46).

Mechanical comparison: linked and non-linked

Comparing linked and non-linked prostheses can teach us something about how constrained knee prostheses function. First, both are constrained to a similar degree to varus and valgus forces. Secondly, both resist anterior and posterior tibial dislocation, although the non-linked designs on average would permit slightly greater excursions before constraint occurred than would hinges. The two types differ profoundly on a third item, freedom of rotation. The rotating hinges claim that they have overcome the previous high loosening rates of hinged prostheses by permitting rotational freedom, which exceeds physiologic rotation in the knee by several orders of magnitude 19). If however hinges loosen at a greater rate than the constrained condylar devices, which are often highly constrained to rotation, then we conclude that rotational constraint is not the major cause of loosening in linked devices. The actual basis for the rotating hinge design is a fallacy. The fourth type of constraint is resistance to hyperextension.

The hyperextension stop distinguishes linked from non-linked constrained devices. Hinged arthroplasties, whether rotating or not, provide a solid mechanical end point to extension. The Guepar prosthesis, amongst others, featured a synthetic pad to cushion the blow of impact. Non-linked constrained devices do not have such stops against hyperextension. Once the limits of extension are reached, the prosthesis is free to hyperextend, but the joint is stabilized by the intact posterior structures. The arthroplasty that is performed with a hinge specifically to treat recurvatum, either in the arthritic primary or revision, is doomed to rapid failure.

Constraint is never the whole answer, the deforming forces have to be eliminated

Constraint, even when used appropriately, is never the complete solution to the problem of instability. Just as ligaments or mechanically constrained devices confer stabilizing forces, there are always destabilizing forces in the joint that favor deformity and instability. While the knee may unpredictably experience sudden forces, the most persistently destabilizing force is malalignment. We have long recognized that varus alignment creates huge compressive forces in the medial compartment of the knee that lead to subsidence of bone, loosening and accelerated polyethylene wear. Valgus alignment, classically associated with patellar tracking problems, creates potent tensile forces in the medial collateral ligament that may result in instability. Plastic deformation of the MCL is probably the most disabling pathology of the valgus knee.

Valgus malalignment of the primary or revision knee arthroplasty also creates huge forces in a constrained prosthesis that may result in loosening of the device from bone or outright breakage of the implant. Deformation of the tibial spine in a constrained condylar device exposed to such forces may lead to recurrent instability (fig. 4).

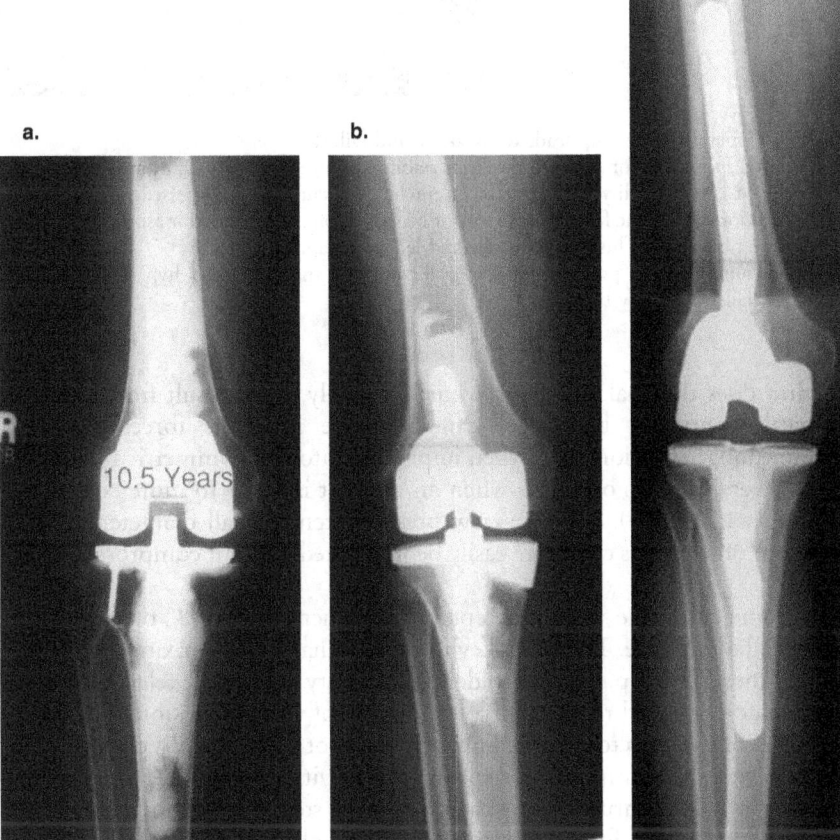

Fig. 4 – Stem extensions.
a. Fully cemented stem extensions. These are non-modular and were intended to be fully cemented. While the fixation is excellent, the limb is in jeopardy if this prosthesis ever needs to be removed.
b. Primary total knee arthroplasty for remote septic arthritis. Stability and bone quality were concerns and so additional fixation was required. Antibiotic was added to the cement and extending stems far into the medullary canals were avoided in the event of recurrent infection. This is probably the longest fully cemented stem extensions that should be considered.
c. A revision knee arthroplasty for loosening and osteolysis. A posterior stabilized knee prosthesis has been implanted with uncemented, offset stem extensions on both the tibia and femur. Note that the tibial stem offset has been placed medially with the component lateral. This matches the usual asymmetry of the tibia. The femoral component has also been placed laterally to enhance patellar tracking and a 200mm stem has been employed to enter the middle of the diaphysis. The desired valgus alignment has been achieved with excellent fit of the stems in the intramedullary canal.

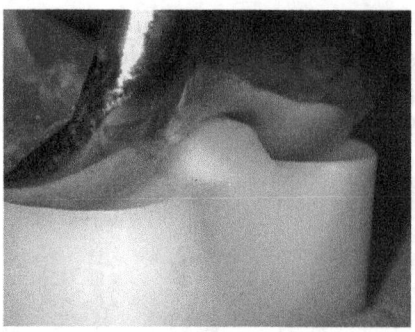 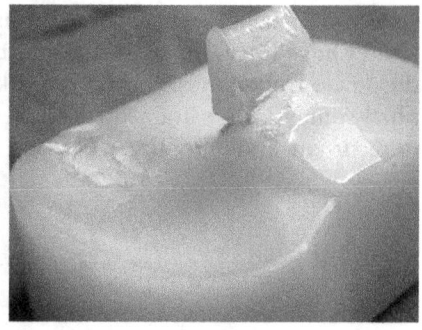

a.   b.

Fig. 5 – Hyperextension stop leads to breakage and failure.
a. Retrieved specimen from a failed posterior stabilized polyethylene implant, in a patient who developed late instability after knee replacement. As recurvatum progressed in this patient, the anterior edge of the femoral component began to contact the anterior aspect of the polyethylene tibial post. This rapidly broke and led to instability.
b. Broken anterior tibial post. Any mechanical constraint that provides a hyperextension stop usually fails rapidly by breakage.

How does this malalignment occur? Certainly it can result from errors in surgical technique, but there can be more insidious forces at work. Intramedullary fixation rods, when implanted into the asymmetric tibia, often lie in several degrees of valgus when an attempt is made to more completely fill the canal (fig. 5). More narrow press fit stems, small diameter press fit stems, or offset stems can more easily be implanted without compromising alignment.

In some cases, the usually acceptable alignment of 6 to 8° of valgus may prove to be excessive. The usual key to these scenarios lies proximal and distal to the knee. The hip, with an older arthroplasty that has a relatively valgus neck shaft angle, will require but a few degrees of valgus to restore the mechanical axis of the limb to neutral. Similarly, the foot with a tibialis posterior tendon rupture, so common amongst patients with valgus knee deformities, transfers a medial thrust to the knee with each step. These conditions of the hip and knee create forces that are strong enough to dislocate a constrained implant, linked or non-linked.

Surgical technique: How do we know when and how much constraint to use? How much conformity?

Knee prostheses range from completely non-conforming rounded femoral condyles on flat tibial articulations to linked non-rotating hinges. Both extremes have been abandoned for virtually all clinical applications. Some failed knee arthroplasties can be revised with simple primary components if adequate bone is present. Neither augments nor stems are necessary, and normal soft tissues stabilize the arthroplasty. While the posterior cruciate ligament is rarely normal at the time of revision, a cruciate retaining prosthesis can nonetheless be employed for revisions if the remaining soft tissues are well balanced. This means equality between flexion and extension gaps as well as between medial and lateral collateral ligaments. The prosthesis with relative conformity and without a posterior cruciate ligament can be made to function, much as the original Total Condylar I functioned. The surgeon's task, however, is easier at revision surgery if some benign constraint is employed, in the form of posterior stabilization.

The classic prosthetic design that provides posterior stabilization has been the Insall-Burstein Posterior Stabilized prosthesis. It was introduced in 1978 as an adjunct to the Total Condylar. It has been used frequently by many surgeons for primary and revision surgery. Numerous clinical studies confirm its efficacy in long-term clinical studies without increased loosening rates. The particular constraint that it imparts to posterior tibial dislocation would seem to be without negative effect.

Other designs have been introduced with alternate means of mechanically resisting posterior tibial dislocation. Some, with a third runner located between the femoral condyles have been abandoned. Others, with a higher anterior lip on the tibial component to resist posterior subluxation have seen limited use and with shorter follow-up. They do not replicate femoral roll back, but rather limit the undesirable femoral roll "forward".

The decision over constraint only becomes a true concern when there is a potential price to pay in terms of durability of the arthroplasty because of constraint. Constrained devices, whether linked or non-linked may be expected to loosen at a higher rate. How do we know when to select a constrained device?

When to use constraint: Technique for revision knee arthroplasty in three steps

A revision knee arthroplasty may be planned and executed by following three phases or steps. While other approaches to revision arthroplasty may well be described, this sequential approach acknowledges the importance of alignment, stability and joint line position. The technique was first published in 1991 and has been refined through a decade of implementation (40-42). In following these three steps a surgeon may encounter two situations where constraint, as provided by non-linked devices may be indicated.

Step 1 focuses on reestablishing the tibial platform as a foundation for the knee, largely because the tibial articular surface is always part of the functioning arthroplasty. In flexion it articulates with the posterior femoral condyles and in extension with the distal femoral condyles. No attempt is made in step 1 to select a tibial articular polyethylene or establish a joint line. Plans are made for the eventual reconstruction of bone defects, but for the moment a trial tibial component is inserted and the surgeon can progress to step two.

Step 2 involves stabilizing the flexion gap *i.e.* stabilizing the knee at 90° of flexion. This is the phase where the most difficult conceptual and technical work is accomplished. It is often useful to remember three goals to accomplish in this phase:

a. establish the correct axis of femoral component rotation, parallel to the transepicondylar axis;

b. select a femoral component that is large enough to stabilize the knee in flexion, resisting all impulses to simply choose a component that fits the residual bone:

c. ensure that the selected femoral component combined with a tibial articular polyethylene creates a joint line that resides at an appropriate level. In general terms, if there is no contracture of the patellar tendon, it will be satisfactory to establish the joint line so that it is inferior to the inferior pole of the patella.

Step 3 is comparatively easy. The femoral component is seated either more proximally or distally to stabilize the knee in extension, avoiding both flexion contracture and recurvatum. It is distinctly unusual to resect additional distal femoral bone in a revision, but far more common to add to the distal femoral condyles with modular augments or allograft.

Two decision points

The majority of revision knees will now be stable and mobile with trial components in place and with a posterior-stabilized articulation. Conventional collateral ligament releases may be necessary to correct deformity. Two situations may arise however where these three steps have failed to create a stable and mobile arthroplasty:

1. flexion-extension gap inequality that cannot be balanced;
2. varus-valgus instability due to collateral ligament incompetence.

The former situation arises when the flexion gap sags open symmetrically or asymmetrically and would require an inordinately thick tibial polyethylene insert in conjunction with an oversized femoral component to achieve stability. This thickness of tibial insert could not easily be accommodated in extension without resecting distal femoral bone and elevating the joint line. The femoral component would overhang the medial and lateral femur. The surgeon must recognize in this setting that the problem is soft tissue failure.

The second decision point arises when the knee cannot be stabilized in extension due to collateral ligament failure, usually on the medial side. As progressively thicker tibial polyethylene is inserted in the joint, the intact posterior structures tighten and a flexion contracture ensues without having stabilized the joint to varus and valgus stresses.

These two situations are the mechanically specific indications for constraint. Not all knees that appear to have failed badly will fall into this category. For many "bad looking knees", reconstruction of bone defects will restore tension to good ligaments, and most revision cases can be treated with a posterior-stabilized articulation. The reflex to choose a constrained device because the knee looks bad is misguided.

Alternative to constraint

Any constraint may be undesirable for some patients, in particular the young or active individual. There are no well established techniques to stabilize the unstable knee without resorting to constraint. Some work has been done however on collateral ligament advancements and reconstructions to eliminate or reduce the dependence on mechanical constraint (22,39).

Revising the failed hinge

The difficulties with a failed hinge revolve around destruction of bone and the challenge of extracting a well fixed, cemented stem when a hinge prosthesis has broken. The classic appearance of the failed hinge, far more common in the 1970's and early 80's was of a thin, sclerotic and expanded cortex resulting from a hinge stem that had been moving like a "windshield wiper" inside the medullary canal. At times it seems that the only recourse would be to recement another hinge, perhaps with a longer stem in the same position. Given the bone compromise, this revision can be expected to fail even more quickly posing an even greater problem. Revision of a hinge with another hinge is unlikely to be successful (17).

Ironically, the hinge prosthesis often protects whatever collateral ligaments may have been present at the time of the original surgery. They are usually spared by the constrained articulation and in most cases a hinge can successfully be revised to either a non-constrained or certainly non-linked prosthesis.

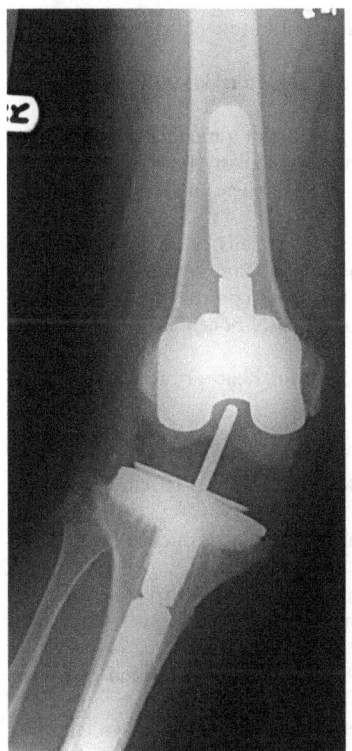

Fig. 6 – Unstable, constrained prosthesis.
Radiograph of an unstable constrained knee prosthesis. The usual contributing factors are complete soft tissue failure and malalignment. Decreased valgus alignment combined with soft tissue reconstruction or ligament allograft may be successful. While a hinge will provide immediate stability, it too will fail in time.

The unique challenge that these failures present to the surgeon is extensive destruction of the medullary canal, which cannot be easily reconstructed with modular or custom components. In some cases structural allograft will be required. In others, where an intact, though thin and sclerotic, tube of bone is present, impaction grafting of particulate allograft has been effective. In three of the senior author's (KGV) cases, the internal bone has been reconstituted and a narrow diameter medullary component cemented into the bone, with pressurization techniques borrowed from hip arthroplasties (fig. 6).

Conclusion

The least constrained prosthesis should be used in knee arthroplasty surgery. Constraint is always undesirable but at times necessary. Non-linked constrained devices are preferred over linked constrained or hinged implants. There are very specific mechanical indications for constrained implants and they are not simply indicated by the severity of the appearance of the failed primary.

References

1. Accardo NJ (1982) Noiles knee replacement prodedure: A six-year experience. Orthop Trans 6: 436-7
2. Accardo NJ, Noiles DG, Pena R et al. (1979) Noiles total knee replacement prodedure. Orthopedics 2: 37-45
3. Barrack RL (2001) Evolution of the rotating hinge for complex total knee arthroplasty. Clin Orthop 392: 292-9
4. Barrack RL, Lyons TR, Ingraham RQ et al. (2000) The use of a modular rotating hinge component in salvage revision total knee arthroplasty. J Arthroplasty 15: 858-66
5. Berman AT, O'Brien JT, Israelite C (1996) Use of the rotating hinge for salvage of the infected total knee arthroplasty. Orthopedics 19: 73-6
6. Blauth W, Hassenpflug J (1990) Are unconstrained components essential in total knee arthroplasty? Long-term results of the Blauth knee prosthesis. Clin Orthop 258: 86-94
7. Bohm P, Holy T (1998) Is there a future for hinged prostheses in primary total knee arthroplasty? A 20-year survivorship analysis of the Blauth prosthesis. J Bone Joint Surg 80B: 302-9
8. Chotivichit AL, Cracchiolo A III, Chow GH et al. (1991) Total knee arthroplasty using the total condylar III knee prosthesis. J Arthroplasty 6: 341-50
9. David HG, Bishay M, James ET (1998) Problems with the Rotaflex: A 10-year review of a rotating hinge prosthesis. J Arthroplasty 13: 402-8
10. Donaldson WF III, Sculco TP, Insall JN et al. (1988) Total condylar III knee prosthesis: Long-term follow-up study. Clin Orthop 226: 21-8
11. Easley ME, Insall JN, Scuderi GR et al. (2000) Primary constrained condylar knee arthroplasty for the arthritic valgus knee. Clin Orthop 380: 58-64
12. Engelbrecht E, Heinert K (1988) Experience with a surface and total knee replacement: further development of the model St. Georg. In: Niwa S, Paul JP, Yamamoto S (eds). Total knee replacement. Tokyo: Springer-Verlag, 257-73
13. Goldberg VM, Figgie MP, Figgie HE III et al. (1988) The results of revision total knee arthroplasty. Clin Orthop 226: 86-92
14. Hanssen AD, Trousdale RT, Osmon DR (1995) Patient outcome with reinfection following reimplantation for the infected total knee arthroplasty. Clin Orthop 321: 55-67

15. Hartford JM, Goodman SB, Schurman DJ *et al.* (1998) Complex primary and revision total knee arthroplasty using the condylar constrained prosthesis: an average 5-year follow-up. J Arthroplasty 13: 380-7

16. Hohl WM, Crawford E, Zelicof SB *et al.* (1991) The total condylar III prosthesis in complex knee reconstruction. Clin Orthop 273: 91-7

17. Inglis AE, Walker PS (1991) Revision of failed knee replacements using fixed-axis hinges. J Bone Joint Surg (Br) 73: 757-61

18. Insall JN, Tria AJ (1979) The Total condylar knee prosthesis type II. Presented at the Annual Meeting of the American Academy of Orthopaedic Surgeons, San Francisco, CA

19. Kabo JM, Yang RS, Dorey FJ *et al.* (1997) *In vivo* rotational stability of the kinematic rotating hinge knee prosthesis. Clin Orthop 336: 166-76

20. Kavolus CH, Faris PM, Ritter MA *et al.* (1991) The total condylar III knee prosthesis in elderly patients. J Arthroplasty 6: 39-43

21. Kester MA, Cook SD, Harding AF *et al.* (1988) An evaluation of the mechanical failure modalities of a rotating hinge knee prosthesis. Clin Orthop 228: 156-63

22. Krackow KA (1990) The technique of total knee arthroplasty. St. Louis, CV Mosby

23. Lachiewicz PF, Falatyn SP (1996) Clinical and radiographic results of the Total Condylar III and Constrained Condylar total knee arthroplasty. J Arthroplasty 11: 916-22

24. McPherson EJ, Vince KG (1993) Breakage of a Total Condylar III knee prosthesis. A case report. J Arthroplasty 8: 561-3

25. Nieder E (1991) Schittenprothese, rotatioskinie und scharnieprothese Modell St. Georg und Endo-Modell: Differentialtherapie in der primaren kniegelenkalloarthroplastik. Orthopade 20: 170-80

26. Rand JA (1991) Revision total knee arthroplasty using the total condylar III prosthesis. J Arthroplasty 6: 279-84

27. Rand JA, Chao EY, Stauffer RN (1987) Kinematic rotating-hinge total knee arthroplasty. J Bone Joint Surg 69A: 489-97

28. Rickhuss PK, Gray AJ, Rowley DI (1994) A 5-10 year follow-up of the Sheehan total knee endoprosthesis in Tayside. J R Coll Surg Edinb 39: 326-8

29. Rinta-Kiikka I, Alberty A, Savilahti S *et al.* (1997) The clinical and radiological outcome of the rotating hinged knee prostheses in the long-term. Ann Chir Gynaecol 86: 349-56

30. Rosenberg AG, Verner JJ, Galante JO (1991) Clinical results of total knee revision using the Total Condylar III prosthesis. Clin Orthop 273: 83-90

31. Scott CE, Heiner J, Worzala FJ *et al.* (1996) Condylar failure of the Lacey Rotating-Hinge total knee. J Arthroplasty 11: 214-6

32. Sculco TP (1989) Total condylar III prosthesis in ligament instability. Orthop Clin North Am 20(2): 221-226

33. Shaw JA, Balcom W, Greer RB III (1989) Total knee arthroplasty using the kinematic rotating hinge prosthesis. Orthopedics 12: 647-654,1989

34. Shindell R, Neumann R, Connolly JF *et al.* (1986) Evaluation of the Noiles hinged knee prosthesis: A five-year study of seventeen knees. J Bone Joint Surg 68A:579-85

35. Smilowicz M (1996) Total knee joint replacement with a rotating hinge endoprosthesis in light of late results. Chir Narzadow Ruchu Ortop Pol 61: 409-13

36. Springer BD, Hanssen AD, Sim FH *et al.* (2001) The kinematic rotating hinge prosthesis for complex knee arthroplasty. Clin Orthop 392: 283-91

37. Vaczi G, Udvarhelyi I, Sarungi M (1997) Comparison of results of different types of knee arthroplasties. Arch Orthop Trauma Surg 116: 177-80

38. Vince KG (1994) Evolution of total knee arthroplasty. In: Scott WN (ed). The knee. St-Louis: CV Mosby, 1045-78

39. Vince KG (1997) Collateral ligament reconstructions in difficult primary and revision total knee arthroplasty. Presented at the Annual Meeting of the American Academy of Orthopedic Surgeons, San Francisco, CA

40. Vince KG (2001) Revision knee arthroplasty. In: Chapman MW (ed) Chapman's Orthopedic Surgery. Philadelphia: Lippincott, Williams and Wilkins, 2897-936

41. Vince KG (2001) Revision knee arthroplasty: How I do it? In: Insall JN, Scott WN (eds) Surgery of the Knee: Philadelphia: Churchill Livingstone, 1958-66

42. Vince KG (2001)Technique of three-step revision total knee arthroplasty. In: Harner CD, Vince KG, Fu FH (eds) Techniques in knee surgery. Philadelphia: Lippincott Williams and Wilkins: 291-304

43. Vince KG, Long W (1995) Revision knee arthroplasty. The limits of press fit medullary fixation. Clin Orthop 317: 172-7

44. Walker PS, Emerson R, Potter T *et al.* (1982) The kinematic rotating hinge: Biomechanics and clinical application. Orthop Clin North Am 13: 187-99

45. Walldius B (1957) Arthroplasty of the knee joint using endoprosthesis. Acta Orthop Scand (suppl) 24: 19-24

46. Westrich GH, Mollano AV, Sculco TP *et al.* (2000) Rotating hinge total knee arthroplasty in severely affected knees. Clin Orthop 379: 195-208

47. Wilkinson JM, Douglas DL (1994) Rotaflex total knee arthroplasty: a report of two prosthetic failures at the hinge mechanism. J R Coll Surg Edinb 39: 375-6

Two-stage reimplantation for infected total knee arthroplasty – Results at 5-year follow-up

A. Ferreira, G. Gacon

Introduction

Because of management difficulties and medicolegal implications, infection of a total knee prosthesis is the most dreaded complication. Incidence of infection varies according to series, but it is consistently higher than that reported in total hip arthroplasty. The published rates range from 1.3 to 5%. During the 1998 AAOS Meeting, Hanssen and Rand (17) reported a 2.5% infection rate in 18,749 TKAs performed between 1969 and 1996. Infection rate was 2% in patients who had not had prior knee surgery (16,035 TKAs).

Although the exact treatment protocol is still under debate, the method of treatment itself was defined by Insall as early as 1983 (22). Today, two-stage reimplantation (removal of the implant followed by reimplantation) with extensive tissue resection at the time of removal is considered the treatment of choice, with a 4 to 8-week interval of intravenous antibiotic therapy (double or triple) between the two stages.

The present series shows the evolution of the outcome at a longer follow-up, and stresses the problems of durability of the results and definition of the healing criteria.

Patients

The initial series involved 29 patients (20 female, 9 male) with septic knee prostheses (27 TKAs, 2 UKAs, performed by 3 surgeons). The index procedures had been performed between 1986 and 1994. At the time of primary implantation, the average age of patients was 70 years (46 to 83 years); at the time or revision, it was 75.5 years. All the patients but one (with rheumatoid arthritis) had been essentially managed for osteoarthritis of the knee. Only sliding knee prostheses and UKRs were considered; hinged knees were excluded.

19 patients had had an infection within 12 months of the operation: an acute infection in 9 and a chronic infection in 10. 10 patients had had a late infection: a chronic infection in 6, a sudden sepsis in 4.

11 patients had had a surgical treatment prior to removal of the prosthesis:

– arthroscopic lavage (4);
– aspiration / lavage (4);

– exploratory arthrotomy (1);
– synovectomy (1);
– arthrolysis for painful stiff knee (1).

All these procedures had failed to clear up the infection; however, in all the cases but one, cultures of specimens had allowed identification of the involved organism.

15 of the 29 patients had none of the risk factors described by De Cloedt (9); the other patients had one or several risk factors, including:

– rheumatoid arthritis (RA) (1);
– previous local surgery (1);
– ASA Grade III or IV (American Society of Anaesthesiology) (3);
– immunodeficiency (1);
– prior knee replacement (7: 5 sliding TKRs, 1 medial UKR, 1 lateral UKR).

Infection diagnosis had been based on the criteria defined by Hannsen and Rand (18): clinical picture and / or same organism identified at least twice in a culture, histological confirmation of the infection using synovial biopsy, presence of a fistula, or unequivocal anatomic conditions.

In 23 of these 29 patients, one organism at least had been identified: coagulase-negative staphylococcus (12), coagulase-positive staphylococcus (8): 1 staphycoccus aureus, 2 streptococci, 2 acinetobacters, 1 pseudomonas, 1 peptococcus, 1 gemella morbidum (anaerobic streptococci). In 7 patients, other organisms were associated, once with staphylococcus aureus and 4 times with coagulase-negative staphylococcus. 3 organisms were methi-resistant: 1 staphylococcus epidermidis, and 2 staphylococci aureus.

Two-stage reimplantation was performed in all the patients, with an interval of double or triple intravenous antibiotic therapy. Mean time to reimplantation was 8.45 weeks (2 to 24 weeks). In all the cases but one, reimplantation was performed with a cemented sliding prosthesis. Antibiotic impregnated bone cement (Gentallin) was used in 25 patients. Antibiotics were continued for 2 to 6 months (maximum) after reimplantation. The first stage consisted of removal of all the components, joint debridement and synovectomy, insertion of a Gentallin loaded cement "spacer" (plus Gentallin beads in 6 cases). During the interval between the two stages, the patients were non-weight bearing and no mobilisation was attempted. The second stage consisted of reimplantation with a total knee prosthesis (patellar component was left in place in 20 patients); in total, 4 hinged knees, 13 posterior stabilized (PS) stemmed prostheses, 12 PS stemless prostheses were implanted.

At an average follow-up of 3.5 years, 24 reimplantations (82.7%) were successful. However, two patients had to be reoperated on for persistent pain. In one case, a one-stage revision was performed for iterative loosening and revealed the presence of staphylococcus epidermidis; infection was considered to be medically cured at review (one year later). In the other case, joint debridement was performed 5 months after reimplantation and revealed the presence of streptococcus D; infection was also considered to be cured at review (10 months later), but the patient had a very poor functional result. Therefore, primary healing was achieved in 22 patients.

As regards functional results, the average Hungerford score was 75.6/100 with 6 excellent results, 10 good, 6 fair and 2 poor. The average ISK score was 80.7/100 for physical examination, and 70/100 for function. Average flexion was 95° (range, 30°-120°).

Five patients (17.3%) with persistent signs of infection who had had an arthrodesis (except one who was lost to follow-up) were considered failures. One of them had died 5 months after the procedure, 2 arthrodeses were still ununited at 12 months. Union had been achieved in one patient only.

A certain number of interesting conclusions were drawn from this study:

– diagnostic value of the inflammatory assessment based on both ESR and CRP. White blood cell count was judged of little value;

– diagnostic value of 3-phase scintigraphy in case of a negative result, since its negative predictive value is considered to be close to 100%;

– clinical diagnosis was sometimes difficult in chronic cases because such symptoms as pain, increased local heat, or functional disorders may be misinterpreted as being signs of infection;

– aspiration for culturing of organisms (if any) was advocated. In contrast, the anatomico-pathological examination that was performed in 13 patients was not significant, except in 2 patients;

– influence of risk factors (particularly previous surgery) was noteworthy; this might bring to question the conservative operative treatments that are proposed to arthritic patients (e.g., arthroscopic lavage);

– the 82.7% success rate was similar to that reported in the literature, and was attributed to the Insall two-stage treatment method (22);

– no correlation was found between the nature of the organism or time on onset of the infection and healing rate;

– among the 5 failures, one risk factor at least was found in 4 cases, and 3 knees had had prior arthroplasty. Other factors might explain these failures, such as the use of double instead of triple antibiotic therapy, and in one case, failure to identify the organism;

– two questions remained unanswered: 1) what should be the optimal interval between the two stages, 2) was it more appropriate to immobilize the knee or, on the contrary, to mobilise the knee using special "spacers";

– at last, infections due to coagulase-negative staphylococcus occurred, whereas this used to be considered a cutaneous saprophyte organism.

Review

At the 1998 review, 2 of the 28 remaining patients had died.
The 26 patients were:

– either clinically evaluated, based on biological results (16);
– interviewed by phone, based on biological results (8);
– or lost to follow-up (2).

Endpoints used for evaluation of the result included:

– clinical and biological healing;
– residual range of motion;

– IKS score for the patients that could be examined;
– patient satisfaction.

X-rays were taken in all the patients that were clinically reviewed: plain AP and lateral roentgenograms and tangential views for the patella.

Results

At review, the average follow-up was 62.3 ± 33 months (5 years and 2 months).

Infectious results

Among the 5 failures recorded at the first review, one patient was lost to follow-up (patent failure; patient was re-operated on in another center), and another one had died 5 months after the arthrodesis.

At the 5-year follow-up:

– 1 sound union has had a favourable outcome (normal biological results);
– 1 arthrodesis that had failed to unite eventually united at 34 months (subnormal biological results);
– 1 arthrodesis is still ununited and the biological analysis confirms the presence of infection.

Among the 24 patients that are considered completely healed (82.7% of the initial series):

– 2 have died. One was still considered completely healed at the last follow-up visit; the other one had to be reoperated on for recurrent infection and had his knee prosthesis replaced in one stage. It is a late septic failure;
– 1 patient is lost to follow-up so that results cannot be analysed;
– 1 patient had recurrence of his infection and had to be re-operated on. An arthrodesis was performed, and union took place in 6 months. It is a late septic failure;
– 1 female patient was not reoperated on, but still has disturbed biological results and severe functional impairment and pain. It is a late septic and mechanical failure;
– 1 patient never had recurrence of his infection, but had a rupture of his extensor mechanism 5 years after the reimplantation. He underwent surgical repair with retention of his knee prosthesis. All intraoperative biopsy specimens were normal and the patient healed uneventfully. It is a late mechanical failure;
– 18 patients are considered clinically healed. However, 7 of them still have subnormal biological results, with increased ESR as compared to the same-age referential, and with CRP equal to the reference value or 5mg higher. One of them has a poor functional result.

Thus, at 5 years – excluding the patient who is lost to follow-up – results are as follows:

– 3 late failures (10.7%); one of the patients has recently died;
– 5 patent failures (17.9%) are confirmed; one of the 3 arthrodeses has eventually healed, and 1 patient had died prior to the first review;

– 20 patients had confirmed healing, but one of them died and another one experienced a mechanical complication. Therefore, at the last follow-up, healing rate is 71.4%;

– as regards the 5 arthrodeses, 3 out of 4 (75%) are considered sound unions at the last follow-up.

Functional results

Functional results have been analysed in 16 clinically evaluated patients:

– mean flexion is 97° ± 25° (range, 60° to 120°); it was 95° at the first review (range, 40° to 120°);

– mean extension lag is 4°±3°.

14 of these 16 patients had had an osteoclasis or elevation of the anterior tibial tuberosity. The patient who had suffered a secondary rupture of the extensor mechanism had not had elevation of the tibial tuberosity during reimplantation.

The mean IKS score was 78/100 for physical examination and 71/100 for function.

Radiological results

No signs of loosening have been found in the 13 healed patients who have been clinically evaluated and have not been reoperated on. Since no goniometry was performed at review, no mechanical axis measurements are available.

Analysis of radiolucencies (12 cases, 8 of which had been noted during the first follow-up visit) is difficult: 10 patients still suffer daily diffuse knee pain (radiological correlation is uncertain).

Because of the small size of the sample and the absence of goniometry, no comparison has been made regarding the different types of revision implants used (2 hinged knees, 7 PS stemmed prostheses, 4 PS stemless prostheses).

Subjective results

Only 15 patients (62.5%) claim to be satisfied with their results; none of the patients is very satisfied, 5 (20.8%) are disappointed, and 4 (16.7%) are dissatisfied.

Specific point

Risks factors

In the initial series, 6 patients had at least 2 or even 3 risk factors (as described by De Cloedt) (5).

One of them has died (considered to be completely healed at the last follow-up visit). 2 only are cured at 5-year follow-up (one of them suffered a secondary rupture of the extensor mechanism).

The other 3 cases are failures (1 is lost to follow-up), one of which occurred after the first review.

At last, in the 6 patients, 4 had already had a total knee prosthesis (3 of them are failures).

In contrast, the patient with rheumatoid arthritis who had two additional risk factors is cured.

Overall, 50% of the patients are cured, but only 33% of them have good biological and functional results.

The 8 cases with only one risk factor include:

– 2 failures (1 prior TKR);
– 1 death following failure and reoperation with arthrodesis;
– 5 complete healings (62.5%) (infection cured, function restored).

The 15 cases with no initial risk factor include:

– 1 patient lost to follow-up;
– 1 patient considered to be cured , but with severe functional impairment;
– 3 failures, 1 of which occurred after the first review.

11 out of 14 patients (78.6%) have been cured of their infection. However, only 10 of the knees (71.4%) have been rated good because one knee has a poor functional result.

Uni-compartmental knee replacement

In the initial series, 2 patients had had an infected unicompartmental knee prosthesis (no prior knee surgery). Both patients who were revised to a TKR and had recurrence of the infection are biologically healed, but one of them has a poor functional result (60° flexion, continual pain, IKS functional score of 60 points).

Prior prosthesis

7 patients had had a prior prosthesis that had been revised to a TKR which got infected:

– 2 UKRs: 2 healings (100%), but 1 poor functional result;
– 5 TKRs: 1 healing (20%), 4 failures;
– in total: infection cured in 42.9% of the cases, no major functional impairment in 28.6%.

Previous surgery

In the 13 patients who had had surgical treatment (meniscectomy, high tibial osteotomy, arthroscopy, or internal fixation of the upper end of the tibia) prior to the primary implantation: 8 (61.6%) are cured of their infection, 7 of whom (53.9%) have no major functional impairment.

Late failures

There are no typical features. 2 patients had no initial risk factor, and 1 had only one risk factor (previous surgery). The 3 organisms were all different (1 staphylococcus aureus, 1 staphylococcus epidermidis, 1 gemella morbidum). Only 1 of the patients had had surgical treatment (synovectomy) before removal of the implant, and 1 had had his prosthesis replaced in one stage shortly after the initial reimplantation.

Surgical treatment prior to two-stage reimplantation

In the 11 patients who were surgically managed with arthroscopy, articular lavage or puncture, there were 4 failures, 1 of which occurred late. Healing rate is 63.4%.

Analysis of interval between the two stages

In the initial series, the average interval between the two stages was 8.8 ± 4.4 weeks (range, 4 to 16 weeks) for the 5 failed cases, and 8.45 ± 4.7 weeks for the whole series. When taking into account the 3 late failures, the average interval remains the same: 8.75 ± 3.9 weeks (range unchanged).

The 2 patients who had the shortest intervals (respectively 2 and 3 weeks) have had no recurrence of the infection.

Age range at implantation of the septic prosthesis

Failures mainly occurred in patients who were generally younger than the average age of the patients in the whole series: 66.8 ± 12 years at the first review, and 68.4 ± 9.8 years at the current review, versus 70 years in the whole series.

Unidentified organisms

The involved organisms were not identified in 6 patients. This resulted in 2 immediate failures (1 patent failure in a patient who was lost to follow-up, and 1 solid fusion at 34 months), 1 late failure (prosthesis was retained), and 3 healings. At present, there are 50% good results.

Discussion

Comparison with data from the literature

Success rate

Although results in this series deteriorated with time (from 82.7% to 71.4%), they remain consistent with those reported in other series (Rasul (34): 71% at 2 years).

Bose (5) reported 0% failure in 18 cases at 3-year follow-up, with a mean range of motion of 109° and an IKS score of 90 points, like Whiteside (39) (1 failure in 34 patients, which occurred 8 years after reimplantation). But, in 1983, Insall (22) reported 9 good results in 11 reimplantations (81.8%), then, in 1990, with Windsor (40), 89.5% of good results (4 failures: 1 recurrent infection and 3 new infections), and at last, in 1996, with Goldman (15), 91% of good infectious results at 7.5 years, and 81.5% of good infectious and mechanical results, with a predictive survivorship curve of 77.4% at 10 years.

In 1991, Bengston (2) reported 75.7% of good results at 6 years in a series of 107 one-stage or two-stage replacements (he did not make any difference between the two methods). According to him, 34% only of these prostheses function normally.

In 1993, Hanssen and Rand (18) reported 33.7% failure, and therefore, only 66.3% of good results in a series of 66 patients evaluated at 52-month follow-up. One-third (11.2%) of these failures were due to recurrent infection.

In 1998, Hirakawa (20) published his 5-year results which are very similar to those in our series, using the same treatment protocol: 80% of success where infection was due to relatively weak organisms (coagulase-negative staphylococcus, streptococcus), 71.4% of polymicrobial infection, and 66.7% where infection was due to methi-resistant staphylococcus aureus. The success rate fell from 82% in patients who initially had knee osteoarthritis to 54% in patients with rheumatoid arthritis. At last, good results were achieved in patients who had not had prior knee surgery; only 41% of good results were achieved in multiply operated patients.

More recently, in 1999, Brandt (6) (Mayo Clinic) reported on a series of 38 two-stage reimplantations (16 TKRs, 22 THRs) for treatment of infection due to staphylococcus aureus. The recurrence rate at an average of 1.4 year after reimplantation was 2.6% (1 case only). However, statistically, the estimated recurrence rate at 5 years is 2.8%.

This means that results are bound to deteriorate with time. Later than 5 years after reimplantation, the average rate of good results ranges from 90 to 66% according to studies. Therefore, the question is: what is the definition of complete healing and when is a patient considered to be cured? In our series, recurrent infection has resulted in 10% increase in the failure rate, with only 18 months of additional follow-up. In view of this, biological and clinical assessments should be performed once a year for at least 5 years, and probably longer.

Assuming that a patient is cured using only one biological criterium is too hazardous. However, bone scintigraphy will provide significant information only if the immediate postoperative course is normal; furthermore, it is very much controversial, due to its low specificity. Only its negative predictive value is interesting. Periodical monitoring of CRP which is more sensitive than ESR seems justified, because it returns to normal 14 days after the arthroplasty, according to Kolstad (23) (versus 4 months for ESR), and 21 days after the arthroplasty, according to Hanssen et Rand (17). But, in the end, time test is the crucial factor.

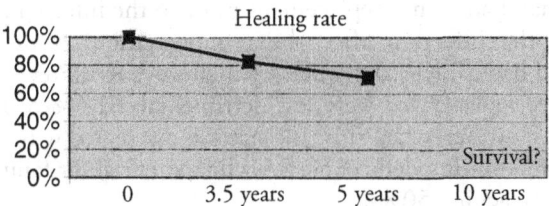

In contrast, as regards failures, results tend to improve over time (except for one patient who is lost to follow-up and whom management is unknown). At 3.5 years, only 1 out of 4 arthrodeses had united, whereas at 5 years, sound union is achieved in 3 out of 4. One just needs to be patient. However, achieving bony fusion does not mean that infection is cured. This long healing time is indicative of poor bone quality at the implantation site. Furthermore, these results should be compared with those of resection arthroplasty which we have no experience with.

Functional outcome

It depends on infectious results. Any patient who complains of persistent pain has a poor functional result, and this is confirmed by a low IKS score. However, the results that have been achieved, particularly regarding mean flexion (slightly less than 100°), are very much comparable to those of aseptic revision knee arthroplasty. Furthermore, no significant deterioration of the functional result is noted at 3.5- to 5-year follow-up. Nevertheless, the low satisfaction rate (62.5%) confirms that this complication does prejudice the results.

This finding contrasts with that of Barrack and Engh (1) who compared two series of revision TKAs (125 cases) using the same implant: 99 cases were treated for aseptic loosening, and 26 for infected TKR after a two-stage reimplantation. In the second group of patients, pre– and postoperative functional results (ROM and KSCS score) were less satisfactory than those achieved in the first group (90° versus 99°; score of 115 points versus 135); however, patients were equally satisfied with their results at 3-year follow-up. Reasons for aseptic revision included established loosening, osteolysis or partial instability of the implant. These complications sometimes occurred quite early, which may explain why the patients did not readily accept to undergo revision surgery.

Influence of risk factors (RF)

Risk factors are critically important: there are 78.6% of good results with 0 risk factor, 62.5% with 1 RF, and 50% with 2 or 3 RFs. Results remain unchanged when the functional score is taken into account: 71.4%, 62.5% and 33%, respectively.

Furthermore, previous surgery has been shown not only to increase the risk of sepsis after a TKA, but also to compromise healing after the infection, particularly if prior surgery was a primary implantation. In our series, 4 of the 7 patients who had had a knee replacement prior to the infected prosthesis had recurrence of the infection after the reimplantation. 3 of them healed (42.9%): 1 had had a TKR, the other 2 patients a UKR. Previous procedures other than knee replacement were less detrimental: 61.6% of healing at the last follow-up. However, when this risk factor is associated with other medical risks (ASA score, immunodeficiency, RA), the potential for failure is dramatically increased (reaching 50%).

In this regard, the Altemeier classification is most interesting. Candidates to surgery are classified in four types:

– Type I: no previous surgery at the operative site;
– Type II: previous surgery or puncture at the operative site, no infection;
– Type III: prior infection at the operative site, that is cured;
– Type IV: active infection.

This classification, which is used for the definition of patients at risk in the study of nosocomial infections, is perfectly suited to implant surgery, and should be taken into consideration together with the ASA score at the time of decision making.

Mechanical results

Only one patient had a severe mechanical complication. Another one has a poor functional result. All the other patients have a fair but satisfactory functional result (62.5% satisfied patients). Therefore, in our series, the infectious result appears to be the most important factor in influencing the mid-term outcome.

Surgical treatment prior to two-stage reimplantation

In our series, it was systematically followed by a two-stage reimplantation. Having no record of healed cases, we are not in a position to discuss the possible therapeutic advantages of such treatment. However, in 1990, Schoifet and Morrey (35) reported 77% of failure at 8.8-year follow-up, which they attributed to the time to surgery (more than 21 days) and to the type of organism involved. In our patients, the average success rate is lower when surgical procedures have been performed (63.4% versus 71.4% in the whole series).

Because these procedures delay the final management of infection, they may have been a factor of poor prognosis.

Questions at issue

One- or two-stage reimplantation?

This study confirms the advantage of performing a two-stage reimplantation for infected total knee replacement, with an intravenous antibiotic therapy between the two stages. Considering that infectiologists are strongly opposed to one-stage reimplantation (bacteriological sterilization is impossible in the presence of a foreign body which recreates the favourable conditions for the growth of germs), one may wonder if it can still be considered a sound alternative. Most authors will agree that this method is justified only in early infections which are rapidly managed, if possible within 2 to 3 weeks from onset. Still, results remain uncertain; furthermore, in view of the failure rate in two-stage reimplantations, it does not seem to be a reasonable option.

Salvage procedures?

Similarly, arthroscopic lavage (Waldman (38) reported 62% of failure in 16 cases, although debridement was performed less than 7 days after onset of infection) or arthrotomy (Brandt and Hanssen (7) reported 69% of failure at 2-year follow-up in 30 cases, failure probability dramatically increasing when surgery was performed later than 2 days after onset of infection), even when performed at an early stage, are of little value, except when infection is due to a weak germ or if poor patient's general condition precludes major surgery.

Furthermore, our study shows the little value of procedures such as synovectomy or articular / arthroscopic lavage once infection has broken out. Mont and Hungerford (32) use these techniques before the 30th postoperative day (100% of success) or the 30th day following the first signs of infection (71% of success). According to Teeny (37), one should not wait more than 2 weeks.

Length of interval between the two stages?

One important issue in two-stage reimplantation is the length of interval between the two stages. Besides the fact that the knee is immobilized and the patient is sent to a rehabilitation center (although home postoperative care solutions are being developed), this phase is detrimental to the functional outcome of the operated knee. This is confirmed by the low ISK score and poor flexion results. Infectiologists believe that this interval may be decreased by using strong and broad-spectrum antibiotic therapies, provided that the knee joint is free of any foreign material. In any case, our study confirms that extension of the interval is not a crucial factor in healing, since healings occurred with short intervals and failures with relatively longer intervals (however, this analysis does not allow for medical elements such as the type of organism or nature of the antibiotic therapy). Length of interval is also dependent on the method of determination of infectious sterilization and its reliability. Are CRP and ESR rating, as well as bone scintigraphy sufficient? Should one wait until levels return to normal? Can second stage be scheduled, based exclusively on the quality of antibiotic therapy? At last, a short course of antibiotics is only conceivable with so-called sensitive germs. Study of microbial ecology shows that there is presently a lower incidence of staphylococcus aureus, and emergence of germs that have long been considered cutaneous saprophyte organisms and may resist antibiotics.

What type of spacer?

The necessity of maintaining a sufficient interval between the two stages poses the problem of insertion of a joint spacer which generally consists of antibiotic impregnated bone cement (most often Gentallin) and is run down by infectiologists. The current tendency is towards a more mobile articulating knee spacer. In 1995, Hofmann (21) used this type of construct in 25 patients and achieved an HSS score of 87/100 at 30-month follow-up, with a mean range of motion between 5° and 106°. The goal of this device is of course to maintain adequate flexion and ligament balance.

Fehring (12) compared the results achieved with this mobile spacer (cement spacer) in 30 patients versus a fixed spacer in 25 patients. The recurrent infection rate was similar (7% versus 12%), HSS score was identical (83 versus 84 points), but flexion was improved (105° versus 98°), and above all, there was no bone loss. Bone loss issue with fixed spacers had previously been studied by this team in 1997 (Calton (8)). In 25 patients who were immobilized for 6 weeks, the average tibial bone loss was 6.2mm in 40% of the cases, and femoral bone loss 12.8mm in 44%, particularly where a small size spacer was used or in the absence of cemented intramedullary stem.

Implantation of special metal devices is very questionable because foreign bodies are known to be very attractive to germs. As a matter of fact, the procedure can be compared to a one-stage reimplantation and is therefore criticisable. However, quite recently, Haddad (16) reported on a series of 45 patients reviewed at 4 years in whom he used a Prostalac® spacer (association of antibiotic impregnated bone cement with a small metal / PE contact surface) with good results: only 1 recurrent infection, good HSS score, preservation of range of motion. The main complications were due to reversible impairment of the extensor mechanism.

In conclusion, all these series show that joint mobilisation has no detrimental effects in infected cases.

Implantation of gentamicin-impregnated beads has no proven efficacy, although Nelson (30), in 1993, stated that it had a higher therapeutic efficiency than simple debridement with parenteral antibiotic therapy.

Reimplantation criteria

Reimplantation can take place only after healing has been achieved. But, presently, there are no reliable healing criteria (normal CRP and ESR rates are necessary, yet not sufficient). Bone scintigraphy is very controversial. Only immediate Technetium-99m skeletal angioscintigraphy has some value, but it is associated with numerous false positives and false negatives due to the fact that it is performed shortly after the operation. Gallium scintigraphy has a relatively good positive predictive value because it shows the inflammatory sites that are related to the presence of leucocytes; however, it has no specific bone affinity. So it is with techniques using Indium 111. At last, LeukoScan (very expensive) is made from a mouse antibody binding to leucocyte receptors with high affinity; however, it is very difficult to reproduce, due to the risk of patient's immunological reaction. PET (positron emission tomography) imaging seems more promising. It is able to detect the presence of 18-fluoro-desoxy-glucose in activated cells (tumor or infection) with a sensitivity and specificity of more than 90%; there is no interference with metal, and it provides correct differentiation of bone and soft tissue infection.

This may require obtention of new specimens either by percutaneous puncture or during secondary surgery (as second-look surgery in cancer patients) with articular lavage and synovectomy. Della Valle (10) performed an intraoperative anatomicopathological study in a series of 64 reimplantations, with bacteriological cultures being systematically performed for comparison. The criterium retained for infection was the presence of 10 polynuclears per field in multicellular areas (negative predictive value of 95%; 98% specificity). In contrast, the positive predictive value was only 50% with a low sensitivity (25%). Bacteriological assessment remains indispensable.

Now, how long should one wait, considering that there are some very slow-growing organisms? A minimum of 3 weeks seems reasonable. In this case, can the spacer be removed? This implies that a strict physical therapy protocol is followed in order to maintain adequate ligament tension and joint space. Should bacteriological results be positive, a further relatively long course of antibiotics will be necessary. Will it be shorter if there is no foreign body as recommended by infectiologists?

The future diagnostic solution will likely rely on immunology: detection of CNA gene (collagen adhesine gene) in staphylococcus aureus strains by PCR (polymerase chain reaction), as studied by Montanaro (28). CNA was found in 29% of the staphylococcus aureus strains (35), 83% of which were able to produce slime allowing adhesion to host tissue. This method is probably the most promising one; however, despite a very high sensitivity (nearly 100% according to Gaston and Simpsom [14]), it is associated with a number of false positives (47% specificity). Ratiq (31) used an ELISA test for diagnostic serology of coagulase-negative staphylococcus (detection of a specific glycolipid antigen). There was a significant difference in IgG and IgM levels between a population of 32 infection-free patients and 15 patients with an infected knee replacement. Unfortunately, for the moment, this test cannot be performed intraoperatively.

Prevention of infection

In view of this, besides treatment of infection, prevention seems indispensable as emphasized by Mathieu (25). Prevention must take into account both the patient's condition and the numerous associated risk factors. It means fighting against nosocomial infections and using appropriate antibiotic prophylaxis. Any postoperative complications (i.e., wound haematoma, wound dehiscence, permeable drainage...) should be closely monitored, but in no case will they justify a prophylactic antibiotic therapy, blindly initiated.

When infection breaks out, diagnosis must be established as early as possible. Early, good quality articular puncture results are more critically important than clinical problems, biological tests, or bone scintigraphy. In this respect, PCR (polymerase chain reaction) for detection of DNA polymerase in joint fluid (Mariani (24), Gaston [14]) seems most promising. Similarly, one must emphasize the importance of obtaining good quality bacteriological specimens that should be analysed by a highly competent microbiological laboratory, to ensure identification of a greater number of organisms. Precise identification of germs is a prerequisite to good healing (50% of failure in our series where a germ failed to be identified).

Conclusion

In conclusion, one can say that the "ideal" case for achieving correct healing in infected knee arthroplasty is a patient:

– with a UKR rather than a TKR (hinged knees are even worse than resurfacing implants);

– who has not had previous surgery;

– with good general condition and no specific risk factor;

– who has been managed early;

– who has been managed with two-stage reimplantation and careful joint debridement, and has not undergone surgery during the interval between the two stages;

– in whom the involved organism has been rapidly identified and is sensitive to strong antibiotics, allowing reduction of the interval.

In any event, whatever the type of patient, this study prompts us to always have a cautious prognosis because recurrent failures may eventually lead to radical procedures. In this respect, arthrodesis (or resection arthroplasty?) is a reasonable alternative, if not satisfactory.

This study does not include analysis of technical difficulties in these challenging revisions (which reopens the debate with regard to "spacers"…), type of cement to be used, use of cementless implants as advocated by Whiteside (39), or possible need for bone grafting. However, experience with allografts (source of infection) in tumor surgery is not inciting. Elevation of the anterior tibial tuberosity is most often required, due to knee ankylosis that occurs during the interval between the two stages. It is interesting to note that the only major mechanical complication occurred after reimplantation using a standard approach.

At last, the social cost of septic revisions, although very difficult to estimate, is quite high. It ranges from US\$ 60,000 to US\$ 100,000 (Bengston [3]). Hebert (19), in 1996, said that this cost was about 3 to 4 times higher than that of a primary replacement and twice as high as that of aseptic revision. Unfortunately, this economic argument may be an additional unfavourable factor in management of these patients, independent of the health care center.

References

1. Barrack RL, Engh G, Rorabeck C *et al.* (2000) Patient satisfaction and outcome after septic versus aseptic revision total knee arthroplasty. J Arthroplasty, 2000, 15(8): 990-3
2. Bengston S, Knutson K, Lindgren L (1989) Treatment of infected knee arthroplasty. Clin Orthop 245, 173-8
3. Bengston S (1993) Prosthetic osteomyelitis with special reference to the knee, risks, treatment and costs. Ann Med (Finland) 25(6) 523-9
4. Bengston S, Knutson K (1991) The infected knee arthroplasty A 6 year follow up of 357 cases. Acta Orthop Scand 62 (4): 301-11
5. Bose WJ, Gearen PF, Randall JC *et al.* (1995) Long-term outcome of 42 knees with chronic infection total knee arthroplasty. Clin Orthop 319: 285-96
6. Brandt CM, Duffy MC, Berbari EF *et al.* (1999) Staphylococcus aureus prosthetic joint infection treated with prosthesis removal and delayed reimplantation arthroplasty. Mayo Clin Proc (United States) 74(6): 553-8
7. Brandt CM, Sistrunk WW, Duffy MC *et al.* (1997) Staphylococcus aureus prosthetic joint infection treated with debridment and prosthesis retention. Clin Infect Dis, 1997, 24(5), 914-9
8. Calton TF, Fehring TK, Griffin WL (1997) Bone loss associated with the use of spacer blocks in infected total knee arthroplasty. Clin Orthop 345: 148-54
9. De Cloedt Ph, Emery R, Legaye J *et al.* (1994) Les prothèses totales de genou infectées. Orientation du choix thérapeutique Rev Chir Orthop 80: 626-33
10. Della Valle CJ, Bogner E, Desai P *et al.* (1999) Analysis of frozen sections of intraoperative specimens obtained at the time of reoperation after hip or knee resection arthroplasty for the treatment of infection. J Bone Joint Surg (Am) 81-5: 684-9
11. Della Valle CJ, Scher DM, Kim YH *et al.* (1999) The role of intraoperative Gram stain in revision total joint arthroplasty. J Arthroplasty 14(4): 500-4
12. Fehring TK, Odum S, Calton TF *et al.* (2000) Articulating versus static spacers in revision total knee arthroplasty for sepsis. The Ranawat award. Clin Orthop 380: 9-16
13. Gacon G, Laurençon M, Van De Velde D *et al.* (1997) Réimplantation en deux temps pour infection après arthroplastie du genou. Rev Chir Orthop 83: 313-23
14. Gaston P, Emmanuel FXS, Beggs I *et al.* (2001) Universal PCR to detect infection in preoperative aspirates of failed joint replacements. Early results. 20th annual meeting of the European Bone and Joint Infection Society, Paris, 17-19 may 2001
15. Goldman RT, Scuderi GR, Insall JN (1996) Two-stage reimplantation for infected total knee replacement. Clin Orthop 331: 118-24
16. Haddad FS, Masri BA, Campbell D *et al.* (2000) The Prostalac functional spacer in two-stage revision for infected knee replacements. Prosthesis of antibiotic-loaded acrylic cement. J Bone Joint Surg (Br) 82-6: 807-12
17. Hanssen AD, Rand JA (1998) Evaluation and treatment of infection at the site of a total hip or knee arthroplasty. J Bone Joint Surg (Am) 80-A: 910-22
18. Hanssen AD, Rand JA, Osmon DR (1994) Treatment of the infected total knee arthroplasty with insertion of another prosthesis The effect of impregnated bone cement. Clin Orthop 309: 44-55
19. Hebert CK, Williams RE, Levy RS *et al.* (1996) Cost of treating and infected total knee replacement. Clin Orthop 331: 140-5
20. Hirakawa K, Stulberg BN, Wilde AH *et al.* (1998) Results of 2-stage reimplantation for infected total knee arthroplasty. J Arthroplasty 13(1): 22-8
21. Hofmann AA, Kane KR, Tkach TK *et al.* (1995) Treatment of infected total knee arthroplasty using an articulating spacer. Clin Orthop 321: 45-54
22. Insall JN, Thompson FM, Brause BD (1983) Two-stage reimplantation for the salvage of infected total knee arthoplasty. J Bone Joint Surg (Am) 65 (3): 1087-88
23. Kolstad K, Levander H (1995) Inflammatory laboratory tests after joint replacement surgery. Ups J Med Sci (Sweden) 100(3): 243-8
24. Mariani BD, Martin PS, Levine HJ *et al.* (1996) The Coventry award polymerase chain reaction detection of bacterial infection in total knee arthroplasty. Clin Orthop 331: 11-22

25. Mathieu M (1995) Prothèses totales de genou infectées. In: Conférence d'enseignement de la SOFCOT 55: 57-62. Expansion scientifique française.
26. Mont MA, Waldman B, Banerjee C *et al.* (1997) Multiple irrigation, debridement, and retention of components in infected total knee arthroplasty. J Arthroplasty (United States), 12(4): 426-433
27. Mont MA, Waldman BJ, Hungerford DS (2000) Evaluation of preoperative cultures before second-stage reimplantation of a total knee prosthesis complicated by infection. A comparison-group study. J Bone Joint Surg (Am), 82-A(11): 1552-7
28. Montanaro L, Arciola CR, Baldassarri L *et al.* (1999) Presence and expression of collagen adhesine gene (cna) and slime production in Staphylococcus aureus strains from orthopaedic prosthesis infections. Biomaterials (England) 20 (20): 1945-9
29. Morrey BF, Westholm MF, Schoifet SD *et al.* (1989) Long-term results of various treatment options for infected total knee arthroplasty. Clin Orthop, 248, 129-8
30. Nelson CL, Evans RP, Blaha JD *et al.* (1993) A comparison of gentamicin-impregnated polymethylmethacrylate bead implantation to conventional parenteral antibiotic therapy in infected total hip and knee arthroplasty. Clin Orthop 295: 96-101
31. Ratiq M , Worthington T, Tebbs SE *et al.* (2000) Serological detection of Gram-positive bacterial infection around prostheses. J Bone Joint Surg (Br) 82-8: 1156-61
32. Rand JA *et al.* (1993) Sepsis following total knee arthroplasty. In: Rand JA. Total knee arthroplasty, New York, Raven Press, 1993
33. Rand JA, Fitzgerald RH Jr (1989) Management of the infected total knee arthroplasty. Orthop Clin North Am 20: 201-10
34. Rasul AT, Tsukayama D, Gustilo RB (1991) Effect of time and depth of infection on the outcome of total knee arthroplasty infections. Clin Orthop 273: 98-104
35. Schoifet SD, Morrey BF (1990) Treatment of infection after total knee arthroplasty by debridement with retention of the components. J Bone Joint Surg (Am) 72 (9): 1383-90
36. Segawa H, Tsukayama DT, Kyle RF *et al.* (1999) Infection after total knee arthroplasty. A retrospective study of the treatment of eighty-one infections. J Bone Joint Surg (Am) 81-10: 1334-45
37. Teeny SM, Dorr L, Murata G *et al.* (1990) Treatment of infected knee arthroplasty. Irrigation and debridement versus two-stage reimplantation. J Arthroplasty (United States) 5(1): 35-39
38. Waldman BJ, Hostin E, Mont MA *et al.* (2000) Infected total knee arthroplasty treated by arthroscopic irrigation and debridment. J Arthroplasty 15(4): 430-436
39. Whiteside LA (1994) Treatment of infected total knee arthroplasty. Clin Orthop 299; 118-24
40. Windsor RE, Insall JN, Urs WK *et al.* (1990) Two-stage reimplantation for the solvage of total knee arthroplasty complicated by infection. Farther follow-up and refinement of indication. J Bone Surg (Am) 72 (2), 272-8

Osteoarthritis of the knee – Soft tissue defect problems: Prevention and treatment

P. Breton

Introduction

Soft tissue complications after total-knee replacement are variously assessed in the literature. According to the series, they occur between 2 and 12% of the cases (14). These complications can delay reeducation and jeopardize the functional result of arthroplasty. More exceptional osteoarthritis complications will require the removal of prosthetic device that may lead to arthrodesis or even amputation.

The mechanism of onset of partial cutaneous necrosis or wound dehiscence is often due to several factors: knee with previous scars, poor health condition, vascular insufficiency (arterial and venous), smoking habit, rheumatoid arthritis treated by steroids.

The prevention of such complications depends essentially on the careful choice of the surgical procedure especially in the case of revision surgery that requires a comprehensive knowledge of skin vascularization.

The procedure of prior skin expansion may also be proposed.

In view of such complications one should avoid a wait-and-see attitude that may cause the silent onset of a deep-seated necrosis leading to severe periprosthetic infection. Plastic surgeon's opinion is often necessary and will enable to realize in time a medial gastrocnemius muscle flap or a fasciocutaneous flap coverage that will salvage the prosthesis.

Anatomical data

Skin arterial vascularization of the knee (5, 18, 19) is dependent on a deep arterial network issuing from the superficial femoral artery, the popliteal artery and the anterior tibial artery (fig.1). This vascular supply forms the circumpatellar anastomosis which will give off perforating arteries making up a predominant multilayer network in the medial region.

Deep arterial network

The superficial femoral artery

After giving off three or four branches to the muscles, it originates the descending or highest genicular artery. This artery separates from the superficial

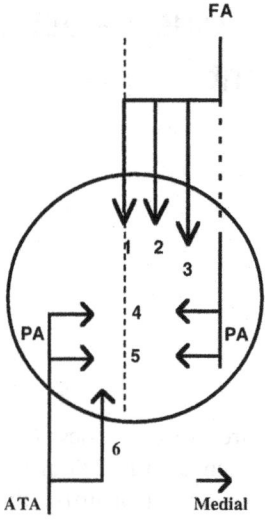

Fig. 1 – Diagram showing the anterior view of arterial vascularization of the knee.
FA: Femoral artery.
PA: Popliteal artery.
ATA: Anterior tibial artery.
1. Anterior genicular artery
2. Medial saphenous artery
3. Descending genicular artery
4. Superior genicular artery (medial and lateral).
5. Inferior genicular artery (medial and lateral).
6. Recurrent tibial artery.

femoral artery above the hiatus adductorius in 80% of the cases (11), sometimes on level with or below the hiatus.

This artery divides into three branches:

– the saphenous artery which courses with the saphenous nerve and gives off 3 to 4 cutaneous branches;

– the anterior genicular artery which runs towards the medial surface of the joint;

– the third collateral is the descending genicular artery which supplies the musculocutaneous region of the vastus medialis muscle.

This division into three branches from the descending genicular artery is observed in 70% of the cases. The collateral arteries arise directly from the femoral artery in 30% of the cases.

The popliteal artery

Five branches that supply the knee joint issue from the popliteal artery: the superior genicular arteries (medial and lateral), the middle genicular artery and the inferior genicular arteries (medial and lateral).

The middle genicular artery supplies the posterior region of the knee, the four other collaterals course around the joint and form the circumpatellar anastomosis.

The anterior tibial artery

The anterior tibial artery gives off the anterior tibial recurrent artery. It splits off from the anterior tibial artery after crossing through the interosseous space and contributes to the peripatellar network.

The circumpatellar anastomosis

This anastomosis issues from the four genicular arteries anastomosing with each other at the anterior surface of the knee ahead of the capsule. This network is supplied with blood by the three collaterals of the femoral artery (anterior genicular artery, descending genicular artery and saphenous artery) and by the recurrent anterior tibial artery.

Superficial arterial network

The penetrating arteries constitute a plexiform network located above the fascia predominant in the medial region.

The teguments of the medial surface of these arteries are mainly vascularized by the descending genicular artery of the knee (issued from the superficial femoral artery) (5). This arterial network is predominant in 71% of the cases. In 29% of the cases, it is supplemented by the medial superior and the medial inferior genicular arteries (5).

In the lateral region, the vascularization is provided by the genicular arteries, the anterior recurrent artery supplies the lateral inferior part of the skin.

On the boundary of the medial and lateral vascular areas, an about 2cm hypovascular band is located on the lateral edge of the patella extending to its inferior part (6) (fig. 2).

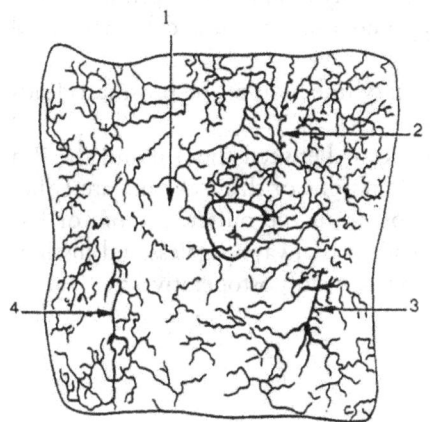

Fig. 2 – Radiography of knee skin (injection in the femoral artery).
1. Lateral hypovascular band.
2. Musculocutaneous penetrating arteries issued from the vastus medialis muscle.
3. Cutaneous branch issued from the saphenous artery.
4. Cutaneous branch issued from the recurrent tibial artery.

Lymphatic draining system

The lymphatic draining system predominates as well on the medial part of the knee since the lateral lymphatic network of the leg joins the medial saphenous network under the tuberosity.

Risk factors

General factors

Risk factors are often intricate and several of them are often found in the same patient considering the indication itself of total knee arthroplasty (1, 6, 8).

The most frequent factors are:

- Advanced age;
- Rheumatoid arthritis, especially in the case of long-term steroid medication (this factor is observed in over one fourth of the complications);
- Arteritis and/or long history of smoking tobacco products (over 20 packs a year);
- Obesity.

Local risk factors

- Knees with previous surgeries (one or several procedures) often presenting with poor tissue healing;
- Local septic history;
- Poor local venous condition (thrombosis history...), lymphedema.

Diagnosis

The occurrence of cutaneous necrosis generally results from primary cutaneous ischemia that may extend deeply and cause wound dehiscence and exposure of joint prosthesis.

However, in 20% of the cases, the primary infection of the prosthesis leads to secondary scar tissue dehiscence (14).

The first signs of cutaneous ischemia occur between the 3rd and the 7th day postoperatively. The cutaneous manifestations of this ischemia are either a white plaque adjacent to the incision or, from the outset, a more or less extensive scabby area (fig. 3). This mechanism is always painless and justifies a very regular examination of the cutaneous aspect, postoperatively.

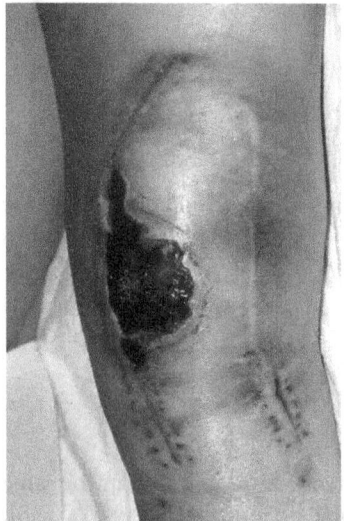

Fig. 3 – Soft tissue necrosis with exposed prosthesis (left knee), the site of the defect is on the medial scar, in the soft tissue area which separates two parallel scars.

The initial evaluation of the infection depth is often difficult. Wise attitude is to wait until the necrotic plaque is totally delimited before realizing necrotic area removal. This procedure must be performed in the operating room and be followed immediately by fasciocutaneous flap or muscle flap coverage.

Prevention

The importance of the preoperative patient's interview and clinical examination (19) must be emphasized: pre-existing scars, sometimes old and hardly visible, must be carefully located and the condition of the skin neighbouring scars meticulously checked.

Infiltrated adipose skin with ecchymotic and telangiectatic aspect is a predisposing factor of delayed healing or possible complication.

In the presence of multiple scars and considering the importance of the medial vascular supply, the most lateral scar possible must be used (19). When a new approach is chosen one must avoid crossing a pre-existing scar or realizing a convergent incision close to that previous scar, thus isolating a soft tissue area that may be the site of a pain zone (we remind that it is difficult to exceed a ratio of length to width greater than 2/1 in leg surgery).

Skin detachment must be as deep as possible in order to preserve the deep arterial anastomosis.

Some surgical procedures have been proposed to lower the risk of soft tissue necrosis during prosthesis insertion: discharge incision, pre-incision and preoperative tissue expansion.

– Discharge incision: such a procedure must be avoided because of the risk of further aggravation of local skin condition. Subsequently, it may jeopardize flap repair procedure.

– Pre-incision: to be realized a few days prior to prosthesis insertion in order to use the "delayed effect" and increase local blood supply. The advantages of such a procedure seem to be quite theoretical. Actually, this technique increases the risk of local infection and does not prevent the onset of a secondary necrosis. Moreover, a necrotic process occurring during pre-incision requires the use of a preliminary flap repair which may subsequently complicate the insertion of the prosthesis.

– Preoperative tissue expansion advocated by Santore and Namba (15, 17) was the subject of several publications: Manifold (12) presents a series of 29 cases of preoperative tissue expansion, including 6 minor complications and 1 failure.

Expansion of the skin around the knee is difficult and Casanova observed, from a series of 103 cases of skin expansion in the lower limb, a complication rate of 19.4% and 5% of complete failure. These complications are the exposure of expansion material, partial or total necrosis and infection. In case of complete failure, postoperative skin condition will be less favourable than before tissue expansion procedure. It will pose a very delicate therapeutic problem and be a definitive contraindication for total knee arthroplasty.

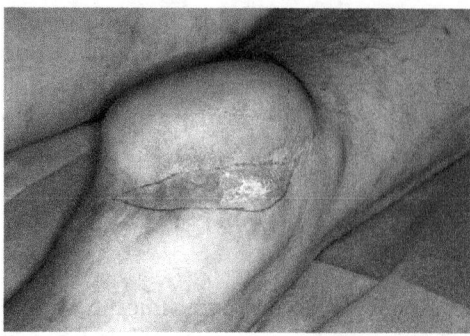

Fig. 4 – Soft tissue expansion realized prior to prosthesis insertion on a scar adherent to the patellar area (left knee).

The indication of skin expansion prior to total knee prosthesis insertion must consequently be established with the greatest caution. Expansion procedure should be realized by an experienced team capable to manage the complications related to this technique (fig. 4).

Tissue expansion is realized over a three-month period and requires two surgical procedures under general anesthesia. A two to three month period prior to orthopedic surgery is necessary. This parameter must be taken into consideration in the careful choice of the indication.

The patient has to be fully informed considering the high complication rate of the procedure.

Management of soft tissue necrosis

In the case of smaller necrotic lesions (less than 3cm in the largest dimension), (fig. 5), several "small" procedures in order to achieve uneventful managed secondary healing include:

– reduction of flexion kinesiotherapy;

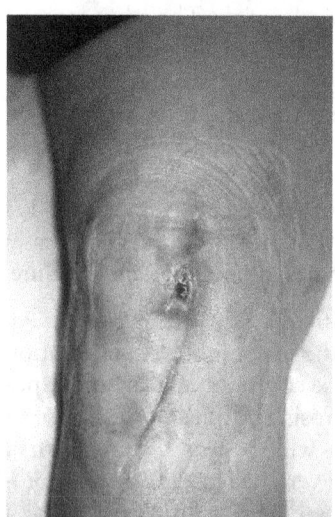

Fig. 5 – Small necrotic wound (left knee) located on the lateral approach (a previous scar is observed on the medial edge).

– daily dressing supervision;
– vasodilator treatment;
– antibiotic therapy discussed in each case;
– resection of necrotic plaque at 8th-10th day then dressing using Calcium Alginate saturated with physiological saline solution.

When the necrotic region is larger (over 3cm maximum), a deep extension can be suspected with a risk of prosthesis exposure. In such cases, debridement in the operating room must be realized in order to evaluate the necessity of local flap use.

In the event of major fast-growing wound separation (often due to primary infection of the prosthesis), revision surgery must be promptly initiated associated with appropriate antibiotic therapy.

Secondary healing after even minimal exposure of prosthetic hardware is illusive. Such a positive evolution can sometimes be observed but it is always a slow process usually obtained at the cost of stiffness of the joint that will reduce the quality of the postoperative result of total knee replacement.

Reconstructive procedures

Three types of flaps can be used: muscle flaps, fasciocutaneous flaps and free muscle transfer. Heterologous grafts have no longer indication.

Muscle flaps

In knee joint repair surgery, they are gastrocnemius muscle rotated flaps (7, 13, 16). The most frequently used is the medial gastrocnemius muscle flap. Coverage will be realized in one-stage procedure or in a secondary surgery. The use of musculocutaneous gastrocnemius flap is possible but the result is not better than coverage with grafted flap; it will even make the procedure more complicated. Muscle flap is raised by posteromedial incision with a superior extremity distant from the operated area and an inferior extremity coming down to the limit of muscular body (fig. 6).

After cleavage of the soleus muscle, a small tendon is left attached to the muscle then separation between the medial gastrocnemius muscle and the lateral gastrocnemius is realized. The muscle is then pedicled on the femoral

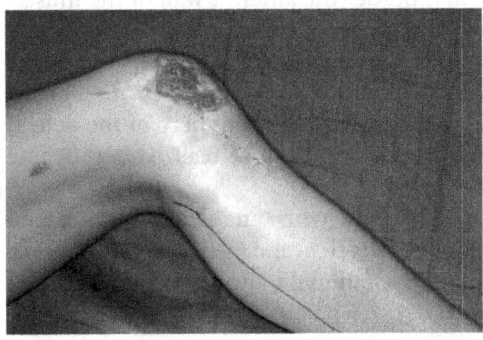

Fig. 6 – Skin incision line for elevation of a medial gastrocnemius muscle flap to cover prepatellar necrotic wound.

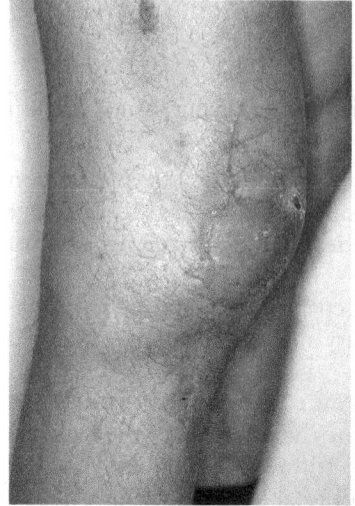

Fig. 7 – Final scar of gastrocnemius muscle flap covered with split skin graft. (Subcutaneous bulging secondary to subskin tunneling of the muscle is clearly visible.)

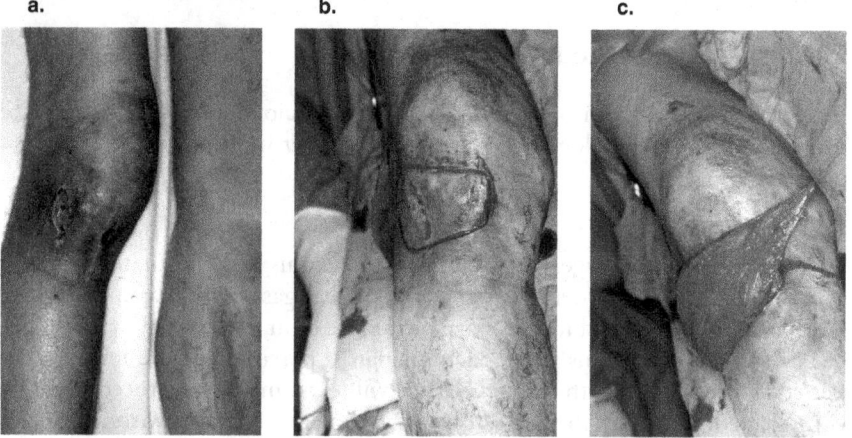

a.   b.   c.

Fig. 8 – Right knee.
a. Bifocal necrosis due to two parallel incisions. Deep lateral necrotic wound.
b. Excision involving the entire soft tissue band located between the two scars.
c. Rotation of the lateral gastrocnemius muscle flap to cover the resected area.

receptor site. The vascular pedicles that border the anterior wall of the muscle do not require visualization. Deep subcutaneous detachment is performed between the donor site and the region to cover. It is often necessary to make cross striations on the anterior fascia of the muscle in order to obtain a better spreading of the muscle flap. The flap is seated at the periphery of the defect. A split dermoepidermal graft taken from the thigh can be realized in the same procedure (fig. 7).

Lateral gastrocnemius flap can be proposed when the defect has a lateral location. The lateral flap covers smaller defects than the medial gastrocnemius. Moreover, its disadvantage is its restricted rotational movement since it crosses outwards the neck of fibula (fig. 8).

Muscular deficit of the leg is minor and usually not perceived by the patient.

Reliability of muscle flap is excellent (about 95%).

Fasciocutaneous flaps

Three types of fasciocutaneous flaps were described for soft tissue coverage of the knee. They are either rotation flaps neighbouring the necrotic region, local pedicled muscle flaps or muscle flaps with identified vascular pedicle.

Local flaps

One of the limits of flap resection is the edge of the necrotic area (fig. 9). The length of the flap must not be over one and a half time its width. Dissection must systematically be realized in the subfascial plane. Soft tissue defect left after flap rotation will be at once covered with split dermoepidermal graft usually taken from the medial surface of the thigh (1, 8, 14).

Lewis (10) described a triangular medial V-Y retroposition flap sutured along the limb of the Y closure (fig. 10).

Fasciocutaneous flaps with local pedicles can be based on the lateral or medial saphenous territory (fig. 11). Sequelae of the donor site can be redu-

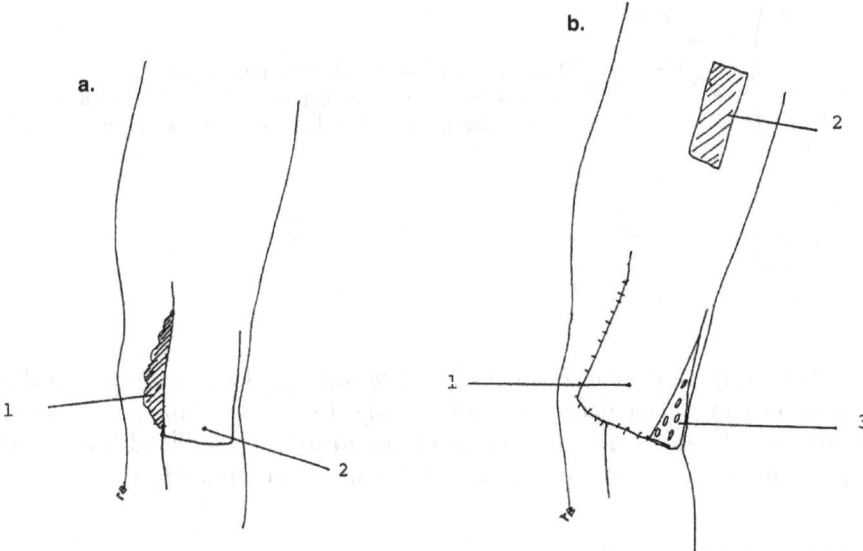

Fig. 9 – Right knee, medial view.
a. 1. Necrotic wound lateral to the scar.
2. Incision line of the fasciocutaneous flap on the medial part of the knee.
b. 1. Flap covering tissue loss.
2. Donor site for dermoepidermal graft taken from the medial surface of the thigh.
3. The graft is covering tissue loss left by the flap transfer.

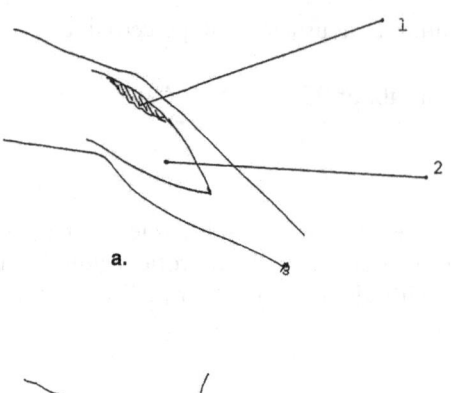

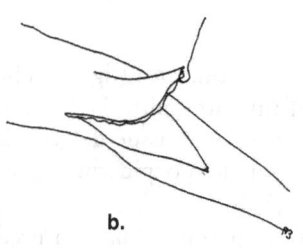

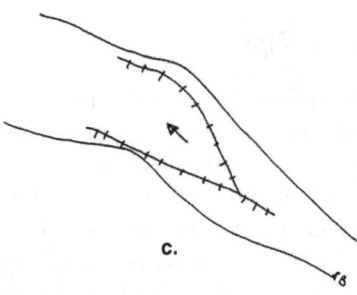

Fig. 10 – Left knee, medial view.
a. 1. Necrotic region.
2. V incision of a medial fasciocutaneous flap.
b. The flap is elevated parallel to the
proximal part of the medial gastrocnemius muscle and at the attachment of the tendons of the sartorius,
gracilis and semitendinosus muscles.
c. V-Y flap closure.

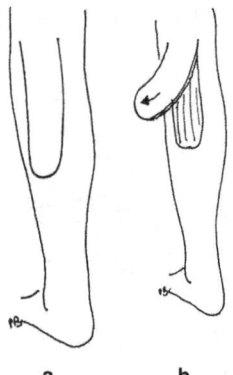

Fig. 11 – Left lower limb, posterolateral view.
a. Incision of the lateral saphenous fasciocutaneous flap.
b. The flap is elevated and covers the tissue loss of the knee.

ced by using a subcutaneous fascial pedicle (fig. 12). Cariou (3) described a
posterolateral fasciocutaneous island flap (fig. 13). The grafting procedure of
this type of flap must be realized according to strict rules, blood being supplied to the flap by the superficial, lateral and median sural arteries.

Pedicled muscle flaps

More recently described, these flaps are pedicled on a richly vascularized zone
previously dissected. Donor site can be chosen in the fibular region requiring
the sacrifice of the fibular artery (9). Baek (2) described the lateral thigh flap
and Malikov (1) the antero-medial neurocutaneous thigh flap; these flaps are
taken from the septal branches of femoral vessels.

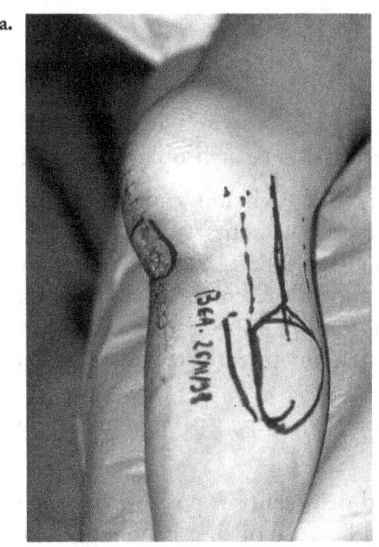
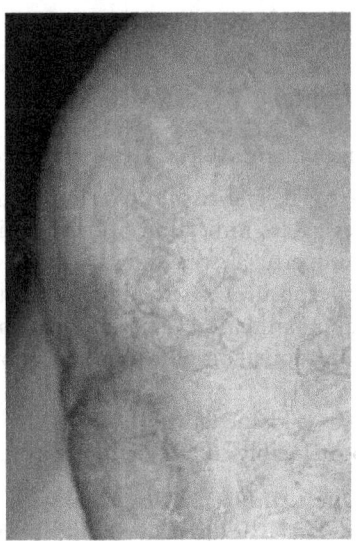

Fig. 12 – Right knee.
a. Small necrotic wound located on the middle of the incision line.
Medial fasciocutaneous flap with subcutaneous pedicle.
b. Result – the donor site received a split skin graft.

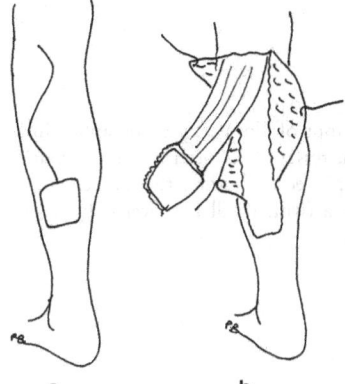

a.   b.

Fig. 13 – Left lower limb, posterolateral view.
a. Incision line of a lateral sural island fasciocutaneous flap.
Curvilinear skin incision allows a wide exposure of the fascia.
Flap design is made parallel to the distal part of the lateral gastrocnemius flap and of the proximal part of Achilles tendon.
b. Elevation of the flap. The aponeurotic pedicle involves the median sural artery (external saphenous artery), the medial sural cutaneous nerve and the small external saphenous vein.

Free flaps (2)

Flaps with minor anastomoses are only indicated in case of failure of a more simple procedure or local flap contraindication. They are generally musculocutaneous flaps. Most of the time, the latissimus dorsi is chosen because of its excellent plasticity, the length of its pedicle that permits distant vascular connection and because of the good reliability of the flap in experienced hands.

Heterologous grafts

Considering the variety of current surgical options, the indication of heterologous grafts must remain exceptional and be used only after failure of a previously described procedure.

Indication

Management of necrotic tissue defect after total knee arthroplasty include:

– superficial tissue loss: local care (Calcium Alginate) and "office procedures". Rare indication of dermoepidermal complementary graft;

– superficial spreading tissue loss without prosthetic exposure (or punctiform exposure): fasciocutaneous rotation flap in preference to an attempt to obtain granulation tissue followed by skin grafting in order to avoid secondary infections complication and allow the patient to early return to reeducation;

– deep tissue loss with prosthetic hardware exposure: gastrocnemius muscle flap preferably to fasciocutaneous flap.

Direct suture for closure of wide wound dehiscence is possible in only few cases. Such a procedure should be avoided because of the risk of aggravation of devascularization and tissue loss enlargement (fig. 14).

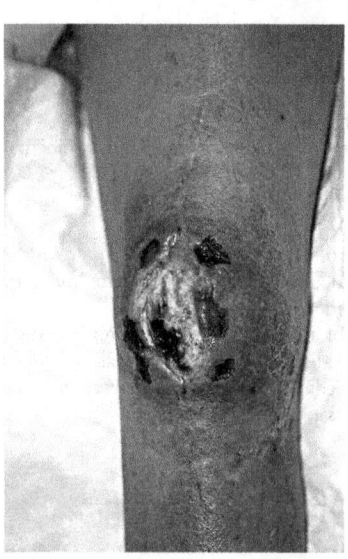

Fig. 14 – Attempt of closure by tissue approximation using mattress sutures after necrotic wound. Failure of the procedure leading to enlargement of the necrotic area (which will be covered by a gastrocnemius flap).

Conclusion

Soft tissue necrosis after total knee arthroplasty is a rare complication. It can be feared in patients with particularly underlying often associated medical conditions.

Long-term results of these coverage procedures are good with 80 to 85% of salvage of the prosthesis in cases of tissue necrosis observed in the most recent series (1, 4).

These techniques of reconstructive surgery must be known by orthopedic surgeons: they can help guide the choice of the approach, avoid inappropriate postoperative procedures and enable to undertake early management of complications which is the only guarantee of an excellent final result.

In high-risk patients, the plastic surgical service is consulted in order to guide the surgical incision and, if necessary, when the regional conditions seem favorable, to propose soft tissue expansion.

This therapeutic option must remain exceptional. Postoperative surveillance of soft tissue condition is the key element since management option must be adapted to the severity of tissue complication. This attitude requires a perfect collaboration between the orthopedic team and the plastic surgeons.

References

1. Adam RF, Watson SB, Jarratt JW et al. (1994) Outcome after flap cover for exposed total knee arthroplasties. J Bone Joint Surg 76: 750-3
2. Baek S (1983) Two new cutaneous free flaps: the medial lateral thigh flaps. Plast Reconstr Surg 71: 354 -63
3. Cariou JL, Lambert F, Arcila M et al. (1995) Le lambeau sural postérolatéral en îlot fasciocutané à pédicule aponévrotique proximal. Ann Chir Plast Esthet 40: 148-61
4. Casanova D, Bali D, Bardot J et al. (2001) Tissue expansion of th lower limb: complications in a cohort of 103 cases. Br J plast Surg 54: 310-6
5. Colombel M, Mariz Y, Dahman P et al. (1998) Arterial and lymphatic supply of the knee integuments. Surg Radiol Anat 20: 35-40
6. De Peretti F, Argenson C, Beracassat R et al. (1987) Problèmes artériels et nerveux posés par les incisions cutanées antérieures au niveau de l'articulation du genou. Rev Chir Orthop Suppl II 73: 231-3
7. Gerwin M, Rothaus KO, Windsor RE et al. (1993) Gastrocnemius muscle flap coverage of exposed or infected knee protheses. Clinical Orthop and Related Research 286: 64-70
8. Hallock GG (1990) Salvage of total knee arthroplasty with local fasciocutaneous flaps. J Bone Joint Surg 72 a: 1236-9
9. Ikeda K, Morishita Y, Nakatani A et al. (1996) Total knee arthroplasty covered with pedicle peroneal flap. J Arthroplasty 11: 478-81
10. Lewis VL, Mossie RD, Stulberg DS et al. (1990) The fasciocutaneous flap: a conservatrive approach to the exposed knee joint. Plast Reconstr Surg 85: 252-7
11. Malikov S, Pivalenti, Masquelet AC (1999) Lambeau neurocutané de la face antéro-interne de cuisse à pédicule distal. Étude anatomique et applications cliniques. Ann Chir Plast Esthet 44: 531-40
12. Manifold SG, Cushner FD, Craig-Scott S et al. (2000) Long-term result of total knee arthroplasty after the use of soft tissue expanders. Clin Orthop 380: 133-9
13. Mc Craw JB, Fishman JH, Sharzer LA (1978) The versatile gastrocnemius myocutaneous flap. Plast Reconstr Surg 62: 15-23
14. Nahabedian MY, Orlando JC, Delanois RE et al. (1998) Salvage procedures for complex soft tissue defects of the knee. Clin Orthop Related Res 356: 119-24
15. Namba RS, Diao E (1997) Tissue expansion for staged reimplantation of infected total knee arthroplasty. J Arthroplasty: 471-4
16. Sanders R, O'Neil T (1981) The gastrocnemius myocutaneous flap used as a cover for the exposed knee prosthesis. J Bone Joint Surg 63: 383-8
17. Santore RF, Kaufman D, Robbins AJ et al. (1997) Tissue expansion prior to revision of total knee arthroplasty. J Arthroplasty 12: 475-8
18. Shim SS, Leung G (1986) Blood supply of the knee joint. Chir Orthop Related Res 208: 119-25
19. Younger ASE, Duncan CP, Masri BA (1998) Surgical exposures in revision total knee arthroplasty. J Ann Acad Orthop Surg 6: 55-64

Computer-assisted navigation in total knee replacement

F. Picard, A.M. DiGioia III, D. Saragaglia

Introduction

Technological progress in the electronics and computer fields has resulted in new methods of surgical aid. Indeed, several types of operations in orthopaedic or trauma surgery can now benefit from computer guidance systems. This relates, for example, to assistance in placing total hip or knee replacements, or again, in implementing difficult surgical procedures such as a peri-acetabular osteotomy (12, 20, 23, 31).

Still very confidential until some years ago, computer-assisted surgery has gained an increasing presence on operating tables. This new technology has been variously baptized: "medical robotics", "image-guided surgery", "surgical navigation system", "integrated computerized system", "stereotaxic guidance system", "avant-garde operative guidance system" or, again, "reality-improving system" (12, 13, 14, 23). We will adopt the following definition: "computer-assisted orthopaedic surgery is the use of a computer tool to help the orthopaedic surgeon plan and carry out a surgical act."

The idea of a robot, complex and fallible, operating in the place of a surgeon, justly disturbs patient and surgeon alike and has rendered "suspect" any concept of computerization around the surgical act. It is certain that the level of complexity of analysis, adaptation and performance by man can in no way be matched by any system of artificial intelligence. This technology, consequently, must be seen as a new tool, certainly a very elaborate one, but one which is simple to use and which makes it possible to improve preoperative planning and guarantee the anatomical result of a surgical action and if possible, to minimize the most invasive and costly elements of each operation. The purpose is also to improve the surgeon's performance, by increasing his accuracy of course, but first and foremost by reinforcing the reproducibility of the act and therefore of the results (fig. 1).

Most equipment used in this technology comes from the mechanical industries (robotics), or the imaging industry (computer-assisted tomography). This technology has been used for a long time for certain surgical specialties, such as neurosurgery and craniofacial surgery. Orthopaedic surgery is even better suited to this new approach, because it is practiced on a rigid structure, name-

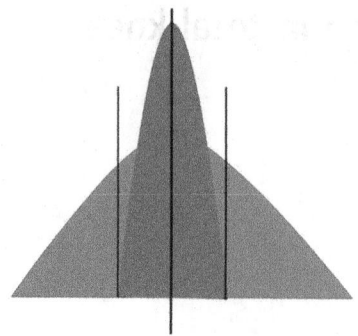

Fig. 1 – Schematic representation of total knee replacement results. The goal is to reduce the dispersion of the results by concentrating the Gauss curve around the ideal result and by eliminating the extremes, i.e., the potential bad results.

ly, the bone. Compared with "soft tissues", the bone is only very slightly deformable. This property makes it possible to fix trackers to a bone, trackers which can then be monitored with great precision when the bone is mobilized.

A scientific demonstration of the utility, safety and ergonomics of this technology is essential. The very encouraging results of comparative studies (conventional techniques versus computer-assisted surgery) and retrospective studies of certain systems have made it possible to attenuate the natural reluctance of user-clinicians and to advance toward products increasingly better adapted to their expectations.

Like all modern science, medicine must adapt to the demands of progress and improve its performance in terms of quality and even of "productivity" which are imposed by the rising costs of health care. Uniting the best of man and the best of the machine should lead to ever simpler and more efficient systems, in order to progress even further in terms of quality of treatment for the benefit of the patient (table I) (39).

Table I – Capacities of man and of the machine

Man	Machine
• Doctor-patient relationship • Medical knowledge and experience (non-exact science) • Thoughtful adaptation to unforeseen situations • Very fine and complex sense of touch • Combination of several senses (touch, sight...) • Agility in using instruments • Dexterity in using both hands in a coordinated way	• Precision of execution (emitters and sensors) • Capacity of collecting and analyzing a large number of data • Capacity of collecting and analyzing • Rapidity of execution • Repeatability of the quality of work executed • Possibility of performing micro-surgery • Repeatability of the quality of work • Possibility of combining several techniques (graphics, detection of movement or of forces...)

We shall first of all discuss the clinical interest of this technology and then the classification of existing systems and will then describe the different concepts used in the field of knee replacement surgery, stressing the advantages, the drawbacks and the prospects for all of these systems. Finally, we will conclude this article.

Clinical interest

General principles and points of interest of this technology in current orthopaedic surgery

The best means of pinpointing the potentialities of computer-assisted surgery is to analyze the different phases of traditional surgery and to determine its limitations or constraints (table II).

Table II – The different phases of the surgical procedure (21, 30, 38, 45)

Preoperative planning phase	Surgical phase	Postoperative phase
Interpretation of patient clinical and anatomical data	Integration of patient clinical and anatomical data in the surgical context	Evaluation of clinical and anatomical data of the surgical act

Preoperative planning

During the past two decades, a considerable amount of development has taken place in the fields of computer-assisted tomography, magnetic resonance and ultrasonography (15). These new techniques have made possible decisive advances, particularly in medical diagnosis and prognosis. In the field of orthopaedics, these images have considerably improved the visualization and the assessment of complex anatomical structures such as the spine, the pelvis or again, the peripheral joints and their contents, such as the knee.

Nevertheless, this progress (15) notwithstanding, this accuracy of preoperative images, however, sophisticated they may be, has not made possible an equally clear-cut improvement of preoperative planning. Radiographic images are still frequently offered to the surgeon as a series of two-dimensional images and it is the surgeon himself who mentally performs the three-dimensional (3D) integration of the CT-scan or MRI data, which he will subsequently interpret, in order to define his therapeutic process. We are working in a subjective field, dependent on the expertise and experience of the surgeon, which is becoming increasingly problematical in our litigious society.

Similarly, just as an aircraft pilot enters his flight plan data into his onboard computer in order to make his flying as safe as possible, computer-assisted surgery makes it possible to integrate pre-operative imaging or guidance data, to store them, to compare them, to analyze them in a reliable and repeatable manner, regardless of the surgeon, thanks to software adapted to the surgical procedure.

Surgical phase

In the practice of surgery, the use of robotic or navigation systems, whether based on imaging or not, goes beyond novelty or technical improvement of the mechanical or computer type. It entails a new concept of reflection about, and organization of, the surgical act, thanks to the use of a tool which makes possible the creation of a reliable and direct link between preoperative planning and the process of surgery. Computerized navigation makes it possible to assist the surgeon during the surgical operation by means of the integration of the preoperative examination (and planning) into the peri-operative data. It has the capacity of measuring and locating all the tools currently used in day-to-day surgical practice and to locate them spatially with respect to osseous structures on which the surgeon is working. Lastly, it provides powerful instruments capable of recording in real time, all information likely to improve the precision of surgical act.

This new technology thus creates a new approach to surgical operations. It makes it possible, for example, to refine bone cut orientation or implant size calculation. It is also possible to simulate joint amplitudes and indeed to re-establish measurement gap following the introduction of a prosthesis.

Postoperative phase

These systems are very useful, because they make it possible to assess a surgical technique and to keep an objective trace of that technique, particularly in the event of a dispute.

They make possible an objective monitoring, in the short-, medium- and long-term, of postoperative results. Measurable and quantifiable data are always simpler than subjective information contributed by the patient and / or the surgeon. The correlation between the anatomical results of a surgical operation and its clinical results is, and will remain, very impartial, since it can be clearly assessed.

Lastly, this technology makes it possible to test a piece of equipment extremely objectively and will assist in adjusting the different instruments or procedures involved in a surgical act.

Summary

Computer-assisted orthopaedic surgery (CAOS) has developed along different lines:

– improve the quality and quantity of information prior to surgery, in order to optimize its prognosis: this is *planning / simulation;*

– improve the interaction between information obtained prior to the operation and information obtained during the operation: this is *navigation;*

– improve the accuracy of the performance of the instruments performing the surgical act: this is *robotization.*

Each line, or combination of lines, has as a goal:

– specifying preoperative reference landmarks and measurements more objectively;

– improving the placement of an implant in order to reduce its wear and to increase its stability;

– improving the function of a joint directly or indirectly involved in the operation (better planning, more accurate orientation or implant level, for example);

– improving the adjustment between the implant and the bone which receives it, in order to reduce the likelihood of loosening and of surgical revisions;

– improving the visibility of unexposed anatomical components;

– documenting an operation (in a manner similar to that of photographing an injured meniscus during an arthroscopy, it is possible, thanks to this technology, to document each phase of the operation);

– reducing the invasive character of certain surgical acts;

– trying to reduce the most "aggressive" factors for the patient or the surgeon (X-rays for instance).

Goals and principles of computerized systems in knee arthroplasty

Since the 1970's, a period of real blossoming of prosthetic knee surgery, progress in this field has increased continually. Aging of the population and technological improvements have naturally increased the volume of implants (7).

Limitations of the traditional technique

Nevertheless, some 10 to 15% of all these prostheses require in the more or less long term a surgical revision (3). The functional requirement of patients, the increasingly strict cost control of every surgical operation and pressure by insurance companies to "guarantee the results of these operations", all these factors have led surgeons and health maintenance organizations to become interested in the overall quality of results. It is estimated that in 1997, 1 to 2.5% of the gross national product of the United States, Canada, Great Britain, France and Australia was spent on the treatment of musculo-skeletal problems (1)!

Whatever the model of the implanted prosthesis may be, inevitable factors must be controlled to ensure the best possible anatomical and functional result. The principal success factors are perfect patient selection, suitable choice of the implant, the prosthesis placement quality and the surgical follow-up of the patient.

As regards the quality of prosthesis placement, two factors must be particularly well controlled during the operation, namely, the making of bone cuts and knee ligament balance. These two imperatives of prosthetic surgery indisputably condition the functional results in the short term and the survival of the implants in the long term.

Bone cuts

In spite of the improvements in mechanical instrumentation facilitating the carrying out of these acts, bone cuts and ligament balance still remain largely dependent on the experience and know-how of the operating surgeon (17). However, even the most experienced professionals recognize their limits, but also the weaknesses of implant instrumentation (19, 32, 33, 34) Vince (50) has shown that in the majority of cases of loosening of prostheses, the loosening occurs where the prosthesis is varus-oriented. Bargren (3) noted a failure rate of 67% in the case of knees with a varus-oriented prosthesis, as against 29% for knees in neutral position. Ritter (46) has presented a shorter life curve for poorly centered and poorly balanced knee prostheses, as compared with prostheses said to be well centered.

Accordingly, one of the difficulties is the carrying out of perfect bone cuts. In theory, it is necessary to control seven cut orientations, five of the femur, one of the tibia and one of the patella (which is a large number compared with prosthetic hip surgery). Although modern instrumentation makes it possible to cut several parts of the bone simultaneously (for example the anterior and posterior sides of the femur) thus limiting the grossest errors, difficulties of orientating the implant remain. These difficulties concern both the frontal / sagittal plane, as well as the transversal plane (implant rotation) (5, 8).

Ligament balance

All surgeons practicing prosthetic knee surgery know how delicate it is to obtain this balance, even with experience (9, 28) The improved understanding of the physiopathology of the prostheticized knee has led manufacturers to increase the complexity and the quantity of instrumentation. This is advantageous neither for the patient (liberation of metallic particles during manipulation of the instrumentation), nor for society (instrumentation costs).

Preoperative radiological examinations

In order to prevent perioperative errors, numerous authors have insisted on and specified radiological planning protocols for these operations. In spite of this, incorrect placement of the implant occurs daily (34). Rigorously following a well-constructed protocol does not offset the inaccuracy of radiological angles. The difficulty of using radiological reference points during the operation and the uncertain nature of these reference points, either because they are located deep in the patient's anatomy (in the coxo-femoral joint, for example), or because of the absence of a constant and reliable reference landmark (particularly in the case of the knee), obviously restricts the ability to interpret these data.

Within the framework of a prospective study which we conducted in order to determine the best criterion of analysis for comparing a traditional technique with a computerized one, we reviewed most of the radiological results quoted in the literature between 1975 and 1995, of a mixture of prostheses (47). We noted that the average frontal femoro-tibial angle after the implantation of various prostheses was 181.37° (1.37° valgus), with a standard deviation of 3.3° (42). It is found that the average alignment of all these prostheses (a mixture of numerous models) is very acceptable. This may partly explain why the results of prosthetic knee surgery are overall satisfactory and that in the USA, for example, the number of knee replacements now exceeds the number of hip replacements (1). These are, however, series which most frequently originate in centers specializing in knee surgery. Now, the majority of knee implants (80%) are fitted by orthopaedic surgeons who are not hyper-specialists and who fit no more than twenty implants a year (32) A recent study carried out in Canada found rates of revision of between 4.2% and 8% (7).

Accordingly, the majority of studies confirm what Insall wrote in 1976 namely that "the majority of failures can be attributed to poor ligament balance or to incorrect alignment." Laskin confirmed this in 1989, saying that "the number of radiological sign of loosening is greater in the case of non-aligned prostheses, than in the case of aligned ones and the difference is statistically significant."

Principal objectives of computerized systems in knee arthroplasty

The results of the traditional technique explain the need to increase even further the accuracy, the regularity and the means of control of the surgical act. Hungerford wrote that "after all, the most important things in prosthetic surgery of the knee are the human brain and eye" (22). Thanks, in particular, to the progress of computerization, the machine has exceeded human capacities in many fields, particularly in the techniques of measurement, control and objectivity in assessing results. Now, the improvements to be made today in the prosthetic replacement of the knee appear to be more concerned with the optimization of the technique, rather than the quality of the implants themselves. Technological developments such as computer-assisted surgery will make it possible to assess results and implants more objectively. This impartial analysis of the computerized tool makes it possible to identify the problems clearly and will contribute to resolving them more efficiently.

These computerized systems have, first and foremost, already made it possible, or will, to use directly and to the full, all preoperative information during a surgical operation. This interactive control of the surgical act increases the chances of a successful implant.

Classification

Given the systems which are currently under development, or which are already being used in the field of the knee, we have elected to classify the systems of computer-assisted surgery as follows (43):

Robotic assistance systems

These are active, semi-active or "passive" mechanical instruments controlled by computer, which most frequently make use of preoperative medical imaging data in order to perform their task.

Active robot

It is able to perform a specific surgical task such as the drilling or the cutting a bone, without the intervention of the surgeon Robodoc® and Caspar® belong to this category) (2, 4).

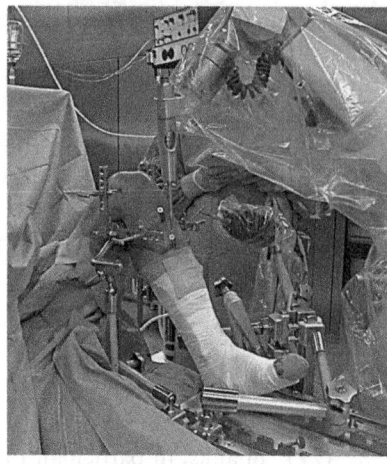

Fig. 2 – Caspar®: robot used for placing TKR (ACL reconstruction on this picture).

Semi-active robot

It is able to perform a limited specific surgical task, through the hand of the surgeon who guides it and via the computer software, which controls it (fig. 3) (10).

"Passive" robot

It is able to perform a specific non-decisive surgical task, for example the mechanized orientation of a cutting guide, or the orientation of a drilling guide. The final (active) action of performing a bone cut or drilling is performed by the surgeon (fig. 4) (37).

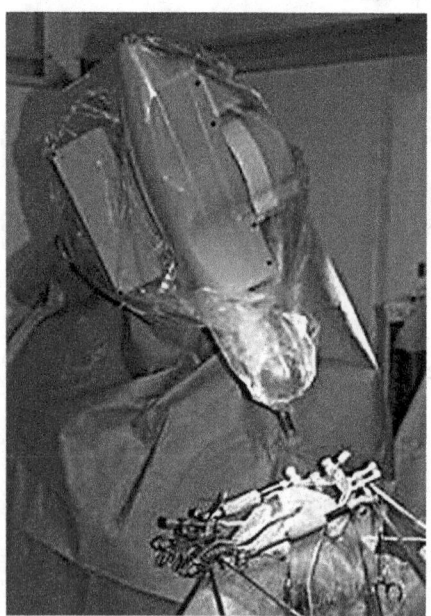

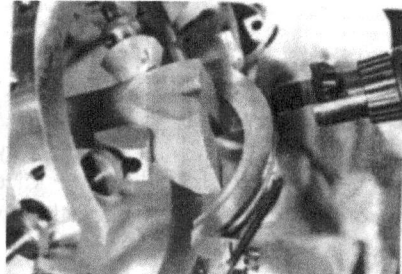

Fig. 4 – An example of a "passive" robot.

Fig. 3 – An example of a semi-active robot (Acrobat® courtesy of J. Cobb).

Navigation systems

These are systems of computer-assisted surgery which make it possible to orient and to guide the surgical procedure. They are able to provide the surgeon with anatomical and radiographic images, graphs controlled by graphic software, values which are relevant to the surgical context (such as, for example, an angle between two axes) or a combination of all these elements, in real time and to do so with great accuracy. These systems may be divided into two categories: those using a preoperative model and those using an intraoperative model.

System with a preoperative model

This is a system of navigation, which functions via the capture of a large set of preoperative data, most frequently imaging data (CT-scan or MRI). This acquisition of anatomical data makes it possible to construct preoperative models which are specific or non-specific to a patient.

Patient-specific models

This system uses the patient's own anatomical data. The taking of a series of preoperative images makes it possible to reconstruct the patient's anatomy. These images will be used for surgical guidance during an operation (fig. 5).

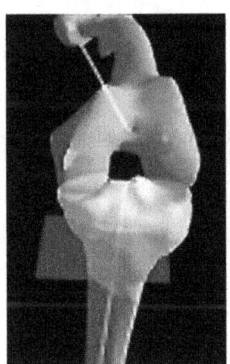

Fig. 5 – Computerized system using patient-specific imagery. The visible image is the 3-D reconstruction of the patient's scan.

Non patient-specific models

This system uses anatomical data not originating from the patient. Thanks to computerization, it is now possible to construct generic forms of bones or joints from several specimens (bodies, dry bones or CT-scan), which will be used during a surgical operation and applied as best as possible to the patient's anatomy. This type of system appears to be extremely promising in all second operation reconstruction cases (revision of knee prosthesis). These generic anatomical data can be "glued" to the anatomy of the patient, facilitating the reconstruction of the knee (fig. 6) (18).

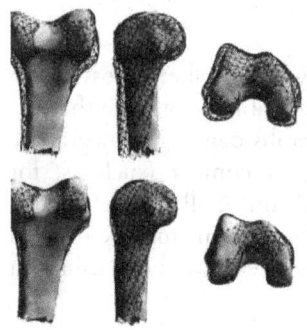

Fig. 6 – Computerized system using non-patient-specific imagery.

Intraoperative model systems

This is a system which only uses data obtained during the operation. This system is divided into two types, according to whether it uses or does not use medical imaging during the surgical procedure (27, 41).

Image-using system

This is a navigation system which uses images obtained during the surgical procedure (e.g., fluoroscopy) (fig. 7).

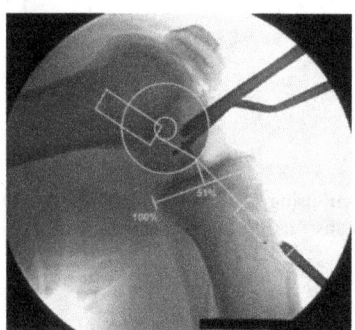

Fig. 7 – System using an image-based intraoperative model.

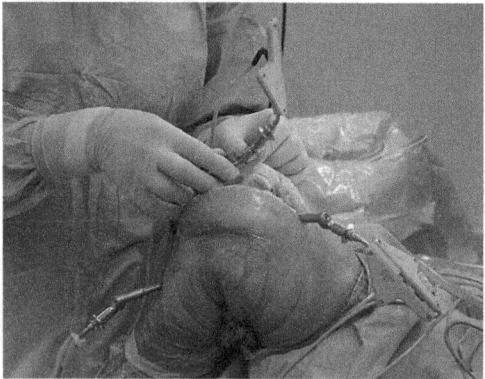

Fig. 8 – System using an intraoperative model without image.

Non-image-using system

This is a navigation system which does not use medical imaging during the surgical operation. In this case, the surgeon accurately determines the reference landmarks which he requires in order to carry out a procedure that will be described in detail in the continuation of this exposé (fig. 8).

Navigation system for implanting total knee replacements: different concepts

Among the navigation systems currently under development, two methods have already given proof of clinical feasibility: navigation systems using a preoperative model (CT-scan imaging) and navigation systems with an intraoperative model (without CT or fluoro-based images).

Computer-assisted image-guided surgery

Introduction

Orthopaedic surgery adapts very well to computer-assisted image-guided technology because of the "relatively rigid" character of the bone. In fact, many orthopaedic surgical procedures involve the "shaping" of the bone by means of various tools. As opposed to the case of ligaments or tendons, an operation on the bone brings about only a slight modification of its anatomical structure. For example, the bone cut of the distal femur in order to implant a knee prosthesis does not fundamentally modify either the femur's shape or the rest of its structure.

Moreover, imaging, since Roentgen, has demonstrated its interest in the field of orthopaedics and computerized image manipulation and has made better surgical planning possible. In parallel, the improvement in the processing of images and of signals has made possible the performance of complex tasks. It is, for example, possible to make the preoperative images (and planning) correspond very clearly and reproducibly to the real anatomy of the patient on which the surgeon performs his work. Accordingly, this makes it possible, on the one hand, to copy the exact preoperative planning on the intraoperative anatomy of the patient and, on the other hand, to control the anatomy modified by surgery by using the same imaging data recorded prior to the operation.

Computer-assisted image-using surgery makes available a new range of sophisticated orthopaedic tools. These are tools of planning, simulation (virtual training) and navigation (comparable to the GPS system installed in certain vehicles).

Clinical and technical stages of these systems

A system of image-guided computer-assisted surgery consists of two components: planning and navigation (40).

The system of preoperative planning makes it possible to optimize the surgical plan.

The patient benefits from a lower leg CT-scan which integrates the joints of the hip and the ankle (approximately 120 cross-sections). These data are transmitted either by the internal communication network, or by disk to a computer workstation. A technician then manually reconstructs the bone in three dimensions, reviewing all the osseous cross-sections. He traces the contours of the bone which he follows with the computer mouse, clicks and records the contour which is of interest to him. Thanks to these images, it is possible to reconstruct a virtual 3-D model of the bones.

Thanks to a sophisticated computer program, the surgeon places the virtual prosthetic implants of his choice on this model, optimizing the positions of these implants with respect to the bone model. Certain systems make it possible to plan the ideal position and size of the prosthesis. Simulation of joint amplitudes following virtual implantation of the knee prosthesis is in the process of development. Once the surgeon has obtained the ideal plan, he records and transmits it to the operating room computerized workstation (fig. 9).

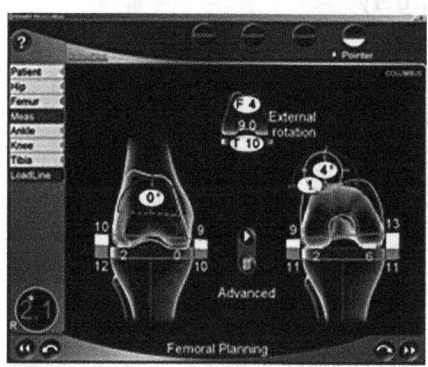

Fig. 9 – An interface used in intraoperative planning.

The intraoperative navigation system requires implementing complex computerized procedures (invisible to the surgeon), which makes it possible to match preoperative imaging and patient anatomy. Thanks to graphic interfaces, this navigation system makes it possible to monitor, in real time, the anatomy of the patient and its planning, as well as the surgical instruments, all of which are equipped with trackers.

Material and methods

We are going to describe the material needed for the functioning of these systems and the methods of utilization. We are not going to describe the specificities of the imaging equipment (CT-scan or MRI), which might complicate this expose.

Material

• Trackers

These are fundamental elements of these navigation procedures. The principle of these components is their ability to locate at any moment all or a part of the anatomical structures in which the surgeon is interested (fig. 10)

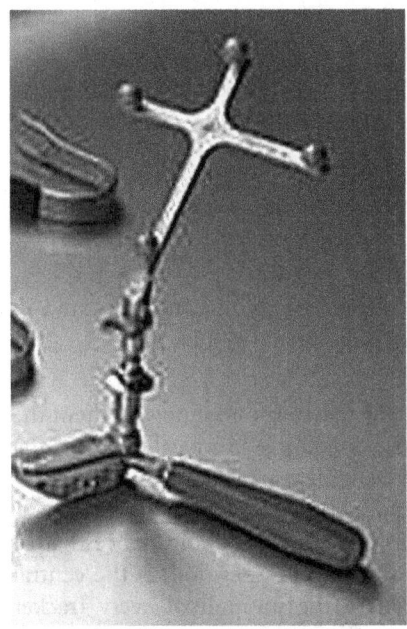

Fig. 10 – Passive infrared tracker.

The trackers (which are also called "rigid bodies" or DRB-Dynamic Reference Base), are attached to the bone by screws or other fittings able to be solidly fixed into the bone. The trackers which are at present available (and suitable for surgical use) are either infrared or electromagnetic.

Physically, these trackers consist of three parts:

– a support structure (plastic or metal), of a variable geometry (plane, cubical...);

– emitters (infrared LED or electromagnetic). To be located spatially, an infrared tracker must contain several emitters (at least three);

– most frequently, connecting cables (which connect these emitters to each other and to a central control unit). The presence of connecting cables between emitters and the central control unit indicates that they are active emitters. These active emitters actively transmit an infrared or an electromagnetic signal.

It should in fact be added that so-called passive infrared "emitters", which do not need to be connected with the control unit, do exist. In this case, the localizer is able to determine the spatial positions of these emitters (reflecting spheres) simply by displaying them. New trackers called active, without cables, have also recently been developed. The major drawback of these infrared active or passive trackers is, of course, the fact that they must be ongoingly viewed by the localizer in order to be located spatially, which is not the case with electromagnetic trackers.

• Sensor or palpator or pointer or probe

This is a metal or plastic object in the form of a pen. Its ergonomic form makes it possible for the user to point very accurately to a particular anatomic tracker (similar to the palpator used in arthroscopy). The tip of the stylus is

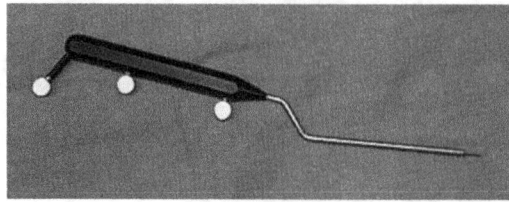

Fig. 11 – Passive infrared tracker on a sensor.

tapered and resistant. The handle of this stylus contains one or more trackers. Once the sensor has been calibrated, the tip of the stylus can be located in space by the localizer with accuracy to the millimeter (fig. 11).

• Localizer

This electronic measuring instrument is able to determine at any moment the spatial position of several trackers (several tracker-equipped surgical instruments) with a very high degree of accuracy (100 measurements per second and an accuracy of less than 1 millimeter!). It receives signals from trackers which flash (infrared signals) and then calculates the position of each emitter and hence that of each tracker. It transmits information about a tracker's position to the central control unit, which updates the calculation of the position of every tracker (fig. 12).

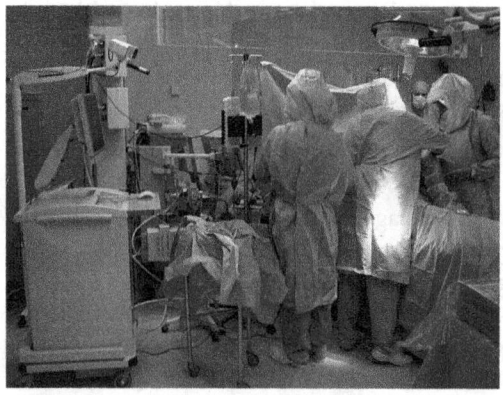

Fig. 12 – Optotrak® localizer (Northern Digital Inc., Waterloo, Ontario, Canada), courtesy of Anthony DiGioia.

Several types of localizers are currently available. Two are already used regularly in orthopaedic surgery; these are optical and electromagnetic. Others are being developed, such as, for example, acoustic devices.

The optical system consists of two or three cameras and functions as a camera. This means that there is a field of visibility and a variable degree of accuracy, depending on the distance separating it from the object to be monitored. The advantage of this type of system is its very high degree of accuracy (< 0.1mm at 2 meters of distance for a certain camera!). The major drawback is the fact that the trackers must always be visible.

The electromagnetic tracker does not have this drawback of an optical tracker because it does not need to be monitored by a camera. The drawback is

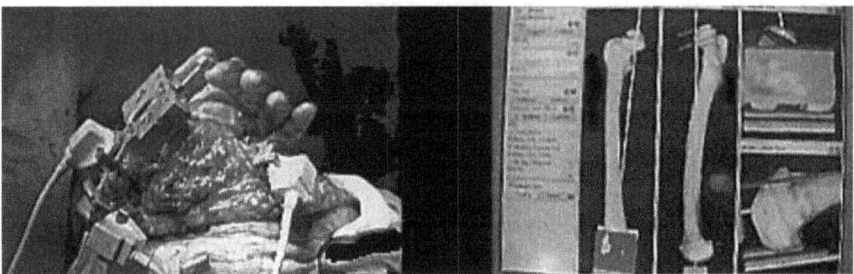

Fig. 13 – System using electromagnetic trackers (Navitrak®, OrthoSoft).

the fact that these trackers are very sensitive to the "metallic" environment of operating rooms, which may alter the device's measurements (fig. 13).

• Central control unit

This is the electronic "brain" of the tracking system to which are connected the connecting cables of each tracker. It controls the switching sequence of the emitters of each tracker. The succession of these flashes is sensed by the localizer to which it is connected. Following a calculation, the control unit determines the exact position of every emitter and hence that of every tracker.

Thanks to this system, any movement of the bone is very accurately monitored by the said tracker, as is a signal from an aircraft by a control tower.

• Computer

This is the brain which coordinates all the components of the system. It controls and records all information required for the correct functioning of the system as a whole.

In the beginning, the workstations were massive. With the progress of technology, these computers are becoming smaller and more powerful. We shall not discuss operating systems (Windows, Unix...), which make it possible for programs to run, this not being our subject.

• Remote control pedal

These pedals are very similar to those which surgeons know and use regularly to operate the electrical scalpel or electrocoagulation or mechanical arthroscopy instruments. These pedals make possible the remote control of the system, theoretically without the intervention of an operating room technician. The surgeon moves to and fro within the program by means of the control pedal, as when remote controlling a television set. Other remote controllers are in use, such as virtual mouse or tracker with controller.

• Graphical interface

Graphical interfaces are displayed on the computer screen in order to inform the surgeon about the action that he is about to undertake. Several interfaces have been created which represent the anatomical image of the patient or, again, interfaces which are very similar to what now exists in well-known programs such as Microsoft Word, which make it possible to move "to

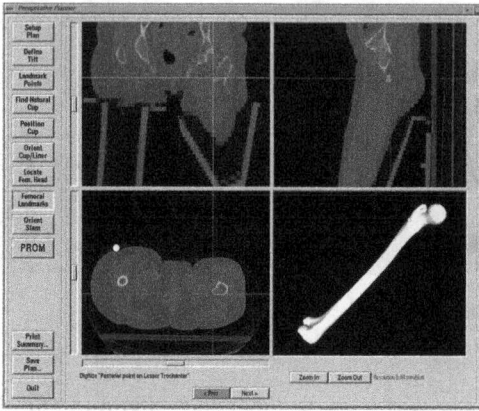

Fig. 14 – Example of a graphical interface.

and fro" within the program. The computer transmits information to the screen in the form of images, graphs or figures, which inform the surgeon about the position of an instrument, or furnish the operation plan in real time and with great accuracy. Certain systems are equipped with touch screens, a feature not always well accepted by orthopaedic surgeons (fig. 14).

• New graphical interfaces: "image overlay"

These interfaces can take various forms, but recently may also be present on integrated screens. Such a screen is a transparent screen, which can be superimposed on the operative area in which the surgeon is working and through which he is able to see, in real time, the patient's osseous anatomy. These images originate in the preoperative CT-scan reconstruction of the patient. Screen and patient are each equipped with a tracker, in such a way that any movement of one with respect to the other is monitored by the localizer. The images projected on the screen by means of an optical process are accurately superimposed on the patient's anatomy. This image is "glued" to the patient, irrespective of the surgeon's angle of vision. Eyeglasses using similar principles have also been developed (fig. 15).

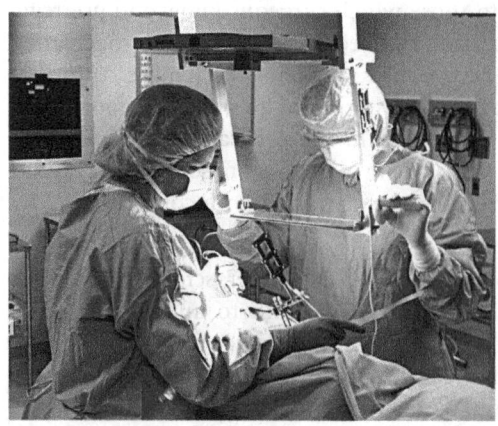

Fig. 15 – New graphical interface known as "image overlay".

Methods

• Matching images

This is without a doubt one of the most important principles of this technology. The development of this procedure has been fundamental to the progress of computer-assisted surgery and to the transmission of planned data to the operative site. The principle is that of putting the preoperative images (reconstruction in 3-D) of the patient's anatomy during a surgical operation into correspondence (or coincidence) with millimeter accuracy. Several procedures for achieving this aim have been developed (fig. 16).

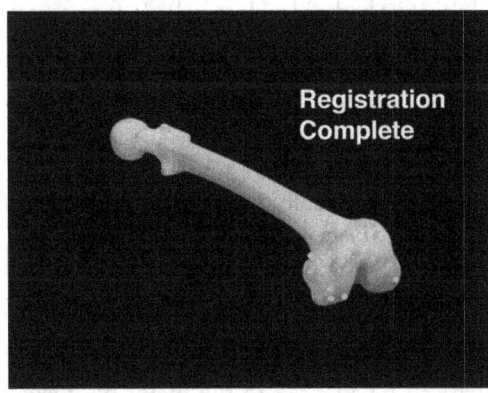

Fig. 16 – Matching procedure. The spots are anatomical landmarks matching with 3D CT preoperative femur.

Early systems used rigid reference fiducials which were fixed into the patient's bone prior to the taking of preoperative images. These metal reference points are anchored in the bone prior to the taking of the image and necessitate the making of several incisions (most frequently under local anesthesia). The advantage of this technique is its accuracy; the drawback, obviously, is that it requires an additional surgical operation.

Another strategy consists in the use of a small number of specific landmarks on the bone which serve as reference points and are used in the procedure of image correspondence (matching of preoperative images with intraoperative anatomy). This method is interesting, because it does not require any prior operation, but has the drawback of being dependent on the surgeon as regards determining the specific landmarks.

The most recent developments of these computerized and mathematical procedures make it possible to bring about the said correspondence solely by the shape of the bone itself. During the surgical operation, a series of points and surfaces are sensed using the pointer described earlier. These points and surfaces generate a three-dimensional model. By means of a mathematical and statistical calculation, the computer will search out the ideal solution for placing the said intraoperative model into correspondence with the preoperative 3-D model with millimeter accuracy (3-D reconstruction of image sections carried out on the said patient). These methods represent a major advance, because they avoid both the drawbacks linked to the determination of specific points and to the surgical nature of their acquisition.

• Object localization

Any object or surgical instrument equipped with a tracker can be monitored during a surgical operation. It is, for example, possible to know the precise orientation of a cutting guide or a drilling guide with respect to the patient's anatomy.

Example of the system using a preoperative model

We are going to describe a typical system of this category, the KneeNav™ (CASurgica Inc, Pittsburgh, PA, USA). This system was developed at the Medical Robotics and Computer-assisted Surgery Center in Pittsburgh (Carnegie Mellon University and UPMC Shadyside Hospital). It forms part of the second generation of the system developed at Pittsburgh after HipNav™ (Hip Navigation). It is a multi-application system, which makes it possible to guide by imaging total knee replacement and anterior cruciate ligament reconstruction operations (44).

Prior to the surgical act, a series of section images (CT-scan and in the future, MRI) are acquired. These images will serve for preoperative planning. Systems based on imaging such as CASPAR (Robot, OrthoMAQUET, Germany) or Robodoc (ISS, USA) make possible the planning of the position of the prosthetic implant (position, size, orientation). These data are then used during the operation.

The navigation module (KneeNav™) for total knee replacement uses a special calibration instrument which can be adapted to the majority of existing instrumentation. It is a resistant, rectangular metal plate, which simulates a saw blade and can be slipped into all traditional cut "guide slots". This plate has two advantages: one, the surgeon can, at any moment, measure the angles he wishes to measure while placing the guides and, two, it can be used with practically any type of mechanical instrumentation. In addition, this plate can be applied to the surface of the bone cut in order to control its orientation.

Graphical interfaces enable a surgeon to control all operation actions, such as the orientation of the cut (angle, distances, cut heights) or, again, ligament balance (laxity angles, or joint amplitudes, for example).

Other very similar systems have been developed in Canada (Navitrak™, Orthosoft. Inc, Montreal, Canada) and are already in clinical use. Other companies have also followed up these concepts. The drawback of the system resides in the fact that it requires, as do all image-based systems, a series of CT-scan images, which is not customary in total knee replacement surgery, and the presence of a technician to organize and transmit these images.

Navigation systems using an intraoperative model without images

Clinical and technical stages of these systems

In preceding chapters, we saw that the techniques of computer-assisted surgery used medical imaging both in the case of medical image-guided navigation techniques as well as in the case of robotic techniques. A new concept has been developed over the past few years whose basic principle is that of not using medical imaging.

From information obtained directly from the patient's anatomy and analyzed during the surgical operation, the surgeon will be guided by the computerized system. In this type of system there is no preoperative planning.

Material and methods

Material

The material used in this approach does not differ in any way from that of other navigation systems. In fact, it consists essentially of a localizer, opto-electronic trackers, a central tracker control unit and, of course, a computer.

The most important instrument in this type of approach is the pointer (fitted with a tracker), whose characteristics we described earlier. The next paragraph will enable us to describe the methods of its use.

Methods

• Calibration principles

To be used during the surgical act, this pointer must be calibrated. Thanks to specific algorithms, the computer will calculate the space coordinates of the tip of this pointer with respect to the trackers (infrared emitters) fixed on the pointer.

In order to calibrate this sensor, another reference tracker is required. This other tracker is usually fixed in the bone and exposed to face the localizer. A small depression is machined in this maker and to serve for the calibration of the sensor. The surgeon or instrument technician orients the sensor trackers towards the localizer and carefully places its point at the bottom of the depression of the other tracker. Next, a slow and regular circular movement is applied to the said sensor for approximately 30 seconds. Simultaneously, the computer records the position of the tracker fixed into the bone and the position of the sensor describing the circular movements and finally calculates the coordinates of the center of the sphere described by the probe. The center of the sphere is of course the point of the probe (fig. 17).

Thus, any ensuing spatial movement of the pointer opposite the localizer provides information on the exact position of the tip of the pointer. The cali-

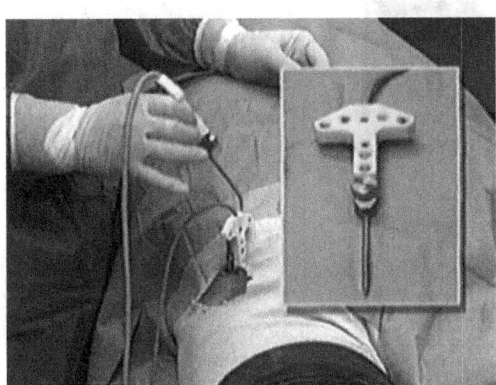

Fig. 17 – Probe calibration technique.

bration is now carried out "in the factory" on commercial systems (this is pre-calibration). The surgeon then performs only a control of the calibration by designating a predefined point (for example a part of a reference tracker of the operative area).

• Using pointer and trackers

Thanks to this pointer, the surgeon will be able to record the relevant landmarks of the anatomy which will be useful to him during the surgical act he performs.

– Collecting a point

How, for example, should the exact position of the internal tibial spine of the knee be registered? For this, it is sufficient to place a tracker on the tibial bone segment and then to calibrate the pointer with respect to the tibial tracker, using the procedure explained earlier. Thus, the localizer and then the computer simultaneously detect the position of the pointer in relation to the tibial tracker and it only remains to place the tip of the pointer on the tibial spine and to register this position, in order to locate it very accurately. By means of this procedure, the computer determines the position in space of the tibial spine in relation to the fixed tracker, regardless of the tibia's position.

– Collecting several points

Let us take the example of the tibial surface around the tibial spine. The sensor is applied to the different points of the tibial surface and the position of its point is registered whenever so desired. The registration of these points is carried out by the subsequent depression of the control pedal which the surgeon implements when the tip of pointer has become stabilized. The computer collects a series of points, which, once they are interconnected by a specific computerized algorithm, will make it possible to construct the virtual surface around the tibial spine with respect to the tibial tracker. Dessenne (J. Fourrier University of Grenoble, France) has described the principles of this technique for knee ligamentoplasty. Subsequently, Marwan Sati (Institut Muller in Berne, Switzerland) used the identical principles (fig. 18) (11, 24, 48).

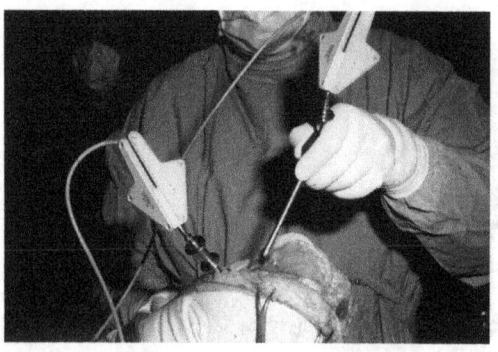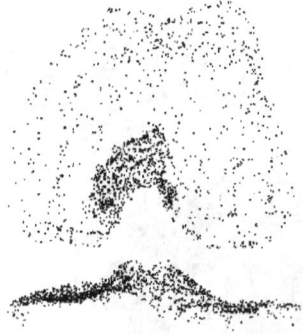

Fig. 18 – Using the probe as a "brush".

The sensing of several osseous surfaces can "virtually design" the proximal surface of the tibia and the distal surface of the femur. This is one of the principles of the Stryker® system (29).

– Registration of the spatial coordinate of the "kinematic centers" and of the reference axes

We have just seen how to register relevant points and anatomical surfaces "directly" during a surgical operation. Picard and Leitner (Grenoble, France) worked out new concepts of registering relevant anatomical points indirectly during a surgical operation (35). To illustrate this category, we will present the principles of the Orthopilot™ system (Aesculap/ B. Braun, Germany), which was the first that could be used in this application (49) in the operating room. The earlier knee roboting systems of Kienzle and Stulberg (Northwestern University, Chicago, IL, USA) (25), Matsen *et al.* (Seattle, WA, USA) (37) and Marccacci *et al.* (Instituti Orthopaedici Rizzoli, Italy) (16, 36) had remained at the laboratory prototype stage. This technique makes it possible to calculate the spatial coordinates of kinematic and anatomic landmark centers of the lower member, in order to control its alignment during the placement of knee prostheses.

Trackers are fixed into each bone segment of the lower member (iliac crest, lower end of the femur, upper end of the tibia) and another tracker is attached to the back of the foot by means of an elastic band. The passive mobilization of every joint (hip, knee and ankle) makes it possible to record the movement of one tracker in relation to the other around the mobilized joint. A specific algorithm has been developed for calculating a "center of these joints" after recording the location of the two trackers (fig. 19).

Every "rotational center or centroid" of each joint of the lower member can be located and controlled by anatomic landmarks: the "mechanical" axis of the femur between the center of the femoral head and the center of the knee and the "mechanical" axis of the tibia between the center of the knee and the center of the ankle.

Redundant methods of control using the principles of direct palpation of anatomical points are also used to verify the correct position of these centers

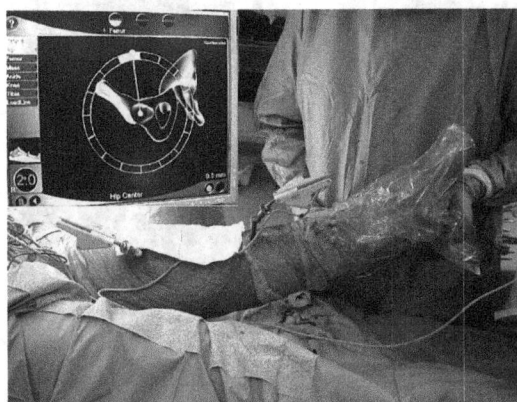

Fig. 19 – Technique for capturing hip joint center.

and these axes. When the calibration phase of the lower member has been completed, the joint centers and, most importantly, the lower member axes are determined virtually in relation to the patient's anatomy.

• Instrument orientation

Surgical instruments are next equipped with trackers and then calibrated before or during the surgical operation. Any movement of these instruments opposite the localizer will be monitored in real time and may be compared with previously determined anatomical points or axes.

Advantages and drawbacks

Advantages

This is a rapid and efficient guidance aid, without the drawbacks of pre- or intraoperative imaging (additional cost, radiographic irradiation, space requirement, length of the procedure, the need of the presence of a technician in the operating room, the possibility of an error of manipulation…). This type of system makes it possible to control accurately the placing of surgical instruments in relation to the patient's anatomy.

This technique meets the requirements of safety and sterility of orthopaedic surgery. Because its use is relatively easy, it only extends operating time very slightly. It is a lightweight system, requiring little space, whose principles are intuitive and as easy to use as a home computer. The use of current material makes it possible for the surgeon always to control the procedure more objectively. He can revert to a traditional technique in the event of an irregularity of result or functioning. The initial results reported in the literature note an improvement in postoperative radiological alignments of total knee repla-

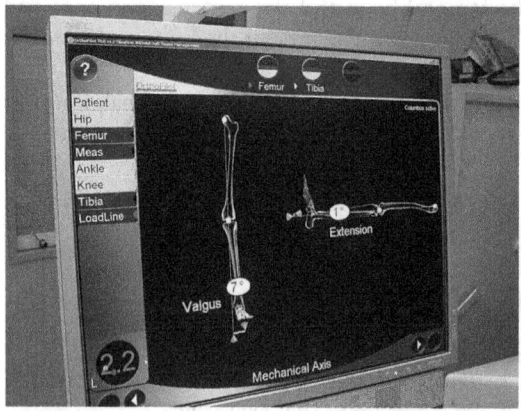

Fig. 20 – Control of lower member alignment in the Orthopilot system (Aesculap / B Braun, Germany).

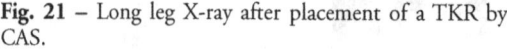

Fig. 21 – Long leg X-ray after placement of a TKR by CAS.

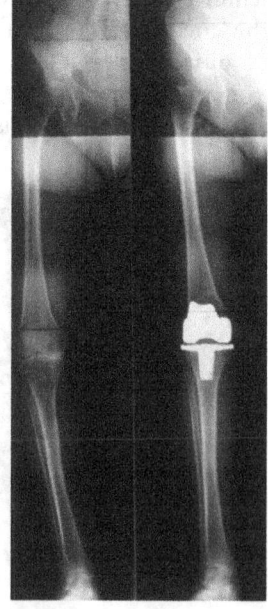

cements using this system, which would represent one of the objectives of this technology (47) (fig. 21).

The information being collected directly from the patient during the operation, a large number of potential and / or cumulative errors (linked to the processing and transmission of images in techniques based on imaging) are avoided. This modular technique may be applied to different types of surgery and of surgeon.

Drawbacks

The gain in accuracy and objectivity of the orientation of instruments undeniably represents an improvement over the traditional technique. Nevertheless, the determination of the relevant preoperative anatomical trackers is still surgeon-dependent as against techniques using the image. It is the surgeon who will palpate the relevant anatomical landmarks, which in theory may represent a source of error. In addition, the absence of preoperative planning certainly constitutes a weakness.

It remains to be seen what degree of accuracy must at present be sought. Currently, traditional techniques make it possible to obtain good results. However it has clearly been shown that, for example, gross errors of alignment of knee prostheses due to technical difficulties or to errors of judgment have proved prejudicial to the long-term results given by these prostheses.

On the other hand, the beneficial results of a perfect anatomical adjustment of implants have not given proof of any significant improvement in longevity using this technique. It is always a question of knowing the threshold of tolerance of poor positioning or of poor ligament balance.

We are nevertheless of opinion that a simple technique, which avoids the grossest errors of alignment or balancing, is certainly useful, in particular to surgeons who carry out relatively few operations. Research on the subject of technology, especially in medicine, must take into account all clinical and economic contingencies to create systems which are useful, capable of being integrated into the operating room, accepted by surgeons and beneficial for the patient and society.

Conclusion

The principal imponderable of this new technique is that of knowing if better anatomical results are going to improve long-term results for patients. On the clinical level, although accuracy is a very important "empirical factor" in the implantation of a knee replacement, the relationship between the adjustment of the prosthesis and the long-term clinical results using these systems has not yet been demonstrated. This question was among the first to be asked on the subject of the robot in orthopaedic surgery, which did not form part of our statement.

On the socio-economic level, the perfect planning of the operation, the elimination or the reduction of traditional mechanical equipment and perhaps longer lasting qualities of prostheses could represent substantial long-term economies. A reliable and robust tool, ensuring the safety of the surgical act, is a plus factor which will rapidly progress from being superfluous to being essential, not only for the sake of the comfort of the act, but first and foremost, in order to meet the requirements of accuracy of a modern society which is subject to strict regulations by insurance companies and to legal pressures.

Lastly, the potential and the implications of computer-assisted orthopaedic surgery as regards both diagnosis and therapy remain to be discovered. Increasingly evolved systems will probably make it gradually possible to extend their application to the complete field of orthopaedic surgery, as well as to that of traumatology.

This technology creates new research and teaching tools which will make it possible to increase understanding of the still poorly mastered field of orthopaedic surgery. It can be expected that it will be possible, in the near future, to completely simulate a surgical act and to establish its bone, ligament, muscular and functional consequences beforehand. This is a new means of exploration, which will in due course redefine the surgery of tomorrow.

However, just as we are far from letting ourselves fly in an aircraft controlled solely by computer, we cannot rely on a "robot surgeon" without human control. Surgical navigation remains a technique which is at present more acceptable than a robot and is undoubtedly better suited to the requirements of orthopaedic surgeons. The doctor-patient relationship and a perfect mastery of medical knowledge and of the surgical act will always remain an essential factor in better patient care and in giving ideal treatment. The computerization of surgery has supplemented and not replaced the practitioner.

References

1. Ayers DC, Dennis DA, Johnson NA *et al.* (1997) Common Complications of Total Knee Arthroplasty. J Bone Joint Surg 79-A(2): 278-311
2. Bargar WL, Bauer A, Borner M (1998) Primary and Revision Total Hip Replacement Using the Robotic System, 354, 82-91
3. Bargren JH, Blaha JD, Freeman MAR (1983) Alignment in Total Knee Arthroplasty: Correlated Biomechanical and Clinical Observations. Clin Orthop 173: 178-83
4. Bauer A (2000) Robot-Assisted Total Hip Replacement in Primary and Revision Cases. Operative Techniques in Orthopaedics 9-13, Vol 10, N° 1 (January)
5. Berger RA, Crosset LS, Jacobs JJ (1998) Malrotation Causing Patellofemoral Complications After Total Knee Arthroplasty 356: 144-53
6. Bettega G, Leitner F, Raoult O, *et al.* (2000) Computer-Assisted Orthognathic Surgery: Consequences of Clinical Evaluation. Springer Publisher, 1008-18
7. Coytes PC, Hawker G, Croxford R (1999) Rates of Revision Knee Replacement in Ontario, Canada, 81-A(6): 773-82
8. Dejour H, Deschamps G (1989) Technique opératoire de la prothèse totale de genou. In: Prothèses totales du genou. Cahier d'Enseignement de la SOFCOT, n° 35: 13-24
9. Dejour H, Neyret P, Boileau P (1994) Anterior Cruciate Reconstruction Combined with Valgus Tibial Osteotomy. Clin Orthop Relat Res 299: 220-8
10. Delp SL, Stulberg SD, Davies B, *et al.* (1998) Computer-Assisted Knee Replacement. Clin Orthop Relat Res 354: 49-56
11. Dessenne V, Lavallee S, Julliard R, *et al.* (1995) Computer-Assisted Knee Anterior Cruciate Ligament Reconstruction: First Clinical Tests. Journal of Image Guided Surgery 1: 59-64

12. DiGioia AM, Jaramaz B, Blackwell M, *et al.* (1998) Image Guided Navigation System to Measure Intra-operatively Acetabular Implant Alignment. Clin Orthop and Relat Res 355: 8-22

13. DiGioia AM, Jaramaz B (1999) Computer-Assisted Tools and Interventional Technologies, The Lancet, 354

14. DiGioia AM, Jaramaz B, Nikou C *et al.* (2000) Surgical Navigation for Total Hip Replacement with the use of HipNav Orthopaedic Techniques in Orthopaedics, 3-8, Vol 10, N° 1(January)

15. Duncan JS, Ayache N (2000) Medical Image Analysis: Progress over Two Decades and the Challenges Ahead. IEEE Transactions on Pattern Analysis and Machine Intelligence, 23(1): 85-105

16. Fadda M, Bertelli D, Martelli S, *et al.* (1997) Computer-Assisted Planning for Total Knee Arthroplasty. In First Joint Conference of CVRMed and MRCAS, Grenoble, France: Springer: 619-28

17. Feng EL, Stulberg SD, Wixson RL (1994) Progressive Subluxation and Polyethylene Wear in Total Knee Replacements with Flat Articular Surfaces. Clin Orthop Relat Res 299: 60-71

18. Fleute M, Lavallee S, Julliard R (1999) Incorporating a statistically-based shape model into a system for computer-assisted anterior cruciate ligament surgery. Medical Image Analysis, Oxford University Press, volume 3: 209-22

19. Freeman MAR (1997) Soft Tissues: A Question of Balance. Knee Arthroplasty: Technique & Management Issues. Orthopaedics: 1-6

20. Ganz R, Klaue K, Vinh JW, *et al.* (1988) A New Periacetabular Osteotomy for the Treatment of Hip Dysplasia, Clin Orthop, 232: 26-36

21. Girardi FP, Cammisa JR, Sandhu HS, *et al.* (1999) The Placement of Lumbar Pedicle Screws Using Computerized Stereotactic. J Bone Joint Surg 81-B: 825-9

22. Hungerford DS, Krackow KA (1985) Alignment in Total Knee Replacement. Clin Orthop 192: 23-33

23. Jaramaz B, DiGioia A, Blackwell M *et al.* (1998) Computer-Assisted Measurement of Cup Placement in Total Hip Replacement, 354: 70-81

24. Julliard R, Lavallee S, Dessenne V (1998) Computer-Assisted Reconstruction of the Anterior Cruciate Ligament. Clin Orthop Relat Res 354: 57-64

25. Kienzle TC, Stulberg SD, Peshkin M *et al.* (1996) A Computer-Assisted Total Knee Replacement Surgical System Using a Calibrated Robot Orthopaedics. In Computer Integrated Surgery, Cambridge, Massachusetts, The MIT Press. RHTaylor Editor: 409-16

26. Kikinis R, Gleason PL, Moriarty TM, *et al.* (1996) Computer-Assisted Three Dimensional Planning for Neurosurgical Procedures. Neurosurgery, 38(4): 640-51

27. Klos TVS, Habets RJE, Banks A, *et al.* (1998) Computer Assistance in Arthroscopic Anterior Cruciate Ligament Reconstruction. Clin Orthop and Relat Res 354: 65-9

28. Krackow KA (1991) Proximal Realignment During Total Knee Arthroplasty of the Valgus Knee. Clin Orthop 273: 9-18

29. Krackow KA, Serpe L, Phillips MJ, *et al.* (1999) A New Technique for Determining Proper Mechanical Axis Alignment during Total Knee Arthroplasty. Orthopedics, 22 (7): 698-701

30. Laine T, Schlenkza D, Makitalo K, *et al.* (1997) Improved Accuracy of Pedicle Screw Insertion with Computer-Assisted Surgery. Spine 22(11): 1254-8

31. Langlotz F, Bachler R, Berlemann U *et al.* (1998) Computer Assistance for Pelvic Osteotomies. Clin Orthop and Relat Res 354: 92-102

32. Laskin RS (1984) Alignment of the Total Knee Components. Orthopaedics 7, 62

33. Laskin RS (2000) Controversies in Total Knee Replacement, Oxford University Press

34. Laskin RS (2000) Total Knee Instruments: You Can't Go on Autopilot! Orthopedics 23: 993-994, September 2000

35. Leitner F, Picard F, Minfeld R, *et al.* (1997) Computer-Assisted Knee Surgical Total Replacement. In First Joint Conference of CVRMed and MRCAS, Grenoble, France Springer: 629-38

36. Marcacci M, Tonet O, Megali G, *et al.* (2000) A Navigation System for Computer-Assisted Unicompartmental Arthroplasty. MICCAI 2000, Pittsburgh, Springer Publisher, 1152-7

37. Matsen FA, Garbini JL, Sidles JA, *et al.* (1993) Robotic Assistance in Orthopaedic Surgery (A proof of principle using distal femoral arthroplasty). Clin Orthop Relat Res 296, 178-86

38. Merloz P, Tonetti J, Pittet L, *et al.* (1998) Pedicle Screw Placement Using Image Guided Techniques. Clin Orthop and Relat Res 354: 39-48

39. Muir P, DiGioia A, Jaramaz B (2000) Computer-Assisted Orthopaedic Surgery: Tools and Technologies in Clinical Practice, 17(5), 34-43

40. Nolte LP, Ganz R (eds.) (1999) Computer-Assisted Orthopedic Surgery, Seattle. Toronto, Bern, Hogrefe & Huber Publishers

41. Ozanian TO, Phillips R (2000) Image Analysis for Computer-Assisted Internal Fixation of Hip Fracture. Medical Image Analysis, 4, 137-59

42. Picard F, Leitner F, Saragaglia D, *et al.* (1997) Mise en Place d'une Prothèse Totale du Genou Assistée par Ordinateur: À propos de 7 implantations sur cadavres. Rev Chir Orthop, 83, Suppl. II, 31

43. Picard F, Moody J, Jaramaz B *et al.* (2000) A Classification Proposal For Computer-Assisted Knee Systems in MICCAI 2000, Pittsburgh , Springer Publisher: 1145-51

44. Picard F, Moody J, Martinek V *et al.* (2000) A Computer-Assisted ACL Reconstruction System. Assessment of two Techniques of Graft Positioning in ACL Reconstruction. MICCAI 2000, Pittsburgh , Springer Publisher: 1136-44

45. Rampersaud YR, Foley KT (2000) Image-Guided Spinal Surgery. Operative Techniques in Orthopaedics, 64-8, Vol 10, N° 1(January)

46. Ritter MA, Faris PM, Keating EM *et al.* (1994) Postoperative Alignment of Total Knee Replacement: its effects on survival. Clin Orthop 299: 153-7

47. Saragaglia D, Picard F, Chaussard C, *et al.* (2001) Mise en place des prothèses totales du genou assistée par ordinateur : comparaison avec la technique conventionnelle. Rev Chir Orthop 87: 18-28

48. Sati M, Staubli HU, Bourquin Y, *et al.* (2000) Clinical Integration of Computer-Assisted Technology for Arthroscopic Anterior Cruciate Ligament Reconstruction. Operative Techniques in Orthopaedics, 40-9, Vol 10, N° 1(January), 2000

49. Stulberg SD, Picard F, Saragaglia D (2000) Computer-Assisted Total Knee Arthroplasty. Orthopaedic Techniques in Orthopaedics, 25-39, Vol 10, N° 1 (January)

50. Vince KG (1993) Principles of Condylar Knee Arthroplasty: Issues Evolving. Chapter 30: 315-24

Conservation of posterior cruciate ligament in fixed-bearing total knee replacement

J.Y. Nordin, Guepar Group

Conservation of the posterior cruciate ligament (PCL) in fixed-bearing total knee replacement is still very controversial (30, 38). The following will be reviewed hereafter:
- anatomy, physiology, and presence of PCL in a diseased knee joint;
- theoretical and practical advantages and drawbacks of PCL retention;
- technical difficulties in cruciate-retaining total knee arthroplasty;
- results of cruciate-retaining total knee replacement (TKR).

Anatomy, physiology, and presence of PCL in a diseased knee joint

PCL is the strongest ligament in the knee. It consists of two bundles which originate from the inferior portion of the lateral aspect of the medial femoral condyle, within a curvilinear area. There is more than 15mm from the inferior portion of this area to the cartilage rim of the condyle. PCL is 38mm long. Its tibial attachment begins on the posterior surface of the proximal tibia and extends to the superior portion of the popliteal surface of the tibia, within the proximal most part of the tibia (27). This anatomic location allows retention of PCL insertions during the distal femoral cut and proximal tibial cut. In cruciate-retaining knee designs, the tibial cut is directed inferiorly and posteriorly, reproducing the posterior slope of the tibia while preserving the middle and posterior portions of the PCL. Elasticity of the posterior cruciate ligament has been studied by Kennedy (40) who found that the percentage of elongation for both bundles is 28.3% and 24% respectively. Race and Amis (59) consider that PCL (length, 32.8 ± 1.95mm) is the knee ligament with the highest ultimate strength; the maximum linear elongation of its anterior bundle is 12.8 ± 5.9 %. This elasticity is a definite advantage in total knee arthroplasty.

The PCL is tight in flexion and lax in extension. Biomechanically, the PCL acts in synergy with the anterior cruciate ligament (ACL) and the lateral ligamentous structures. This role will inevitably be affected by the absence of the ACL as illustrated by Freeman (25): cruciates are like the two shanks of scissors which cannot work independently. In flexion, it prevents posterior translation of the tibia and promotes femoral rollback on the tibia, thus increasing quadriceps lever arm. It further acts as a joint stabilizer in the AP plane, mainly in flexion, in cases where the lateral ligamentous structures are overstretched (56). Resection of the PCL brings the collateral ligaments to a more vertical position and increases the joint space (more in flexion: 2 to 4mm on average, than in extension).

Whereas the ACL is often absent or deficient in degenerative, inflammatory or post-traumatic knee pathologies amenable to total knee replacement, it must be pointed out that in Scott's series (1982), the PCL was present in 99% of the knees, and in Aubriot's series, it was normal in 71% of the knees or subnormal in 22%. Even in rheumatoid patients, Sledge and Walker (37) found functional posterior cruciate ligaments in more than 2,000 knees; only in 3 cases the PCL was absent, and in other 3 cases it had to be sacrificed to correct an irreducible flexion contracture.

The mechanical benefits of PCL in knees with degenerative or inflammatory joint disease are very much debated. The impact of ageing of PCL has been emphasized by Aglietti, Caton, and Goutallier (28) who noted histological changes to the PCL whenever the ACL was deficient or absent, which is generally the case in these pathologies. However, this criticism should also apply to collateral ligaments, and yet, their function as postoperative stabilizers of knee prostheses has never been called into question.

Theoretical and practical advantages and drawbacks of PCL retention

Retention of the PCL has many theoretical advantages:

– The PCL promotes femoral rollback which results in increased flexion, provided that physiological conditions are good and implant design, particularly the tibial component, is appropriate. It further increases the quadriceps lever arm by 20 to 30%, which increases knee extension power that is particularly useful where prior patellectomy has been performed. However, Huang (35) and Bolanos (12) did not note any difference in muscle power between cruciate-retaining and cruciate-sacrificing prostheses;

– The PCL takes up most of shear forces in flexion, thus decreasing the amount of shear forces transferred to the prosthesis and, of course, to the bone-cement interface, which reduces the potential for loosening;

– According to Andriacchi (2) and as suggested by the works of Mihalko, Miller and Krackow (53, 54) on fresh cadaver specimens, PCL maintains a balanced flexion space at 90° and increases AP stability of the prosthetic knee. Once ACL and menisci have been excised and one centimeter of the proximal tibia has been resected, resection of the PCL results in increased flexion gap at 90° with a mean distraction space of 5.26 ± 1.9mm;

– The PCL is a very important stabilizer of the knee in the AP plane. This is confirmed by the fact that after release of the medial ligamentous structures and resection of the PCL, valgus laxity is 6.9° in extension and 13.4° at 90° of flexion. In contrast, when the PCL is retained, the same release will only result in 5.2° of laxity in extension and 8.7° in flexion. Similarly, after release of the lateral ligamentous structures and resection of the PCL, varus laxity is 8.9° in extension and 18° in flexion, whereas when the PCL is retained, the same release produces only 5.4° of laxity in extension and 4.9° at 90° of flexion. Therefore, the PCL acts as a third centrally positioned collateral ligament that limits varus-valgus movements (1) mainly in flexion, but also in extension, which likely explains the low rate of postoperative instability in cruciate-retaining total knee arthroplasty, except in the rare instances where capsuloligamentous structures on the convex side are severely overstretched;

– The PCL prevents posterior translation of the tibia in flexion (posterior drawer) since it is tight in flexion;

– The PCL helps maintain the instant center of rotation and therefore automatic external rotation and patellar tracking;

– The PCL resists lateral lift-off of the tibial component when loaded in flexion, and varus shift in a correctly aligned knee. As a result, stresses on the medial tibiofemoral compartment and at the tibial bone-cement prosthesis interface are reduced. If large contact areas are maintained, there is no increase in stresses on the PE tibial bearing or PE tibial component;

– Retention of the PCL improves knee proprioception. As a matter of fact, although Barrett (5), Franchi (24), and then Fuchs (26) claimed that the number of receptors in the posterior cruciate ligament is reduced in the elderly and even lower in the arthritic patient, Del Valle (16) demonstrated in his immuno-histochemical analysis the presence of mechanoreceptors in PCL even in arthritic patients. Warren (77) emphasized the role of PCL in knee proprioception, contrary to Cash (14), Lattanzio (45), Simmons (65), and Laskin (43) in rheumatoid knees. In spite of these conflicting opinions, it seems logical to consider that maintenance of proprioception, even attenuated, is far more preferable to loss of proprioception from resection of the PCL.

Knee replacement must provide restoration of the preoperative PCL tension and native ligament's orientation. This is why the geometry of components is of paramount importance. Walker and Garg (75) showed that a taut PCL leads to decreased flexion, and that some factors improve flexion. The most important factor, as emphasized by Whiteside (79), is restoration of the preoperative posterior tibial slope. Singerman (66) also stressed its influence on PCL strain and its impact on flexion, even with variations as small as 5-8°. Conversely, severe increase in the tibial slope may lead to anterior subluxation of the tibia if the ACL is absent (according to Migaud [52]), and to severe wear of the posterior aspect of the tibial component (according to Besson [10]). Booth (11) pointed out the significant influence of postoperative joint line level on PCL function: any change greater than 4mm in the joint line position is detrimental to kinematics of a cruciate-retaining knee prosthesis, whereas a posterior stabilized prosthesis can cope with a change greater than 8mm. One easily understands the critical importance of using a rigorous surgical technique and accurate instruments. Emodi (21) also agrees with this. However, restoring PCL to normal tension is difficult. Incavo (36), in his cadaver study, achieved restoration of adequate tension and near normal femoral rollback in only 2 out of 8 cases, whereas Mahoney (48) did not. Kim's analysis (41) is in agreement with this. Udomkiat (69) achieved restoration of a physiological femoral rollback in only 2 out of 10 cases in cruciate-preserving total knee arthroplasty, and noted anterior translation of the femur during flexion in the other cases.

Excessive PCL tightness causes anterior subluxation and anterior lift-off of the trial tibial component; Ritter (60), Worland (83), Arima (4), Hofmann and Pace (31), as well as Whiteside (78) suggested partly releasing the PCL to preserve the benefits of cruciate retention. In contrast, in Besson's study (10) involving 44 Miller Galante cruciate-retaining prostheses, posterior laxity was evaluated using Telos™ arthrometer, and functional results were compared with those in a control series; the conclusion was that where the PCL is not tight enough and posterior laxity is equal to or greater than 5mm, an average of 9.8 points decrease in the HSS score is noted.

To achieve all this, particularly restoration of near normal knee kinematics using the adaptive capacity of the PCL within physiological limits, and despite the absence of the ACL, the design of the prosthesis must be well thought out and feature a truly diverging femoral component, and a tibial component that is asymmetric in all three planes (17, 68, 70, 71). One cannot evaluate the results of a cruciate-retaining TKR and possibly compare them with those of other knees, not knowing its design (*i.e.*, tibiofemoral and patellofemoral joint design and contact areas).

One of the drawbacks of PCL retention is a potential inefficiency or secondary failure which sometimes leads to instability and pain.

Laskin (43) compared the results achieved in three series of total knee replacements with a mean follow-up of 8.2 years (minimum, 6 years). The first series consisted of 98 knees with rheumatoid arthritis (RA) managed with cruciate-retaining TKRs. The second series consisted of 80 RA knees managed with posterior stabilized TKRs, and the third one included 599 arthritic knees (OA knees) managed with cruciate-retaining TKRs. In the first series, there was more than 10mm of posterior laxity in 50% of the knees and recurvatum in 13%. In the second series, there was more than 10mm of posterior instability in 1% of the knees, but no recurvatum. In the third series, there was more than 10mm of posterior laxity in 14% of the knees and recurvatum in 0.2%. This study suggests that PCL attrition occurs and may lead to secondary rupture; attrition is more significant in RA knees than in OA knees, whereas posterior stabilized prostheses prevent recurvatum while minimizing potential for posterior laxity.

In one of his presentations during a SOFCOT meeting, Huten also emphasized the potential for secondary laxity with Wallaby 1 cruciate-retaining total knee prostheses, particularly in rheumatoid patients.

Montgomery and Goodman (55), in 150 cruciate-retaining total knee arthroplasties, reported 3 secondary ruptures of the PCL leading to instability.

Shai's study (63) involved 61 press-fit cruciate retaining total knee replacements in 38 patients, with a mean follow-up of 11 years. No patient was lost to follow-up. 14 patients died. Results suggest a very mild impairment of the PCL function: 1 knee had 5° of hyperextension with occasional instability, and 4 asymptomatic knees had 3° of hyperextension. Two knees were revised, one for synovectomy, and the other one for a patellar problem, but none for posterior instability.

Practical advantages of PCL retention

– In the majority of cases, retention of the PCL allows maintenance of the joint line level, provided that the amount of bone removed from the distal femur corresponds to the thickness of the prosthetic condyles, thus avoiding the risk of patella baja as often seen in posterior stabilized TKA.

– Decreased tightness of collateral ligaments in flexion as compared to PCL-sacrificing TKA.

– Lower incidence of instability and prosthetic dislocation than in posterior stabilized TKA (34, 46, 64, 76).

– Patellar clunk syndrome (8, 47) which is due to wedging of a suprapatellar fibrous nodule into the intercondylar notch is only exceptionally observed in cruciate-retaining TKA, whereas the rate of occurrence in posterior stabilized TKA ranges from 1 to 3.5%.

– The design of the femoral component usually makes it possible to perform retrograde femoral nailing for treatment of a supracondylar fracture (a currently very popular technique for treatment of fractures after total knee arthroplasty).

– Krackow (42) claimed that retention of the PCL simplifies soft tissue balancing since in TKA indications, its length is almost unchanged and can be used as a reference for ligament balancing, thus avoiding notable changes to the joint line. But this assumption was questioned by Sorger (67).

– As regards *in vivo* analysis of knee kinematics, Andriacchi's study (in 1982) (1) showed the advantage of retaining the PCL for stair climbing, which was confirmed in Dorr's study (20) in 1988. Kelman (39) showed the advantage of retaining the PCL both for stair climbing and stair descending. Migaud (51) studied in 1995 the behaviour of 19 total knee replacements of four different designs (Hermes which retains both cruciates, Osteonics which retains the PCL and has a relatively constrained tibial component, Miller Galante which retains the PCL and has a flat tibial design, IBS posterior stabilized total knee prosthesis). His results show that retention of both cruciates does not have any positive influence on knee kinematics (particularly automatic external rotation), and that prostheses which retain the PCL provide higher flexion ROM during walking and stair climbing / descending than those which sacrifice the PCL, although the difference is not significant.

Technical difficulties in cruciate-retaining total knee arthroplasty

As Hungerford and Krackow with the PCA knee and Whiteside with his own designs, for many years, surgeons of the Guepar Group have tremendously expanded the indications for PCL retention.

In a knee with mild bone deformity and good range of motion, the femoral cuts are generally performed before the tibial cut. The distal femoral cut is referenced off the more prominent distal condyle and removes an amount of bone that corresponds to the thickness of the femoral component. The posterior femoral cut is referenced off the anterior surface of the distal femur, in the supratrochlear area. Owing to the offset design of femoral components, the amount of bone removed from the posterior femoral condyles corresponds exactly to the thickness of the posterior part of the femoral component, which places the femoral component in external rotation. Some cutting guides are designed to provide a 3° externally rotated femoral cut. Otherwise, the amount of external rotation depends on anatomic conditions; in a valgus knee, there will be a necessary trade-off between the Whiteside line, the transepicondylar axis, the posterior condyle line, and even the tibial cut (in cases where the tibial cut has been performed first to balance the knee in flexion). The tibial cut slopes posteriorly between 3° and 5°, rarely 7°, to reproduce the preoperative posterior tibial slope of the patient's knee.

An irreducible varus deformity is generally not a problem; as a matter of fact, convex-side laxity is a rare occurrence. In knees with severe fixed varus deformities, after release of superficial MCL from its tibial attachment in continuity with the periosteum, hamstring tendons, semimembranosus and posteromedial corner, possibly the posteromedial capsule, and exceptionally, the popliteus and soleus arch, the PCL may be overly tensioned and restrict range of motion. Some authors suggested performing true PCL lengthening. As a matter of fact, in our technique, we often perform partial release of the anterior fibers of the PCL at the tibia at the same time as we remove the resected tibial bone fragment. We do not systematically try to keep a small island of bone to protect the proximal anterior insertion of the PCL. This reduces the risk of complete detachment of the ligament or fracture-avulsion of the distal insertion of the PCL. But on the other hand, in flexion, the PCL loses the "reflection pulley" formed by this bony island. The tibial cut is performed with reference to the lateral tibial condyle. Reconstruction of the medial bone loss is sometimes necessary to preserve integrity of the PCL fibers; this is performed using bone grafts, a metal augment, or even cement if it is a small-size bone defect.

An irreducible valgus deformity is technically challenging, particularly if there is convex-side laxity. In the most severe cases, a lateral approach is used (Keblish technique). One critical technical point is reconstruction of the knee with reference to the medial tibiofemoral compartment. Lateral release procedures which used to be performed during the first surgical step are now performed in two stages: mild release at the beginning of the procedure, adjusted according to the tests performed in extension and flexion; fine-tuning after insertion of the trials. Release of lateral capsuloligamentous structures involves the tensor fascia lata which is released from its insertion on Gerdy's tubercle, taking care to maintain continuity with the fascia of the leg; it is rarely lengthened by making multiple incisions or so-called scarifications, or a true Z lengthening at the distal thigh. Release of the LCL and popliteus, more rarely the biceps femoris and lateral capsule, is necessary, especially if one selectively evaluates the structures which prevent correction of the valgus deformity in extension and flexion. Burdin's technique (13) is effective in relieving tension on the LCL and popliteus through release of their combined insertion attached to a bone block that is moved to the cutaneous aspect of the lateral femoral condyle and fixed with a screw, after correction of the valgus deformity.

The distal femoral cut is equal to the thickness of the prosthetic condyles and is referenced off the medial femoral condyle. The posterior femoral cuts are performed, based on the previously mentioned criteria. The lateral tibial condyle may need to be reconstructed with bone grafts or a metal augment. Sometimes, in severe valgus deformities, distal and even posterior femoral bone defects also need to be reconstructed on the lateral side, since the distal femoral cut is referenced off the medial femoral condyle and removes an amount of bone that is equal to the thickness of the femoral component. Whiteside (80) made a publication in 1999 in which he claimed that in 231 knees with valgus deformities of up to 45°, 13 only could not be managed with a cruciate-retaining prosthesis and received a posterior stabilized implant. He further emphasized that in valgus deformities greater than 25°, tibial and femoral bone grafts were used in many cases, 100% of the time sometimes in the most severely affected knees.

One of the major issues when implanting a cruciate-retaining TKR in a severe fixed valgus deformity is overstretching of the medial capsuloligamentous structures which may require tightening of the superficial MCL, using various tricks such as: bone block with the attached femoral insertion of PCL, reattached and secured with screws or staples; tightening of MCL on the proximal tibia; suturing of MCL using the overlapping technique. But of course, despite the stabilizing effect of the PCL, all these techniques carry a risk of secondary laxity. In view of the difficulty to correct a valgus deformity after extensive lateral release, and the risk of secondary laxity, surgeons often prefer to use a posterior stabilized knee (more or less constrained) rather than a cruciate-retaining knee.

In flexion contractures greater than 25°, restoration of full extension may require more than simple capsular release, resection of posterior osteophytes, and a thicker distal femoral cut flush with the condylar insertions of the PCL. In this situation, rather than lengthening the PCL (a possible option), implanting a posterior stabilized prosthesis seems more appropriate (11).

It must be reminded that PCL retention requires careful assessment of its status: if too lax, a thicker tibial insert must be used; if too tight, it must be released, at least partly. Should rupture or detachment of the PCL occur intraoperatively, an ultracongruent tibial insert (32) can be used in preference to a posterior stabilized prosthesis.

In conclusion, we can say that, most of the time, PCL retention is technically possible in total knee arthroplasty. In knees with severe fixed valgus deformities, particularly with overstretched medial capsuloligamentous structures, in knees with fixed varus deformities, and in knees with flexion contractures greater than 25°, the use of a posterior stabilized prosthesis is more reasonable and sometimes necessary (Pereira [58]).

Results of cruciate-retaining total knee replacement

To be in a position to support PCL retention, one must keep in mind the excellent results reported in Insall's series of cruciate-sacrificing TKRs which are the "gold standard" in total knee arthroplasty.

The published results of some series of cruciate-retaining TKRs show survivorship rates and good / very good results which compare favourably with those in cruciate-sacrificing TKRs:

– AGC (Anatomic Graduated Components): Meding (44) published in 2001 the 10-year results of 387 TKRs with a tibial insert only 4.4mm thick. Using revision or loosening as the endpoint, the survivorship rates were 98.7%, 95.4%, and 94.3% at 5 years, 10 years, and 15 years, respectively;

– Vazquez-Vela Johnson (72) studied patient demographics as a predictor of the ten years survival rate in 562 primary TKRs implanted from November 1986 to September 1990. The overall results showed a survival of 96.8% at 14 years with 1.44% lost to follow-up. The best results were seen in non-obese women with osteoarthritis who were less than 60 years of age in whom there was 10 years follow-up of 99.4%; the worst results were observed in obese men with osteoarthritis who were less than 60 years: 10 years survival of 35.7%;

– Berend and Ritter (7) highlighted 4 distinct failures mechanisms in tibial component revision after reporting a survival rate of this implant of 98.9% at 10 and 15 years with no knees revised for PE wear or osteolysis;

– Meding (50) published a series of 212 TKR in rheumatoid arthritis. Excluding infections and failed metal-backed patellas the survival rate at 10, 15 and 20 years were 99.5%, 97.9% and 96.5% respectively;

– GENESIS: Laskin (44) studied 100 total knee replacements for treatment of osteoarthritis, with a 10-year follow-up. The PCL was excised in 44 knees for combined flexion contracture and frontal deviation greater than 15-20°. The survivorship rate was 96% in cruciate-retaining TKRs, with a mean ROM of 117°, 76% of excellent results, and 20% of good results. In contrast, the 56 cruciate-sacrificing posterior stabilized TKRs had a survivorship of 97%, with 114° of flexion, 75% of excellent results, and 23% of good results;

– KALI (Guepar Group): in a series of 698 TKRs, using all indications for revision surgery, except sepsis, as the endpoint, the survivorship rates were 96%, 90% and 86% at 10 years, 12 years, and 15 years, respectively;

– KINEMATIC: In 1998, Ansari (3) reported the results achieved in 445 TKAs: survivorship rate was 96% at 10-year follow-up, using revision or indication for revision as the endpoint; there were 84% of excellent and good results (according to the HSS score); mean ROM was 100°. In 1999, Ewald (19) evaluated the results of 306 TKRs with a mean follow-up of between 10 and 14 years: the survivorship rate was 96%, and there were 81.3% of excellent and good results. In 2001, Sextro (62) published the 15-year results of 168 Kinematic I knees implanted at the Mayo Clinic: mean HSS score was 87.9; the survivorship rate was 88.7% (excluding infections), and mean flexion was 106°;

– KINEMAX: Wright (84) reported a series of 523 knees which had primary TKR between January 1988 and April 1991. The mean age of the patients at time of the surgery was 69 years. The probability of survival at 10 years was 96.1% with revision for any reason as the end point and 97.2% when only aseptic failures were considered;

– MILLER GALANTE: Berger (9) compared 172 Type I TKRs with a mean follow-up of 11 years versus 109 Type II TKRs with a 9-year follow-up.

The differences essentially involved the tibiofemoral compartment and resulted in an increase in the 10-year survivorship rate from 84.1% to 100%. This shows that sometimes the outcome of total knee arthroplasty is not related to retention or sacrifice of the PCL;

– NATURAL KNEE: Hoffman (32) reported a series of 176 uncemented prostheses out of 300 TKRs with a mean follow-up of 12 years. The survivorship rate, including revision for infection and simple tibial insert replacement, was 93.4%, or 95.1% when excluding these two criteria; mean flexion was 120°;

– ORTHOLOC I (porous coated knee, without metal-backed patellar component): in 2001, Whiteside (81) reported a survivorship rate of 98.6% at 18-year follow-up in a series of 265 prostheses, 5 of which had been lost to follow-up. Mean flexion was 112°;

– PRESS FIT CONDYLAR CRUCIATE RETAINING:

• Rodricks (61) reported 160 consecutive TKRs with this device implanted between 1986 and 1989 with mean age of the patients being 70.5 years at the time of index procedure. At mean of 15.8 years the overall survival rate of the knee was 91.5% with revision for any reason and 97.2% with aseptic loosening as estimate the end point;

• Fehring (23) studied the factors influencing wear and osteolysis in this type of prosthesis. For the 1,287 of 2,016 knees with more than 5 years follow-up, the prevalence of wear-related failure was 8.3%. The 13-year survivorship for all patients was 82.6%. It was impossible to identify one factor as the defining reason for these wear-related failures;

• Dixon (19) reported a consecutive series of 139 TKAs performed by one surgeon. The survival rate without revision or a need for any reoperation was 92.6% at 15 years;

• Vessely (73) reviewed 1,008 consecutive TKRs from January 1987 to August 1989. Mean follow-up of living patients with their TKA components in situ (244 patients, 331 knees) was 15.7 years. Survivorship at 15 years for revision for any reason, revision for mechanical failure, and revision for aseptic loosening were 95.9%, 97.0%, and 98.8% respectively;

– PROFIX Cementless: Hardeman (29) reported a consecutive series of 115 TKRs. The estimate of implant survival at 10 years was 97.1%;

– TOTAL CONDYLAR (cruciate-retaining design): Ritter (60) evaluated a series of 394 prostheses followed for 1 to 18 years (mean, 8 years): the survivorship rate was 96.8% at 12-year follow-up;

– WALLABY I (assymetrical and divergent femoral condyles as well as asymmetrical plateaus): Witwoët and GUEPAR (82) evaluated the results of a prospective series of the first 425 TKRs implanted from December 1992 to February 1995. Mean patient age at implantation was 70.5 years. 315 prostheses were followed for more than 5 years (5-9 years) with mean follow-up of 6.3 years. Prosthesis survival at 8 years was 97.7% considering all reasons for prosthesis removal and 98.5% for removal for aseptic loosening.

Dejour (15), Pagnano (57), Vinciguerra (74), published comparative studies of two series of cruciate-retaining and cruciate-sacrificing prostheses. The clinical and / or radiological results did not show any significant difference in favor of cruciate-retaining prostheses. Becker's study (6) involving 30 patients with a cruciate-retaining prosthesis on one side and a cruciate-substituting prosthesis on the contralateral side, did not show any significant difference at 5-year follow-up.

Conclusion

Retaining or sacrificing the PCL is above all a matter of personal convictions, and practical and theoretical benefits, most of which have not been contradicted by clinical experience despite paradoxical anterior femoral translation during deep flexion commonly observed by Dennis and Komistek (18) in PCL staring, TKA. Although the retained PCL does not consistently reproduce the femoral rollback on the tibia, it seems to decrease the incidence of prosthetic instability. On the other hand, PCL retention carries the risk, although rare, of secondary rupture. Different views regarding retention or sacrifice of the PCL in fixed-bearing knee designs are perfectly acceptable, even though from a technical standpoint, almost every knee is amenable to cruciate-retaining TKA if performed by a surgeon who has enough experience to expand its indications.

But a longer follow-up will be necessary to check the validity of the cruciate-retaining option, particularly as regards quality of fixation and polyethylene wear, provided that prosthetic components have an appropriate design.

References

1. Andriacchi TP, Galante JO, Fermier RW (1982) The influence of total knee replacement design on walking and stair climbing. J Bone Joint Surg 64-A: 1328-35
2. Andriacchi TP, Galante JO (1988) Retention of the posterior cruciate in total knee arthroplasty. J Arthroplasty 3 oct suppl. 13-9
3. Ansari S, Ackroyd CE, Newman JH (1998) Kinematic posterior cruciate ligament-retain total knee replacements. A ten-year survivorship study of 445 arthroplasties. Am J Knee Surg 11 (1): 9-14
4. Arima J, Whiteside LA, Martin JW et al. (1998) Effect of partial release of the posterior cruciate ligament in total knee arthroplasty. Clin Orthop 353: 194-202
5. Barrett DS, CobbAG, Bentley G (1991) Joint proprioception in normal osteoarthritic and replaced knees. J Bone Joint Surg 73-B: 53-6
6. Becker MW, Insall JN, Faris PM (1991) Bilateral total knee arthroplasty. One cruciate retaining and one cruciate substituting. Clin Orthop 271: 122-4
7. Berend ME, Ritter MA, Meding JB et al. (2004) Tibial component failure mechanisms in total knee arthroplasty. Clin Orthop Relat Res Nov (428): 26-34
8. Beight JL, Binnan Yao, Hozack WJ et al. (1994) The patellar clunk syndrome after posterior stabilized total knee arthroplasty. Clin Orthop 299: 139-42
9. Berger RA, Rosenberg AG, Barden RM et al. (2001) Long-term follow-up of the Miller-Galante total knee replacement. Clin Orthop 388: 58-67
10. Besson A, Brazier J, Chantelot C et al. (1999) Laxity and functional results of Miller-Galante total knee prosthesis with posterior cruciate ligament sparing after a 6-year follow-up. Rev Chir Orthop 85: 797-802
11. Booth RE Jr (1999) The price of PCL retention in TKA is too high. Orthopedics 12: 1125

12. Bolanos AA, Colizza WA, McCann PD *et al.* (1998) A comparison of isokinetic strength testing and gait analysis in patients with posterior cruciate-retaining and substituting knee arthroplasties. J Arthroplasty 13: 906-15

13. Burdin P (1996) L'équilibre ligamentaire dans les prothèses de genou.Ann Orthop Ouest 28:19-30

14. Cash RM, Gonzalez MH, Garst J *et al.* (1996) Proprioception after arthroplasty: role of the posterior cruciate ligament. Clin Orthop 331: 172-8

15. Dejour D, Deschamps G, Garotta L *et al.* (1999) Laxity in posterior cruciate sparing and posterior stabilized total knee prostheses. Clin Orthop 364: 182-93

16. Del Valle ME, Harwin SF, Maestro A *et al.* (1998) Immunohistochemical analysis of mechanoreceptors in the human posterior cruciate ligament: a demonstration of its proprioceptive role and clinical relevance. J Arthroplasty 13, 8: 916-22

17. Dennis DA, Komistek RD, Colwell CE *et al.* (1998) *In vivo* anteroposterior femorotibial translation of total knee arthroplasty: a multicenter analysis. Clin Orthop 356: 47-57

18. Dennis DA, Komistek RD, Mahfouz MR *et al.* (2003) Multicenter determination of *in vivo* kinematics after total knee arthroplasty. Clin Orthop Relat Res Nov (416): 37-57

19. Dixon MC, Brown RR, Parsch D *et al.* (2005) Modular fixed-bearing total knee arthroplasty with retention of the posterior cruciate ligament. A study of patients followed for a minimum of fifteen years. J Bone Joint Surg Am March 87(3): 598-603

20. Dorr LD, Ochsner JL, Gronley J *et al.* (1988) Functional comparison of posterior cruciate-retained versus cruciate-sacrificed total knee arthroplasty. Clin Orthop 236: 36-43

21. Emodi GJ, Callaghan JJ, Pedersen DR *et al.* (1999) Posterior cruciate ligament function following total knee arthroplasty: the effect of joint line elevation. Iowa Orthop J 19: 82-92

22. Ewald FC, Wright RJ, Poss R *et al.* (1999) Kinematic total knee arthroplasty: A 10- to 14-year prospective follow-up review. J Arthroplasty 14 (4): 473-80

23. Fehring TK, Murphy JA, Hayes TD *et al.* (2004) Factors influencing wear and osteolysis in press-fit condylar modular total knee replacements. Clin Orthop 428: 40-50

24. Franchi A, Zaccherotti G, Aglietti P (1995) Neural system of the human posterior cruciate ligament in osteoarthritis. J Arthroplasty 10: 679-82

25. Freeman MA, Railton GT (1988) Should the posterior cruciate ligament be retained or resected in condylar nonmeniscal knee arthroplasty? The case for resection. J Arthroplasty 3 Suppl: 3-12

26. Fuchs S, Thorwesten L, Niewerth S (1999) Proprioceptive function in knees with and without total knee arthroplasty. Am J Phys Med Rehabil 78: 39-45

27. Girgis FG, Marshall JL, Al Monajem ARS (1975) The cruciate ligaments of the knee joint. Clin Orthop 106: 216

28. Goutallier D, Allain J, Le Mouel S *et al.* (1998) Évaluation de l'état histologique du ligament croisé postérieur en fonction de l'état macroscopique du ligament croisé antérieur : Intérêt pour l'indication des prothèses conservant le ou les ligaments croisés. Rev Chir Orthop 84 suppl 2: 30

29. Hardeman F, Vandenneucker H, Van Lauwe J *et al.* (2006) Cementless total knee arthroplasty with Profix: a 8- to 10-year follow-up study. Knee December 13(6): 419-21; Epub 2006 Oct 24

30. Hirsch HS, Lotke PA, Morrison LD (1994) The posterior cruciate ligament in total knee surgery. Save, sacrifice, or substitute? Clin Orthop 309: 64-8

31. Hofmann AA, Pace TB (1994) Cruciate ligament retention in total knee arthroplasty. Knee surgery. Edited by Fu FH, Harner CD, Vince KG. Williams & Wilkins. Vol 2: 1313-20

32. Hofmann AA, Tkach TK, Evanich CJ *et al.* (2000) Posterior stabilization in total knee arthroplasty with use of an ultracongruent polyethylene insert. J Arthroplasty 15: 576-83

33. Hofmann AA, Evanich JD, Ferguson RP *et al.* (2000) Ten to 14-year clinical follow-up of the cementless natural knee system. Clinical Orthopaedics 388: 85-94

34. Hossain S, Ayeko C, Anwar M *et al.* (2001) Dislocation of Insall-Burstein II modified total knee arthroplasty. J Arthroplasty 16: 233-5

35. Huang CH, Lee YM, Liau JJ et al. (1998) Comparison of muscle strength of posterior cruciate-retained versus cruciate-sacrificed total knee arthroplasty. J Arthroplasty 13: 779-83

36. Incavo SJ, Johnson CC, Beynnon BD *et al.* (1994) Posterior cruciate ligament strain biomechanics in total knee arthroplasty. Clin Orthop 309: 88-93
37. Insall JN (1984) Surgery of the knee. Churchill Livingstone New York, Edinburgh, London, and Melbourn
38. Insall JN (1998) Presidential adresss to the Knee Society. Choices and compromises in total knee arthroplasty. Clin Orthop 226: 43-8
39. Kelman GJ, Biden EN, Wyatt MP *et al.* (1989) Gait laboratory analysis of a posterior cruciate-sparing total knee arthroplasty in stair ascent and descent. Clin Orthop 248: 21-5
40. Kennedy JC, Hawkins RJ, Willis RB *et al.* (1976) Tension studies of human knee ligament. J Bone and Joint Surg (Am) 58: 350-5
41. Kim H, Pelker RR, Gibson DH *et al.* (1997) Rollback in posterior cruciate ligament-retaining total knee arthroplasty. A radiographic analysis. J Arthroplasty 12: 553-61
42. Krackow KA (1990) The surgical procedure of total knee arthroplasty. In: Krakow KA (ed) Total Knee Arthroplaty. CV Mosby, Philadelphia: 168-237
43. Laskin RS, O'Flynn HM (1997) The Insall Award. Total knee replacement with posterior cruciate ligament retention in rheumatoid arthritis. Problems and complications. Clin Orthop 345: 24-8
44. Laskin RS (2001) The genesis total knee prosthesis: a 10-year follow-up study. Clinical Orthopaedics 388: 95-102
45. Lattanzio PJ, Chess DG, MacDermid JC (1998) Effect of the posterior cruciate ligament in knee-joint proprioception in total knee arthroplasty. J Arthroplasty 13: 580-5
46. Lombardi AV, Mallory TH, Vaughn BK (1993) Dislocation following primary posterior-stabilized total knee arthroplasty. J Arthroplasty 8: 633-9
47. Lucas TS, DeLuca PF, Nazarian DG (1999) Arthroscopic treatment of patellar clunk. Clin Orthop 367: 226-9
48. Mahoney OM, Noble PC, Rhoads DD *et al.* (1994) Posterior cruciate function following total knee arthroplasty. A biomechanical study. J Arthroplasty 9: 569-78
49. Meding JB, Ritter MA, Faris PM (2001) Total knee arthrosplasty with 4.4mm of tibial polyethylene: 10-year follow-up. Clinical Orthopaedics 388: 112-7
50. Meding JB, Keating EM, Ritter MA *et al.* (2004) Long-term follow-up of posterior cruciate retaining TKR in patients with rheumatoid arthritis. Clin Orth 428: 146-52
51. Migaud H, Gougeon F, Diop A *et al.* (1995) Kinematic *in vivo* analysis of the knee: a comparative study of 4 types of total knee prostheses. Rev Chir Orthop 81: 198-210
52. Migaud H, de Ladoucette A, Dohin B *et al.* (1996) Influence of posterior tibial slope on anterior tibial translation and mobility after a non constrained total knee arthroplasty. Rev Chir Orthop 82: 7-13
53. Mihalko WM, Krackow KA (1999) Posterior cruciate ligament effects on the flexion space in total knee arthroplasty. Clin Orthop 360: 243-50
54. Mihalko WM, Miller C, Krackow KA (2000) Total knee arthroplasty ligament balancing and gap kinematics with posterior cruciate ligament retention and sacrifice. Am J Orthop 29: 610-6
55. Montgomery RL, Goodman SB, Csongradi J (1993) Late rupture of the posterior cruciate ligament after total knee replacement. Iowa Orthop J 13: 167-70
56. Newmann A (1993) Postoperative return of motion in MCL/ACL injuries. The effect of MCL rupture location. Ann J Sports Med 21 1: 20-5
57. Pagnano MW, Hanssen AD, Lewallen DG *et al.* (1998) Flexion instability after primary posterior cruciate retaining total knee arthroplasty. Clin Orthop 356: 39-46
58. Pereira DS, Jaffe FF, Ortiguera C (1998) Posterior cruciate ligament-sparing versus posterior cruciate ligament-sacrificing arthroplasty. Functional results using the same prosthesis. J Arthroplasty 13: 138-44
59. Race A, Amis AA (1992) Mechanical properties of the two bundles of the human posterior cruciate ligament. Trans Orthop Res Soc 17: 124
60. Ritter MA, Berend ME, Meding JB *et al.* (2000) Long-term follow-up of anatomic gratuated components posterior cruciate-retaining total knee replacement. Clinical Orthopaedics 388: 51-7
61. Rodricks DJ, Patil S, Pulido P *et al.* (2007) Press-fit condylar design total knee arthroplasty. Fourteen- to seventeen-year follow-up. J Bone Joint Surg Am January 89(1): 89-95

62. Sextro GS, Berry DJ, Rand JA (2001) Totol knee arthroplasty using cruciate-retaining kinematic condylar prosthesis. Clinical Orthopaedics 388: 33-40
63. Shai PA, Scott RD, Thornill TS (1999) TKR with PCL retention in rheumatoid arthritis, problems and complications. Clin Ortho 367: 96-106
64. Sharkey PF, Hozack WJ, Booth RE et al. (1992) Posterior dislocation of total knee arthroplasty. Clin Orthop 278: 128-33
65. Simmons S, Lephart S, Rubash H et al. (1996) Proprioception following total knee arthroplasty with and without the posterior cruciate ligament. J Arthroplasty 11: 763-8
66. Singerman R, Dean JC, Pagan HD et al. (1996) Decreased posterior tibial slope increases strain in the posterior cruciate ligament following total knee arthroplasty. J Arthroplasty 11: 99-103
67. Sorger JI, Federle D, Kirk PG et al. (1997) The posterior cruciate ligament in total knee arthroplasty. J Arthroplasty 12: 869-79
68. Stiehl JB, Komistek RD, Dennis DA (1999) Detrimental kinematics of a flat on flat total condylar knee arthroplasty. Clin Orthop 365: 139-48
69. Udomkiat P, Meng BJ, Dorr LD et al. (2000) Functional comparison of posterior cruciate retention and substitution knee replacement. Clin Orthop 378: 192-201
70. Uvehammer J, Karrholm J, Brandsson S (2000) In vivo kinematics of total knee arthroplasty: Concave versus posterior stabilized tibial joint surface. J Bone Joint Surg (Br) 82-B: 499-505
71. Uvehammer J, Karrholm J, Brandsson S et al. (2000) In vivo kinematics of total knee arthroplasty: flat compared with concave tibial joint surface. J Orthop Res 18: 856-64
72. Vazquez-Vela Johnson G, Worland RL, Keenan J et al. (2003) Patient demographics as a predictor of the ten-year survival rate in primary total knee replacement. J Bone Joint Surg Br January 85(1): 52-6
73. Vessely MB, Whaley AL, Harmsen WS et al. (2006) The Chitranjan Ranawat Award: Long-term survivorship and failure modes of 1,000 cemented condylar total knee arthroplasties. Clin Orthop Relat Res November 452: 28-34
74. Vinciguerra B, Pascarel X, Honton JL (1994) Results of total knee prostheses with or without preservation of the posterior cruciate ligament. Rev Chir Orthop 80: 620-5
75. Walker PS, Garg A (1991) Range of motion in total knee arthroplasty, a computer analysis. Clin Orthop 262: 227-35
76. Wang CJ, Wang HE (1997) Dislocation of total knee arthroplasty. A report of 6 cases with 2 patterns of instability. Acta Orthop Scand 68: 282-5
77. Warren PJ, Olanlokun TK, Cobb AG et al. (1993) Proprioception after knee arthroplasty. Clin Orthop, 297: 182-7
78. Whiteside LA, Saeki K, Mihalko WM (2000) Functional medical ligament balancing in total knee arthroplasty. Clin Orthop 380: 45-57
79. Whiteside LA, Amador DD (1988) The effect of posterior tibial slope on knee stability after ortholoc total knee arthroplasty. J Arthroplasty 3 suppl: 51-7
80. Whiteside LA (1999) Selective ligament release in total knee replacement of the knee in valgus. Clin Orthop 367: 96-106
81. Whiteside LA (2001) Long-term follow-up of the bone-ingrowth ortholoc knee system without a metal-backed patella. Clinical Orthop 388: 77-84
82. Witvoet J, Huten D, Groupe GUEPAR et al. (2005) Mid-term results of Wallaby I posterior cruciate retaining total knee arthroplasty: a prospective study of the first 425 cases. Rev Chir Orthop December 91(8): 746-57
83. Worland RL, Jessup DE, Johnson J (1997) Posterior cruciate recession in total knee arthroplasty. J Arthroplasty 12: 70-3
84. Wright, RJ, Sledge CB, Poss R et al. (2004) Patient-reported outcome and survivorship after kinemax total knee arthroplasty. J Bone Joint Surg (Am) 86A(11): 2464-70

Substitution of the posterior cruciate ligament in total knee arthroplasty: Advantages and pitfalls

H. Migaud, F. Tirveilliot, J. Girard

Introduction

The substitution of Posterior Cruciate Ligament (PCL) was introduced during the mid seventies by Insall with the IB II Postero-Stabilized (PS) which demonstrated an improvement in kinematics and function by comparing with the Total Condylar PCL sacrificing (37). Thereafter, during the eighties, the preservation of PCL was promoted, in theory to improve knee kinematics (range of flexion in stairs, quadriceps efficiency) and subsequently the knee function (2). In spite of excellent results usually reported with PS prostheses (37, 64), the popularity of PCL sparing designs increased until the late eighties when some adverse effects were highlighted: instability (21), wear (9, 78), and patello-femoral disorders (8). The number of reports advocating PCL substitution increased after 1990 and the popularity of PCL sparing designs decreased in parallel, particularly when *in vivo* kinematics of TKA retaining the PCL was identified as abnormal by comparing with older PS designs (19, 75, 77, 82). However, some questions remain concerning PCL sacrifice or substitution: Are theoretical advantages of PCL retaining effective? Which adverse effects should we be aware of with PCL retaining? Which are the advantages of PCL substitution (postero-stabilised or deep-dished)? The aim of the present paper is to investigate these topics in order to give consistent arguments to support the PCL substitution. We will focus on five headings which had been considered in the past as major arguments to preserve the PCL:

1) Proprioception in TKA;
2) Ligament balance, tibial slope and joint line height;
3) TKA kinematics;
4) TKA and wear;
5) Function with PCL sparing and PS designs in TKA.

The analysis of these five headings will demonstrate the reasons for PCL retaining were not well founded and subsequently we will identify arguments issued from long-term clinical experience to support the PS designs. Among the PS designs the place for ultracongruent (deep-dished) designs will be discussed.

Proprioception in TKA

The favorable effect of PCL retaining to improve proprioception after TKA is widely discussed. First, one should consider the PCL retained in elderly arthritic knees is quite different from the native and healthy ligament. Franchi *et al.* (25) reported that there were less receptors (reduction by 50%) in the PCL of arthritic knees and that the number of receptors decreased according to the age of the patient. In clinical studies, Fuchs *et al.* (26) and Barrett *et al.* (5) confirmed this assertion as they observed a reduction of proprioception in arthritic knees with or without arthroplasty.

The interest of PCL retaining to improve proprioception remains controversial in many clinical studies. Some reports demonstrated no difference between PCL retaining and PS designs (13, 26, 46), while some observed an advantage for PCL retaining (87), and finally others identified an advantage for PS designs (71). The high level of controversies makes questionable the efficiency of PCL retaining to improve proprioception. Moreover, one should consider the alteration of the PCL structure related to the knee pathology particularly in case of rheumatoid arthritis (44). Likewise, retaining of PCL appears more uncertain when ACL is macroscopically abnormal, this last feature is very frequent and indicates severe microscopic alteration of PCL as reported by Goutallier *et al.* (29).

In conclusion, retaining PCL in TKA to improve proprioception remains non-consistent and has not been clearly confirmed in clinical studies. This hypothetical advantage remains too low in comparison to adverse effects related to PCL sparing. A PS design exposes to a theoretical lower proprioception but seems less technical demanding and finally is a reasonable solution in terms of proprioception since the patients in whom TKA is implanted had previous disturbance of proprioception related to age and pathological condition.

Ligament balance, tibial slope and joint line height

If the PCL is preserved, the restoration of an adequate tension and orientation is necessary so that the ligament could improve knee stability and kinematics (51). Incavo *et al.* (36) demonstrated the low tolerance of PCL tension related to tibial slope and joint line position. Even in a controlled experimental implantation of TKA, Incavo *et al.* (36) obtained only 2 correct tensions for PCL and 1 physiological femoral rollback out of 8 knees. Mahoney *et al.* (51) were unable to reproduce *in vitro* the normal PCL strain after insertion of a PCL retaining TKA. These results make questionable the ability of surgeons to obtain a favorable PCL tension in arthritic deformited knees. These difficulties to restore adequate PCL tension had been suspected by Insall in 1988 (38), they were confirmed thereafter in clinical studies:
1) Udomkiat *et al.* (81) obtained a physiological femoral rollback in only 2 out of 10 PCL sparing TKA but in 8 out of 10 postero-stabilised TKA. Moreover, they observed an abnormal anterior femoral displacement instead of rollback during flexion in 8 of the PCL sparing prostheses;
2) Booth (10) supported that, to obtain a TKA with physiological function,

the joint line position should not be modified over 4mm when retaining PCL and up to 9mm when the PCL is substituted. This underlined the ability of PS designs to be implanted in a larger number of situations particularly in case of severe deformation or in every situation which exposes to modifications of the joint line position. Even with low modifications of tibial height, inside the limits defined by Booth (10), Emodi *et al.* (21) clearly demonstrated that PCL tension could increase or decrease producing a lower knee function (8). A tibial resection over 10mm make questionable the PCL preservation as advocated by Freeman et Railton (24), considering the distal part of the PCL insertion on the tibia is extended 8 to 10mm below the tibial plateau (10).

A modification of the tibial slope during prosthetic implantation could modify PCL tension when preserved, it also means that respect of the preoperative tibial slope is necessary when the PCL is retained. If the tibial slope is reduced by TKA implantation, the range of flexion could be reduced (72). On the contrary, an increase of the tibial slope or the respect of an excessive preoperative tibial slope (over 10°) could produce an anterior tibial subluxation in weight bearing (fig. 1) when PCL is retained (ACL sacrificed) (56). Finally it could drive to catastrophic wear of the posterior aspect of tibial polyethylene (fig. 1) (8, 9). Moreover, one should also consider the risk for an error in tibial slope modification since:

1) a modification of the tibial slope is very sensitive as 3° represent 1/3 of the mean posterior slope (12);

2) the current instrumentation are not so accurate to determine during surgery the slope of the proximal tibial resection (12, 56);

3) an error in the horizontal orientation of the tibial resection guide (external or internal rotation) could drive to an additional error in the slope of the tibial resection.

In some circumstances the PCL preservation appear as an "impossible challenge":

1) a preoperative tibial slope over 15° (56) (fig. 1);

2) preoperative fixed flexion deformity over 15° (24, 68).

In such situations a PS design should be preferred as it is easier to implant and more secure concerning the control of knee laxity and prevention of wear.

In vivo assessment of femoro-tibial laxity after TKA implantation confirmed the difficulties to restore an adequate PCL tension. Waslewski *et al.* (88), out of 202 TKA, identified 8% of abnormal frontal and sagittal laxity just after implantation of PCL sparing prostheses. They related this result to an elevation (mean 10.3mm vs. 5mm elevation in the series) of the joint line which could release the PCL tension. They advise to avoid joint line elevation and consequently recommend to increase tibial resection that could also drive to distal PCL section. Finally if the PCL tension has to be respected, the risk of error appears undoubtedly too high to accept in many situations the PCL preservation. It's also possible to decide not to respect PCL physiological tension, considering this has a low influence on functional score or prosthetic survival. This was denied by Besson *et al.* (8) which identified a wide range of posterior laxity (0 to 10mm) assessed by Telos™ in 44 PCL sparing Miller-

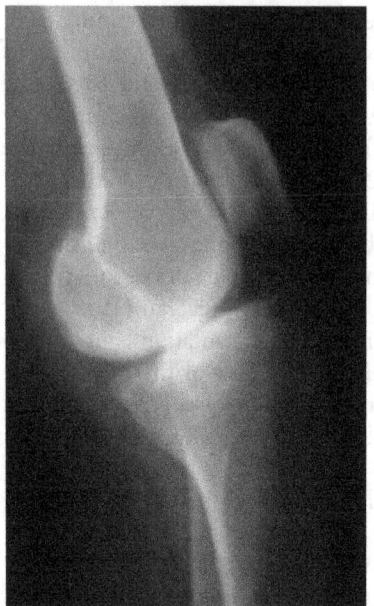
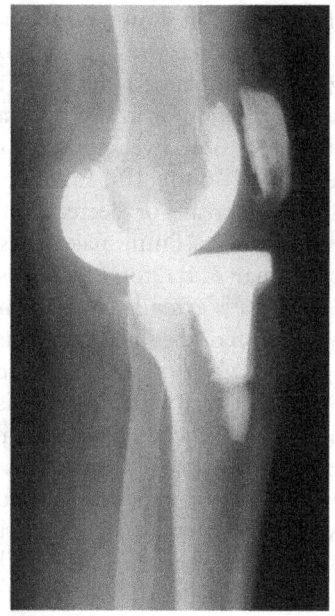
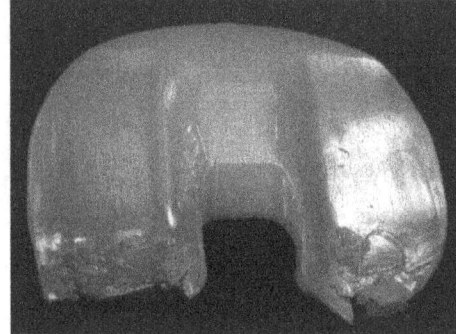

Fig. 1 – Adverse effect of a severe posterior tibial slope on behaviour of a PCL retaining TKA.

a. Preoperative lateral view of an osteoarthritic knee with 19° posterior tibial slope.

b. The Osteonics™ (Stryker) PCL sparing was implanted with reduction of posterior tibial slope. In spite of the decrease in tibial slope, the TKA demonstrated an anterior tibial subluxation in weight bearing (excessive PCL tension?)

c. The revision was performed after 5 years. On the retrieved tibial component a severe posterior wear was identified

Galante TKA. They related a decrease by 9.8 points of HSS knee score when posterior laxity was 5mm or more (8), underlining the necessity to respect PCL tension. Another solution if PCL appears too tight during surgery is to perform a partial PCL recession (92). It seems there is no long-term adverse effect of such procedure (4, 92), but no study demonstrated the ability of surgeons to determine the exact recession to restore an acceptable PCL tension. In conclusion, it appears more convenient to substitute the PCL in order to throw away the difficult problem of PCL tension adjustment

During the eighties, Krackow (42) advocated the PCL preservation to make simpler the ligament balance. This was justified considering:

1) the low influence of arthritic deformities on PCL length (by comparison with collateral ligaments);

2) the favorable effect of PCL which could be a reference for collateral ligament balance avoiding the large modifications of joint line position.

This opinion was not supported by Pagnano *et al.* (59), which related to
PCL sparing some instability in flexion. *In vitro*, an adequate ligament balancing during TKA is easier to obtain after PCL resection (73). Sorger *et al.* (73)
explained the majority of TKA designs use symmetrical femoral condyles,

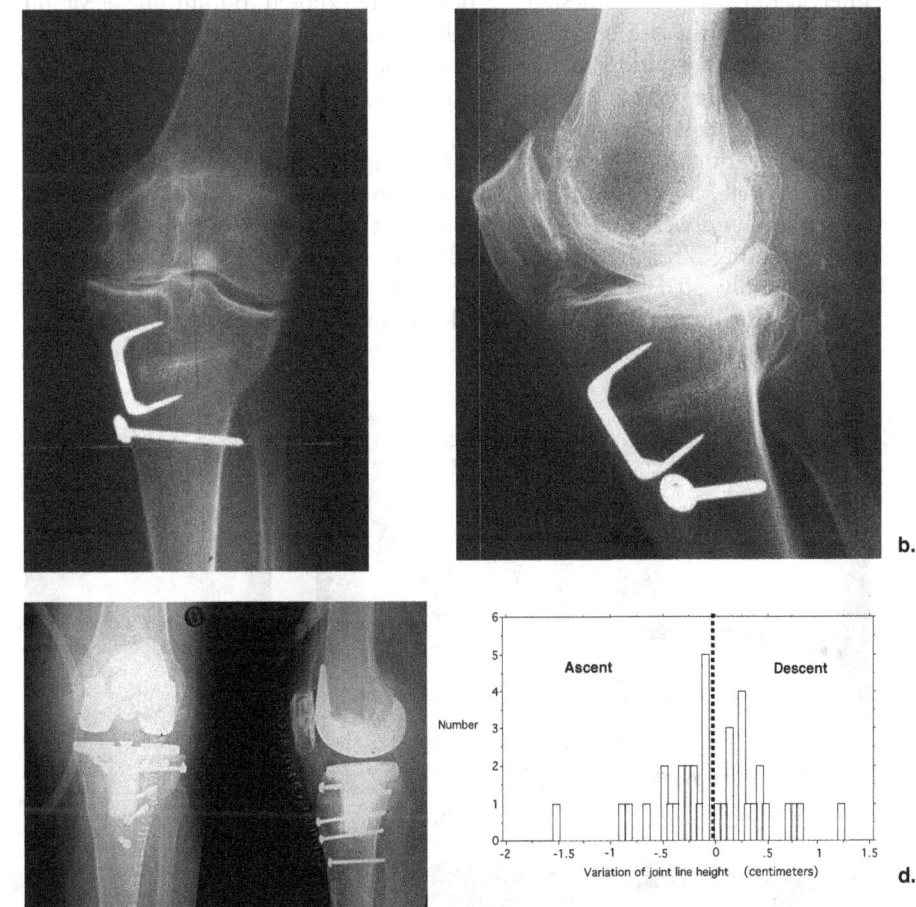

a.

b.

c.

d.

Fig. 2 – Interest of ending the procedure by distal femoral preparation and the use of a tensor
to adjust gap between flexion and extension with a PS TKA.
a. and b. AP and lateral view of an osteoarthritic knee, failure of a previous tibial osteotomy.
There is valgus deformity and severe patella infera.
c. Postoperative AP and lateral view showing there was only slight joint line elevation but correction of patella infera. An anterior tibial tubercle elevation was performed during surgical
approach because of preoperative stiffness (preoperative ROM = -15° to 75°). The prosthesis
(HLS™ PS, Tornier) uses a final distal femoral cut and a tensor to avoid joint line elevation
and to harmonize gap between flexion and extension.
d. Evolution of joint line height after implantation of 50 consecutive PS HLS™ prostheses
using a tensor and ending by distal femoral cut. The mean joint line elevation is slight: 2.6mm
± 0.5mm (range: 15mm ascent to 12mm descent).

which have low compatibility with PCL preserving. They advocated the PCL substitution unless using a TKA with non-symmetrical femoral condyles. Likewise, Dejour *et al.* (17) supported the PCL sacrifice facilitates the ligament balance, considering the PCL could impair the control of an adequate balance; since it is the first ligament drive under tension, it could hide some defaults in the collateral ligament balance. These authors confirmed this (17) with the same TKA design with or without PCL retaining: the control of laxity was definitely better with the PS design. PS designs are exposed to joint line elevation (57), however the use of a tensor and the practice of the distal femoral cut ending bone preparation could resolve this problem (17) (fig. 2 and 11).

If the PCL tension is adequate without excessive posterior tibial slope and with a correct collateral ligament balance, at least a PCL retaining TKA would be a knee with chronic anterior laxity (33) (fig. 3). The adverse effects of this laxity are well known for the cartilage, and undoubtedly should be considered for survival and wear of a TKA. Likewise, the control of posterior laxity with PCL retaining TKA is uncertain with long follow-up. Matsuda *et al.* (53) reported only 50% of satisfactory control of posterior laxity with Miller-Galante prostheses. To reduce the risk for anterior instability, some authors (89) propose to use congruent tibial polyethylene, but this could drive to an

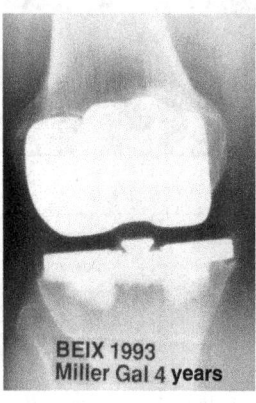
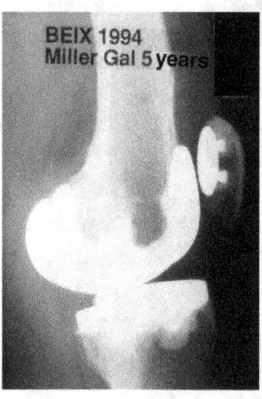
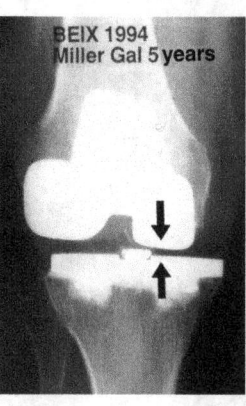

a.   b.   c.

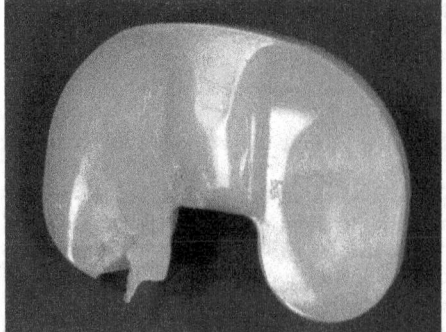

d.

Fig. 3 – Deleterious effect of anterior tibial laxity on polyethylene after 5 years of follow-up with a PCL retaining Miller-Galante™ TKA (Zimmer).

a. AP standing view after 4 years of follow-up. There was no evidence of wear.

b. and c. AP and lateral weight bearing views at 5 years follow-up. A severe wear (arrows) was identified on AP indicating revision surgery. On lateral view an anterior tibial subluxation was diagnosed instead of a slight posterior tibial slope.

d. Tibial insert retrieved after 5 years showing severe wear of the posterior aspect of the polyethylene.

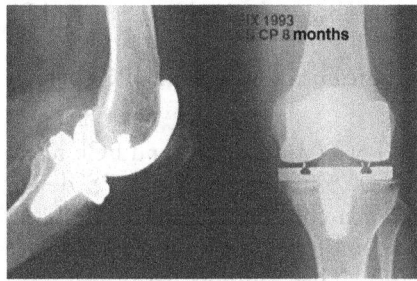

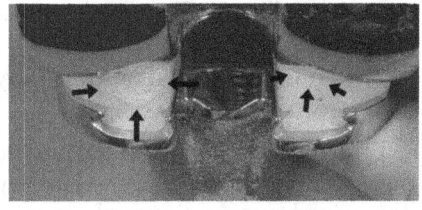

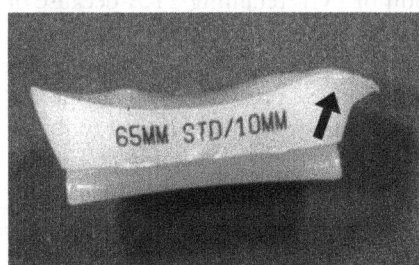

Fig. 4 – Increase in congruency with PCL retaining could produce wear of the posterior lip of the polyethylene insert.
a. AP and lateral view of a LCS™ PCL (DePuy) retaining meniscal bearing. Revision surgery was indicated after 4 years of follow-up because of pain related to possible tibial loosening (radiolucent line under tibial tray) and non-resurfacing of the patella.
b. and **c.** Wear and deformation of the posterior lip of the polyethylene insert (arrows), more severe on the medial compartment. PCL was present and do not appeared to tighten at revision.

excessive constraint on the posterior aspect of polyethylene (fig. 4) and could reduce the ability of femoral rollback which is a major goal of PCL retaining. In clinical studies, the survival of PCL retaining with congruent designs (3, 66) is higher than with flat designs (8). However the increase of congruency makes questionable the role of PCL retaining, as this design is not so far of the original Total Condylar which could function as well with (28) or without PCL (65). To prevent the chronic anterior laxity with cruciate retaining prostheses, another solution is to spare both cruciate ligaments (15). Cloutier (14) with the same TKA design underlined the retention of PCL alone gave lower functional results than retention of both cruciate ligaments.

In conclusion, the risk of anterior instability or inadequate PCL tension or abnormal rollback makes the PCL retaining questionable. Moreover, like reported Takatsu *et al.* (79), keeping physically the PCL do not mean retaining function of the PCL considering the ACL resection and the modification of joint line or articular geometry induced by the TKA.

TKA kinematics

One of the major reasons for PCL preservation was the respect of femoral rollback and the axial rotation (tibial internal rotation) during flexion (2). However, Freeman et Railton (24) make questionable this advantage considering this movement depends not only on PCL preservation but also on the other knee ligaments and upon all on the shape of the femoral condyles. This was confirmed by *in vivo* kinematics studies:

1) Dennis *et al.* (19) demonstrated the preservation of PCL authorized abnormal antero-posterior displacement of the femoral condyles (roll-forward

instead of rollback). The best kinematics was observed with bicruciate and PS designs;

2) Kim *et al.* (41) demonstrated any significant rollback with a PCL retaining prosthesis.

By comparing *in vitro* different designs (PS, PCL retaining, and PCL resection without substitution), Mahoney *et al.* (51) confirmed the PS design determined the most normal kinematics when considering femoral rollback. The PCL retaining could drive to femoral roll-forward but also to excessive rollback as reported by Whiteside *et al.* (90). These authors performed 25% of PCL partial release during implantation of PCL retaining TKA because of an "excessive femoral rollback". This could indicate an excessive PCL tension, but upon all confirmed the difficulties to adjust PCL tension in many situations. It appears more secure to use a mechanical procedure (PS design) in order to obtain in almost all the situations a well-controlled femoral rollback.

The report of Andriaccchi *et al.* (2) in 1982 was the starter for PCL retaining designs as it supported the PS TKA had lower kinematic results particularly in stairs. However one should consider that some of the cruciate retaining TKAs analyzed by Andriacchi *et al.* (2) were Cloutier bicruciate TKAs. Later Cloutier (14) himself reported better results in stairs with the Cloutier bicruciate instead of the same design retaining only the PCL. The favorable effect of PCL retaining on kinematics had not been widely demonstrated:

1) Kelman *et al.* (40) reported the PCL retaining improved kinematics of the Total Condylar design;

2) Dorr *et al.* (20) demonstrated higher performance on level walking for PS design and slight difference in favor of PCL retaining in stair climbing;

3) Wilson *et al.* (91) reported the kinematics with PS design was as good as with PCL retaining and superior to that of PCL sacrificing TKA;

4) Migaud *et al.* (55) observed no gain in kinematics with PCL retaining designs. The worst performances were observed with a PCL retaining flat on flat design (fig. 5). Moreover, wide variations of movements were observed for each type of TKA (bicruciate, PCL congruent, PCL flat on flat, PS) suggesting the kinematics depends not only on TKA designs but also on patient-related factors. In this last study none of the TKAs were able to reproduce the range of movements of a control group instead of unilateral pathological knee. It was surprising to observe axial rotations for each of the PS highly congruent designs (fig. 6);

5) Nilsson *et al.* (58) reported poor kinematics with the Miller-Galante™ (Zimmer) and the LCS New Jersey™ (DePuy) particularly regarding screw home axial rotation in spite of PCL retaining designs.

In conclusion PCL retaining gave little kinematic improvement and was not consistent in the majority of clinical studies. One should also determine if a prosthetic knee has to reproduce the kinematics of a healthy knee:

1) the anomalies in proprioception and muscle function induced by the pathological condition may not authorize such result in a large population;

2) the artificial prosthetic bearing surfaces are probably not able to assume the kinematics usually applied to native cartilage (fig.7);

3) the knee kinematics involves a lot of functions (mechanical axis, ligaments,

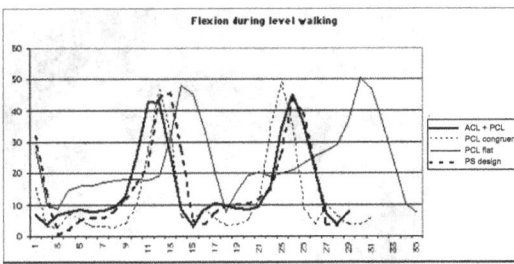

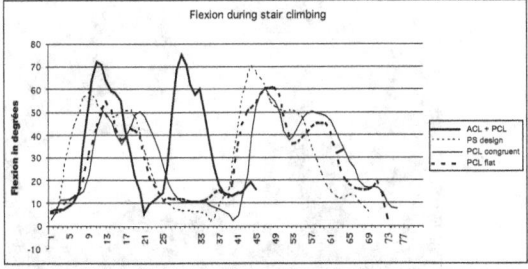

Fig. 5 – Range of flexion of four types of TKA during level walking and stair climbing (bicruciate, PCL retaining with congruent polyethylene, PCL retaining with flat polyethylene, PS). Kinematics was recorded with a 6° freedom electromagnetic-goniometer. The PCL retaining did not increased the ranges of flexion during level walking or stair climbing. Only the bicruciate TKA retaining demonstrated an increase of the range of flexion particularly in stairs. Axial rotation was recorded for each of the PS instead highly congruent (Insall Burstein II™ [Zimmer]).
a. On level walking there were slight differences between bicruciate, PCL congruent, and PS. Only the PCL flat demonstrated a longer stance phase.
b. The bicruciate demonstrated the highest range of flexion. There were no obvious differences between PCL congruent and PS. Only the PCL flat demonstrated reduced range of flexion during stair climbing

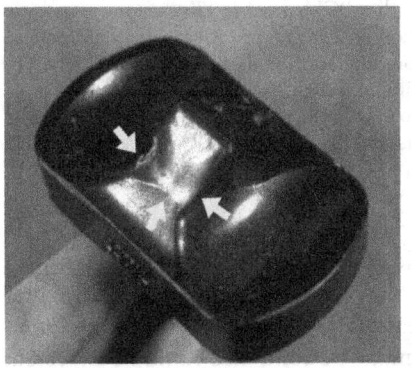

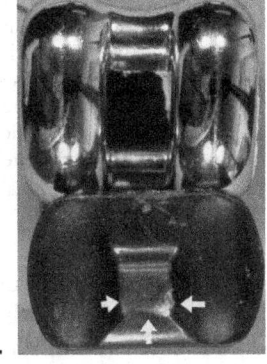

Fig. 6 – Axial rotation might be observed with PS congruent TKA. Retrieved components (Insall-Burstein™ PS [Zimmer]) after 8 years, because of late infection.
a. There was no wear of the congruent tibial polyethylene. A slight wear (arrows) on the posterostabilizing device suggested this prosthesis demonstrated axial rotation.
b. Aspect of the postero-stabilizing design. The femoral box induced wear on the tibial "spine". The rounding of the anterior aspect of the "spine" (arrows) suggested the prosthesis demonstrated axial rotation.

proprioception, shape of the articular surfaces) which cannot be all replaced during TKA implantation. Particularly knee kinematics depends mainly on the shape of the articular surfaces whose are different from one patient to another. Consequently the replacement by "one shape of prosthetic surface" may not be able to authorize normal kinematics (83). This suggests this is more secure to "enforce" a knee kinematics by means of mechanical system (i.e., postero stabi-

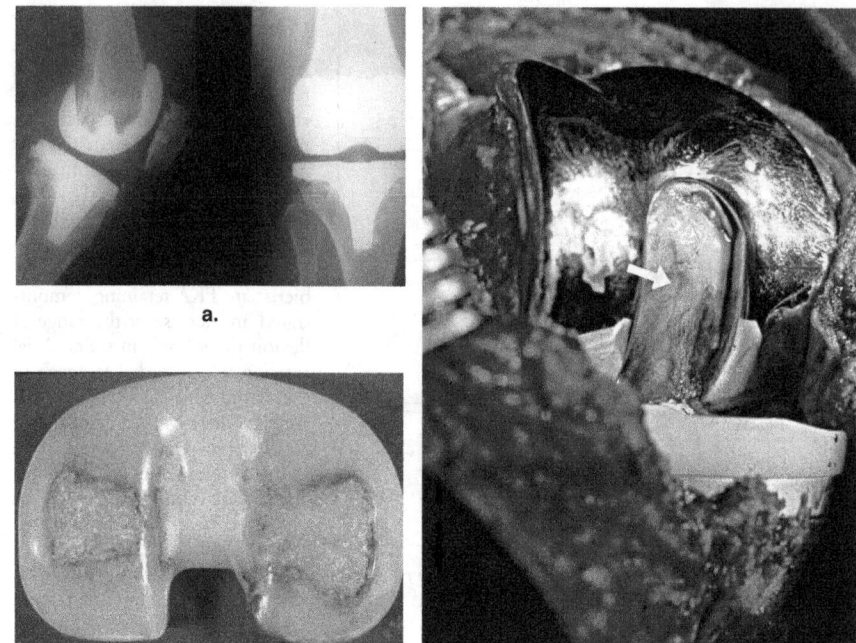

Fig. 7 – Severe wear of the tibial polyethylene with a PCL retaining TKA after 8 years.
a. AP and lateral view of an Osteonics™ (Stryker) PCL retaining. Aseptic loosening of the three components (extended radiolucencies without migration) indicated revision surgery. The position of the components was acceptable in spite of a slight patella infera.
b. Intraoperative view of the revision. The PCL (arrow) was present and did not appear too tighten.
c. Instead of a correct positioning of the implants and the efficiency of PCL a severe symmetric wear of the polyethylene was diagnosed.

lization) than to expect a normal kinematics with a non-constrained design with the help of cruciate ligaments whose function is probably impaired by the previous pathological condition. For these reasons a PS design should be preferred even if in few circumstances a lower kinematic performance could be expected, at least the mean kinematics would be acceptable in the majority of knees.

TKA and wear

Retention of PCL in TKA was promoted to protect the bone fixation with or without cement. (41). With PS designs all the constraints from the femur distribute directly to tibial bone interface, on the contrary with PCL retaining the ligament acts as a bypass for a large part of constraint (42). However, this theoretical advantage was not confirmed in clinical studies, the rate of loosening was quite similar when comparing the PCL congruent and PS designs, but significantly higher for PCL retaining non congruent.

The protection of bone fixation was not observed with PCL retaining and the occurrence of severe wear demonstrated the low mechanical bypass per-

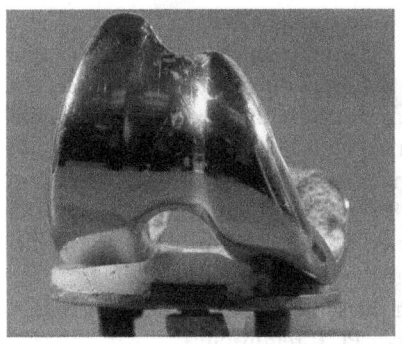
a.

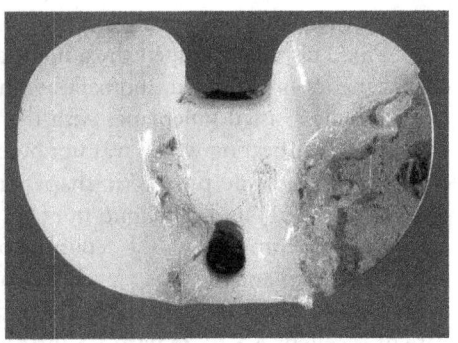
b.

Fig. 8 – Poor manufacturing of PCL retaining PCA™ (Howmedica-Stryker) components (thin polyethylene, heat-treated polyethylene, low congruent) driving to severe wear after 8 years of follow-up.

formed by the PCL (fig. 7). Many arguments have been advanced to explain the higher frequency of wear with PCL retaining TKA:

1) Overtension in PCL and / or excessive tibial slope, which could explain the excessive wear of the posterior aspect of tibial polyethylene (22, 55, 78);

2) The abnormal antero-posterior displacement of the femur instead of an harmonious rollback which could explain an overstress of polyethylene (76);

3) Factors related to the prosthetic designs: femoro-tibial low congruency which overstressed the polyethylene, default in polyethylene structure, low thickness of polyethylene (27) (fig. 8). Finally none of this problems were discussed for PS prostheses since early and severe wear was never observed with such designs (16).

Function with PCL sparing and PS designs in TKA

Function and kinematics are not correlated since excellent functional scores could be observed instead of severe kinematics anomalies related to PCL retaining:

1) Udomkiat *et al.* (81) observed comparable Knee Society score (KS) between PS and PCL designs in spite of the absence of femoral rollback in 80% of PCL retaining prostheses;

2) Nilsson *et al.* (58) reported excellent Knee score with Milller-Galante™ (Zimmer) and LCS™ (Depuy) TKA instead of obvious kinematics anomalies.

The advantage of PCL retaining to improve specific features of function remain controversial:

1) Bolanos *et al.* (11) and Huang *et al.* (35) comparing PCL retaining and PS observed no difference in terms of muscle strength (quadriceps and hamstrings) tested by isokinetic device nor electromyographic waveforms during level walking and stair climbing;

2) Dennis *et al.* (18) reported the PCL retaining TKA demonstrated lower range of flexion (103°) in active weight bearing by comparison with PS designs

(113°) (instead of the same range of motion in non-weight bearing (123° PCL and 127° PS). This demonstrated the amplitude of motion may not be used because of kinematics or muscular anomalies with PCL retaining designs. Likewise, the mechanically assisted kinematics with the PS design authorized an effective roll-back in weight bearing which was not observed with PCL retaining designs;

3) With the same prosthetic shapes (matching for PS and PCL retaining) Pereira *et al.* (61) and Vinciguerra *et al.* (85) observed any difference in HSS knee score by comparing PCL retaining or PS design. Both underlined the difficulties to implant the PCL sparing designs without functional benefit;

4) Dejour *et al.* (17) demonstrated with the same prosthetic design a higher rate of excellent KS score with PS instead of PCL retaining;

5) Shoji *et al.* (69) and Becker *et al.* (6) reported no difference in the ability to practice stair climbing in patient with bilateral TKA (one retaining and one sacrificing PCL). Finally most of the studies in favor of PCL retaining are *in vitro*, but this advantage is not confirmed in the majority of clinical *in vivo* studies.

The improvement of range of motion by means of femoral rollback was a major reason for PCL retaining. However, this was not confirmed *in vivo* as reported by Hirsch *et al.* (32) who observed no advantage of PCL retaining to improve range of motion, the best results being observed for the Insall-Burstein II™ (Zimmer). The absence of femoral rollback identified in the majority of *in vivo* investigation of PCL retaining designs may explain this result. The increase of range of motion is a current challenge of TKA, but in most clinical studies only the preoperative range of motion govern consistently the mobility at follow-up. With modern TKA designs the retaining of one or two cruciate ligaments will probably has little influence on the range of mobility. The range of motion with PCA™ (Howmedica-Stryker) retaining the PCL was 107° (27), 107° with the Cloutier™ (Zimmer and Hermes Ceraver) bicruciate prostheses (15), 114° with another bicruciate design (62), 108° with the HLS PS™ (Tornier) (17), 112° with an ultracongruent PCL sacrificing designs (33). A mechanically controlled kinematics (femoral rollback with PS) is probably more efficient than PCL retaining to improve the range of motion, but undoubtedly this has less influence than preoperative mobility (17). The mechanically assisted kinematics with PS designs appear more secure as in some reports of PCL retaining TKA the range of mobility decreased after surgery: Besson *et al.* (8) reported loss of 9.4° after implantation of Miller-Galante™ (Zimmer) prostheses with a mean range of motion at follow-up of 102.6°. Such significant decrease in range of motion has never been reported with PS designs. Consequently even if the theoretical mobility authorized by PS designs is lower, it appears as a reasonable solution to permit a satisfactory range of motion in the majority of knees.

The advantages of ultracongruent deep-dished components

The functional results of ultracongruent and PS designs are comparable in primary surgery (45) or in revision surgery (33). The absence of bone resection to admit the PS device makes the surgery simpler and authorizes bone saving (49). On the other hand, *in vivo* kinematics of ultracongruent TKA is not well known.

It should be preferable to control the femoral rollback with a PS mechanical device instead to leave it under the control of antero-posterior polyethylene lips as reported by Matsuda et al. (54). Moreover, if the congruency is excessive the femoral rollback could be extremely low. Matsuda et al. (54) demonstrated in vivo a low femoral rollback with ultracongruent TKA and also underlined such design needs more quadriceps force to extend the knee by comparison with PS designs. However ultracongruent components should be considered as they avoid specific complications related to PS designs (patellar clunk syndrome, dislocations) and it permits the load distribution to a larger surface of postero-substitution build with polyethylene. Likewise ultracongruent components authorize osteosynthesis of distal femoral fractures by means of retrograde nails.

Finally ultracongruent designs bring some advantages without short-term pitfalls. But the kinematics of such design is not as good as for the original PS designs. One should be aware of the increase in load transfer and the increase in femoro-tibial area of contact related to ultracongruency which could drive to osteolysis or tibial loosening, even if these complications had not been related by now with such designs.

Specific adverse effects related to PS designs

The posterior dislocation is a rare but serious pitfall of postero-stabilized TKA. The rate of posterior dislocation ranges from 0.2% (34) to 4.9% (48). To explain this complication, the PS design was firstly suspected (47, 48), but other reasons had been pointed out: patellar dislocation (67), revision surgery (67), and excessive range of flexion (48). Finally the prosthetic design was definitively involved as emerged a higher rate of dislocations with the Insall Burstein II™ (Zimmer) prosthesis (34, 48). A subsequent modification of this design was introduced in 1990, allowing an acceptable rate of dislocation remaining at 0.2% (34). Dislocations are also identified with PCL retaining design but at a lower rate (67, 86), they are related to progressive lengthening of PCL. This complication has probably been overestimated for PS designs and related to the introduction of the primary pattern of the IB-II prosthesis. A careful attention in PS design components could maintain this complication at an extremely low level.

Patellar clunk syndrome was first reported with Total Condylar™ (Howmedica and Zimmer) and PS designs. The rate of this complication varies from 1% (7) to 3.5% (50). Many authors had looked for the predisposing factors, but finally only the PS design was significantly involved. Among the PS designs, the Insall-Burstein was specifically incriminated because of the shape of junction between the condyles and the trochlear groove (50). In fact, many other PS designs do not produce a rate of clunk syndrome exceeding 1% (50). According to Lucas et al. (50), this complication must not be overrated since the arthroscopic treatment is simple (no complications) and efficient (100% success). Likewise, PCL retaining designs are not free of this complication which was diagnosed in 4% by Shoji et al. (70) with the AGC™ prosthesis (Biomet) with or without resurfacing of the patella.

PS designs have been reported to have a higher incidence of patellar complications: patellar fractures (1 to 3.3% related to primary or revisions TKA

[30, 80]), clunk syndrome (1% [7] to 3.5% [50]). The Insall-Burstein designs (I and II) were pointed out because of fair trochlear design and poor instrumentation for patellar preparation. One should also consider the PCL retaining designs are not free of extensor mechanism complications: Johnson et Eastwood (39) identified 25% of patellar complications (fracture or subluxation) with the Kinematics™ (Howmedica) PCL sparing TKA. With a precise attention to patello-femoral preparation, Larson et Lachiewicz (43) demonstrated the rate of patellar complications could significantly decrease even with an old PS design like the Insall-Burstein (1% of patellar fracture, no clunk, no subluxation, 10% was anterior knee pain and only 1% severe).

Joint line elevation is frequently opposed to PS designs, considering that PCL when preserved protects from this complication since its tension avoid the outcome of and excessive femoro-tibial gap. However, the joint line elevation remains moderate with PS designs: between 5 and 7mm for most of the studies related to Insall-Burstein II™ (Zimmer) TKA (50, 80). The consequences of a slight joint line elevation are demonstrated *in vitro* (52) (limitation of range of motion, ligament tightening), but few studies report adverse effects in clinics: Partington *et al.* (60) identified a threshold of 8mm before the joint line elevation had consequences on function. This last value is over the mean elevation reported for PS designs explaining the low consequences of a slight elevation when a PS prosthesis is implanted. Both to avoid such complication and to obtain a good ligament balance, a tensor should be used with PS designs as reported by Dejour *et al.* (17).

Severe wear is uncommon with PS designs as reported by Colizza *et al.* (16), on the contrary the TKA PCL retaining demonstrated a higher rate (27, 31) particularly with poor manufacturing or thin insert of tibial polyethylene (31). Wear of the PS mechanism had been highlighted in retrieval studies (63) but is not a main problem in clinical series (fig. 6 and 9) (17) even after 15 years of follow-up (74).

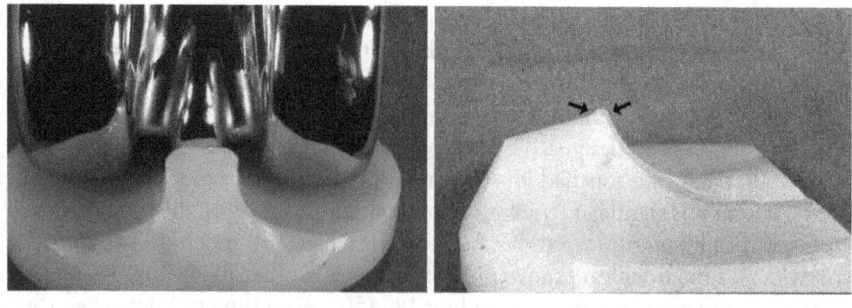

a.   **b.**

Fig. 9 – The wear of the postero-stabilizing systems is uncommon and slight after mid-term follow-up.
a. AP view of the HLS PS™ (Tornier) prosthesis. A third condyle substitute PCL after 35° of flexion by contact with a congruent groove of the polyethylene.
b. Lateral view of a retrieved component after 6 years of follow-up. The wear was slight and mainly consisted in limited cold deformation (arrows).

Conclusion

The long-term clinical studies of TKA showed excellent results for almost all PS and also for some of the PCL retaining designs with 10-year survival exceeding 95% (65, 74). PCL sparing was promoted to decrease load on tibial interface and subsequently to decrease the rate of tibial loosening (42), but this was not widely

a.

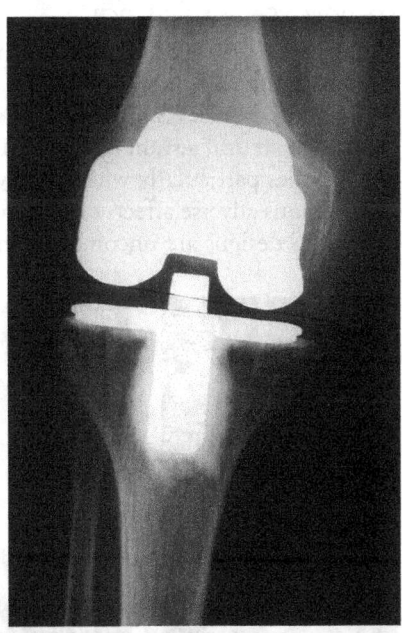
b.

c.
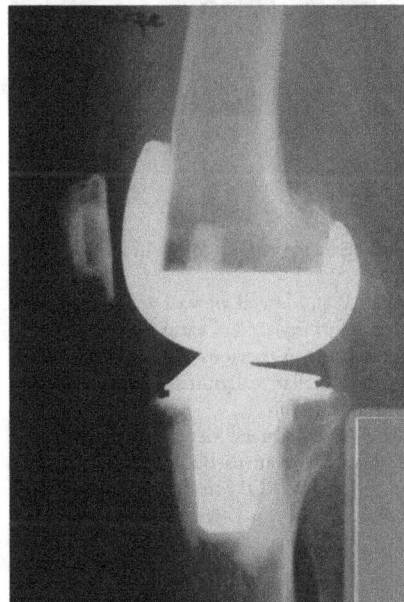

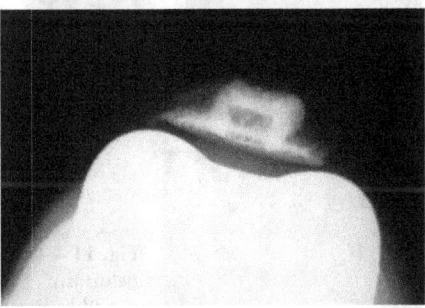
d.

Fig. 10 – Long-term follow-up (18 years) of a PS design. Install Burstein II™ (Zimmer) implanted because of osteoarthritis.

a. and **b.** AP stress view in valgus and varus by means of Telos™ at 150 Newton. There was no evidence of wear or abnormal laxity. Any radiolucency was identified.

c. and **d.** Lateral view and axial patello-femoral view. Any radiolucency was observed. The joint line and patellar positions were good.

demonstrated in clinical studies after 10 years of follow-up (64). Moreover, short-term failures were reported with PCL retaining with low congruent designs (8, 27). When looking to long-term results of PCL retaining, the excellent results are almost reported with highly congruent designs (23, 28, 89), which makes questionable the interest of PCL retaining. In fact, with the Total Condylar design, the rate of success is similar with or without PCL retaining underlining the interest of design instead of ligament retain (92% of success without PCL for Aglietti *et al.* (1), 96 % of success with PCL retaining for Ritter *et al.* (66)). When detailing survival rates over 10 years, the PCL congruent designs had remarkable results (23, 28, 84), but the 15 years survival give a little advantage to the PS design (fig. 10): 94% with the Insall PS (23) vs. 62% with PCL conforming design (84).

The theoretical advantages of PCL retaining had not been confirmed in clinical studies particularly when follow-up exceeds 10 years. On the other hand, some serious adverse affects of PCL retaining were highlighted where as the pitfalls of PS designs are uncommon and in the majority slight and do not com-

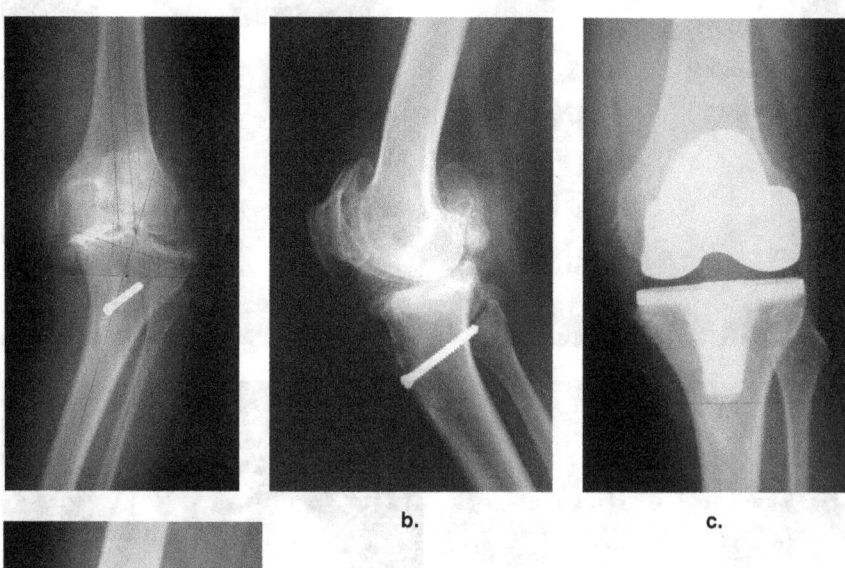

a.

b.   c.

Fig. 11 – The PS prostheses are simpler to use in case of severe deformity.

a. and b. Preoperative AP and lateral view of an osteoarthritic knee with severe varus deformity (25° of varus between mechanical axes of tibia and femur). A previous tibial tubercle osteotomy was performed for patellar realignment. Severe decrease in ROM = -20° to 80° of flexion.

c. and d. Postoperative AP and lateral view. Good radiological positioning of the implants without patella infera. The severity of the deformity and the limited ROM made questionable PCL retaining.

d.

promise the TKA behaviour. In some rare and special situations the cruciate retaining can make the function slightly better than PS designs, particularly with bicruciate (15, 62), however this is much more technical demanding. But for the majority of knees a PS design bring to an excellent result with long-term survival exceeding 95%. For PCL retaining the "price to pay is definitely too high" to hypothetical kinematics advantages which have in fact no consistent effect for the patient. The place for bicruciate TKA is certain because it brings true functional benefits to the patient without abnormal kinematics but the indications are limited to few primary knees with intact ACL and low deformity. The indications for PS designs are large without limitation (fig. 11), and can be extended to rheumatoid arthritis in which the rate of instability (posterior and recurvatum) appears too high when PCL is retained (44).

References

1. Aglietti P, Buzzi R, De Felice R, Giron F (1999) The Insall-Burstein total knee replacement in osteoarthritis: a 10-year minimum follow-up. J Arthroplasty 14: 560-5.
2. Andriacchi TP, Galante JO, Fermier RW (1982) The influence of total knee replacement design on walking and stair climbing. J Bone Joint Surg 64-A: 1328-35
3. Ansari S, Ackroyd CE, Newman JH (1998) Kinematic posterior cruciate ligament-retaining total knee replacements. A 10-year survivorship study of 445 arthroplasties. Am J Knee Surg 11: 9-14
4. Arima J, Whiteside LA, Martin JW et al. (1998) Effect of partial release of the posterior cruciate ligament in total knee arthroplasty. Clin Orthop 353: 194-202
5. Barrett DS, CobbAG, Bentley G (1991) Joint proprioception in normal osteoarthritic and replaced knees. J Bone Joint Surg 73-B: 53-6
6. Becker MW, Insall JN, Faris PM (1991) Bilateral total knee arthroplasty. One cruciate retaining and one cruciate substituting. Clin Orthop 271: 122-4
7. Beight JL, Binnan Yao, Hozack WJ et al. (1994) The patellar clunk syndrome after posterior stabilized total knee arthroplasty. Clin Orthop 299: 139-42
8. Besson A, Brazier J, Chantelot C et al. (1999) Laxity and functional results of Miller-Galante total knee prosthesis with posterior cruciate ligament sparing after a 6-year follow-up. Rev Chir Orthop 85: 797-802
9. Blunn GW, Joshi A, Minns RJ et al. (1997) Wear in retrieved condylar knee arthroplasties. A comparison of wear in different designs of 280 retrieved condylar knee prostheses. J Arthroplasty 12: 281-90
10. Booth RE Jr (1999) The price of PCL retention in TKA is too high. Orthopedics 12: 1125
11. Bolanos AA, Colizza WA, McCann PD et al. (1998) A comparison of isokinetic strength testing and gait analysis in patients with posterior cruciate-retaining and substituting knee arthroplasties. J Arthroplasty 13: 906-15
12. Brazier J, Migaud H, Gougeon F et al. (1996) Méthodes de mesure radiographique de la pente tibiale. Analyse de 83 genoux témoins. Rev Chir Orthop 82: 195-200
13. Cash RM, Gonzalez MH, Garst J et al. (1996) Proprioception after arthroplasty: role of the posterior cruciate ligament. Clin Orthop 331: 172-8
14. Cloutier JM (1991) Long-term results after non-constrained total knee arthroplasty. Clin Orthop 273: 63-5
15. Cloutier JM, Sabouret P, Deghrar A (1999) Total knee arthroplasty with retention of both cruciate ligaments. A nine to eleven-year follow-up study. J Bone Joint Surg 81-A: 697-702
16. Colizza WA, Ninsall JN, Scuderi GR (1995) The posterior stabilized total knee prosthesis. Assessment of polyetylene damage and ostelolysis after a ten-year minimum follow-up. J Bone Joint Surg 77-A: 1317-20.
17. Dejour D, Deschamps G, Garotta L et al. (1999) Laxity in posterior cruciate sparing and posterior stabilized total knee prostheses. Clin Orthop 364: 182-93

18. Dennis DA, Komistek RD, Stiehl JB *et al.* (1998) Range of motion after total knee arthroplasty: the effect of implant design and weight-bearing conditions. J Arthroplasty 13: 748-52

19. Dennis DA, Komistek RD, Colwell CE *et al.* (1998) *In vivo* anteroposterior femorotibial translation of total knee arthroplasty: a multicenter analysis. Clin Orthop 356: 47-57

20. Dorr LD, Ochsner JL, Gronley J *et al.* (1988) Functional comparison of posterior cruciate-retained versus cruciate-sacrificed total knee arthroplasty. Clin Orthop 236: 36-43

21. Emodi GJ, Callaghan JJ, Pedersen DR *et al.* (1999) Posterior cruciate ligament function following total knee arthroplasty: the effect of joint line elevation. Iowa Orthop J 19: 82-92

22. Fehring TK, Valadie AL (1994) Knee instability after total knee arthroplasty. Clin Orthop 299: 157-62

23. Font-Rodriguez DE, Scuderi GR, Insall JN (1997) Survivorship of cemented total knee arthroplasty. Clin Orthop 345: 79-86

24. Freeman MA, Railton GT (1988) Should the posterior cruciate ligament be retained or resected in condylar non-meniscal knee arthroplasty? The case for resection. J Arthroplasty 3 Suppl: 3-12

25. Franchi A, Zaccherotti G, Aglietti P (1995) Neural system of the human posterior cruciate ligament in osteoarthritis. J Arthroplasty 10: 679-82

26. Fuchs S, Thorwesten L, Niewerth S (1999) Proprioceptive function in knees with and without total knee arthroplasty. Am J Phys Med Rehabil 78: 39-45

27. Gacon G, Coillard JY, Barba L *et al.* (1995) Non cemented primary PCA total knee prosthesis. A five to nine year follow-up. Rev Chir Orthop, 81: 510-3

28. Gill GS, Joshi AB, Mills DM (1999) Total condylar knee arthroplasty. 16- to 21-year results. Clin Orthop 367: 210-5

29. Goutallier D, Allain J, Le Mouel S *et al.* (1998) Évaluation de l'état histologique du ligament croisé postérieur en fonction de l'état macroscopique du ligament croisé antérieur: Intérêt pour l'indication des prothèses conservant le ou les ligaments croisés. Rev Chir Orthop 84 suppl 2: 30

30. Grace JN, Sim FH (1987) Fracture of the patella after total knee arthroplasty. Clin Orthop 230: 168-75

31. Hirakawa K, Bauer TW, Yamaguchi M *et al.* (1999) Relationship between wear debris particles and polyethylene surface damage in primary total knee arthroplasty. J Arthroplaty 14: 165-71

32. Hirsch HS, Lotke PA, Morrison LD (1994) The posterior cruciate ligament in total knee surgery. Save, sacrifice, or substitute? Clin Orthop 309: 64-8

33. Hofmann AA, Tkach TK, Evanich CJ *et al.* (2000) Posterior stabilization in total knee arthroplasty with use of an ultracongruent polyethylene insert. J Arthroplasty 15: 576-83

34. Hossain S, Ayeko C, Anwar M *et al.* (2001) Dislocation of Insall-Burstein II modified total knee arthroplasty. J Arthroplasty 16: 233-5

35. Huang CH, Lee YM, Liau JJ *et al.* (1998) Comparison of muscle strength of posterior cruciate-retained versus cruciate-sacrificed total knee arthroplasty. J Arthroplasty 13: 779-83

36. Incavo SJ, Johnson CC, Beynnon BD *et al.* (1994) Posterior cruciate ligament strain biomechanics in total knee arthroplasty. Clin Orthop 309: 88-93

37. Insall JN, Lachiewicz PF, Burstein AH (1982) The posterior stabilized condylar prosthesis: a modification of the total condylar design. J Bone Joint Surg 64-A: 1317-23

38. Insall JN (1988) Presidential adresss to the Knee Society. Choices and compromises in total knee arthroplasty. Clin Orthop 226: 43-8

39. Johnson DP, Eastwood DM (1992) Patellar complications after knee arthroplasty. A prospective study of 56 cases using the Kinematic prothesis. Acta Orthop Scand 63: 74-9

40. Kelman GJ, Biden EN, Wyatt MP *et al.* (1989) Gait laboratory analysis of a posterior cruciate-sparing total knee arthroplasty in stair ascent and descent. Clin Orthop 248: 21-5

41. Kim H, Pelker RR, Gibson DH *et al.* (1997) Rollback in posterior cruciate ligament-retaining total knee arthroplasty. A radiographic analysis. J Arthroplasty 12: 553-61

42. Krackow KA (1990) The surgical procedure of total knee arthroplasty. In: Krakow KA (ed) Total Knee arthroplaty. CV Mosby, Philadelphia, 168-237

43. Larson CM, Lachiewicz PF (1999) Patellofemoral complications with the Insall-Burstein posterior-stabilized total knee arthroplasty. J Arthroplasty 14: 288-92

44. Laskin RS, O'Flynn HM (1997) The Insall Award. Total knee replacement with posterior cruciate ligament retention in rheumatoid arthritis. Problems and complications. Clin Orthop 345: 24-8

45. Laskin RS, Maruyama Y, Villaneuva M *et al.* (2000) Deep-dish congruent tibial component use in total knee arthroplasty: a randomized prospective study. Clin Orthop 380: 36-44

46. Lattanzio PJ, Chess DG, MacDermid JC (1998) Effect of the posterior cruciate ligament in knee-joint proprioception in total knee arthroplasty. J Arthroplasty 13: 580-5

47. Lecuire F, Jaffar-Bandjee Z (1994) Posterior luxation of the tibia on total knee prosthesis: apropos of 6 cases. Rev Chir Orthop 80: 525-31

48. Lombardi AV, Mallory TH, Vaughn BK *et al.* (1993) Dislocation following primary posterior-stabilized total knee arthroplasty. J Arthroplasty 8: 633-9

49. Lombardi AV, Mallory TH, Waterman RA *et al.* (1995) Intercondylar distal femoral fracture: an unreported complication of posterior-stabilized total knee arthroplasty. J Athroplasty 10: 643-9

50. Lucas TS, DeLuca PF, Nazarian DG *et al.* (1999) Arthroscopic treatment of patellar clunk. Clin Orthop 367: 226-9

51. Mahoney OM, Noble PC, Rhoads DD *et al.* (1994) Posterior cruciate function following total knee arthroplasty. A biomechanical study. J Arthroplasty 9: 569-78

52. Martin JW, Whiteside LA (1990) The influence of joint line position on knee stability after condylar knee arthroplasty. Clin Orthop 259: 146-56

53. Matsuda S, Whiteside LA, White SE *et al.* (1997) Knee kinematics of posterior cruciate ligament sacrificed total knee arthroplasty. Clin Orthop 341: 257-66

54. Matsuda S, Miura H, Nagamine R *et al.* (1999) Knee stability in posterior cruciate ligament retaining total knee arthroplasty. Clin Orthop 366: 169-73

55. Migaud H, Gougeon F, Diop A *et al.* (1995) Kinematic *in vivo* analysis of the knee: a comparative study of 4 types of total knee prostheses. Rev Chir Orthop 81: 198-210

56. Migaud H, De Ladoucette A, Dohin B *et al.* (1996) Influence of posterior tibial slope on anterior tibial translation and mobility after a non-constrained total knee arthroplasty. Rev Chir Orthop 82: 7-13

57. Mihalko WM, Miller C, Krackow KA (2000) Total knee arthroplasty ligament balancing and gap kinematics with posterior cruciate ligament retention and sacrifice. Am J Orthop 29: 610-6

58. Nilsson KG, Karrholm J, Gadegaard P (1991) Abnormal kinematics of artificial knee. Roentgen sterophotogrammetric analysis of 10 Miller-galante and 5 New Jersey LCS knees. Acta Orthop Scand 62: 440-6

59. Pagnano MW, Hanssen AD, Lewallen DG *et al.* (1998) Flexion instability after primary posterior cruciate retaining total knee arthroplasty. Clin Orthop 356: 39-46

60. Partington PF, Sawhney J, Rorabeck CH *et al.* (1999) Joint line restoration after revision total knee arthroplasty. Clin Orthop 367: 165-71

61. Pereira DS, Jaffe FF, Ortiguera C (1998) Posterior cruciate ligament-sparing versus posterior cruciate ligament-sacrificing arthroplasty. Functional results using the same prosthesis. J Arthroplasty 13:138-44

62. Pritchett JW (1996) Anterior cruciate-retaining total knee arthroplasty. J Arthroplasty 11: 194-7

63. Puloski SK, McCalden RW, MacDonald SJ *et al.* (2001) Tibial wear in posterior statbilized arthroplasty. An unrecognized source of polyethylene debris. J Bone Joint Surg 83-A: 390-7

64. Ranawat CS, Hansraj KK (1989) Effect of posterior cruciate sacrificing on durability of the cement-bone interface: a nine-year survivorship study of 100 total condylar knee arthroplasties. Clin Exp Rheumatol 7 suppl 3: 149-52.

65. Ritter MA, Campbell E, Faris PM *et al.* (1989) Long-term survival analysis of the posterior cruciate condylar total knee arthroplasty. A 10-year evaluation. J Arthroplasty 4: 293-6

66. Ritter MA, Herbst SA, Keating EM *et al.* (1994) Long-term survival analysis of a posterior cruciate-retaining total condylar total knee arthroplasty. Clin Orthop 309: 136-45

67. Sharkey PF, Hozack WJ, Booth RE *et al.* (1992) Posterior dislocation of total knee arthroplasty. Clin Orthop 278: 128-33

68. Shoji H, Solomonow M, Yoshino S et al. (1990) Factors affecting postoperative flexion in total knee arthroplasty. Orthopedics 13: 643-9
69. Shoji H, Wolf A, Packard S et al. (1994) Cruciate retained and excised total knee arthroplasty. A comparative study in patients with bilateral total knee arthroplasty. Clin Orthop 305: 218-22
70. Shoji H, Shimozaki E (1996) Patellar clunk syndrome in total knee arthroplasty without patellar resurfacing. J Arthroplasty 11: 198-201
71. Simmons S, Lephart S, Rubash H et al. (1996) Proprioception following total knee arthroplasty with and without the posterior cruciate ligament. J Arthroplasty 11: 763-8
72. Singerman R, Dean JC, Pagan HD et al. (1996) Decreased posterior tibial slope increases strain in the posterior cruciate ligament following total knee arthroplasty. J Arthroplasty 11: 99-103
73. Sorger JI, Federle D, Kirk PG et al. (1997) The posterior cruciate ligament in total knee arthroplasty. J Arthroplasty 12: 869-79
74. Stern SH, Insall JN (1992) Posterior stabilized prosthesis. J Bone Joint Surg 74-A: 980-6
75. Stiehl JB, Voorhorst PE, Keblish P et al. (1997) Comparison of range of motion after posterior cruciate ligament retention or sacrifice with a mobile bearing total knee arthroplasty. Am J Knee Surg 10: 216-20
76. Stiehl JB, Komistek RD, Dennis DA (1999) Detrimental kinematics of a flat on flat total condylar knee arthroplasty. Clin Orthop 365: 139-48
77. Stiehl JB, Komistek RD, Cloutier JM et al. (2000) The cruciate ligaments in total knee arthroplasty: a kinematic analysis of 2 total knee arthroplasties. J Arthroplasty 15: 545-50
78. Swany MR, Scott RD (1993) Posterior polyethylene wear in posterior cruciate ligament-retaining total knee arthroplasty. A case study. J Arthroplasty 8: 439-46
79. Takatsu T, Itokazu M, Shimizu K et al. (1998) The function of posterior tilt of the tibial component following posterior cruciate ligament-retaining total knee arthroplasty. Bull Hosp Jt Dis 57: 195-201
80. Tria A, Harwood DA, Alicea JA et al. (1994) Patellar fracture in posterior stabilized knee arthroplasties. Clin Orthop 199: 131-8
81. Udomkiat P, Meng BJ, Dorr LD et al. (2000) Functional comparison of posterior cruciate retention and substitution knee replacement. Clin Orthop 378: 192-201
82. Uvehammer J, Karrholm J, Brandsson S (2000) In vivo kinematics of total knee arthroplasty: Concave versus posterior stabilized tibial joint surface. J Bone Joint Surg (Br) 82-B: 499-505
83. Uvehammer J, Karrholm J, Brandsson S et al. (2000) In vivo kinematics of total knee arthroplasty: flat compared with concave tibial joint surface. J Orthop Res 18: 856-864
84. Van Loon CJ, Wisse MA, De Wall Malefijt MC et al. (2000) The kinematic total knee arthroplasty. A 10 to 15-year follow-up and survival analysis. Arch Orthop Trauma Surg 120: 48-52
85. Vinciguerra B, Pascarel X, Honton JL (1994) Results of total knee prostheses with or without preservation of the posterior cruciate ligament. Rev Chir Orthop 80: 620-5
86. Wang CJ, Wang HE (1997) Dislocation of total knee arthroplasty. A report of 6 cases with 2 patterns of instability. Acta Orthop Scand 68: 282-5.
87. Warren PJ, Olanlokun TK, Cobb AG et al. (1993) Proprioception after knee arthroplasty. Clin Orthop 297: 182-7
88. Waslewski GL, Marson BM, Benjamin JB (1998) Early, incapacitating instability of posterior cruciate ligament-retaining total knee arthroplasty. J Arthroplasty 13: 763-7
89. Weir DJ, Moran CG, Pinder IM (1996) Kinematic condylar total knee arthroplasty. A 14-year survivorship analysis of 208 consecutive cases. J Bone Joint Surg 78-B: 907-11
90. Whiteside LA, Saeki K, Mihalko WM (2000) Functional medical ligament balancing in total knee arthroplasty. Clin Orthop 380: 45-57
91. Wilson SA, McCann PD, Gotlin RS et al. (1996) Comprehensive gait analysis in posterior-stabilized knee arthroplasty. J Arthroplasty 11: 359-67
92. Worland RL, Jessup DE, Johnson J (1997) Posterior cruciate recession in total knee arthroplasty. J Arthroplasty 12: 70-3

Fixation with or without cement in total knee arthroplasty

J. Bellemans

Introduction

Cemented total knee arthroplasty has been considered by the majority of knee surgeons as the gold standard in total knee arthroplasty. Over the years, improvements in surgical technique, component design, and cement technology, have lead to the situation where long-term success of total knee arthroplasty is no longer determined by the durability of the fixation, but rather by wear-related issues.

Likewise, uncemented total knee arthroplasty has gained popularity, based upon an increased knowledge of the process of osseo-integration of cementless components, in combination with excellent long-term clinical success rates.

In this chapter an overview is given on both methods of fixation, focusing on the biomechanical aspects, clinical results, and surgical technique.

Cemented TKA

Many people today consider cemented total knee arthroplasty as the gold standard, based upon its published success rates. The prevalence of good and excellent results with cemented total knee arthroplasties has been reported to be 88 to 95%.

With revision used as the endpoint, a survival rate of 90 to 95% at 10 to 15 years has been noted, in one recent report with the longest follow-up so far eve 91% at 21 years (1, 3). Cement fixation has proven to perform well in TKA regardless of prosthetic design, with comparably low loosening rates for PCL-retaining designs, PCL-sacrificing designs, and posterior stabilised designs (4, 10).

Weir *et al.* reported a loosening rate of 2.9% in 208 PCL-retaining Kinematic[R] condylar knee replacements with a mean follow-up of 12 years (8), while Emmerson *et al.* have published a 2.7% loosening rate in 109 posterior cruciate substituting Kinematic[R] stabilizer knees at a mean follow-up of 12.7 years (4).

Vince, Insall and Kelly reported on 4 cases (3.1%) with component loosening in their 10 to 12-year results with the PCL-sacrificing Total Condylar Prosthesis®, and attributed the 3 tibial loosenings to technical errors due to inadequate alignment and soft tissue balance (6).

Since these publications, others have reported comparable loosening rates using different designs (1, 10).

Polymethylmetacrylate (PMMA) bone cement can therefore be considered as an adequate anchoring substance for knee arthroplasty components, being able to withstand the applied loads for a relatively long period.

Cementing knee arthroplasty components is a relatively easy and reproducible technique, and has the advantage that minor irregularities in the prepared bone surfaces can be filled, making a precise bone preparation less critical with regard to implant fixation.

Despite all these satisfactory clinical data, a number of potential downsides associated with the use of cement have however been noted in the past as well.

Bone cement is prone to fatigue failure and is a poor transmittor of tensile and shear stress (11, 12). Although this is the biggest disadvantage of bone cement, it is not its only drawback (table I).

Bone cement is brittle, it is a potential source for third body wear, and it can cause massive osteolysis (13, 15).

During its polymerisation phase, cement is cytotoxic and heat necrosis of the underlying bone can occur due to high temperture generation (16, 19).

In a study using transoesophageal echocardiography, bone cement has been suggested to contribute to the formation of venous clot and the intraoperative embolic insult by activation of the coagulation cascade (20).

Cadaver studies have shown that cement increases the risk for femoral stress shielding in total knee arthroplasty (21).

Furthermore, PMMA cement has been found to impair chemotaxis, phagocytosis, and killing ability of polymorphonuclear leucocytes, increasing the susceptibility to infection (22, 24).

The cementing technique itself is not free of problems either: inadequate and asymetric pressurization (tibial component), inadequate cement thickness (femoral component), periprosthetic cement extrusion (patellar components), inadequate porosity due to inadequate mixing, inadequate cleaning of the bone surface with residual blood or bone marrow contaminating the interface, all seem to be inevitable occurrences associated with cementing total knee implants (25, 26).

Table I – Negative factors attributed to cement fixation

– Fatigue failure
– Poor transmission of tensile stress
– Poor transmission of shear stress
– Brittleness
– Third body wear
– Osteolysis
– Cytotoxicity
– Heat necrosis of bone
– Stress shielding
– Wedge sign
– Loosening
– Cement extrusion and impingement
– Impairement of chemotaxis
– Inhibition of phagocytosis
– Increased susceptibility to infection
– Increased thromboembolic activation

All these above mentioned shortcomings of cement have however not lead to substantial clinical problems in the past, and the majotity of knee surgeons both in Europe and the U.S.A. therefore continue to prefer cemented over cementless fixation for TKA components.

Biomechanical aspects

Much of our current knowledge on the specific characteristics of the ideal cement mantel for TKA components is based upon what we know from hip arthroplasty.

Although the situation in knee arthroplasty is completely different with regard to cement fixation, it is clear that a number of well established facts can be extrapolated from cemented hip arthroplasty. For example, it may be clear that bone cement after mixing must result in a homogenous product with low porosity. Vacuum mixing of bone cement reduces its porosity as compared with hand mixing, and also improves the fracture toughness and fatigue resistance (27).

A number of other important cement parameters specific for knee arthroplasty have however received very little scientific attention so far.

In hips it is generally accepted that the cement mantle thickness should at least be 2mm (28). Whether this is true for knees as well, is not known. In fact, in most cemented femoral components one will never reach this thickness, due to the precise fit which is generally achieved.

On the tibial side the situation is even more unclear for the surgeon, since he has the possibility to cement the baseplate alone, or cement the keel as well.

Bert and McShane noted increased micromotion when fin-keeled baseplates were fixed with cementation of the baseplate alone, compared to combined baseplate and stem cementation. Only when the cement mantle under the baseplate reached the thickness of 3mm, excellent stability of the implant was seen regardless of stem cementation (29).

These findings were confirmed in a clinical study by Lombardi *et al.* who noted a 9% aseptic failure rate in baseplate alone cemented knees, versus no failures in the baseplate plus keel cemented group, using an identical design (Maxim®, Biomet) (30).

Surgical technique

Successful cement fixation depends upon the ability for the cement to penetrate into the cancellous bone. It is therefore recommended that the resected bone surfaces are thoroughly cleansed with pulsed lavage to remove bone debris, blood, and fat particles.

Ritter *et al.* have demonstrated that such preparation of the bone surface is more important than how the cement is placed, with no significant difference between finger-packed versus pressure-injected groups (31).

Our cementing technique is based upon the technique described by the school of Insall (32).

The components are cemented sequentially, using one batch of cement in its doughy state. Sclerotic areas are drilled with a 2.5mm drill to allow cement interlocking.

The tibial component is cemented first, by applying cement onto the undersurface of the baseplate, and around the keel if this is possible with the keel configuration. Additionally, cement is placed upon the proximal tibial surface. The tibial component is introduced using a slap-hammer, and any excess cement is removed using a small curette.

Next, cement is applied upon the resected distal femur in a "horseshoe" fashion, but not on the posterior surface (32). On the femoral component, cement is placed on the posterior condyles only (fig. 1)

The femur is introduced using a slap-hammer, guiding the component somewhat into extension. This manoeuvre will assure correct positioning along the resected anterior plane and will avoid the tendency for a slight flexion positioning.

The appropriate tibial trial insert is then inserted, the knee is brought into full extension, and stabilized in neutral rotation by the scrub nurse holding the foot. Excess cement is removed using the small curette.

Finally, the patella is cemented by applying cement on the undersurface of the component and on the resected patellar bone, but only to such extent that the peg holes remain visible for easy introduction. The patellar component is inserted, clamped, and excess cement is removed. Only when the cement has completely hardened, the knee is flexed again, and extruded cement is removed using an osteotome, taking care to avoid free cement particles entering the joint.

Recently a number of additional techniques to improve cement intrusion have been reported, based upon the creation of a negative pressure (33, 34). Negative pressure intrusion is an alternative cementing technique for the tibial baseplate that uses a suction canula in the proximal tibia to remove excess fluid and fat, providing a dry and clean bone surface for optimal cement penetration (fig. 2).

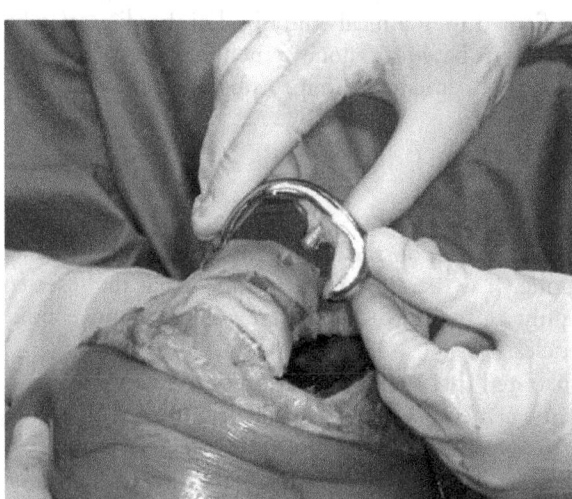

Fig. 1 – Cementing technique for the femoral component (see text).

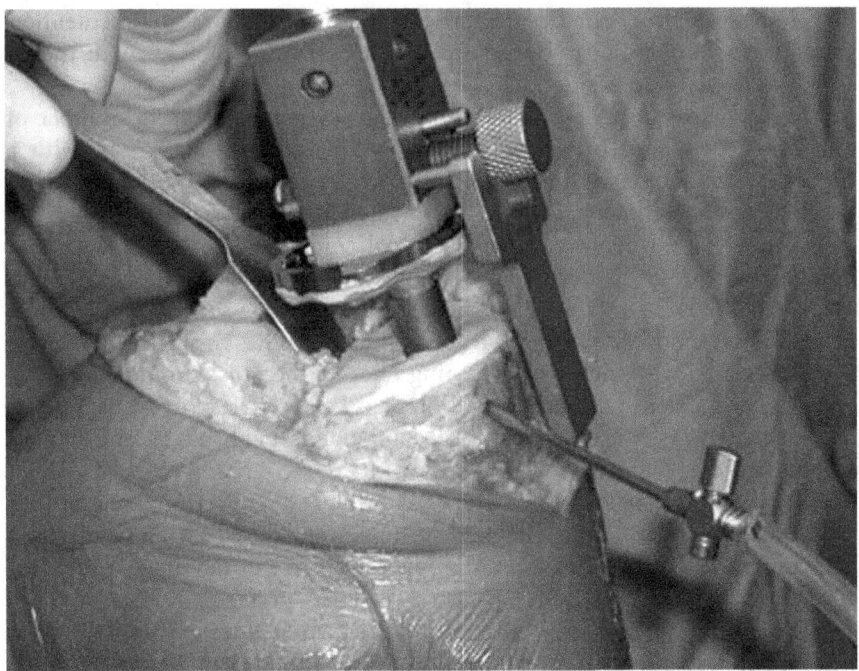

Fig. 2 – "Negative pressure intrusion" technique for the tibial component, using an intra-osseous suction canula.

Banwart *et al.* (33) demonstrated a tighter cement-bone composite using this technique, while Norton and Eyres (34) noted significantly higher cement penetration with this technique compared to conventional cementation, regardless of whether or not a tourniquet was used.

Uncemented TKA

Opponents of cemented total knee arthroplasty have argued that the above mentioned disadvantages associated with the use of PMMA cement can be avoided by using cementless fixation.

This option has become increasingly attractive since published series of uncemented TKA have become available, showing that at least equal results can be obtained both in the short and longer term as those using cement.

Scott *et al.* have reported a 95% component survivorship at 7 to 11-year follow-up in 212 knees using cementless fixation of the Natural-knee system (35).

Using revision as an end point, Whiteside has reported an overall survival rate of 94% at 10 years in 163 knees with the uncemented Ortholoc I knee (36).

Buechel published an overall survivorship rate of 95% at the 12 year interval for the cementless LCS-knee in 158 cases (37).

Sorrells *et al.* have reported a 93% survivorship at 13-years follow-up in 417 patients (38).

These reports can not be disregarded and they do show that cementless total knee arthroplasty can be as successful as cemented total knees at the 10 to 15-year follow-up evaluation.

Opponents of uncemented TKA have however argued that a number of negative papers have been published regarding uncemented knees, with a higher incidence of component loosening, radiolucencies, and osteolysis compared to cemented knees.

Rosenberg *et al.* reported a higher tibial component loosening rate in a comparative prospective study on the Miller-Galante uncemented versus cemented knee (39). Other uncemented knee designs such as the Porous-Coated Anatomic knee (PCA) (40, 42) and the AGC knee (43), have also been associated with increased loosening rates on the tibial components.

A higher incidence of radiolucent lines has been reported by some authors at the interface of uncemented tibial components in the PCA and Miller-Galante system (39, 41).

Other people however have seen no differences concerning radiolucent lines in studies comparing cemented versus uncemented fixation of identical implant types, or even a significantly higher number of radiolucent lines for the cemented group (44, 45).

Osteolysis has been associated with uncemented knee arthroplasty in a number of systems, such as a PCA knee, the Miller-Galante prosthesis, the Synatomic prosthesis, and the Arizona prosthesis (46, 48), but has also been reported for cemented knee components (49, 51).

Nevertheless, the problems of loosening, radiolucent lines and osteolysis that were observed in several uncemented knee systems can not be denied. They are however the consequence of not applying techniques or design features that are necessary for obtaining successful results with uncemented total knee arthroplasty.

The criteria for successful uncemented TKA are today well established. They include:

1) the presence of an appropriate contact between the implant and the underlying bone;

2) rigid initial fixation of the prosthetic components;

3) the presence of an appropriate porous coating.

Appropriate contact implant-bone

Several authors have shown that optimal integration of uncemented arthroplasty components requires the presence of an interface gap that is smaller than 0.5mm (52, 54).

Using modern instrumentation systems the operative accuracy for the femoral side has been reported to range between 0.5 and 0.8mm (55, 57) and between 1 to 2.4mm for the tibial side (56, 58).

Meticulous surgical technique and extremely accurate instrumentation are therefore of uppermost importance when performing uncemented total knee arthroplasty.

It is not surprising that many of the early generation uncemented knee systems were associated with increased loosening rates, especially at the tibial components, since they were inserted using instruments and surgical techniques that were not capable of reproducing the accuracy required for successful uncemented fixation, resulting in interface gaps larger than 0,5mm.

Using a precise surgical technique together with modern and more accurate instruments, these problems can be avoided.

The use of autologous bone grafts or hydroxyapatite coatings can further enhance the osseo-integration process.

Hofmann *et al.* have reported on the use of cancellous bone paste on the cut surface of the tibia and the femur to augment ingrowth, using autograft bone obtained from the cut surface of the tibial wafer using the patellar reamer (59).

Using this technique exellent clinical results were noted at 7 to 11 years of follow-up, with consistent and abundant bone ingrowth in as high as 40% of the pore volume. (59, 60)

The same effect has been noted for hydroxyapatite coatings based upon their osteoconductive characteristics, making the magnitude of the bone-implant interface gap less critical.

Soballe *et al.* have shown that unloaded hydroxyapatite-coated titanium plugs became osseointegrated even in the presence of 1mm interface gaps, while uncoated implants did not under these circumstances (61). These data were confirmed in other studies using hip and knee arthroplasty components in animal models, showing significantly higher bone ingrowth and bone ongrowth for hydroxyapatite-coated implants on histomorphometric analysis (62, 63, 65).

Hydroxyapatite coatings therefore seem to be most benefical in situations with relatively large (> 0.5mm) interface gaps between the implant and the bone.

An important concern however is the desintegration of hydroxyapatite coatings over time.

Although some resorption or dissolution is of course essential to trigger the basic osteoconductive effect of hydroxyapatite coatings, fast or complete desintegration could theoretically lead to loss of integration and component loosening over time (64, 68).

Long-term clinical data are therefore necessary to determine whether hydroxyapatite can serve as a substitute to precise surgical technique in obtaining a close implant-bone contact.

Rigid initial fixation

Stable initial fixation is another prerequisite for successful integration of uncemented components.

Excessive interface motion has been shown to lead to the formation of a fibrous connective tissue layer, while bone ingrowth has been noted in mechanically stable implants (69, 70). Achieving initial mechanical stability and thus minimizing micromotion is therefore a prime consideration in uncemented total knee arthroplasty. Relative displacement less than 150μm of motion has been found to be consistent with osseo-integration (69, 70).

Rigid initial fixation with micromotion less than 150μm does not seem to be a problem for the femoral component in TKA, since it provides adequate intrinsic resistance to rigid body motion by virtue of its shape and box-like configuration. Press fitting the anterior and posterior condylar surfaces increases the frictional forces and tends to immobilize the femoral component. The anterior and posterior surfaces tend to resist antero-posterior translation, flexion-extension tilt and rotation. The routine use of metaphyseal lugs or pegs distally further prevents mediolateral tilt, mediolateral translation and rotation (71).

For the tibial component however, obtaining rigid fixation is more problematic.

Tibial trays fixed with simple interference fit peg fixation have been shown to move 400 to 800μm, with or without additional fixation of a central screw (72, 73). Tibial trays fixed with a central cylindrical stem alone, show an initial micromotion of 200 to 400μm, which is still too high for reliable integration.

The addition of cruciate-shape blades to such a stem further inhibits micromotion, but still in the region of 150 to 200μm (74).

Volz *et al.* and Miura *et al.* have shown that when tibial trays are fixed with four screws, micromotion is between 100 to 200μm, which might be compatible with osseointegration (73, 75). Adding a central stem to the four screws does not seem to improve micromotion in tibial bone with good quality, but can lead to substantially less micromotion in osteopenic bone (76, 77).

The routine combination of four screws and a central stem for fixation of uncemented tibial components therefore seems to be the best choice for controlling micromotion (fig. 3).

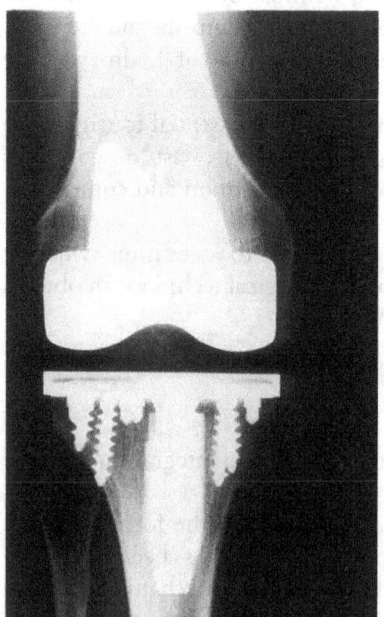

The addition of interference pegs might be additionally beneficial, as has been shown by Natarajan *et al.*, who reported relative tangentinal displacements as high as 200μm when subjecting tibial components to compressive loads (78).

Such tangentinal displacement is the consequence of the variation in elastic modulus between the metal tibial tray and the underlying bone, and can be reduced substantially by the use of interferences pegs. As stated above, these pegs do not influence the rigid body motion, which is to be controlled by screws and an additional stem.

Fig. 3 – Rigid component fixation and precise surgical fit are two important prerequisites for successful uncemented TKA.

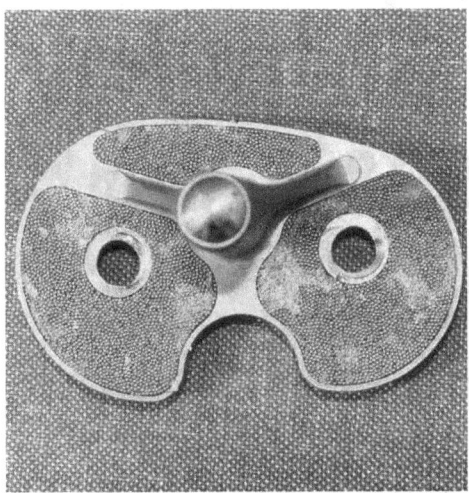

Fig. 4 – Many " first generation" cementless knees were inserted with poor initial fixation, leading to the formation of a fibrous connective tissue layer and an increased risk for loosening.

In view of these data, it is again not surprising that an increased prevalence of radiolucent lines and an increased number of tibial component loosenings have been reported in many of the early and even current uncemented knee designs, as a consequence of the poor initial fixation options available for the tibial component in these systems, resulting in micromotion exceeding 150μm. (fig. 4).

Using components with an adequate initial fixation can however avoid these problems.

Appropriate porous coating

The third prerequisite for successful uncemented total knee arthroplasty is the presence of an appropriate porous coating on the component surface.

The effective pore size of the coating should be between 50 and 400μm for reliable cementless integration (79).

Titanium versus cobalt chrome alloy, or beads versus fiber structure appear not to be very important issues. Continuity of the coating, however, is. Smooth metal bridges separating the porous coating are a pathway for debris migration, while a uniform continuous coating can effectively seal off the interface, even if that interface is occupied entirely by fibrous tissue.

Protection of the implant-bone interface by the fibrous tissue mantle that penetrates the porous coating is a well-documented phenomenon (79, 81).

Further evidence concerning this was provided by Whiteside, who reported a 0% incidence of osteolysis in the uncemented Ortholoc knee when a continuous porous coating was applied, versus a 17% incidence of osteolytic lesions when a porous coating interrupted by smooth metal bridges was used on the same system (82) (fig. 5).

With a limited distribution of porous coating, particles can enter the implant-bone interface and metaphyseal bone by way of the unbonded inter-

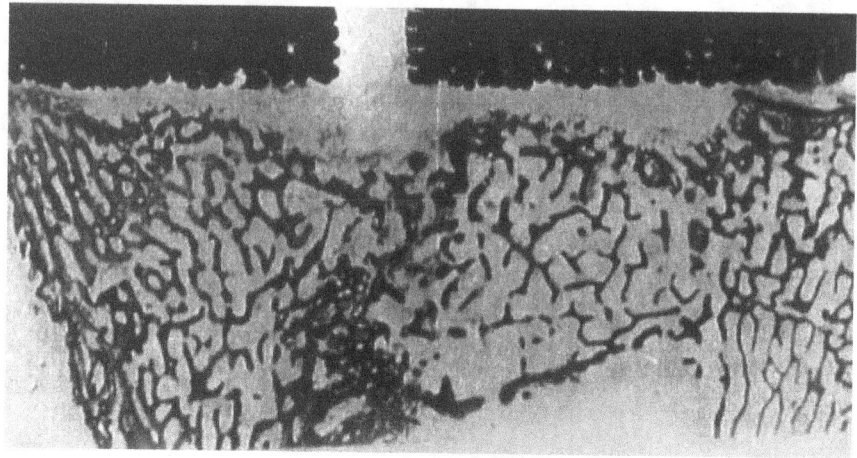

Fig. 5 – Undersurface of a revised uncemented tibial component with osteolysis, clearly showing the smooth metal bridges separating the porous coating, which act as a pathway for debris migration.

face between the smooth metal and bone. The development of osteolysis is not a direct function of the absence of cement, but is related to other variables that have been associated with first generation total knee replacements, such as polyethylene quality and articular surface design (83).

It is therefore not surprising that osteolysis has also been noted with cemented components as well (49, 51).

For the same reason it is not surprising that many of the early cementless knees, with a high potential for debris generation due to poor articular surface design and polyethylene quality, in combination with the presence of smooth metal bridges separating the porous coating, have been associated with osteolysis.

This however can be minimized when modern designs with more confirming surfaces in combination with an appropriate continous porous coating are used.

Conclusion

Several authors have shown that both cemented and uncemented total knee arthroplasty can be successful at the 10 to 15 years follow-up.

The potential disadvantages associated with the use of polymethylmetacrylate cement have not tempered the enthusiasm based upon the clinical results. Cement therefore remains the gold standard for a number of surgeons, also because of its more "forgiving" nature with regard to surgical technique.

Meticulous surgical technique is an important prerequisite for successful uncemented TKA, together with two other aspects: rigid initial fixation and the presence of an appropriate porous coating on the implant.

Failure to comply with these criteria has lead to a number of negative reports in the past concerning cementless fixation of knee arthroplasty components.

Surgeons who do use the techniques necessary for uncemented TKA, together with an appropriate design, can achieve the same excellent results as with cemented TKA, giving their patients the additional benefit of a biological and durable cement-free interface.

References

1. Stern S, Insall J (1992) Posterior stabilized prosthesis. Results after follow-up of nine to twelve years. Journal of Bone and Joint Surgery 74-A: 980-6
2. Font-Rodriguez D, Scuderi G, Insall J (1997) Survivorship of cemented total knee arthroplasty. Clinical Orthopaedics and Related Research 345: 79-86
3. Ranawat C, Flynn W, Saddler S et al. (1993) Long-term results of the total condylar knee arthroplasty : a 15-year survivorship study. Clinical Orthopaedics and Related Research 286: 94-102
4. Emmerson K, Moran C, Pinder I (1996) Survivorship of the kinematic stabiliser total knee replacement. A 10 to 14-year follow-up study. Journal of Bone and Joint Surgery 78-B: 441-5
5. Scott R (1996) Posterior cruciate ligament retaining designs and results. In: Current concepts in primary and revision total knee arthroplasty. Eds. Insall J, Scott W, Scuderi G, 37-40. Lippincott-Raven, Philadelphia
6. Vince K, Insall J, Kelly M (1989) The total condylar prosthesis:10 to 12-year results of a cemented knee replacement. Journal of Bone and Joint Surgery 71-B: 793-7
7. Ranawat C, Boachie-Adjei O (1988) Survivorship analysis and results of total condylar knee arthroplasty. Eight to twelve year follow-up period. Clinical Orthopaedics and Related Research 226: 6-13
8. Weir D, Moran C, Pinder I (1996) Kinematic condylar total knee arthroplasty: 14-year survivorship analysis of 208 consecutive cases. Journal of Bone and Joint Surgery 78-B: 907-11
9. Schai P, Thornhill T, Scott R (1998) Total knee arthroplasty with the PFC system. Results at a minimum of 10 years and survivorship analysis. Journal of Bone and Joint Surgery 80-B: 850-8
10. Gill G, Joshi A, Mills D (1999) Total condylar knee arthroplasty: 16 to 21-year results. Clinical Orthopaedics and Related Research 367: 210-5
11. Lewis G (1997) Properties of acrylic bone cement : state of the art review. Journal of Biomedical Materials Research 38: 155-82
12. Spector M (1992) Biomaterial failure. Orthopaedic Clinics of North America 23: 211-7
13. Jones L, Hungerford D (1987) Cement disease. Clinical Orthopaedics and Related Research 225: 192-203
14. Isaac G, Wroblewski B, Atkinson J et al. (1990) Source of the cement within the Charnley hip. Journal of Bone and Joint Surgery 72-B: 149-50
15. Jasty M, Jiranek W, Harris W (1992) Acrylic fragmentation in total hip replacements and its biological consequences. Clinical Orthopaedics and Related Research 285: 116-28
16. Oates K, Barrera D, Tucker W et al. (1995) In vivo effect of pressurization of polymethyl methacrylate bone cement. Biomechanical and histologic analysis. Journal of Arthroplasty, 10: 373-81
17. Savarino L, Stea S, Ciagetti G et al. (1995) Microstructural investigation of bone-cement interface. Journal of Biomedical Materials Research 29: 701-5
18. Kindt-Larsen T, Smith D, Jensen J (1995) Innovations in acrylic bone cement and application equipment. Journal of Applied Biomaterials, 6: 75-83
19. Liu Y, Park J, Njus G et al. (1987) Bone particle-impregnated bone cement : an in vitro study. Journal of Biomedical Materials Research 21: 247-61

20. Berman A, Parmet J, Harding S et al. (1998) Emboli observed with use of transesopheal echocardiography immediately after tourniquet release during total knee arthroplasty with cement. Journal of Bone and Joint Surgery 80-A: 389-96

21. Seki T, Tashiro T, Omori G et al. (1998) Microstrain on the cortex and within the bone of the distal femur with cemented and uncemented femoral components in total knee arthroplasty. Proceedings of the 44th Annual Meeting of the Orthopaedic Research Society: 699

22. Petty W (1978) The effect of methylmetacrylate on bacterial phagocytosis and killing by human polymorphonuclear leukocytes. Journal of Bone and Joint Surgery 60-A: 752-7

23. Petty W (1978) The effect of methylmetacrylate on chemotaxis of polymorphonuclear leukocytes. Journal of Bone and Joint Surgery 60-A: 492-8

24. Hanssen A, Rand J (1998) Evaluation and treatment of infection at the site of a total hip or knee arthroplasty. Journal of Bone and Joint Surgery 80-A: 910-22

25. Otani T, Fujii K, Ozawa M et al. (1998) Impingement after total knee arthroplasty caused by cement extrusion and proximal tibiofibular instability. Journal of Arthroplasty, 13: 589-91

26. Sambatakakis A, Wilton T, Newton G (1991) Radiographic sign of persistent soft-tissue imbalance after knee replacement. Journal of Bone and Joint Surgery 73-B: 751-6

27. Graham J, Pruitt L, Ries M et al. (2000) Fracture and fatigue properties of acrylic bone cement. The effects of mixing method, sterilization treatment, and molecular weight. Journal of Arthroplasty, 15: 1028-35

28. Schmidt J (1998) The cemented prosthesis: what is sure, what is open? In: Walenkamp G. (ed) Biomaterials in surgery. Thieme, Stuttgart: 48-51

29. Bert J, McShane M (1998) Is it necessary to cement the tibial stem in cemented total knee arthroplasty? Clinical Orthopaedics and Related Research 356: 73-8

30. Lombardi A, Mallory T, Gunderson R et al. (1998) Surface cementation of the tibial component in total knee arthroplasty. 65th Annual Meeting of the American Academy of Orthopaedic Surgeons, New Orleans, 19-23 February

31. Ritter M, Herbst S, Keating M et al. (1994) Radiolucency at the bone cement interface in total knee replacement. Journal of Bone and Joint Surgery 76-A: 60-5

32. Insall J, Scuderi G (2001) Acrylic cement is the method of choice for fixation of total knee implants. In: Laskin R. (ed) Controversies in total knee replacement. Oxford University Press, New York: 163-72

33. Banwart C, McQueen D, Friis E et al. (2000) Negative pressure intrusion cementing technique for total knee arthroplasty. Journal of Arthroplasty, 15: 360-7

34. Norton M, Eyres K (2000) Irrigation and suction technique to ensure reliable cement penetration for total knee arthroplasty. Journal of Arthroplasty, 15: 468-74

35. Scott D, Hofmann A, Thach T et al. (1997) Seven to eleven year experience with cementless fixation using the Natural knee. Proceedings of the 64th Annual Meeting of the American Academy of Orthopaedic Surgeons: 353

36. Whiteside L (1994) Cementless total knee replacement. 9 to 11-year results and 10-year survivorship analysis. Clinical Orthopaedics and Related Research 309: 185-92

37. Buechel F (1994) Cementless meniscal bearing knee arthroplasty: 7 to 12-year outcome analysis. Orthopaedics, 17: 833-6

38. Sorrells B, Voorhorst P, Greenwald S (1999) The long-term clinical use of a rotating platform mobile bearing TKA. Proceedings of the 66th Annual Meeting of the American Academy of Orthopaedic Surgeons: 228

39. Rosenberg A, Barden R, Galante J (1990) Cemented and ingrowth fixation of the Miller-Galante prosthesis. Clinical and roentgenographic comparison after 3 to 6 years follow-up studies. Clinical Orthopaedics and Related Research 260: 71-9

40. Moran C, Pinder I, Lees T et al. (1991) Survivorship analysis of the uncemented porous-coated anatomic knee replacement. Journal of Bone and Joint Surgery 73-A: 848-57

41. Collins D, Heim S, Nelson C et al. (1991) Porous-coated anatomic total knee arthroplasty: A prospective analysis comparing cemented and cementless fixation. Clinical Orthopaedics and Related Research 267: 128-36

42. Eskola A, Vahvanen V, Santavita S et al. (1992) Porous-coated anatomic knee arthroplasty. Three year results. Journal of Arthroplasty, 7: 223-8

43. Nielsen P, Hansen E, Rechangel K (1992) Cementless total knee arthroplasty in unselected cases of osteoarthritis and rheumatoid arthritis. A 3-year follow-up study of 103 cases. Journal of Arthroplasty, 7: 137-43

44. Rand J (1991) Cement or cementless fixation in total knee arthroplasty. Clinical Orthopaedics and Related Research 273: 52-62

45. McCaskie, Deehan D, Green T et al. (1998) Randomised, prospective study comparing cemented and cementless total knee replacement. Journal of Bone and Joint Surgery 80-B: 971-5

46. Lewis P, Rorabeck C, Bourne R (1995) Screw osteolysis after cementless total knee replacement. Clinical Orthopaedics and Related Research 321: 173-7

47. Peters P, Engh G, Dwyer K et al. (1992) Osteolysis after total knee arthroplasty without cement. Journal of Bone and Joint Surgery 74-A: 864-76

48. Kim Y, Oh J, Oh S (1995) Osteolysis around cementless porous-coated anatomic knee prosthesis. Journal of Bone and Joint Surgery 77-B: 236-41

49. Robinson E, Mulliken B, Bourne R et al. (1995) Catastrophic osteolysis in total knee replacement. A report of 17 cases. Clinical Orthopaedics and Related Research 321: 98-105

50. Ries M, Guiney W, Lynch F (1994) Osteolysis associated with cemented total knee arthroplasty. A case report. Journal of Arthroplasty, 9: 555-8

51. Ezzet K, Garcia R, Barrack R (1995) Effect of component fixation method on osteolysis in total knee arthroplasty. Clinical Orthopaedics and Related Research 321: 86-91

52. Carlsson L, Rostlund T, Albrektsson B et al. (1988) Implant fixation proved by close fit cylindrical implant-bone interface studies in rabbits. Acta Orthopaedica Scandinavica, 59: 272-5

53. Sandborn P, Cook S, Spires W et al. (1988) Tissue response to porous coated implants lacking initial bone apposition. Journal of Arthroplasty, 3: 337-46

54. Dalton J, Cook S, Thomas K et al. (1995) The effect of operative fit and hydroxyapatite coating on the mechanical and biological response to porous implants. Journal of Bone and Joint Surgery 77-A: 97-110

55. Otani T, Whiteside L, White S (1993) Cutting errors in preparation of femoral components in total knee arthroplasty. Journal of Arthroplasty, 8: 503-10

56. Dueringer K, Stalcup G (1995) Bone cut accuracy and flatness from milling and sawing. A comparative study. Zimmer Inc

57. Lennox D, Cohn B, Eschenroeder H (1998) The effects of inaccurate bone cuts on femoral component position in total knee arthroplasty. Orthopedics, 11: 257-60

58. Toksvig-Larsen S, Ryd L (1991) Surface flatness in orthopedic bone cutting. Transactions of the Orthopaedic Research Society, 16: 497

59. Hofmann A, Murdock L, Wyatt R et al. Total knee arthroplasty: 2 to 4 year experience using an assymetric tibial tray and a deep trochlear-grooved femoral component. Clinical Orthopaedics and Related Research 269: 78-88

60. Scott D, Hofmann A, Thach T et al. (1997) Seven to eleven year experience with cementless fixation using the Natural knee. Proceedings of the 64th Annual Meeting of the American Academy of Orthopaedic Surgeons: 353

61. Soballe K, Hansen E, Brockstedt-Rasmussen H et al. (1990) Hydroxyapatite coating enhances fixation of porous coated implants : a comparison in dogs between press fit and non interference fit. Acta Orthopaedica Scandinavica 61: 299-306

62. Geesink R (1989) Experimental and clinical experience with hydroxyapatite coated hip implants. Clinical Orthopaedics and Related Research 291: 239-42

63. Munting E (1996) The contribution and limitation of hydroxyapatite coating to implant fixation. International Orthopaedics 20: 1-6

64. Bauer T (1993) The histology of HA - coated implants. In: Hydroxyapatite coatings in ortopaedic surgery (eds. Geesinck R. and Manley M), pp. 305-318. Raven Press, New-York

65. Bellemans J (1997) Osseo-integration in porous coated knee arthroplasty. The sheep stifle joint as in vivo evaluation model. Ph.D. Dissertation, Katholieke Universiteit Leuven, Belgium: 56-127

66. Bloebaum R, Beeks D, Dorr L (1994) Complications with hydroxyapatite particulate separation in total hip arthroplasty. Clinical Orthopaedics and Related Research 298: 19-26

67. Le Geros R, Dalculsi G, Orly I *et al.* (1992) Formation of carbonate apatite on calcium phosphate materials: dissolution/precipitation processes. In : Bone-bonding biomaterials, pp. 201-12, Read Healthcare Communications, Leiderdorp

68. Soballe K, Overgaerd S (1996) The current status of hydroxyapatite coating of prostheses. Journal of Bone and Joint Surgery 78B: 689-91

69. Burke D (1991) Dynamic measurements of interface mechanics *in vivo* and the effect of micromotion on bone ingrowth into a porous coated surface device under controlled loads *in vivo*. Transaction of the Orthopaedic Research Society, 16: 103

70. Pilliar R, Lee J, Maniatopoulos C (1986) Observations on the effect of movement on bone ingrowth into porous-surfaced implants. Clinical Orthopaedics and Related Research 208: 108-13

71. Rosenberg A, Galante J (1994) Cementless total knee arthroplasty. In "Knee surgery" volume II, (eds. F.Fu, C.Harner, K.Vince) pp. 1367-1383, Williams Wilkins, Baltimore

72. Shimagaki H, Bechtold J, Sherman R, Gustilo R (1990) Stability of initial fixation of the tibial component in cementless total knee arthroplasty. Journal of Orthopaedic Research 8: 64-71

73. Volz R, Nisbet J, Lee W *et al.* (1988) The mechanical stability of various noncemented tibial components. Clinical Orthopaedics and Related Research 226: 38-42

74. Walker P, Hsu H, Zimmerman R (1990) A comparative study of uncemented tibial components. Journal of Arthroplasty, 5: 245-53

75. Miura M, Whiteside L, Easley J *et al.* (1990) Effects of screws and a sleeve on initial fixation in uncemented total knee tibial components. Clinical Orthopaedics and Related Research 259: 160-68

76. Lee R, Volz R, Sheridan D (1991) The role of fixation and bone quality on the mechanical stability of tibial knee components. Clinical Orthopaedics and Related Research 273: 177-83

77. Yoshii J, Whiteside L, Milliano M *et al.* (1992) The effect of central stem and stem length on micromovement of the tibial tray. Journal of Arthroplasty7: 433-8

78. Natarajan R, Andriacchi T (1988) The influence of displacement incompatibilities on bone growth in porous tibial components. Transaction of the Orthopaedic Research Society 13: 331

79. Bobyn J, Jacobs J, Tanzer M *et al.* (1995) The susceptibility of smooth implant surfaces to peri-implant fibrosis and migration of polyethylene wear debris. Clinical Orthopaedics and Related Research 311: 21-39

80. Engh C, Zettl-Schaffer K, Kukita Y *et al.* (1993) Histological and radiographic assessment of well functioning porous-coated acetabular components. Journal of Bone and Joint Surgery 75-A: 814-24

81. Ward W, Johnson K, Dorey F *et al.* (1993) Extramedullary porous coating to prevent diaphyseal osteolysis and radiolucent lines around proximal tibial replacements. Journal of Bone and Joint Surgery 75-A: 976-87

82. Whiteside L (1995) Effect of porous coating configuration on tibial osteolysis after total knee arthroplasty. Clinical Orthopaedics and Related Research 321: 92-7

83. Schmalzried T, Callaghan J (1999) Wear in total hip and knee replacements. . Journal of Bone and Joint Surgery 81-A: 115-36

The mobile plateau in total knee arthroplasty

P. Aglietti, A. Baldini

Introduction

Mobile bearing knees are a class of knee prostheses in which a plastic bearing is interposed between the femoral component and the tibial plate, such that the plastic moves with the femur and slides on the plate (48). A lot of different designs of mobile bearing knee prosthesis are being developed today by different companies. This concept was introduced in the late 1970s guided by the purpose of reproducing closer kinematics to the normal knee. The goal of these new designs is to try and solve the problem of polyethylene wear through highly conforming surfaces, replicating meniscal function, while removing constraint in rotation and / or A-P slide. An other objective is to improve knee function and flexion. Both of these objectives relate to the possibility of using these knees in younger and more active patients.

Rotation occurs at the knee during most activities, including walking. It has been calculated in walking volunteers that 5° of internal tibial rotation takes place for a few milliseconds during the stance phase (with load) and 10° of external rotation occur during the swing phase without load (46). A modern knee prosthesis requires at least 12° of rotation to take care also of situations without load (76).

An important feature of physiological knee kinematics is that the posterior cruciate produces a posterior displacement of the femur on the tibia as flexion proceeds, while the relatively greater stability of the medial side of the joint compared with the lateral results in a differential in roll-back, producing tibial internal rotation (6, 61, 73). As flexion progresses, the femuro-tibial contact points move posteriorly, particularly laterally, by a total of 8mm on average through the 0-120° flexion range. In parallel with the posterior displacement of the femur there is an internal rotation of the tibia about its long axis (20). These movements are guided by the PCL only if it is properly tensioned (67).

Classic femoral anatomy describes a decreasing radius for the posterior condyles, but recent studies have shown a constant posterior condylar radius in the order of magnitude of 21 to 23mm for medial femoral condyle (26, 37). Thus a femoral component with a constant sagittal radius would appear to be the most desirable.

It has been postulated that the knee flexes around an axis closely approximating the femoral epicondyles. This axis passes through the centers of the posterior femoral condyles (37) and is always perpendicular to the tibial axis at all degrees of flexion (75). Furthermore, there is a second rotational axis which is approximately parallel to the tibial long axis and medial to the joint center (44).

Since 1976 P Trent and P Walker, using ten fresh autopsy specimens and a pho-
tographic method, observed that the center of transverse rotation of the tibia
was located on the medial aspect of the tibial spine (74). This implies that
during knee motion there are two distinct components: flexion-extension, that
rotates about the transepicondylar axis, and internal-external rotation about a
medially biased tibial axis. Such "compound hinge model" was recently
demonstrated by Churchill *et al.* recording the 3-D tibiofemoral kinematics in
fifteen cadaveric knees tested in simulating squatting using an Oxford rig (21).

Recently Freeman and coauthors studied the shapes and relative movements of the femur and tibia in the loaded and unloaded cadaver and living
knee using MRI and RSA. They found that the combination during flexion
of no anteroposterior movement medially (i.e., sliding) and backward rolling
(combined with sliding) laterally equates to internal rotation of the tibia
around a medial axis with flexion. About 5° of this rotation may be obligatory from 0° to 10° flexion; thereafter little rotation occurs to at least 45°. Total
rotation at 110° is about 20°, most of which can be suppressed by applying
external rotation to the tibia at 90° (35, 36, 41, 53, 57).

Types of mobile bearing knees

Based on the degree of conformity of the articular surface of the mobile bearing these prostheses are divided into two categories: partially conforming and
fully conforming. Another category that has been recently introduced is that
of posterior stabilized meniscal bearing prostheses.

Partially conforming

In this first category the most time-tested design is the **Low Contact Stress
(LCS) total knee system** (DePuy Inc., Warsaw, Indiana, USA) with both the

Table I – Partially conforming mobile bearing knees

Implant type	Manufacturer
Low contact stress (LCS) knee system	DePuy Inc., Warsaw, Indiana, USA
PFC Sigma rotating platform knee system	DePuy Inc., Warsaw, Indiana, USA
Self Aligning (SAL) mobile bearing knee	Sulzer Orthopaedics, Baar, Switzerland
Innex knee system	Zimmer, Warsaw, Indiana, USA
Total articulating cementless knee (TACK)	Waldemar Link, hamburg, Germany
Interax : Integrated secure asymmetric	Howmedica, Rutherford, New Jersey, USA
Total rotating knee (TRK)	Cremascoli, Milan, Italy
Profix total knee system	Smith & Nephew Inc., Memphis, TN, USA
Genesis II Total knee system	Smith & Nephew Inc., Memphis, TN, USA
Minns meniscal knee prosthesis	Zimmer U.K., Swindon, U.K.

rotating platform or the anatomically separated two meniscal bearing knee design. This prosthesis is still the most widely used mobile bearing design and was developed at the end of the 70s by Buechel and Pappas.

In 1977 these authors introduced the first version that was composed of two separated plastic bearings located in curved tracks on the tibial tray. Both cruciates could be preserved. They also pioneered a second version, the one piece plastic bearing rotating platform with a postprojecting below in a hole of the tray to allow for free rotation. When one side of the platform moves backward the other moves forwards which is not physiological but simple and functional. This design is highly congruent in both planes resulting in a large contact area with very low contact stresses and offers stability in the AP direction substituting the function of the PCL. Also the patellar component is of the rotating-bearing type. It was developed in order to maintain a spherical contact area on the medial and lateral facets with the femoral trochlea throughout flexion (12, 55).

Initially the prostheses were used with cement (16), in 1981 non-cemented use was also introduced with the availability of sintered-bead porous coating.

The cemented and uncemented unicompartmental meniscal knee replacement have a reported 91% and 98% of survivorship at ten years respectively (8, 11, 14). At ten years of follow-up the reported survivorship for the cemented bicruciate retaining meniscal bearing design is 90% and for the cementless device 95%. Failure with these devices where observed in cases of previous high tibial osteotomy or tibial plateau fracture (Hamelynck, p.com.). Another cause of failure with these implants was a deficient ACL. In fact, in these cases, early or late rupture of the ACL degrades the arthroplasty to the level of an ACL-deficient knee (13, 16). The cemented and cementless rotating platform have a reported survivorship rate of 97.5% at 10 years of follow-up (9,15). Sorrels evaluated 665 cementless rotating platform consecutively implanted between 1984 and 1995. Survivorship at 11 years was 94.7%, with a revision rate of 2% (65). Callaghan reviewed the results of 119 cemented LCS rotating platform TKRs after 9 to 12-years of follow-up. There were no mechanical failures and none of the components had been revised. The average HSS score was 84 points. Knee flexion was 102° on average at follow-up (18).

Mechanical complications have been identified for meniscal bearings, rotating platforms and rotating bearing patellar replacements (17). These complications include: loosening, bearing dislocation, fracture and wear, patella bearing "spin out" and osteolysis. Meniscal bearing dislocation was seen by Buechel et al. in 1.1% of primary TKRs during FDA clinical trials and was associated with rotatory malposition of the tibial component and poor flexion-extension gaps balance. Meniscal bearing fracture was also seen in 1.1% of primary TKRs and was associated with rotatory malposition of the tibial component, a thin flexible lip on the bearing, poor quality polyethylene and gamma radiation in air sterilization. Severe wear has required bearing exchange or revision in 1% of the cases between 8 and 19 years of follow-up. Rotating platform dislocation was observed in less than 0.5% of primary or multiply operated TKRs and in 5% of revision TKRs over a 12 years period (10). Bert et al. reported a high dislocation rate of 9.3% using rotating platform and PCL-retaining LCS knee replacements (7). Jordan *et al.* in 473 cementless cruciate retaining meniscal bearing LCS, followed for 5 years in average, reported a 3.6% of mechanical failures with 12 polyethylene fractures or dislocations and 5 tibial subluxations secondary to ligamentous instability (45). It was pointed out that such dislocation rates could be caused by failure to obtain a proper flexion-extension knee stability at surgery (12). Rotating bearing patellar replacements dislocated, dissociated, fractured or wore out in less than 1% of all cases over a 20 year period, and patellar component spin out occurred in less than 0.05% of the cases (17).

In vivo kinematic analysis was performed by J Stiehl *et al.* using fluoroscopy and image matching technique in 10 normal patients and in 10 patients with a PCL retaining bimeniscal bearing knee replacement. He observed that the initial contact point in extension is more posterior than normal and beyond 60° of flexion there tends to be anterior femoral translation. Kinematic patterns beyond 60° of flexion tend to be erratic and less reproducible respect to normal knees. 5 of the meniscal bearing knees had anterior sliding of the bearings with flexion, whereas 5 bearings remained stationary in the same position relating to the tibial tray (68).

Additional kinematic analysis by the same authors showed that patients who have had a posterior-cruciate-sacrificing rotating platform have less anteroposterior femorotibial translation during gait, with less variability among patients, than those who have had a fixed-bearing TKR. Femoral lateral condylar lift-off was commonly found after all types of TKR and did not appear to be related by bearing mobility (70, 71, 19).

The **P.F.C. Sigma Rotating Platform (RP) Knee System** (DePuy Inc., Warsaw, Indiana, USA) combines the design and clinical experience of the P.F.C. Sigma fixed bearing and LCS mobile-bearing implants. This system has two rotating bearing versions: "Curved" or "Posterior Stabilised". Each insert rotates around a central stem location as in the LCS rotating platform. Femoral component that articulates with the "Curved" version is the same as in the P.F.C. Sigma cruciate-retaining fixed bearing type, while for the "PS" is the same as in the P.F.C. Sigma cruciate substituting fixed bearing type.

Tibial baseplates are chromium cobalt higly polished 4.8mm thick. All the components of this system are cemented or cementless types. The main difference between older Sigma fixed bearing design and the newer Sigma RP is almost full conformity in both the coronal and sagittal planes. The radii are closely matched to one another (i.e., 1.03:1mm in the coronal plane and 1.02:1 in the sagittal plane).

Peak contact stresses measured using Tekscan through a full range of motion showed an average stress reduction of 4MPa for the P.F.C. "Curved" mobile bearing respect to the "Curved" fixed bearing (23).

Dr Schifrine from Annecy, France reported his experience from 1996 to 1999 of 126 Sigma RP-PS in 115 patients. At a follow-up of 21 months average Knee Society score increased from 42 to 94 points and Function score from 54 to 89. Mean active flexion was 110° preoperatively and 117° postoperatively. Complications were 5 patellar clunks and one case of deep infection (62).

Dr Perka from Berlin, Germany reported his experience with 87 Sigma RP Curved and PS. At a follow up of 12 months average Knee Society score increased from 54 to 90 points and function score from 52 to 81. Mean active flexion was 85° preoperatively and 102° postoperatively. Complications were 1 case of deep infection, 1 major haematoma and delayed wound healing (56).

The **Self Aligning (SAL) mobile bearing knee** (Sulzer Orthopaedics, Baar, Switzerland) designed by Bourne and Rorabeck in 1987 allows limited A-P translation and unlimited rotation thanks to an oval recess in the back surface of the one piece poly that matches a peg on the tibial tray. The femoral component is relatively flat in the coronal surface and has full conformity throughout the first 70-75° of flexion, while the posterior condyles are only partially conforming. The trochlear groove is deep and extended. Right and left femoral components are available. The tibial tray is now of a stiff polished CoCrMo (while in the first version the tray was titanium) with a single peg on the upper surface and two fixation broach pegs with a central stem (two sizes available: 25 or 50mm) on the back-surface. The patella (two sizes available: 25 or 30mm) is a modified dome single pegged and symmetrical but sensitive to position due to a central eminence (9mm thick). Components fixation can be with cement (preferred by the authors) or cementless.

Polyethylene wear study was performed using 3-D measurements referring to some markers in the poly. No detectable wear of both the top surface and the back surface was observed. In 1988 the first 10 SAL knees were implanted. In a multicentric european clinical trial started in 1993, 234 SAL-I knee replacements were followed at 2 and 5 years of follow-up. Preoperative diagnosis was osteoarthritis in 172 patients. Average Knee Society rating score increased from 35 points preoperatively to 84 points at 2 years and 90 points at 5 years of follow-up. Patellar lateral release was performed in 24 (10%) knees. PCL managing included: retention (most of times), recession (10% of the cases) or sacrifice (less than 5%). Revision rate was 5.1%. In 3 cases reoperation was caused by a femoral component loosening; in 2 cases it was caused by vertical patellar fracture (Rorabeck, p. com.).

Kaper *et al.* evaluated 141 patients with osteoarthritis of the knee that underwent 172 total knee replacements using the Self Aligning I TKR. At average follow-up of 5.6 years, clinical results showed a 94% satisfaction rate. Two revision surgeries have been performed for polyethylene wear, with none of the remaining knees showing evidence of discernible wear (40).

The **Innovation Nexus Next Generation (Innex) Knee System** was developed at Wilhelm Schulthess Clinic in Zurich. This system provides fixed and mobile bearing implant versions both with cemented and cementless options.

There are two types of mobile bearings:

1) The "UCOR" (Ultra Congruent Only Rotating) is implanted with sacrifice of the cruciate ligaments and the bearing is a partial conforming rotating platform that rotates around a central post of the tray;

2) The "CR" (Cruciate retaining) allows for posterior cruciate ligament preservation and is free to rotate and glide anteroposteriorly thanks to a slot in the insert undersurface that articulates with a orizontal track guiding mecha-

nism that controls also rotation by a central postprojecting below in a hole of the tray.

The **Total Articulating Cementless Knee (TACK)** (Waldemar Link, Hamburg, Germany) has been implanted since 1990. This prosthesis has right and left femoral components of the total condylar type that articulate with a rotating polyethylene platform. The tibial tray is provided with two semi-circular guides that engage circular tracks on both sides of the platform allowing for free rotational movements in each direction. PCL retention is permitted by a central cut out in the platform and the tibial tray. Back surfaces of tibial and femoral components are composed of a three dimensional grid-like and a hydroxyapatite coating is also available in order to improve cementless fixation.

The **Interax I.S.A. (Integrated Secure Asymmetric)** (Howmedica International, Rutherford, New Jersey, USA) retains high but not full conformity between the spherical distal condyles of the asymmetric femoral component (left and right knees) and the meniscal bearing in extension. In flexion this conformity gradually decreases. The tibial baseplate is symmetrical and has two central posts protruding from the plate with a circular mushroom cap that engages with a T-shaped curved guide track in the inner surface of meniscal bearing that is provided in left and right configuration as determinated by the curve of this track. This confers a medially biased kinematics to the knee (47). This mechanism allows for internal and external rotation of the bearing of 36°, pivoting around a point in the medial compartment and for an AP motion of 14-24mm from extension to flexion (57). Fixation choices include a unique Cast-Mesh ingrowth surface, Cast-Mesh with hydroxyapatite or "Diamond" macro-textured surface for cemented option.

In vivo fluoroscopic evaluation of bearing mobility in 24 patients was conducted at Saarland University by Dr Kohn who demonstrated that in squatting activity from 0 to 90° the average bearing displacement was 2mm.

An ongoing prospective international multicentre clinical study is being conducted at four centres throughout Europe. 153 patients were entered into the trial from November 1995 to April 1997. A mean follow up time of 24 months was available for 57 of these patients. The average age was 68.1 years (range: 32-86) and 79.1% were female. Preoperative diagnosis was osteoarthritis in 84.3%. The prostheses were implanted without cement and approximately two third of the patellae were not resurfaced. Patellar retinacular lateral release was performed in 11.8% of the cases. The PCL was functionally preserved in the majority of cases (97.4%). The Knee score improved from 42.3 at the preoperative assesment (n = 153) to a maximum of 91.5 at the 2-year assessment (n = 57). The function score improved from 44.5 (n = 153) to a maximum of 85.3 at 2-year (n = 57). Range of motion improved form 98.2° (n = 153) to 110.4° at 2-year (n = 57).

D Kohn compared the results of Interax I.S.A. with the Interax fixed bearing version at a follow-up of 12 to 28 months. Pain relief was very similar in both groups. Active flexion at follow-up was in average 105° for the fixed bearing and 110° for the mobile bearing group. Knee scores and functional scores improved similarly in the fixed and in the mobile bearing group. Improvement was more pronounced in the mobile bearing group but was not statistically significant.

Complications encountered in both groups were: early aseptic loosening in two percent of the fixed bearing knees, reoperation for postoperative major haematoma in 3% (fixed) versus 2% (mobile), 4% of patients in both groups had manipulation under general anaesthesia because of impaired functional ROM of less than 90° of flexion three weeks after surgery. Overall complications in both groups were considered comparable (43).

The **Total Rotating Knee (TRK)** (Cremascoli, Milan, Italy) is designed by Prof. Ghisellini who has implanted about 500 of these prostheses since 1992. The TRK is composed of a total condylar type femoral component and a metal tibial tray that is provided with a central post that projects from the center of the plate. Both these components are made of CoCr alloy, for use with or without cement. The patella is an all-poly single pegged dome. There are two types of plastic bearings, each available in five sizes and four thicknesses. The first (R = rotating) has a rounded hole in the undersurface that fits the post of the tray allowing freedom of rotation, this version is indicated for the case of PCL retaining. While the second type (R = rotating and sliding) has a slot allowing 10mm of A-P sliding as well as freedom of rotation, wich is indicated when the PCL is retained. The initial results of F. Ghisellini (Ghisellini, p.com.) are encouraging. Wear testing, performed with a knee-joint simulator, after 4 million cycles showed only little evidence of abrasive and adhesive wear without signs of fatigue wear.

Both the **Profix** and **Genesis II Total Knee Systems** (Smith & Nephew Inc., Memphis, TN, USA) have mobile bearing options. These cruciate preserving TKAs are composed of an anatomic Co-Cr femoral component and a tibial tray which articulates with the polyethylene bearing by a "pin on slot" mechanism allowing the bearing to rotate without AP translation. The femoral components of these systems are also available with the option of Oxidized Zirconium finishing that seems to reduce wear rate by up to 85% in *in-vitro* testing (Smith & Nephew Inc., data on file).

The **Minns meniscal knee prosthesis** (Zimmer U.K., Swindon, U.K.) has a femoral component of the total condylar design and a tibial plateau with dovetail A-P slots, which engage two separate polyethylene "menisci", which allow rolling and sliding movements during flexion. Because the slots are straight and parallel, a single sliding plateau engaged in both slots that only slides during flexion but limits rotation is also available. The two separate menisci design allows 59° of rotation (both internal and external) while the sliding one piece plateau design has torque-rotation characteristics comparable to that of the total condylar design. The tibial tray has a central cut-out to allow the presence of both cruciate ligaments.

Forty patients with a Minns meniscal knee prosthesis were studied by fluoroscopy with spot films taken laterally at four different angles of flexion. In 6 patients the menisci did not seem to move. Menisci starting position relative to the tibial tray showed also variability in single patients. In most of the cases the menisci moved forward during the first 20-30° of flexion and then backward. In some patients the medial meniscus moved more than the lateral one and in others the opposite was seen.

Wear testing was performed on a knee simulator up to a maximum of one million cycles at 3,000N of load and the meniscus top surface. Contact area was studied every 100,000 cycles with Fuji contact films. Minimal wear was observed only after the first 100,000 cycles then it was negligible as the contact area increased.

The review of the first 165 implants at a maximum follow-up of five years were rated excellent and good in 88% of the cases. Bearing dislocations and fractures were an evident problem in the first series (63). Posterior tibial component placement was found to be responsible for bearing fracture because of the high loading on the front of the polyethylene that slided off the tibial plate. The tibial surface cutting guide was modified to include a curved viewing slot that allows to better refer to the anterior tibial cortex avoiding posterior tibial positioning. Bearing dislocations problems are solved by the authors by substituting the meniscal bearing (at surgery or as a revision procedure) with the single sliding plateau (49-51).

Fully conforming

The **Oxford unicompartmental knee replacement** (Biomet Ltd, Bridgend, South Wales, Australia) was the first mobile bearing design to be introduced in the market by Goodfellow and O'Connor (1976) (28). In this design individual femoral and tibial bearing surfaces are replaced on either one or both sides of the joint. The femoral component has a spherical articular surface with a 24mm radius. Free meniscal bearings, spherically concave above and flat below, lie between the flat tibial (five sizes available) and curved femoral (one single size available) component, held in place by their geometry and ligamentous tension (32). The meniscal bearings are provided in many thicknesses from 3.5mm to 11.5mm. The surfaces are congruent throughout the range of motion, thus a contact area of 600mm^2 per condyle is available in all joint positions (29).

Retrieved bearings after a period of use *in vivo* which ranged from 1 to 9 years showed very low penetration wear rates (0.026-0.043mm per year) (4).

Table II – Fully conforming mobile bearing knees

Implant type	Manufacturer
Oxford unicompartmental knee replacement	Biomet Ltd, Warsaw, Indiana, USA
Oxford Total Meniscal Knee (TMK)	Biomet Ltd, Warsaw, Indiana, USA
Rotaglide total knee system	Corin Medical, Cirencester, U.K.
Meniscal Bearing Knee (MBK)	Zimmer, Warsaw, Indiana, USA

The results of this prosthesis are dependent on the function of the ACL. In fact in a description of results of 125 unicompartmental replacements Goodfellow *et al.* reported a failure rate of 8.8% at six years in those with an absent or damaged ACL and of 4.8% in knees with a normal ACL (30). Also in the description of the first 103 cases by Goodfellow this same issue was evident: 16.2% of failure rate in the 37 knees with damaged ACL and 4.8% in 63 knees with both cruciate normal (30). In a later review of 301 patients the survival rate at six years was 95% in knees with normal ACL and 81% in knees with absent or damaged ACL (31). A success rate of 99.1% at 7 years was observed in 121 knees that fulfilled the criteria of intact ACL, normal cartilage in the lateral compartment of the knee and anteromedial osteoarthritis with varus deformity passively correctable to neutral (42).

Svard and Price evaluated a series of 124 Oxford meniscal-bearing unicompartmental arthroplasties carried out for osteoarthritis of the medial compartment. All the knees had an intact anterior cruciate ligament, a correctable varus deformity and full-thickness cartilage in the lateral compartment. 37 patients had died; the mean time since operation for the remainder was 12.5 years (10.1 to 15.6). 6 knees had been revised (4.8%). At 10 years there were 94 knees still at risk and the cumulative survival rate was 95% (confidence interval, 90.8 to 99.3) (72).

The **Oxford Total Meniscal Knee (TMK)** (Biomet Ltd, Bridgend, South Wales, Australia) is available from the year 2000. It follows the design principle of the Oxford Uni employing spherical femoral condyles and matching radii meniscal bearings which offer full area contact throughout the range of motion. The meniscal bearing rotates around a tibial tray retaining post which has a mushroom shape to allow also 4mm of antero-posterior translation and 2mm of medio-lateral movement of the bearing. The tibial component top surface is highly polished and available in seven sizes.

In vitro testing is showing less than 0.1 penetration wear after 4 million cycles with the knee simulator (Biomet inc., data on file).

The **Rotaglide total knee system** (Corin Medical, Cirencester, U.K.) designed in 1986 by Polyzoides and Tsakonas uses a femoral component that maintains the same intercondylar distance and radius of curvature in all the sizes. This feature is represented also on the upper surface of the one-piece polyethylene meniscal component, allowing a contact area of 600mm^2 per condyle maintained almost completely from full extension to flexion and complete matching of all femoral and tibial sizes. The lower surface of the polyethylene platform is flat and glides 5mm in an AP direction and rotates 12.5° each side, on the polished upper surface of the tibial tray. The tibial plateau has two bollards: one in the front, which prevents anterior dislocation while restricting the rotation of the platform and another in the middle of the tray which prevents posterior dislocation. Both components are fixed by a single stem with the addition of two broach pegs for the tibial side, and they are usually implanted with cement (58). Recently is also available a PS version with a post on the meniscal bearing and a cam in the femoral component.

From 1988 to 1998 1,600 patients have been operated by two teams of surgeons. Preoperative diagnosis was osteoarthritis and rheumatoid arthritis. The follow-up ranged between 6 and 10 years. Using the BASK Chart, relief of pain was 97.8% and patient satisfaction was 96%. The average flexion was 115°. All the knees were stable and the average walking distance was 3 kilometers daily for the osteoarthritic patients. Patellar problems occurred in 3.3% of rheumatoid patients and 1.2% of osteoarthritic patients. There was no radiological evidence of polyethylene wear or osteolysis. No tibial component loosening was observed. The revision rate was 0.9% in 1,600 knees for infection, patellar problems and femoral component loosening (59).

The details of the **Meniscal Bearing Knee (MBK)** (Zimmer, Warsaw, Indiana, USA) prosthesis will be developed later in this chapter.

PS-Mobile bearing knees

The **Two Radii Area Contact (TRACK)** mobile bearing total knee replacement (Biomet, Warsaw, Indiana, USA) designed by Draganich and Pottenger and available in the market since 1997. This prosthesis has two areas of tibiofemoral contact. This was obtained by dividing the condylar surface into two sections of different radii of curvature. The larger, centrally located distal radii of curvature is completely congruent with the "inner tracks" of the bearing from 5° of hyperextension through 8° of flexion. The smaller posterior radii of curvature engage the "outer tracks" of the bearing from 8° through 120° of flexion. The posterior shift in tibiofemoral contact at about 8° of flexion reduces the contact area from 1,077mm^2 to 674mm^2 when the outer track becomes the bearing surface and simultaneously the femoral cam engages the post inducing roll-back (24).

Table III – Posterior stabilized mobile bearing knees

Implant type	Manufacturer
Two radii area contact (TRACK)	Biomet, Warsaw, Indiana, USA
HLS-PS mobile	Tornier, Montbonnot, France
Nexgen Legacy-PS Flex Mobile	Zimmer, Warsaw, Indiana, USA
Rotaglide PS	Corin Medical, Cirencester, U.K.
P.F.C. sigma rotating platform PS	DePuy Inc., Warsaw, Indiana, USA

The preliminary results of the first 86 TRACK prostheses reported by the designers showed an HSS clinical score of 85 points in average at one year follow-up (Pottenger, p.com.).

The **HLS-PS mobile** (Tornier, Montbonnot, France) was designed adding a mobile bearing to the HLS-PS Evolution fixed bearing knee. The femoral component has an inner track as cam that articulates with the bearing post with the principle of the "third condyle". The polyethylene bearing is a rotating platform with high conformity on the frontal plane and partial conformity on sagittal plane. The insert rotates with an anterior pivot thanks to a slot in the back surface that articulates with a curved "lip and slide" mechanism projecting from the tray. *In vitro* wear rates were compared between the mobile and the fixed bearing HLS type. At 10 million cycles global wear (weight loss) were 0.011 gr for the mobile type and 0.016 for the fixed bearing type (54).

The **Nexgen Legacy-PS Flex Mobile** (Zimmer, Warsaw, Indiana, USA) was developed for patients with the ability and desire to perform high-flexion activities. It represents the evolution of the Legacy Posterir Stabilized fixed bearing prosthesis and was designed to accommodate resumption of high-flexion daily activities. Extended posterior condyles on the femoral component facilitates tibiofemoral contact to support high flexion up to 155°. Conforming geometry of the femoral component with its articulating surface allows minimal loss of contact area during high flexion. Posterior stabilization offers a predictable roll-back. The spine / cam mechanism was modified in order to deepen posterior clearance and reduce bending moment. The mobile bearing allows 25° of rotation with a central anterior pivot that reduces overhang. Rotation stop prevents "spin out". An anterior cut-out on the tibial articulating surface helps reducing tension and provides greater clearance for the extensor mechanism.

We have had an early experience with this implant in few selected cases (thin, motivated, preoperative flexion > 115°) which showed excellent short-term results with an average flexion at one year follow-up of 127° without any complications (Aglietti, p. com).

Meniscal bearing knee

Design

The concept underlying the design of the M.B.K. prosthesis is to have a complete congruency at all degrees of flexion between the femoral component and the polyethylene insert while allowing rotation and A-P translation between the polyethylene insert and the tibial tray (fig. 1A et 1B). The femoral component has femoropatellar and femorotibial surfaces separated by two condylo-throclear grooves (fig. 2). There are right and left femoral components. The femorotibial surface has complete conformity throughout motion owing to the fixed radius of the posterior femoral condyles. Its magnitude changes with the prosthetic size. The radius ratio is one to one in both the sagittal and frontal planes. The patellar sulcus is deep and prolonged distally. It is slightly displaced laterally to improve patellar tracking. It may accommodate the natural patella.

The profile of the patellar component can be "dome" or "sombrero". The sombrero is more anatomical and fits well in the M.B.K. "friendly" trochlea providing an area contact throughout flexion, but there are some concerns

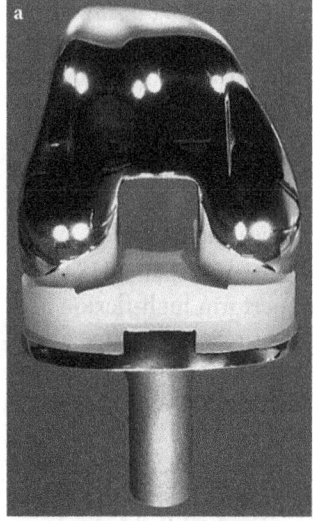
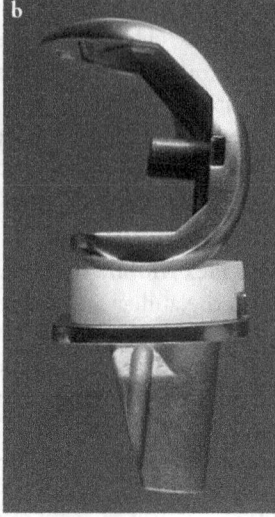

Fig. 1 – Front and side view of the femoral component of the M.B.K, showing the fixed radius of the posterior femoral condyles.

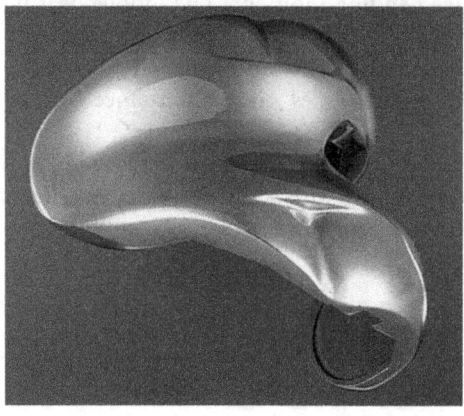

Fig. 2 – The femoral component has a deep and prolonged trochlea. Two condylo-trochlear grooves separate the femorotibial surface and the posterior femoral condyles.

about alignment regarding this design, thus we prefer to routinely use the dome patella that is more tolerant to tilting and, although it provides a point-line contact with the femoral trochlea, wear and deformation in time adjusts the polyethylene surface, providing a large contact area in the positions under high contact stress (25). This behaviour of the polyethylene seems to confer "biological"-like properties to the material ("Bio-poly") (Insall, p. com.).

The tibial tray is a strong CoCr fluted design and is 4mm thick without holes. The polished tibial plate finishing has a low tolerance, in the order of 0.1μ (fig. 3) and has a central D-shaped "mushroom" and an anterior stop. The polyethylene insert engages the mushroom with a "snap on" mechanism (fig. 4). This system allows for 20° of rotation each side and 4.5mm of A-P sliding of the plastic bearing (fig. 5). PCL retention and an anterior lip in the plastic provide for posterior stability. Medial-lateral translocation is prevented by a prominent intercondylar "saddle" of the bearing.

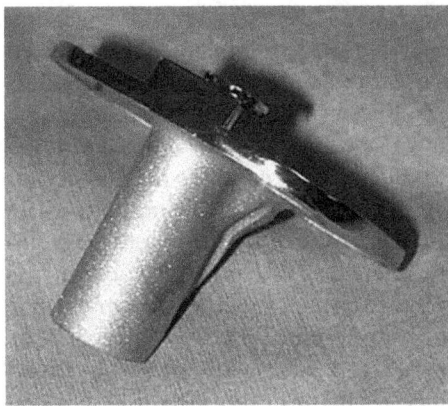

Fig. 3 – Tibial tray fluted design of the M.B.K.

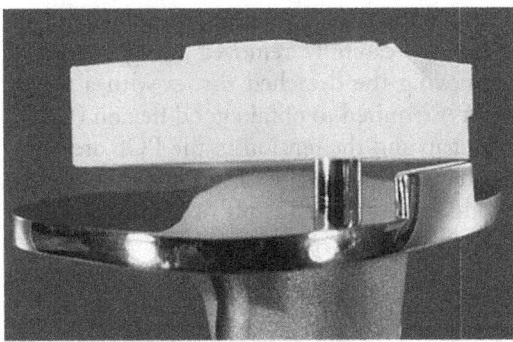

Fig. 4 – The D-shaped mushroom fits into the undersurface slot of the polyehtylene insert with a "snap on" mechanism.

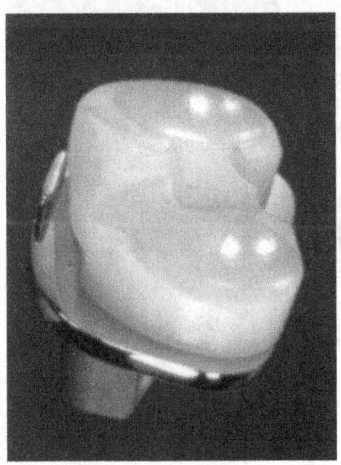

Fig. 5 – Polyethylene insert of the M.B.K. can rotate 20° each side on the tibial tray.

Surgical technique

Through a straight longitudinal anteromedial parapatellar approach we begin the procedure from the femoral cuts using an intramedullary guide for correct valgus alignment but we always double check with an extramedullary rod going 2.5 fingerbreaths medial to the A.S.I.S. This cut has also 3° of flexion in relationship to the distal femoral axis. We used to implant this prosthesis with the epicondylar instrumentary in order to refer to the epicondylar axis as femoral component rotational landmark. Recently we prepare the femur using the "4 in 1" femoral cutting guide that can be automatically adjusted to 3, 5 or 7° of external rotation referencing to the posterior condyles respectively for the varus, valgus and valgus with subluxed patella knee, according to the data published by Griffin *et al.* (33). This guide is adjusted for the antero-posterior resections using anterior and posterior reference. The proximal tibial cut is accomplished using an extramedullary guide trying to remove 10mm of bone from the normal tibial plateau with 4-5° of posterior slope (27, 34, 38). The flexion and extension gaps are established and sized with spacer blocks. In order to achieve the proper PCL balance we perform routinely a PCL recession by subperiosteally peeling it from the tibia (fig. 6) (60).

The osteophytes which are present at the level of posterior femoral condyles and in the notch around the PCL are carefully removed using curved or straight thin osteotomes while removing the detached tissues with a hernia forceps. This kind of posterior work is required to obtain good flexion (fig. 7).

After these resections the flexion gap and the tension in the PCL are assessed using spacers and a trial prosthesis is inserted to ensure that there is no increased tension in the PCL producing anterior lift-off of the tibial insert.

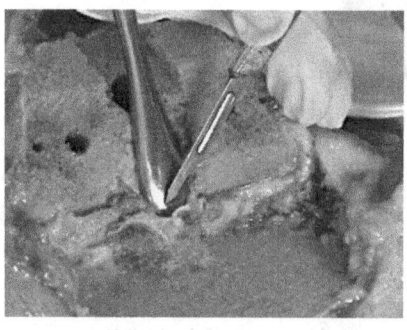

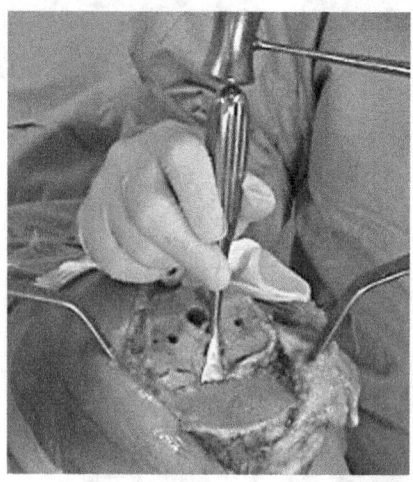

Fig. 6 – PCL subperiosteal recession from the back of the tibia is performed using a small knife and an elevator.

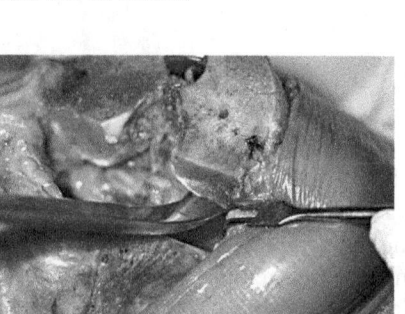

Fig. 7 – Posterior work with a curved osteotome to clean posterior recesses from the osteophytes.

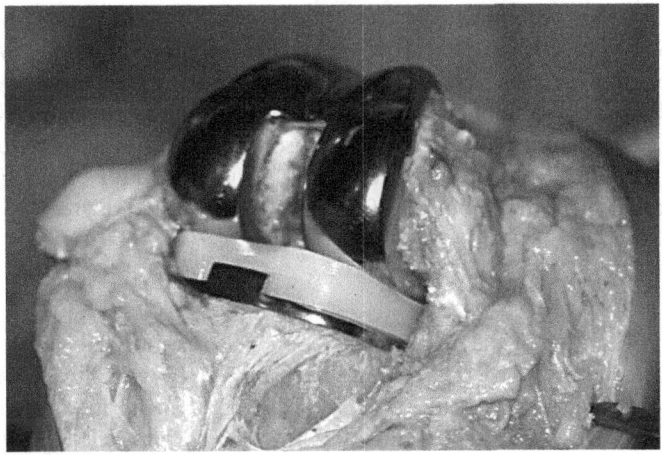

Fig. 8 – Surgical view of an M.B.K. prosthesis implanted in a right knee.

The patella is replaced with an all-poly, three pegged, dome implant. Finally we cement all the components paying attention to remove all excess cement to avoid third body wear (fig. 8).

MBK studies

Contact area measurements

A 3-D finite element study by S. Greenwald reported top and back surfaces stresses and contact areas for a number of mobile bearing tibial inserts of several knee systems, including the M.B.K., with a load of 2,5kN at 0° of flexion. Regarding the M.B.K. he found a top surface total (bicondylar) contact area equal to 530mm^2 and 293mm^2 for the back surface (52). In this study all the analyzed inserts showed lesser contact areas than expected. Most interestingly, the back surface contact areas shows perimeter contact. Subsequent analysis from the same group found different data regarding the MBK top surface total contact area: 358mm^2 in the second analysis and 429mm^2 in the third one.

   Probably the finite element method used leads to excessive artefact problems in this kind of prosthesis. In fact another study by W Walsh and M Harris in Sydney (Walsh, p.com.), using a computerized contact area and pressure measurement system with K-Scan 4000 (Tekscan Inc., South Boston, MA, USA) showed different contact areas and stresses in the M.B.K. 14mm thick polyethylene insert. The K-Scan 4000 system comprises a plastic laminated thin-film (0.1mm), electronic pressure transducer (a sensor with 4,576 sensing elements), hardware and software for an IBM-compatible PC, and a coupler to connect the two. Tests were performed applying loads of 3,600N, 3,240N and 2,880N (equal to 5, 4.5 and 4 times a 73kg body weight) at flexion angles of 0, 30, 60, 90 and 110°. Average stress values resulted in the order of 4MPa for all loads and flexion degrees except for the 110° value (about 7.5MPa). The "peak" contact stresses in compression are below the failure stress of polyethylene for all ranges except for 110° of flexion where the peak stress was 22MPa. The M.B.K. top surface total contact area approximated 800mm² at 0, 30 and 60° of flexion, 700mm² at 90° and 380mm² at 110°. The back surface total contact area profiles at the same degrees of flexion investigated with the ultra super low (USL) Fuji film (Fuji Photo Film Co., Tokyo, Japan) measured about 1,200mm² for each tested degree.

Wear in the laboratory

We believe that one of the theoretical advantages of a mobile bearing prosthesis, in particular of the M.B.K., should be reduction of wear. The issue is complex because there are in reality two surfaces that can produce wear: the top side and the back side. If one considers the wear of an M.B.K., top surface wear should be added to back surface wear. This should be compared to a well established prosthesis with good records for wear, such as the IB-II in an experimental investigation carried out in a special simulator that can reproduce forces and motions of true life in the laboratory.

This is being performed by Prof. P Walker in London. He has conducted 3 series of experiments where he compared 3 sets of M.B.K.s to 3 of IB-IIs each time. Now he is up to 10 million cycles (equivalent to 7-8 years of life) in the knee symulator. In the first group the forces and motions used for the M.B.K. were double the ones for the IB-II. Wear for M.B.K. was more evident. In the second and third group similar forces were utilized. It appeared that the M.B.K. wears less than the IB-II in terms of "penetration" wear, but in terms of "volumetric" wear the M.B.K. wears some 30% more than the IB-II. In fact the M.B.K. produces very little, negligible wear from the top surface (only some burnishing), but more wear from the back surface, with some adhesive and abrasive mechanisms. Delamination wear was not seen (fig. 8).

It might be that the tibial plate finishing requires an extremely low tolerance (better than the order of 0.1μ) or alternatively there might be lubrication problems in the back side which we were not accustomed to see in the fixed bearing knees.

The debris particles produced have also been studied (Pat Campbell, at UCLA). They are in the form of granules (size = <1μ), fibrils (size = 3μ long), flakes (size = 5-10μ long). With the MBK there are less small particles compared to IB-II, and this is favourable because they are more biologically active (like in the hip) (63).

Gait analysis

Gait analysis studies performed by Catani in 1997 compared the behaviour of 10 M.B.K.s and 10 IB-IIs during stairs ascending and descending. The patients were asked to consecutively climb four steps. They were monitorized with surface markers, and their position in the space was assessed by a special setting of cameras connected with a digital device provided with an analyzing data software previously described (3). Simultaneously limb muscles activity was recorded by surface electromyography.

Analysis of the results showed better quadriceps function in the M.B.K. group due to reduction in the extension moment with still good flexion moment. The adduction moment was significantly reduced in the M.B.K. group respect to the IB-II group. This lead to more symmetric load across the joint during almost all the late stance phase of gait with consequent less medial compartment loading. This phenomenon observed in the M.B.K.s could be probably due to external rotation in late stance. In the M.B.K. group the flexion moment during the late stance phase of the gait showed little "bumps" that seem to be related to little sliding movements of the polyethylene insert in the AP direction.

Muscle activities during ascending in both groups demonstrated a prolonged activity of the rectus femoris and of the anterior tibialis throughout the late stance phase. Increased activation of the hamstrings was observed in the M.B.K. group probably as a response to the A-P sliding movements of the bearing. During stairs descending normal patterns were recorded in both groups.

Kinematics

In order to assess the kinematics of the M.B.K., a video fluoroscopic study with a three-dimensional computer assisted matching was carried out by Barrett and Walker in several patients performing the function of climbing a step. The videos were analyzed using an inverse perspective technique that uses image matching. Digital libraries containing three-dimensional computer-assisted design drawings were created. At each increment of flexion, two-dimensional fluoroscopic images were replaced by best fit three-dimensional computer-assisted design drawings found in the libraries as described by Stiehl (68).

There were a lot of individual variations. In general from flexion to extension there was backward sliding of the femur on the tibia first, then as extension occurs climbing the step, there was forward motion of the femur on the tibia, and then, toward terminal extension, a final backward motion of the femur was observed.

Rotational patterns were also variable with individual differences (especially in reaching the neutral position). The internal-external rotation range varied between 6 and 8°. There was terminal external rotation of the tibia like in the normal knee. There was no evidence of lateral condylar lift-off differently from others reports. In fact Stiehl *et al.* using a 3D-CAD iterative modeling method demonstrated a lift-off rate at heel strike in about 50% of 20 LCS cruciate-sacrificing mobile bearing knees (69). Concerning the A-P displacement: these motions were relatively small (1.0-4.5mm, average: 3.1mm), not continuous but usually in short bursts; this is probably due to a frictional force (about 150N) that holds the plastic in place against shear forces generated during the climbing of one step.

Clinical outcomes

Three series of cases have been operated with the M.B.K. prosthesis in Florence. The first series (Mark I) includes 24 patients operated from October 1993 to June 1994. The second series (Mark II) includes 24 cases operated from December 1994 to June 1996. The third series (Mark III or the final version of the prosthesis) includes over 200 cases operated from December 1996 until now.

We prospectively reviewed 120 patients operated with consecutive M.B.K.s performed between December 1996 and May 1999 (2).

The mean follow-up period was 2.5 years (range: 1-4). At follow-up one patient had died and one was bedridden, leaving 118 knees (97 females and 21 males). Mean age at surgery was 71 years. Diagnosis was osteoarthritis in 93% of the cases. The preoperative main deformity was varus in 67%, valgus in 16% and fixed flexion contracture in 11%. The PCL was spared but completely released from the tibia. Lateral retinacular release was performed in 16%.

The Knee Score increased from an average of 38 preoperatively to 94 points at follow-up. There were 95% excellent-good results. Mean postoperative active flexion was 111° (range: 70°-135°). The Functional Score at follow-up increased from 35 to 84. Postoperative A-P drawer was within 5mm in 109 patients, between 5-10mm in 8 and more than 10mm in one. Postoperative varus-valgus rotation was within 5mm in 92% of the patients. Seven patients (5%) reported a feeling of "clicking" in the knee. Asymptomatic patellar crepitus was present in 16 patients. All the knees showed a satisfactory alignment over the mechanical axis (0°+5°). Radiolucent lines were present in 19% of the tibial components and in 11% of the femoral components (image amplifier). We did not observe osteolysis or polyethylene wear by radiological means (fig. 9). The early results of this series are very satisfactory. Long-term advantages of this sophisticated design are still unknown.

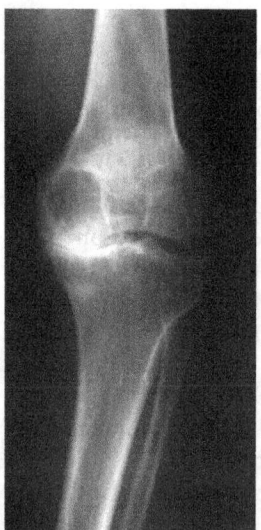
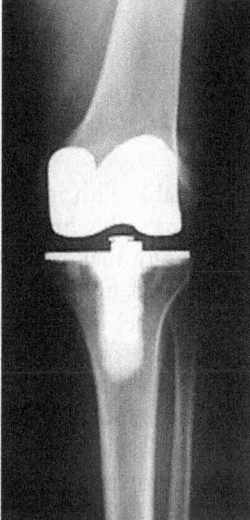

Fig. 9 – a. Preoperative radiograph of a varus osteoarthritic left knee
b. Postoperative radiograph at 1 year of follow-up of an MBK prosthesis.

a.

b.

In another prospective randomised study we compared the postoperative recovery and early results of two groups of patients undergoing Total Knee Arthroplasty: group I included patients with a fixed bearing posterior stabilized prosthesis (LPS), group II received the meniscal bearing prosthesis (M.B.K.) (5). Each group included 100 patients. Preoperative parameters did not differ between the two groups. Body Mass Index averaged 27 in both groups. The PCL was sacrificed and substituted in group I and spared but completely released from the tibia in group II. Accurate posterior recesses work and removal of posterior osteophytes were done in all patients. All patients received the same rehabilitation protocol. Continuous passive motion was used for the first 24 hours postoperatively (0-70°). Evaluation was performed preoperatively, postoperatively at 1 week, 1, 3, 6 and 12 months. Results are shown in table I. No significant differences between the two groups were found. Subjective feeling of clicking in the knee was present in 4 patients (6%) of group I and 6 patients (9%) of group II (n.s.). Using a fixed (PS) or a mobile bearing design didn't seem to influence the short-term recovery and early results after knee replacement.

Table IV – Results of the prospective randomized comparative study of M.B.K. vs Legacy-PS.

Result	1 week		1 month		3 month	
	LPS	M.B.K.	LPS	M.B.K.	LPS	M.B.K.
Maximum flexion	95±6°	91±4°	99±7°	97±8°	109±10°	108±11°
Extension loss	2±2°	2±2°	2±3°	1±2°	1±2°	0±2°
Pain (VAS: 0-10)	3.5±1.9	3.3±1.6	2±1.4	1.8±1.5	0.5±1.2	0.5±1.1

	Preoperative		6 month		12 month	
Knee Score	39±7	43±8	94±4	93±5	95±4	94±3
Maximum flexion	102±7°	99±6°	109±8°	108±9°	114±9°	110±11°

In a third study 3 different knee replacements, with 3 trochlear designs, were prospectively evaluated clinically and radiographically for patellar function and presence of patellar complications (1). They included the IB-I and the IB-II (PCL substituting) and the M.B.K. (PCL recession). The trochlea of the IB-I was short and shallow with an anterior sharp edge of the intercondylar box (later modified to a smoother edge) and the femoral component had a prominent "shoulder". In the IB-II the trochlea was deeper to allow for soft tissue clearance. In the M.B.K. the trochlea was more prolonged, with R and L components and the "shoulder" was less prominent. In all the cases the patella was resurfaced with an all polyethylene dome prosthesis. Knees with tibio-femoral problems were excluded. The demographics and the results and complications are shown in table II. From the data of the present study the following conclusions can be drawn:

1) The most frequent problem was impingement (clunks) with the early version of the IB-I. Smoothening of the anterior edge significantly reduced the incidence of clunks to 5% in the modified IB I;

2) With the IB-II deepening the trochlea for soft tissue clearance improved the degree, not the incidence of clunks (4,5%), compared to the modified IB I;

3) With the M.B.K. clunks were very rare and patellar function improved;

4) Throughout the three series patellar stress fractures and instability were rare and loosening or wear not evident;

5) Normal function (including stairs ascending and descending) can be expected in over 80% of category A patients;

6) Of the various radiological parameters only patella baja correlated with symptoms in the IB prostheses;

7) We still prefer the dome design because is more tolerant and with cold flow may better conform it to the trochlea increasing contact area.

Table V – Patellar functional results and complications after resurfacing in IB-I, IB-II, and M.B.K.

	IB-I	IB-II	M.B.K.
Knees	73	67	61
Average follow-up	6	6	2.5
OA	75%	100% (primary)	92%
AT. release	48%	22%	29%
Anterior pain			
Mild	14%	1.5%	–
Moderate / severe	1.5%	3%	–
Patellar tracking			
Asymptomatic crepitus	23%	21%	16.5%
Clunks (impingement)	21%	4.5%	1.5%
Function			
Average flexion	96°	116°	110°
Normal stairs (Cat. A patients)	64%	81%	81.5%
Complications			
Stress fractures (asymptomatic)	1.5%	–	3%
Patellar instability	1.5%	–	–
Radiology			
Medial tilt > 5°	34%	37%	6.5%
Lateral tilt > 5°	–	8%	23%
Lateral subluxation	1.5%	16%	11.5%
Patella baja (< 40%)	20.5%	7%	11%

Comments

The concept of the mobile bearing knee is intellectually attractive and can potentially reduce the problems of polyethylene wear while improving kinematics and function.

We feel that the Insall-Burnstein posterior stabilized knee will maintain its place in the field of total knee replacement as a "generic" knee to be used by most surgeons in most cases, with a standard technique and reliable long-term results (22, 64, 66). However we think that there is a place for an "high-tech" knee to be used by specialized surgeons, possibly in younger patients with increased demands. This implant should allow improved performance with reduced polyethylene wear. The results of the M.B.K. series are preliminary but promising and require a long-term evaluation. The M.B.K. design offers the advantages of full conformity throughout flexion and the possibility of keeping the PCL and releasing it. It can be used in cases of mild to moderate deformities although in recent times we have expanded the indications to more severe cases.

In summary, the possible theoretical advantages of reducing wear, better knee function and more physiological knee kinematics, expected for this new prosthesis, still need a longer term evaluation. Possible disadvantages could be represented by some mechanical complexity of this sophisticated design, the potential for instability and the higher costs compared to other simpler knee systems.

Fixed bearing knee design have reached their ultimate expression; often, this stage of development indicate impending obsolescence. Mobile bearing knees offers an attractive avenue for future developments (39).

References

1. Aglietti P, Baldini A, Buzzi R et al. (2001) Patella resurfacing in total knee replacement: functional evaluation and complications. Knee Surgery, Sports Traumatology, Arthroscopy 9-S1: 27-33
2. Aglietti P, Baldini A, Vena L.M et al. (2000) Meniscal Bearing Knee (MBK): preliminary results. Presented at European Society of Sports Traumatology, Knee Surgery and Arthroscopy 9th Congress, London, UK, September 16-20
3. Andriacchi TP, Galante JO, Fermier RW et al. (1982) The influence of total knee replacement design on walking and stair climbing. J Bone Joint Surg, 64A: 1328-1335
4. Argenson JN, O'Connor JJ (1992) Polyethylene wear in meniscal knee replacement: a 1-9 year retrieval analysis of the Oxford Knee. J Bone Joint Surg 74B: 228-32
5. Baldini A, Aglietti P, Vena LM et al. (2001) Postoperative Recovery and Early Results: Meniscal Bearing Knee vs Legacy PS. Presented at International Society of Arthroscopy, Knee Surgery and Orthopaedic Sports Medicine Congress, Montreux, Switzerland, May 14-18
6. Barnes CL, Sledge CB (1993) Total knee arthroplasty with posterior cruciate ligament retention designs. In: Surgery of the knee. Insall JN 2nd ed, New York, Churchill Livingstone 815-27
7. Bert JM (1990) Dislocation / subluxation of meniscal bearing elements after New Jersey Low-Contact Stress total knee arthroplasty. Clin Orthop 254: 211
8. Buechel FF, Pappas MJ (1986) The New Jersey Low Contact Stress Knee replacement system: biomechanical rationale and review of the first 123 cemented cases. Arch Orthop. Trauma Surg 105: 197-204
9. Buechel FF, Pappas MJ (1990) Long-term survivorship analysis of the cruciate-sparing versus cruciate-sacrificing knee prostheses using meniscal bearings. Clin Orthop 260; 162-169
10. Buechel FF (1990) Cemented and cementless revision arthroplasty using rotating platform total knee implants: a 12-year experience. Orthop Rev Suppl 71
11. Buechel FF et al. (1991) New Jersey LCS unicompartmental knee replacement: clinical, radiographic, statistical and survivorship analyses of 106 cementless cases performed by 7 surgeons. Food and Drug Administration Panel Presentation. Rockville, Md, August 16
12. Buechel FF, Pappas MJ, Greenwald AS (1991) Evaluation of contact stresses in metal-baked patellar replacements: A predictor of survivorship. Clin Orthop 273: 190-7
13. Buechel FF (1991) Cementless mobile bearing TKR: concepts and 10-year evaluation.

Presented at the 7th Annual Joint Replacement Symposium, Palm Beach, Florida, October 23

14. Buechel FF, Keblish PA, Lee JM et al. (1994) Low contact stress meniscal bearing unicompartmental knee replacement: long-term evaluation of cemented and cementless results. J Orthop Reum 7:31-41

15. Buechel FF (1994) Meniscal bearing knee replacement: development, long-term results, and future technology. In: The Knee, Scott NW ed, New York, Mosby 1157-77

16. Buechel FF (1996) Low-Contact-Stress, meniscal bearing knee replacement. Design concepts, failure mechanisms and long-term survivorship. In: Current concepts in primary and revision total knee arthroplasty Insall JN, Scott WN, Scuderi GR ed, Lippincott-Raven, Philadelphia 47-64

17. Buechel FF (1998) Evolving clinical use of mobile bearing knee design concepts. The complications of long experience. Presented at the 14th annual current concepts in joint replacements symposium, Orlando, FL, Dec. 11

18. Callaghan JJ, Squire MW, Goetz DD et al. (2000) Cemented rotating-platform total knee replacement. A nine to twelve-year follow-up study. J Bone Joint Surg Am 82(5): 705-11.

19. Callaghan JJ, Insall JN, Greenwald AS et al. (2001) Mobile-bearing knee replacement: concepts and results. Instr Course Lect 50:431-49

20. Chao EY, Laughman RK, Schneider E et al. (1983) Normative data of knee joint motion and ground reaction forces in adult level walking. J Biomech 16 (3): 219

21. Churchill DL, Incavo SJ, Johnson CC, Beynnon BD (1998) The transepicondylar axis approximates the true flexion / extension axis of the knee. Personal communication, Knee Society Meeting

22. Colizza WA, Insall JN, Scuderi GR (1995) The Posterior Stabilized total knee prosthesis. Assessment of polyethylene damage and osteolysis after a ten-year minimum follow-up. J Bone Joint Surg 77A:1713-20

23. Dennis DA (2001) Technical aspects of mobile-bearing knee implants. Orthopedics Today, January / February 6-7

24. Draganich LF, Pottenger LA (2000) The TRAC PS mobile-bearing prosthesis: design rationale and in vivo 3-dimensional laxity. J Arthoplasty 15 (1): 102-12

25. Elbert K, Bartel D, Wright TM (1995) The effect of conformity on stresses in dome- shaped polyethylene patellar components. Clin Orthop 317: 71-5

26. Elias SG, Freeman MAR, Gockay EI (1990) A correlative study and anatomy of the distal femur. Clin Orthop 260: 98-103

27. Goldstein SA, Wilson DL, Sostengard DA et al. (1983) The mechanical properties of human tibial trabecular bone as a function of metaphyseal location. J Biomech 16 (12): 965-9.

28. Goodfellow JW, O'Connor JJ (1978) The mechanics of the knee and prosthetic design. J Bone Joint Surg 60B: 385-69

29. Goodfellow JW, O'Connor JJ (1986) Clinical results of the Oxford knee. Clin Orthop 205: 21-42

30. Goodfellow JW et al. (1988) The Oxford Knee for unicompartmental osteoarthritis. J Bone Joint Surg 70B: 692-701

31. Goodfellow JW, O'Connor JJ (1992) The anterior cruciate ligament in knee arthroplasty: a risk factor with unconstrained meniscal prostheses. Clin Orthop 276: 245-52

32. Goodfellow JW, O'Connor JJ (1994) The role of congruent meniscal bearings in knee arthroplasty. In: The Knee. Scott NW ed, New York, Mosby, 1143-56

33. Griffin FM, Insall JN, Scuderi GR (1998) The posterior condylar angle in osteoarthritic knees. J Arthropl 13(7): 812-5

34. Harada Y, Wevers HW, Cooke TDV (1988) Distribution of bone strength in the proximal tibia. J Arthropl 3(2): 167-75

35. Hill PF, Vedi V, Williams A, et al. (2000) Tibiofemoral movement 2: the loaded and unloaded living knee studied by MRI. J Bone Joint Surg 82B: 1196-8

36. Hiwaki H, Pinskerova V, Freeman MA et al. (2000) Tibiofemoral movement 1: the shapes and relative movements of the femur and tibia in the unloaded cadaver knee. J Bone Joint Surg 82B: 1189-95

37. Hollister AM, Jatana S, Singh AK *et al.* (1993) The axes of rotation of the knee. Clin Orthop 290: 259-68
38. Insall JN (1993) Surgical techniques and instrumentation in total knee arthroplasty. In: Insall JN, ed. Surgery of the knee 2nd ed. New York, Churchill Livingstone
39. Insall JN (1998) Adventures in mobile-bearing knee design: a mid-life crisis. Orthopedics 21(9): 1021-23
40. Kaper BP, Smith PN, Bourne RB *et al.* (1999) Medium-term results of a mobile bearing total knee replacement. Clin Orthop 367: 201-9
41. Karrholm J, Brandsson S, Freeman MA *et al.* (2000) Tibiofemoral movement 4: changes of axial tibial rotation caused by forced rotation at the weight-bearing knee studied by RSA. J Bone Joint Surg 82B: 1201-3
42. Keyes GW, *et al.* (1991) Oxford meniscal prosthesis for anteromedial osteoarthritis of the knee and intact ACL. J Bone Joint Surg 73B (Suppl. 2): 140
43. Kohn DM (2001) Tibial bearings mobile versus fixed: A prospective comparative study. Presented at ISAKOS Knee Committee Interim Meeting, Florence, Italy, January, 11-13
44. Kurosawa H, Walker PS, Abe S (1985) Geometry and motion of the knee for implant and orthotic design. J Biomech 18: 487-99
45. Jordan LR, Olivo JL, Voorhost PE (1997) Survivorship analysis of cementless meniscal bearing total knee arthroplasty. Clin Orthop 338: 119-23
46. La Fortune MA, Cavanagh PR, Sommer MS *et al.* (1992) Three dimensional kinematics of the human knee during walking. J Biomech 25: 347-57
47. Martelli S, Ellis RE, Marcacci M *et al.* (1998) Total knee arthroplasty kinematics. Computer simulation and intraoperative evaluation. J Arthropl 13(2): 145-55.
48. Menchetti PPM, Walker PS (1997) Mechanical evaluation of mobile bearing knees. Am J Knee Surg 10(2): 73-82
49. Minns RJ, Eng B, Campbell J (1978) The meniscal testing of a sliding meniscus knee prosthesis. Clin Orthop 137: 268-75
50. Minns RJ (1989) The Minns meniscal knee prosthesis: biomechanical aspects of the surgical procedure and a review of the first 165 cases. Arch Orthop Trauma Surg 108 (4): 231-5
51. Minns RJ, Blamey JM, Blunn GW *et al.* (1994) The polyethylene wear of meniscal bearings in the early Minns meniscal knee replacement. The knee 1: 57-64
52. Morra EA, Postak PD, Greenwald AS (1998) The influence of mobile bearing knee geometry on the wear of UHMWPE tibial inserts: a finite model element study. Presented at the 65th Annual Meeting of the American Academy of Orthopaedic Surgeons, New Orleans, March, 1998
53. Nakagawa S, Kadova Y, Todo S *et al.* (2000) Tibiofemoral movement 3: full flexion in the living knee studied by MRI. J Bone Joint Surg 82B: 1199-200
54. Neyret P (2001) Design Criteria for a PS Knee Rotating Platform. Presented at ISAKOS Knee Committee Interim Meeting, Florence, Italy, January, 11-13
55. Pappas MJ, Makris J, Buechel FF (1987) Biomaterials for hard tissue applications. In: Pizzoferrato P.G. et al editors: Biomaterials and clinical applications: evaluation of contact stresses in metal-plastic knee replacements Amsterdam, Elsevier, 259-64
56. Perka C (2001) A prospective single-center study: durability of the P.F.C. SigmaRP, Orthopedics Today, January / February 2001, 18-9
57. Pinskerova V, Iwaki H, Freeman MA (2000) The shapes and relative movements of the femur and tibia in the unloaded cadaveric knee: a study using MRI as an anatomic tool In: Insall JN, ed. Surgery of the knee, 3nd ed. New York, Churchill Livingstone
58. Polyzoides AJ, Dendrinos GK, Tsakonas H (1996) The Rotaglide total knee arthroplasty. Prosthesis design and early results. J Arthropl 11(4): 453-9
59. Polyzoides AJ, Brooks S, Tsakonas A *et al.* (1999) Design characteristics, experimental work and 10 year clinical experience with a fully conforming mobile bearing knee prosthesis. Presented at: International conference on knee replacement: 1974-2024. ImechE Headquarters, London, U.K, 22-24 April
60. Ritter MA, Faris PM Keating EM *et al.* (1988) Posterior cruciate ligament balancing during total knee arthroplasty. J Arthropl 3(4): 323-6

61. Rovick JS, Reuben JD, Schrager RJ *et al.* (1991) Relation between knee motion and ligament length patterns. Clin Biomechanics 6(4): 213-20
62. Schifrine P (2001) International clinical experience with the P.F.C. SigmaRP. Orthopedics Today, January / February 16-7
63. Schmalzried TS, Jasty M, Harris WH (1992) Periprosthetic bone loss in total hip arthroplasty. Polyethylene wear debris and the concept of the effective joint space. J Bone Joint Surg 74A(6): 849-63
64. Scuderi GR, Insall JN, Windsor RE *et al.* (1989) Survivorship of cemented knee replacement. J Bone Joint Surg
65. Sorrells RB (1996) The rotating platform mobile bearing TKA. Orthop 19(9): 793-6
66. Stern SH, Bowen MK, Insall JN *et al.* (1990) Cemented total knee arthroplasty for gonarthrosis in patients 55 years old or younger. Clin Orthop 260: 124-9
67. Stiehl JB, Komistek RD, Dennis DA *et al.* (1995) Fluoroscopic analysis of the kinematics after posterior cruciate retaining knee arthroplasty. J Bone Joint Surg 77-B: 884-9
68. Stiehl JB, Dennis DA, Komistek RD *et al.* (1997) *In vivo* kinematic analysis of a mobile bearing total knee prosthesis. Clin Orthop 345: 60-6
69. Stiehl JB, Dennis DA, Komistek RD *et al.* (1998) *In vivo* determination of condylar lift off and screw home in a mobile bearing total knee arthroplasty. Presented at the 65th Annual Meeting of the American Academy of Orthopaedic Surgeons, New Orleans, March, 1998
70. Sthiel JB, Dennis DA, Komistek RD *et al.* (1999) *In vivo* determination of condylar lift-off and screw-home in a mobile-bearing total knee arthroplasty. J. Arthroplasty 14(3): 293-9
71. Sthiel JB, Komistek RD, Haas B *et al.* (2001) Frontal plane kinematics after mobile-bearing total knee arthroplasty. Clin Orthop 392: 56-61
72. Svard UC, Price AJ (2001) Oxford medial unicompartmental knee arthroplasty. A survival analysis of an independent series. J Bone Joint Surg 83B: 191-4
73. Thompson WO, Thaete FL, Fu FH *et al.* (1991) Tibial meniscal dynamics using three-dimensional reconstruction of magnetic resonance images. Am J Sports Med 19: 210-6
74. Trent P.S, P.S. Walker, Wolf B (1976) Ligament length patterns, strength, and rotational axes of the knee joint. Clin Orthop 117: 263-70
75. Yoshioka Y, Siu D, Cooke DV (1987) The anatomy and functional axes of the femur. J Bone Joint Surg 69A: 873
76. Walker PS (1993) Design of total knee arthroplasty. In: Surgery of the knee. Insall JN, 2nd ed, New York, Churchill Livingstone, 723-38

Rotation in total knee arthroplasty

M. Bonnin

The rotational positioning of the femoral component in total knee prostheses affects the functional result and the development of tibiofemoral and patellofemoral complications. In the first and oldest method of positioning (1, 2, 11, 26, 48), symmetric posterior condylar resection was performed parallel to the posterior condylar line (PCL) and the femoral component was positioned parallel to this line. Initially this appeared to be a satisfactory and logical option because it placed the femoral component in an anatomic position. However, it did not take account of the fact that total knee arthroplasty is not simple resurfacing, but calls for a certain number of compromises with anatomy and biomechanics where bone resection and femoral and tibial design are concerned. Thus, in this context, apparently anatomic positioning of the femoral component was found to lead to a number of difficulties. Several studies have shown that positioning in external rotation relative to the posterior condylar line was an appropriate option.

Arguments in favour of external rotational positioning

Tibial resection

The angle between the mechanical axis of the tibia (mAT) and the tibiofemoral joint line (tibial angle, TA) varies according to individual morphology. In an individual with a normally aligned knee, where the mechanical axis of the leg passes through the centre of the knee, the tibial varus angle averages 3° (19, 24, 29, 34, 35) (fig. 1 **a.**). This gives an oblique joint line of 3°, tibial varus being compensated by femoral valgus. In total knee replacement, tibial resection perpendicular to the mAT is therefore not anatomic and necessarily involves excessive resection on the lateral side. This deviation from anatomy is compensated in extension by femoral resection, which is perpendicular to the mechanical axis of the femur (mAF), leading to excessive femoral resection on the medial side (fig. 1 **b.**). This is not the case in flexion and there is no automatic correction by posterior femoral resection. Thus, if resection in flexion is carried out parallel to the PCL, with symmetric resection of the posterior condyles, the result is a space which is trapezoid in flexion with a medial compartment which is too tight and a lateral compartment which is too lax (26, 35) (fig. 1 **c.** and 1 **d.**).

There are several ways of compensating for this situation.

Hungerford and Kenna (24, 25) as well as Townley (46) and Krakow (29, 30) advise leaving a certain degree of varus in tibial resection in order to set the tibial component in an anatomic position. They justify this choice by gait studies: as during weight bearing there is a 3° overall adduction of the limb, the joint line remains horizontal although it is 3° varus relative to the mechanical axis of the leg. Hsu (23) confirmed these findings in a radiographic study showing that during weight bearing the joint line forms an angle of 0.4°±1.6 with the horizontal. This option avoids the difficulties related to "non-anatomic" tibial resection but brings up the potential risks related to placing the tibial component in varus (26) (fig. 2).

Insall (26), preferring tibial resection perpendicular to the mAT, advised asymmetric posterior condylar resection, in external rotation relative to the

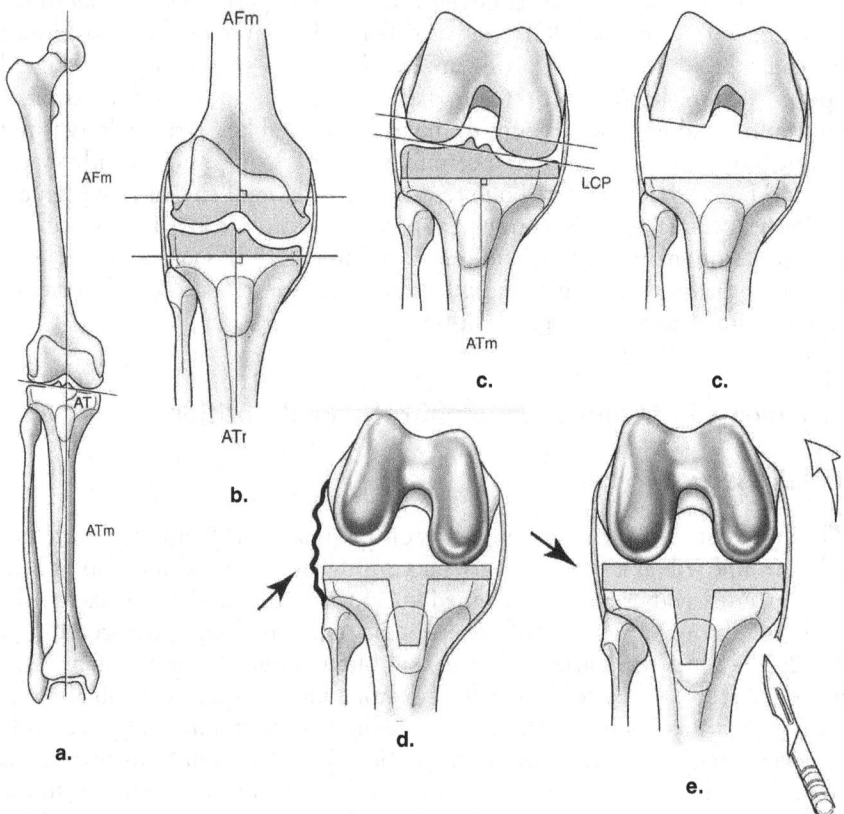

Fig. 1 – a. In a subject with normal alignment, the mechanical axis of the leg passes through the centre of the knee. The joint line is oblique in slight varus (mAT = 87° [19, 24, 29, 34, 35]).
b. Tibial resection perpendicular to the mAT leads to excess lateral resection which is compensated in extension by excess medial resection.
c. In flexion, if posterior condylar resection is parallel to the posterior condylar line (PCL), the flexion space will be trapezoidal with a tight medial compartment and a lax lateral compartment.
d. If the tibial component is adjusted to the medial compartment, the implant will be lax laterally.
e. To block lateral laxity, medial release must be done which will have an effect on extension.

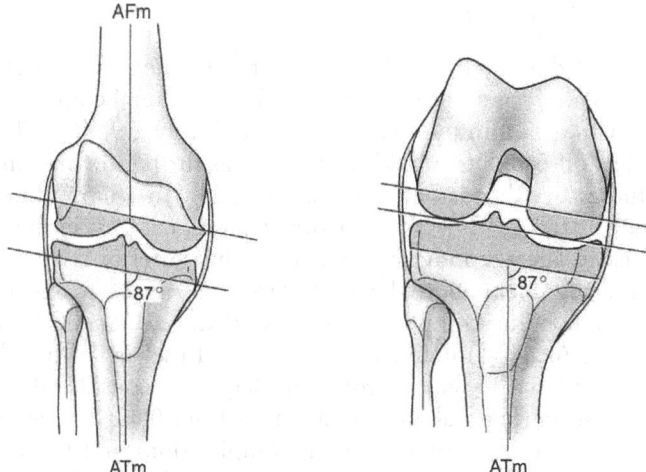

Fig. 2 – Tibial resection is performed with a few degrees of varus. In flexion, posterior condylar resection can be carried out parallel to the PCL. The flexion space will be symmetric.

PCL. He proposed carrying out posterior condylar resection after tautening the ligaments in order to obtain a symmetric flexion space (fig. 3). This option provides a solution to the difficulties of soft tissue balance in flexion while retaining the principle of tibial resection at 90° and being adaptable to each case (35). It raises however the problem of adjusting this rotation since it depends on the state of the ligaments (see below).

A third solution is to release the medial collateral ligament (MCL) in flexion, giving satisfactory soft tissue balance (11). In this option, the problem is merely transferred to extension and soft tissue balance is no longer physiological (fig. 1 **e.**).

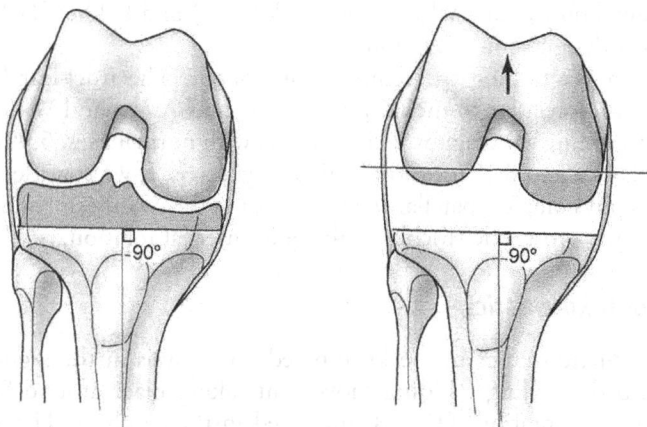

Fig. 3 – Tibial resection is perpendicular to the mechanical axis of the tibia. Posterior condylar resection, performed after tautening the peripheral ligaments, is parallel to tibial resection in order to obtain a symmetric flexion space.

Patellofemoral rotation

Several authors during the 1980s stressed the frequency of patellofemoral complications after total knee replacement if the femoral component was in rotational malposition in internal rotation (9, 16, 33, 39, 40). The influence of rotation on patellofemoral kinematics was further defined in 1993 by *in vitro* studies by Rhoads (41) and Anouchi (3). In 1995 Whiteside (48) and Arima (4) stressed the risk of incorrect rotational positioning in valgus knees related to lateral condylar hypoplasia. The posterior condyle is in fact affected and alignment with the PCL carries a risk of malposition with serious patellofemoral complications. Lastly, the *in vivo* CT studies of Berger (7) and Akagi (1) defined and quantified the risk of patellofemoral complications relative to femoral rotation. Berger (7) considered that overall prosthetic rotation (femoral and tibial) varies from 0° to 10° external rotation in patients without patellofemoral complications and from 1° to 17° internal rotation in the group with complications. In addition, the severity of the complication increases with the increasing degree of femoral internal rotation: 0.8° in simple tilt, 1.8° on average in patellar subluxation, 2.4° in luxation and 3.9° in loosening. For Akagi (1) placing the femoral component in external rotation reduces the rate of lateral flange resection from 34% to 6%.

The decreased rate of patellofemoral complications when the femoral component is placed in external rotation can be explained by:

– Femoral anatomy: the trochlear groove normally lies 2.4mm ± 2.1 lateral to the sagittal plane passing through the centre of the intercondylar notch (12). As this asymmetry of the distal extremity of the femur is not generally reproduced in total knee replacements, the trochlear groove of the implant is *ipso facto* translated internally relative to the bony trochlea. Femoral external rotation is a means of correcting this defect in implant design by artificially superposing the trochlear grooves of the implant and the bone. Rather than correct this phenomenon by external rotation, Laskin (31) and Eckhoff (12) suggest that implant design should be modified;

– Error in positioning the femoral component. The trochlear line is in external rotation relative to the PCL by 3.8° ± 2 for Arima and Whiteside (4) and even according to Akagi by 7° in patients with normal axes, 5.9° for those with a varus axis and 8.1° for those with a valgus axis. If we consider that this line reflects physiological patellar tracking, setting the prosthesis parallel to the PCL places the prosthetic trochlear groove in internal rotation.

Tibiofemoral kinematics

Classic kinematic studies of the knee based on analysis in the sagittal plane have described a rolling / sliding movement taking place around "instantaneous centres of rotation" (17, 18) dispersed in the condyles. Three-dimensional analysis techniques (8) have shown that flexion of the knee occurs around multiple axes. Moreover, classic anatomy describes non-circular posterior condyles with several geometric centres. Elias (13), Hollister (22),

Churchill (10) and Iwaki and Pinskerova (27, 37) have changed this vision of kinematics and functional anatomy. Their anatomic, radiographic, MRI and biomechanical studies have shown that:

1. Condylar curvature beyond the first degrees of flexion is wholly circular, thus laying classic anatomic descriptions open to question;

2. Rolling / sliding is a debatable notion. Medially, the movement is almost entirely a sliding one (96% of the movement according to Pinskerova) with roll-back of the tibiofemoral contact point of only 1.5mm. Laterally, rolling (40% of the movement) occurs essentially between 45° and 120° of flexion;

3. Flexion / extension movements of the knee may be likened to rotation occurring round two axes, one longitudinal parallel to the tibial axis and the other transverse. The transverse axis is the same as the transepicondylar axis for Hollister and oblique by 2.9° ± 1.2° for Churchill (fig. 4).

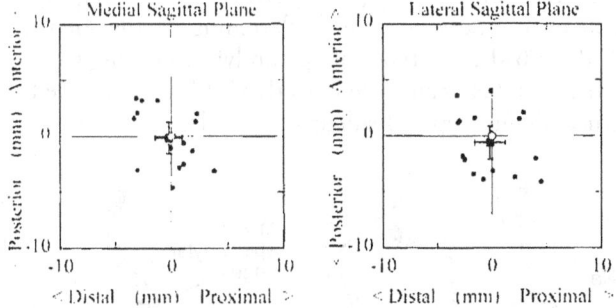

Fig. 4 – Position in a sagittal plane of the transepicondylar axis (dotted line) relative to the optimal axis of the knee in flexion-extension (intersection of the two straight lines), on the two compartments of the knee. Results of 15 cadaver knees (dotted line). Mean TEA (black square) defined with a confidence interval of 95%.
Churchill DL, Incavo SJ, Johnson CC *et al.* (1998) The transepicondylar axis approximates the optimal flexion axis of the knee. Clin Orthop 356: 111-8, fig. 6 p. 116 (reproduced with permission).

These studies naturally lead to the conclusion that setting the femoral component parallel to the transverse axis of flexion / extension of the knee (the transepicondylar axis) is ideal. Moreover, Yoshioka (50) and Stiehl (44) concur with this by showing that the TEA remains perpendicular to the tibial and femoral mechanical axes when the knee is flexed.

Practical anatomic landmarks

We have thus seen that all these clinical, technical and biomechanical arguments are in favour of positioning the femoral component in slight external rotation relative to the PCL in total knee replacement. The degree of rotation and the guides to be used are still debatable. Several anatomic landmarks can be used.

The transepicondylar axis

Anatomy

The epicondyles correspond to the zones of insertion of the collateral ligaments of the knee. The lateral epicondyle forms a prominence on the lateral condyle on which the lateral collateral ligament (LCL) inserts. It is bordered anteriorly by the insertion groove of the popliteal tendon and superiorly and posteriorly by part of the insertion of the lateral gastrocnemius.

The medial epicondyle, which is larger, consists of a horseshoe-shaped ridge with an inferior concavity. The peripheral ridge corresponds to the zone of insertion of the superficial bundle of the medial collateral ligament (MCL) and the central depression (sulcus), at the insertion of the deep bundle of the MCL (6) (fig. 5). For Griffin (21) its diameter is 11.4 ± 1.4mm and the depth of the central sulcus is 1.2 ± 0.4mm. The central sulcus can always be identified in healthy knees on CT scan (6) or MRI (21). However, this is not always possible in arthritic knees because of flattening of the medial epicondyle. Akagi (1, 2) described three types of epicondyle according to the visibility of the central sulcus on CT scan: type I clearly visible sulcus, type II sulcus recognizable with difficulty, type III sulcus not visible.

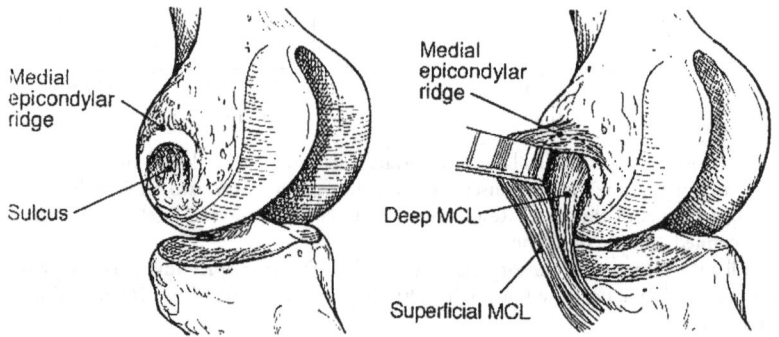

Fig. 5 – Anatomy of the medial epicondyle.
Griffin FM, Math K, Scuderi GR *et al.* (2000) Anatomy of the epicondyles of the distal femur. MRI analysis of normal knees. J Arthroplasty 15: 354-9, fig. 6 p. 357, reproduced with permission.

The transepicondylar axis (TEA) runs between the lateral and the medial epicondyle. Two types of axis have been described depending on the landmark chosen at the level of the medial epicondyle (1, 2, 6, 7) (fig. 6):

– The "clinical" TEA takes account of the most prominent zone (most easily palpable) of the medial epicondyle. This is the anterior prominence seen on CT scan or MRI at 90°. The angle between the clinical TEA and the PCL forms the condylar twist angle (CTA) (50);

– The "surgical" TEA is based on the sulcus of the medial epicondyle. The angle between the surgical TEA and the PCL forms the posterior condylar angle (PCA) (6).

Three authors have compared these three axes (table I). The angle between them varies from 1.2° to 4.9°, the clinical TEA being rotated more externally.

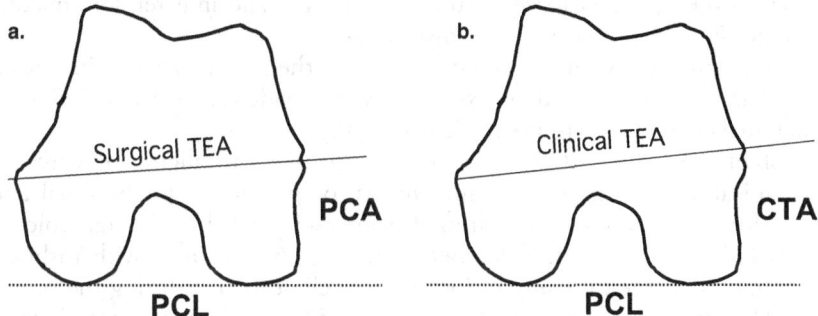

Fig. 6 – The two transepicondylar axes (TEA)
a. Surgical TEA defining the posterior condylar angle (PCA) relative to the posterior condylar line (PCL).
b. Clinical TEA defining the condylar twist angle (CTA) relative to the posterior condylar line (PCL).

Table I – Angle between the transepicondylar axis (TEA) and the posterior condylar line (PCL) in the various series of the literature.

Authors	PCA (°)	CTA (°)	Technique
Yoshioka (50)		men: 5.0±1.8 women: 6.0±2.4	preop CT scan (TKR)
Berger (6)*	men: 3.5±1.2 women: 0.3±1.2	men: 4.7±3.5 women: 5.2±4.1	cadaver study
Arima (4)		4.4±2.9	cadaver study
Poilvache (38)		3.60±2.02	preop measurement (TKR)
Matsuda (32)		6.03±3.6 healthy knees 6.0±2.35 varus knees	MRI volunteers
Griffin (20)	3.7±2.2		preop CT (TKR)
Griffin (21)	3.11±1.75		MRI healthy knees
Akagi (2)	4.2±2.1	6.4±1.4 varus knees 7.2±2 normal axis 8.8±3.2 valgus knees	preop CT (TKR)
Yoshino (49)	3.0±1.6	6.4±1.6	preop CT (TKR)

* Note lower standard deviation for the PCA than for the CTA.

History and clinical applications

The practical value of this landmark in total knee replacement was emphasized for the first time in 1987 by Yoshioka (50). He showed that:

1. The clinical TEA is a crucial landmark in biomechanics as it is perpendicular to the mechanical axes of the leg in flexion and in extension, making it one of the reference axes of the lower limb;

2. The angle between the clinical TEA and the bicondylar line in flexion (condylar twist angle) and in extension varies widely between individuals, which makes the PCL an unreliable landmark.

Yoshioka therefore advised placing the prosthesis in alignment with the mechanical axes of the lower limb, that is, perpendicular to the tibial and femoral mechanical axes in the frontal plane and parallel to the transepicondylar axis in the horizontal plane. Berger in 1993 (6) concurred with Yoshioka but emphasized the difficulty of locating the clinical TEA during the procedure. He noted considerable intra-observer (1.5°) and above all inter-observer (4°) variation in CTA measurement and described the surgical TEA as easier to locate. He advised it should be used to adjust femoral component rotation, considering it of interest only in cases where the PCL cannot be used, in particular implant revision. Stiehl in 1995 (44) confirmed the findings of Yoshioka in an *in vitro* study based on the clinical TEA. This lies perpendicular to the mechanical axis of the femur (a mean of 0.61° varus, ranging from 5.9° varus to 3.7° valgus) and of the tibia, both in extension (mean 0.4° varus, 3.6° varus to 4.2° valgus) and in 90° flexion (mean 0.43° varus, 0.43° varus to 4.2° valgus). Berger in 1998 (7) introduced measurement of the surgical TEA by CT scan and showed the importance of alignment along this axis in order to reduce patellofemoral complications in total knee replacement.

Griffin in 1998 (20) using measurements taken during surgery, showed that the PCA varies considerably, with a mean of 3.7° but with extremes ranging from 0° to 10°. In varus knees the range is 3.3° ± 1.9 and in valgus knees 5.5° ± 2.3. He concluded that it was difficult to select a fixed, universal angle relative to the PCL for all patients, and proposed that the angle should be adjusted during the procedure depending on the surgical TEA. In an MRI study in 2000 (21), he further defined the anatomy of the epicondyles and in particular the greater reliability of the surgical TEA. Akagi (2) in 2001 in a CT study of 111 knees undergoing total replacement found that the sulcus of the medial epicondyle was not visible or was difficult to recognize in 75% of cases. Moreover, he revealed a linear statistical relationship between femoral valgus (anatomic femoral angle) and the CTA when the femoral angle was greater than 9°: the greater the femoral valgus, the greater the CTA. Below 9° of femoral valgus, the CTA was constant at 6°. In this study, the deepest point of the trochlear groove was perpendicular to the clinical TEA, whatever the frontal morphology. The author concluded that the clinical TEA was more reliable and advised adjusting femoral rotation according to preoperative CT measurements of the CTA. Yoshino (49) in 2001 confirmed the difficulty of identifying the sulcus of the medial epicondyle in arthritic knees (it was undetectable in 59% of cases) especially if arthritis was long-standing. He proposed locating it by the surgical TEA in early arthritis but using the CTA as measured on preoperative CT scan in severe arthritis.

Orientation of the TEA relative to the reference axes of the leg

Numerous authors have studied the relationships between the TEA and the PCL in the horizontal plane (table I). However, there are few studies of its orientation in the frontal plane relative to the axes of the femur (table II) or tibia (table III).

Table II – Angle in the frontal plane between the mechanical femoral axis (mFA), anatomic femoral axis (aFA) and transepicondylar axis (+) TEA in varus. Angle between the TEA and the distal condylar line (DCL).

Authors	mAF	aFA	DCL	Reference	Type of study
Hollister (22)		6°±2.4	4.3°±1.0	not given	cadaver
Yoshioka (50)	1°±2.5			clinical TEA	cadaver
Sthiel (44)	0.61°			clinical TEA	cadaver

Table III – Angle between the mecchanical axis of the tibia (mAT) and the transepicondylar axis (TEA).

Authors	mAT in extension	mAT in flexion	Type of study	Reference
Yoshioka* (50)	90°	90°	cadaver	clinical TEA
Hollister (22)	2°±1.2 valgus		cadaver	not given
Stiehl (44)	0.4° varus	0.4° varus	cadaver	clinical TEA

* Study quoted but not published in full.

The anteroposterior axis (Whiteside's trochlear line)

In 1992, Whiteside and McCarthy (47) described their technique of unicompartmental knee arthroplasty, notably the technique of rotational positioning of the femoral component. An intramedullary stem is inserted at the top of the intercondylar notch. The femoral condyle is aligned with the line between this insertion point and the deepest part of the trochlear groove with the knee in 90° flexion. These authors showed that this anteroposterior axis (APA) is perpendicular to the transverse axis of the knee and parallel to the tibial axis. In 1995, Arima and Whiteside (4) described the value of this axis in total knee replacement, particularly in valgus knees since lateral condylar hypoplasia makes the PCL unreliable. In a cadaver study, they showed that the perpendicular to this axis is close to the clinical TEA, with slight internal rotation of 0.6° (mechanical measurement) or 2.6° (radiographic measurement). In this study, there were marked individual variations of the angle between the PCL on the one hand and the TEA or APA on the other (respectively 20° and 11°). These authors advised alignment of the prosthesis with the APA, arguing that it is more easily identified at surgery than the TEA and shows less variability.

Feinstein (15) and Eckhoff (12) in 1996 identified in cadaver studies the orientation of the trochlear groove relative to the reference axes of the femur.

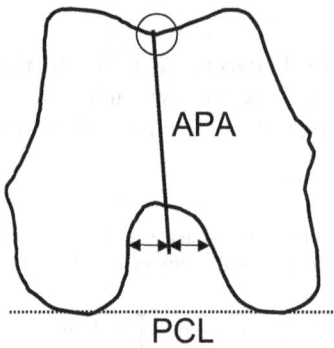

Fig. 7 – The anteroposterior axis (APA) or Whiteside's trochlear line.

It lies 2mm laterally to the sagittal plane passing through the centre of the intercondylar notch. In the frontal plane, it is inclined relative to the mechanical femoral axis, externally by 3.6° ± 0.5 for Eckhoff but internally by 1.4° ± 3.7 for Feinstein (there was however considerable variability in this study, with trochleas external by 6.7° or internal by 7.7°).

Poilvache (38) using measurements made during surgery found a mean angle between the perpendicular to the APA and the clinical TEA of 0.33° ± 2.44 (non-significant mean internal rotation of the trochlea relative to the TEA). He noted however a gender difference, the APA being in 1.2° ± 2.15 internal rotation in men and in 0.41° ± 2.45 external rotation in women. Akagi (2), using preoperative CT scan measurements of arthritic knees, showed that the perpendicular to the APA is nearly always parallel to the clinical TEA (angles of 0.5 ± 1.9, 0.2 ± 1.9 and 0.7 ± 1.8 in varus, normal and valgus knees, respectively).

Techniques for adjusting femoral rotation

The reference anatomic landmark is the transepicondylar axis because it has a constant relationship with the reference axes of the leg and because it corresponds to the flexion-extension axis of the knee. Other landmarks are justified by the fact that they have constant relationships with the TEA and their advocates argue that they are easier to use.

External rotation determined relative to the posterior condylar line

– Principle: the implant is aligned on the TEA and rotated externally relative to the PCL to a predetermined degree. In the literature, the mean angle between the TEA and the PCL has been found to range from 0° to 6°, and this angle is applied to the posterior condylar cutting jig which is supported by the posterior condyles.

– Advantages: this is a simple technique which does not have to be adapted to the various situations encountered at surgery since rotation is determined by the ancillary.

– Disadvantages:

1. The CTA and PCA vary greatly between individuals. It therefore seems difficult to choose arbitrarily a fixed angle relative to the PCL: an angle of 3° may be too much in certain cases and inadequate in others. Akagi (2) advises using a fixed external rotation angle of 6° in arthritic varus knees or knee with normal axes, but recommends preoperative CT scan measurement in markedly valgus knees (see above) (fig. 8);

2. There is an average difference of about 3° between the two TEAs which can be used, and this may be as much as 4.9° (6). In fact, it is difficult to know which axis better reflects the functional axis of the knee.

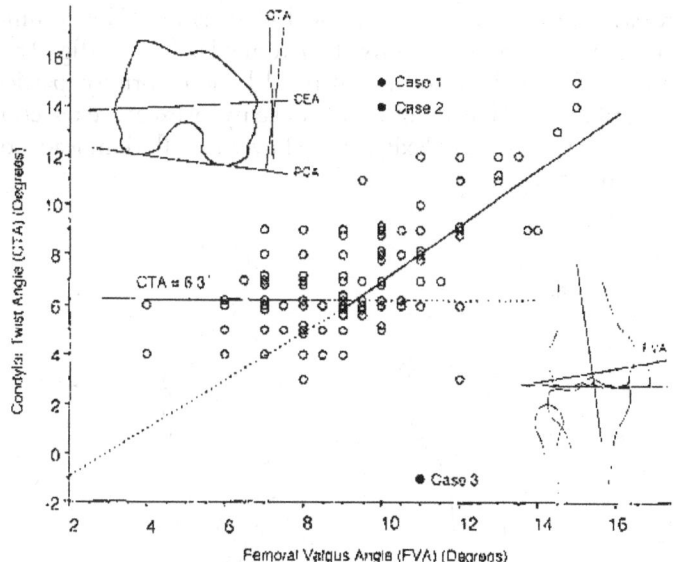

Fig. 8 – Relationship between the condylar twist angle (CTA) and the anatomic femoral angle (AFA). Up to 9° anatomic femoral valgus, the CTA is constant at 6.3°. Over 9° anatomic femoral valgus, the CTA increases.

Cases 1, 2 and 3 were not included in statistical analysis as measurements were biased by osteophytes.

Akagi M, Yamashita E, Nakagawa T *et al.* (2001) Relationship between frontal knee alignment and reference axes in the distal femur. Clin Orthop 388: 147-56, fig. 5, p. 153, reproduced with permission.

Rotation adjusted to the flexion space

– Principle: After resecting the tibia at 90°, posterior condylar resection is carried out parallel to the plane of tibial resection, in 90° flexion, after tensing the collateral ligaments. This technique recreates a symmetric flexion space and thus promotes soft tissue balance.

– Advantages: A simple technique which gives optimal tibiofemoral stability in flexion and avoids lateral lift-off in flexion. Certain authors have recently shown that the functional results of total knee replacement are influenced by this phenomenon which is often difficult to demonstrate (42, 43). Moreover, Attfield has shown that the quality of soft tissue balance improves proprioception after total knee arthroplasty (5).

– Disadvantages:

1. The rotational position depends on the state of the ligaments and this may lead to significant malpositioning, notably in valgus knees with medial laxity. Moreover, resection in flexion is influenced in this technique by the amount of medial release carried out in extension in the first stage: the volume of space will depend on the amount of this release and final femoral positioning depends on this factor. Fehring (14) considers this as an advantage giving in all events a rectangular space. This may be considered as a risk, as ill-judged release can be a cause of rotational malposition. This technique thus necessitates a double check using fixed anatomic landmarks (fig. 9 **a.**);

2. If there is marked constitutional tibial bone deformity, particularly in varus knees, tibial resection at 90° produces laxity by excessive resection on the "healthy" side. This resection laxity, carried over into flexion, leads to rotational malposition (fig. 9 **b.**).

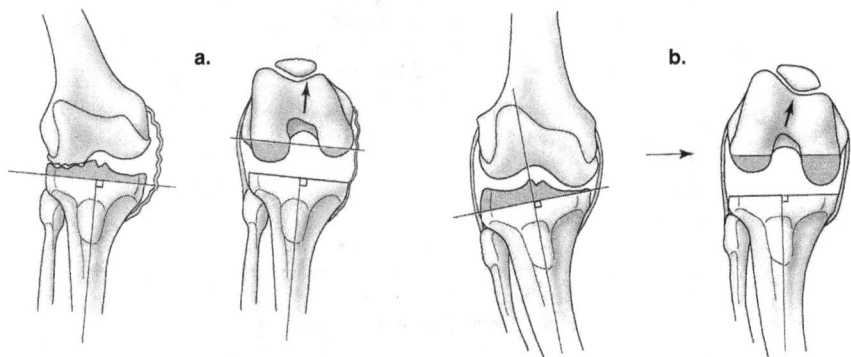

Fig. 9 – Critique of the technique based on the flexion space.
a. If the medial collateral ligament (MCL) is lax, there is the risk that resection will be done in internal rotation.
b. In constitutional varus knees due to tibial varus, laxity of resection is considerable and there is a risk of excessive external rotation.

The transepicondylar axis

– Principle: The posterior condylar cutting jig is rotated in alignment with the TEA and resection is aligned with this axis.

– Advantages: Ideal positioning from the kinematic viewpoint as the prosthesis is in alignment with the flexion / extension axis of the knee.

– Disadvantages:

1. The medial epicondyle is difficult to locate both at surgery (4) and on preoperative CT scan (2) making this measurement unreliable. For Griffin (21) the central hollow of the medial epicondyle can always be identified and its small size makes it a reliable landmark. On the other hand, use of the per-

ipheral ridge is imprecise as its diameter is large and it is difficult to know on palpation whether one is on the anterior, superior or posterior part of the horse-shoe. Poilvache (38) considers it to be the most prominent area of the epi-condyle and the easiest to detect on palpation;

2. Deviation of 3° (up to 4.6°) between the two TEAs has been described in the literature. Some authors consider the surgical axis should be preferred as it is more reliable (21) and corresponds better to the flexion / extension axis of the knee (44). For other authors (2), the clinical axis which is in a constant rela-tionship to the deepest point of the trochlear groove is a landmark of choice;

3. The TEA is assimilated to the flexion / extension axis of the knee by approximation only and so is theoretically debatable (10, 27, 37). For Churchill, however, the angle between these two axes is not significant and the most prominent points of the epicondyles are close to the optimal flexion axis of the knee (0.2mm behind and 0.14mm below on the medial side and res-pectively 0.2mm and 0.6mm on the lateral side). For Pinskerova, flexion / extension takes place along two parallel axes, of which the TEA is the best approximation.

The anteroposterior axis

– Principle: The posterior condylar cutting jig is rotated in alignment with the perpendicular to the anteroposterior axis of Arima and Whiteside. This axis is defined by the line running between the deepest point of the trochlear groove on the knee at 90° and the centre of the intercondylar notch.

– Advantages:

1. A simple technique which can be adapted to the patient's anatomy and is independent of morphological abnormalities, in particular in valgus knees;

2. This line is easily identified at surgery, and according to its advocates there is less risk of error than when using the epicondyles as landmarks;

3. Technique giving alignment on the TEA, as these two lines are practical-ly perpendicular in all studies of healthy knees except that of Feinstein (15).

– Disadvantages:

1. The deepest point of the trochlear groove is sometimes difficult to locate in knees with longstanding patellofemoral arthritis or trochlear dysplasia (37);

2. Even if the mean angle between the APA and the TEA is close to 90°, this varies considerably between individuals, with the deepest point of the tro-chlear groove sometimes in neutral, sometimes in internal, sometimes in external rotation relative to the TEA. Systematic positioning in this alignment can lead to rotational malposition relative to the TEA.

The tibial axis

– Principle: As the mechanical axis of the tibia is perpendicular to the cli-nical TEA (44, 50) the principle is to align posterior condylar resection with the perpendicular to the mAT after adjusting for the part of deformity which is related to wear (fig. 10 a.).

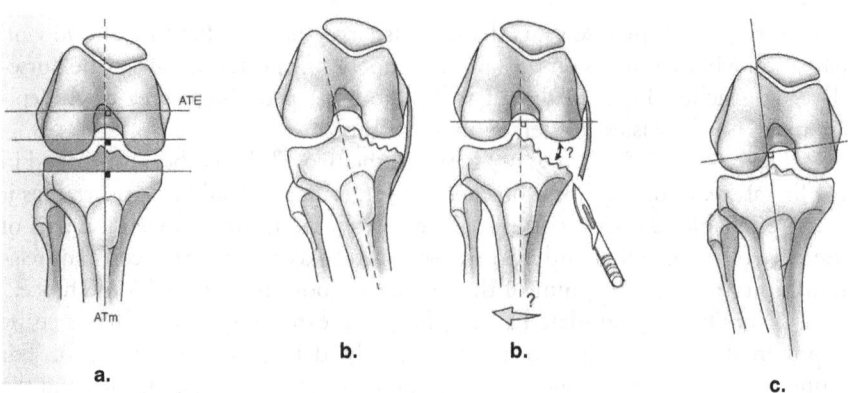

Fig. 10 – Critique of the technique based on the mechanical axis of the tibia.
a. In the absence of marked wear and constitutional deformity, the mechanical axis of the tibia is perpendicular to the transepicondylar axis. Posterior condylar resection, carried out in the first stage, is perpendicular to the tibial axis.
b. If there is marked tibial wear, adjustment is not precise and it may cause rotational malposition.
c. In constitutional varus knees due to tibial varus, positioning may be in excessive external rotation.

– Advantages: A simple and logical method, if one is dealing with knees with normal axial alignment and without wear.

– Disadvantages:

1. There is an element of inaccuracy related to adjustment for bone wear which requires the use of a distractor. Final positioning therefore depends on the state of the ligaments and on evaluation of bone wear by the operator. Posterior wear is particularly difficult to assess on a flexed knee. Adjustment for this wear is thus artificial, especially as the tibial slope and ligament retraction or distension have to be taken into account (fig. 10 **b.**);

2. In constitutional tibial deformity, the alignment error is automatically carried over to posterior condylar resection and so to rotational positioning of the femoral component (fig. 10 **c.**);

3. Only two published studies have determined the angle between the TEA and the mAT (22, 44): neither analyzed this angle in relation to the frontal morphology of the leg and both were based on external anatomic measurements which were therefore imprecise.

Comparative studies and summing-up

Few studies have compared the precision and the results of these various techniques.

Olcott (36) compared methods 1, 2, 3 and 4 and obtained better soft tissue balance by using the transepicondylar axis as a landmark during surgery. Stiehl (45), comparing techniques 2 and 5, obtained better alignment with the TEA using the method based on the tibial axis. Fehring (14), comparing the flexion space obtained with different methods of posterior condylar resection, found that techniques based on the fixed bony landmarks 1, 3 and 4 resulted in a trapezoidal space in 44% of cases. He therefore recommended that resection should be adapted to the flexion space in order to obtain a space which is always symmetric. Katz (28) in an *in vitro* study of non-arthritic knees showed that techniques 2 and 4 were more reliable than the technique based on TEA identification during surgery in terms of soft tissue balance and even of positioning relative to the true axis of the knee. Identification of the TEA during surgery is subject to considerable variability from one operator to another, resulting in this study in external rotational positioning compared with techniques 2 and 4.

At the present time, there seems to be no perfect technique for adjusting femoral component rotation. Techniques which make use of fixed bone landmarks raise the problem of recognition during surgery. Such difficulties of identification occur both for the deepest point of the trochlear groove and for the medial epicondyle. Systematically adjusting rotation according to preoperative CT measurements raises the question of the cost of the investigation and of the choice of bone landmark (medial epicondylar crater or crest).

Moreover, the relationships between the various reference axes (TEA, mAT, and APA) vary greatly from one patient to another. It is true that the deepest point of the trochlear groove and the mechanical tibial axis are generally perpendicular to the transepicondylar axis but is a wide range of values and calculations based on averages carry the risk of malrotation. Akagi thus noted fixed CTA values for varus or neutral femurs with mean values of 6.3° (fig. 8). It should however be noted that in these groups CTA variations ranged from 3° to 10.5°. Similarly, the APA, although generally perpendicular to the TEA, may be in internal or external rotation with individual variations of as much as 11°. Stiehl observed that the TEA is perpendicular to the mechanical axis of the tibia but values ranged from 3.6° varus to 4.2° varus. As for techniques based on flexion space or the tibial axis, they are totally unreliable in constitutional bone deformity or ligament distension.

Table IV – Advantages and disadvantages of femoral rotation adjustment techniques in total knee replacement.

Technique	Advantages	Disadvantages
Fixed RE	Reliable anatomic reference	– Arbitrary choice of RE angle
Flexion space		– Transfers to rotation the constitutional defects of the tibial axis – Errors of ligamentous origin
TEA	Biomechanical reference	– Difficult to identify by operator – Choice between two TEAs
APA	Adapted to patellofemoral rotation	– Identification sometimes unreliable – Individual variations of TEA
Tibial axis		– Transfers to rotation the constitutional defects of the tibial axis – Errors of ligamentous origin

It appears important to be always able to use several landmark techniques in difficult cases and not to be restricted to a single system. Preoperative CT scan in at-risk cases should prevent certain malpositions.

References

1. Akagi M, Matsusue Y, Mata T *et al.* (1999) Effect of rotational alignment on patellar tracking in total knee arthoplasty. Clin Orthop 366: 155-63
2. Akagi M, Yamashita E, Nakagawa T *et al.* (2001) Relationship between frontal knee alignment and reference axes in the distal femur. Clin Orthop 388: 147-56
3. Anouchi YS, Whiteside LA, Kaiser AD *et al.* (1993) The effects of axial rotational alignment of the femoral component on knee stability and patellar tracking in total knee arthroplasty demonstrated on autopsy specimens. Clin Orthop 287: 170-7
4. Arima J, Whiteside LA, McCarthy D *et al.* (1995) Femoral rotational alignment based on the antero-posterior axis, in total knee arthroplasty in a valgus knee. A technical note. J Bone Joint Surg (Am) 77: 1331-4
5. Attfield SF, Wilton TJ, Pratt DJ *et al.* (1996) Soft tissue balance and recovery of proprioception after total knee arthroplasty. J Bone Joint Surg (Br) 78: 540-5
6. Berger RA, Rubash HE, Seel MJ *et al.* (1993) Determining the rotational alignment of the femoral component in total knee arthroplasty using the epicondylar axis. Clin Orthop 286: 40-7
7. Berger RA, Crossett LS, Jacobs JJ *et al.* (1998) Malrotation causing patellofemoral complications after total knee arthroplasty. Clin Orthop 356: 144-53
8. Blankevoort L, Huiskes R, de Lang A (1990) Helical axes of passive knee-joint motion. J Biomech 22: 1219-29
9. Briard JL, Hungerford DS (1989) Patellofemoral instability in total knee arthroplasty. J Arthroplasty 4 Suppl: 87-97
10. Churchill DL, Incavo SJ, Johnson CC *et al.* (1998) The transepicondylar axis approximates the optimal flexion axis of the knee. Clin Orthop 356: 111-8
11. Dejour H, Deschamps G (1989) Technique opératoire de la prothèse totale à glissement du genou. Cahiers d'enseignement de la SOFCOT n° 35
12. Eckhoff DG, Burke BJ, Dwyer TF *et al.* (1996) Sulcus morphology of the distal femur. Clin Orthop 331: 23-8
13. Ellias SG, Freeman MAR, Gokcay EI (1990) A correlative study of the geometry and anatomy of the distal femur. Clin Orthop 260: 98-103
14. Fehring TK (2000) Rotational malalignment of the femoral component in total knee arthroplasty. Clin Orthop 380: 72-9
15. Feinstein WK, Noble PC, Kamaric E *et al.* (1996) Anatomic alignment of the patellar groove. Clin Orthop 331: 64-73
16. Figgie HE, Goldberg VM, Figgie MP *et al.* (1989) The effect of alignment of the implant on fractures of the patella after condylar total knee arthroplasty. J Bone Joint Surg (Am) 71: 1031-9
17. Frain P, Fontaine C, D'Hondt D (1984) Contraintes du genou par dérangement méniscoligamentaires. Étude de l'articulation condylo-tibiale interne. Méthode cinématique expérimentale. Rev Chir Orthop 70: 361-9
18. Frankel VH, Burstein AH, Brooks DB (1971) Biomechanics of internal derangement of the knee. J Bone Joint Surg (Am) 53: 945-62
19. Greenberg RL, Kenna RV, Hungerford DS *et al.* (1984) Instrumentation for total knee arthroplasty. In: Total knee arthroplasty; a comprehensive approach. Hungerford DS, Krackow KA, Kenna RV, Williams and Wilkins, Baltimore, 35-70
20. Griffin FM, Insall JN, Scuderi GR (1998) The posterior condylar angle in osteoarthritic knees. J Arthroplasty 13: 812-5
21. Griffin FM, Math K, Scuderi GR *et al.* (2000) Anatomy of the epicondyles of the distal femur. MRI analysis of normal knees. J Arthroplasty 15: 354-9

22. Hollister AM, Jatana S, Singh AK *et al.* (1993) The axes of rotation of the knee. Clin Orthop 290: 259-68
23. Hsu RWW, Himeno S, Coventry MB *et al.* (1990) Normal axial alignment of the lower extremity and load-bearing distribution at the knee. Clin Orthop 255: 215-27
24. Hungerford QS, Kenna RV (1983) Preliminary experience with a total knee prosthesis with porous coating used without cement. Clin Orthop 176: 95-107
25. Hungerford DS, Krackow KA (1985) Total joint arthroplasty of the knee. Clin Orthop 192: 23-33
26. Insall JN (1984) Total knee replacement. In: Surgery of the knee. Insall JN. Churchill Livingstone, New York: 587-695
27. Iwaki H, Pinskerova V, Freeman MA (2000) Tibiofemoral movement 1: the shapes and relative movements of the femur and tibia in the unloaded cadaver knee. J Bone Joint Surg (Br) 82: 1189-95
28. Katz MA, Beck TD, Silber JS *et al.* (2001) Determining femoral rotational alignment in total knee arthroplasty. J Arthroplasty 16: 301-5
29. Krackow KA (1990) Preoperative assessment: axial and rotational alignment and X-Ray analysis. In: The technique of total knee arthroplasty. Krakow KA, Mosby Company, St Louis: 86-117
30. Krackow KA (1990) Intraoperative alignment and instrumentation. In: The technique of total knee arthroplasty. Krakow KA, Mosby Company, St Louis: 118-67
31. Laskin SR (2000) Flexion space balancing using a prosthesis with asymmetrical posterior femoral condyles without external rotation. Am J Knee Surg 13: 169-72
32. Matsuda S, Matsuda H, Miyagi T *et al.* (1998) Femoral condyle geometry in the normal and varus knee. Clin Orthop 349: 183-8
33. Merkow RL, Soudry M, Insall JN (1985) Patellar dislocation following total knee replacement. J Bone Joint Surg (Am) 67: 1321-7
34. Moreland FR, Bassett LW, Hanker GJ (1987) Radiographic analysis of the axial alignment of the lower extremity. J Bone Joint Surg (Am) 69: 745-9
35. Moreland FR (1988) Mechanism of failure in total knee arthroplasty. Clin Orthop 226: 49-64
36. Olcott CW, Scott RD (1999) Femoral component rotation during total knee arthroplasty. Clin Orthop 367: 39-42
37. Pinskerova V, Iwaki H, Freeman MAR (2001) The shapes and relative movements of the femur and tibia in the unloaded cadaveric knee: a study using MRI as an anatomic tool. In: Surgery of the knee, third edition. Insall JN, Scott WN, Churchill Livingstone, Philadelphia, 255-83
38. Poilvache PL, Insall JN, Scuderi GR *et al.* (1996) Rotational landmarks and sizing of the distal femur in total knee arthroplasty. Clin Orthop 331: 35-46
39. Ranawat CS (1986) The patellofemoral joint in total condylar knee arthroplasty. Pros and cons based on five- to ten-year follow-up observations. Clin Orthop 205: 93-9
40. Rhoads DD, Noble PC, Reuben JD *et al.* (1990) The effect of femoral component position on patellar tracking after total knee arthroplasty. Clin Orthop 260: 41-3
41. Rhoads DD, Noble PC, Reuben JD *et al.* (1993) The effect of component position on the kinematics of total knee arthroplasty. Clin Orthop 286: 122-9
42. Romero J, Binkert C, Braum V *et al.* (2001) Revision total knee arthroplasty for lateral flexion instability due to internal malrotation of femoral component. 5th Congress of the European Federation of National Associations of Orthopaedics and Traumatology (EFORT). Rhodes June 6th
43. Scuderi GR, Insall JN, Komistek RD *et al.* (2001) *In vivo* correlation of condylar lift-off and femoral component alignment during a deep knee bend. Proceedings of the 68th Annual Meeting of AAOS, San Francisco, paper N° 46: 558
44. Stiehl JB, Abbott BD (1995) Morphology of the transepicondylar axis and its application in primary and revision total knee arthroplasty. J Arthroplasty 10: 785-9
45. Stiehl JB, Cherveny PM (1996) Femoral rotational alignment using the tibial shaft axis in total knee arthroplasty. Clin Orthop 331: 47-55
46. Townley CO (1985) The anatomic resurfacing arthroplasty. Clin Orthop 192: 82-96

47. Whiteside LA, McCarthy D (1992) Laboratory evaluation of alignment and kinematics in a unicompartmental knee arthroplasty inserted with intramedullary instrumentation. Clin Orthop 274: 238-47
48. Whiteside LA, Arima J (1995) The anteroposterior axis for femoral rotational alignment in valgus total knee arthroplasty. Clin Orthop 321: 168-72
49. Yoshino N, Takai S, Ohtsuki Y et al. (2001) Computed tomography measurement of the surgical and clinical transepicondylar axis of the distal femur in osteoarthritic knees. J Arthroplasty 16: 493-7
50. Yoshioka Y, Siu D, Cooke TDV (1987) The anatomy and functional axes of the femur. J Bone Joint Surg (Am) 69:873-80

Steps and strategies in the insertion of posterior-stabilized knee replacements

P. Neyret, P. Rivat, T. Aït Si Selmi

Most implant designers and manufacturers nowadays stress the need for careful implant selection, bearing in mind the mechanical, kinematic, and biological properties of the devices. However, little thought appears to be given to the way in which the instrumentation matches the device to be implanted.

This chapter explores the aspects involved in optimizing the actual implantation of a total knee replacement (TKR).

Knee arthroplasty is performed in a sequence of steps or stages. These steps are interlinked: each one may affect the following ones. Also, each implant has its own rules of insertion, which derive from the design of the prosthesis.

Total knee replacement is, thus, an equation with a large number of (sometimes interdependent) variables. The surgeon has to know the chosen implant, and, in the light of this knowledge, determine the variables (such as bone cuts, soft tissue releases, thickness of components) that will allow him or her to obtain the desired result.

One of the factors that may be varied by the surgeon during the actual procedure is the degree of implant constraint. However, this constraint may also be determined by the surgeon prior to the procedure, in which case the other parameters will need to be varied to suit the chosen constraint.

The problem posed by the different steps and stages in the insertion of the different knee replacement systems may also be shown as a circle (fig. 1). This circle may be entered at different points: at the tibial bone cut, the femoral bone cut, dependent or independent cuts, the type of implant, the soft tissue releases, the goal of arthroplasty. All these steps are linked with each other. In total knee replacement, the surgeon needs to decide where he or she will enter the circle, knowing that the entry point will, in turn, affect each one of the other factors involved.

Of late, the circle has been rendered even more complex by the advent of computer-assisted targeting systems, which have changed the rules of the game; by the provision of tibial components with a rotating-platform mobile bearing and by the design of implant systems that do not involve resurfacing of the patella.

Once the entry point has been chosen, total knee replacement proceeds in a sequence of steps, which may, in certain cases, involve trade-offs, and which will, invariably, affect the subsequent steps, and have to be performed in such a way as not to compromise the final outcome.

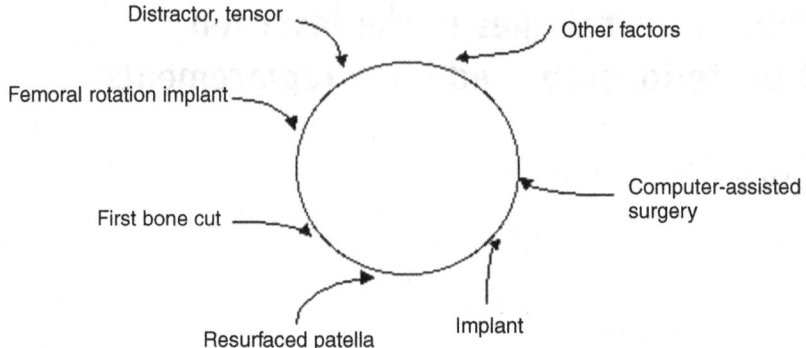

Fig. 1 – Implant insertion is an equation with a large number of (sometimes interdependent) variables.

Definitions

Bone cuts

Bone cuts involve the tibia, the femur, and (where appropriate) the patella.

Except in cases of local bone defects, there will be only one *tibial cut*.

In the *femur, three main cuts* are made: a distal femoral cut, a posterior femoral cut to remove the posterior part of the condyles, and an anterior femoral cut. Additional cuts may be required, in particular anterior and posterior chamfering, or the fashioning of a hole to accommodate the posterior stabilization system or the third condyle.

The *patellar cut* is not a standard feature of total knee replacement. It is required only if a patellar component is to be inserted.

The cuts are made using jigs with slots or guide pins. The actual cutting instrument may be a sawblade or a rotary milling blade guided by the jigs or by a navigation system.

Each cut is defined by its *level*, which is usually referenced to a joint, as well as by its *orientation*. Bone resection that is equal in the frontal or the sagittal plane is known as *symmetrical*, while resection that removes different amounts of bone in the frontal or the sagittal plane is known as *asymmetrical bone resection*.

The soft tissue envelope

The soft tissue envelope (fig. 2) consists of the capsule and the peripheral ligaments. The soft tissue restraints are not confined to the collateral ligaments and the popliteus tendon: they also include the semitendinosus corner and the popliteus corner. The posterior capsular structures and the extensor apparatus, too, are integral parts of the soft tissue envelope, which also includes the retinacula.

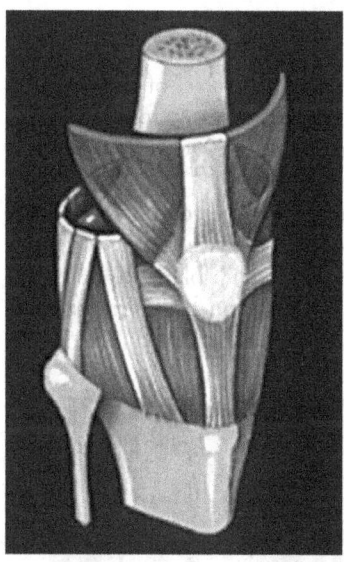

Fig. 2 – The soft tissue envelope is constituted by the collateral ligaments as well as by the patellar tendon.

Dependent and independent cuts – Use of tensor versus spreader

The tibial and femoral cuts may be made independently of each other, in which case they are referred to as independent cuts.

Equally, though, the orientation and the level of the cut made at one level may be linked, through the instrument system, to the cut made in the other bone. In that case, the cuts are considered to be dependent (fig. 3).

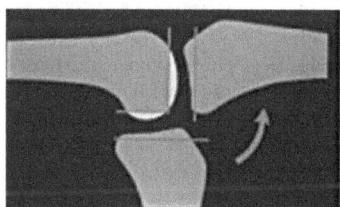 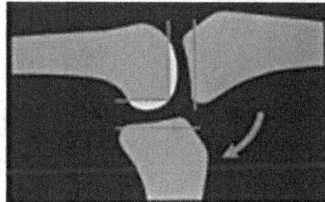

Fig. 3 – Dependent cuts: the different cuts are linked, with regard to their level and orientation, by the instruments used for implant insertion.

The instrument used for adjusting the cut in one bone to the cut in the other bone may be a tensor or a spreader. With most of the instrument systems currently available, the degree of dependence between the cuts will be a function of the instrument, as well as of the soft tissue envelope.

There is a substantial difference between a spreader, which does not distinguish between the medial and the lateral compartment, and a tensor, which treats each side separately.

The spreader serves to keep the bone cuts parallel. If need be, the soft tissues will be adjusted to change the space produced by the bone cuts. The spreader itself allows the height of the cut to be adjusted (fig. 4).

The tensor is used to tension the soft tissue envelope. The orientation of the bone cuts will be a function of this tensioning and of the level of the cut. It is assumed that any ligament releases will have been performed beforehand, and the bone cut will be made as a function of the release achieved and of the tensioning of the ligaments.

There are different models of tensors, which allow the medial and the lateral collaterals to be tensioned individually. Some have two blades that are controlled separately; equally, there are systems in which a blade on a central pivot is pressed against the medial and lateral condylar surfaces. Tensors and spreaders allow the space required by the implant to be simulated (fig. 5).

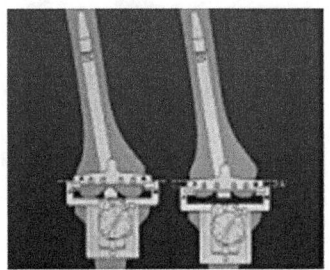 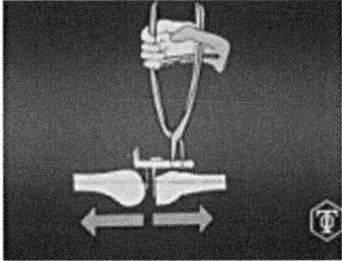

Fig. 4 – The spreader (symmetrical tensor) keeps the bone cuts parallel and allows the level of the cut to be controlled.

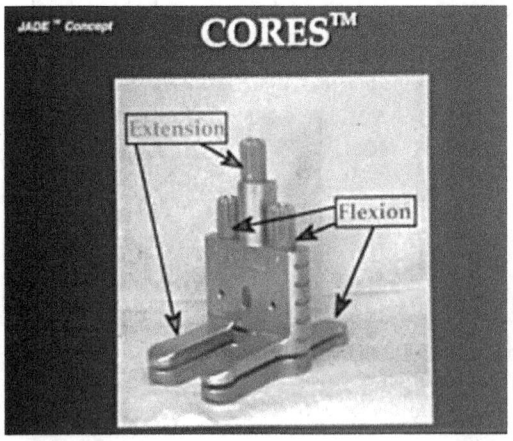

Fig. 5 – The asymmetrical tensor allows the orientation and the level of the cuts to be determined after tensioning of the soft tissue envelope.

Spaces

The cuts made within the soft tissue envelope create spaces – the tibiofemoral space, and the patellofemoral space.

Tibiofemoral space

Throughout the range of movement, there is only one space. For better visualization of the concept, the terms *extension space* and *flexion space* are often

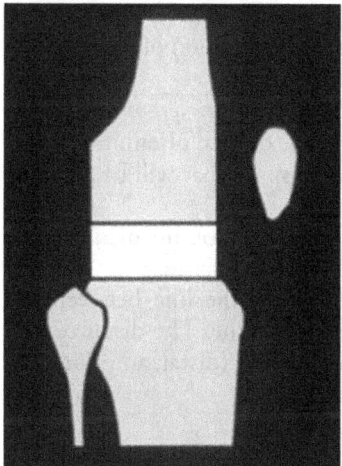

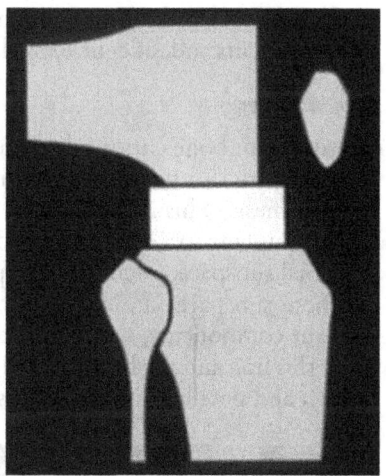

Fig. 6 – Extension space.   **Fig. 7** – Flexion space.

used. The extension space (fig. 6) is defined by the distal femoral cut and the tibial cut. The flexion space (fig. 7) is determined by the posterior femoral cut and by the tibial cut. This distinction is, however, an academic and an artificial one: in actual fact, the two spaces merge into one another.

Patellofemoral space

Throughout the range of movement, there is only one space. As with the tibiofemoral space, it may be more convenient, for descriptive purposes, to refer to an anterior space (10) bounded by the anterior femoral cut (or trochlear cut) on the one hand, and the patellar cut (fig. 8) or the patellar joint surface, on the other hand. Also, the term patellofemoral flexion space has been used, to denote the space between the distal femoral cut and the patellar cut or the patellar joint surface.

It must, however, be borne in mind that, while the knee joint may be subdivided into the above mentioned spaces, it is, in fact, one single entity. The tibiofemoral and patellofemoral spaces are interlinked, and merge as the knee goes through its range of movement. Thus, the distal tibiofemoral space and the patellofemoral flexion space are linked by the distal femoral cut; while the tibiofemo-

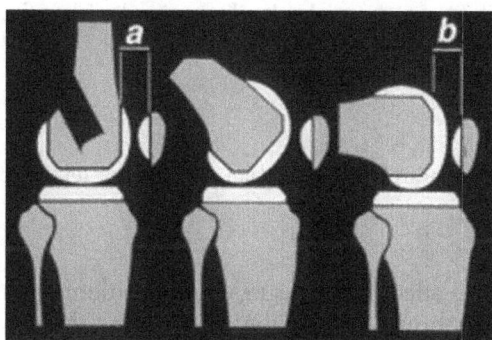

Fig. 8 – The anterior space (**a.**) is bounded by the anterior femoral cut and the patellar cut. The patellofemoral flexion space (**b.**) is bounded by the distal femoral cut and the patellar cut.

ral flexion space and the anterior patellofemoral space are linked by the orientation of the cuts and, of course, by the anteroposterior dimension of the implant.

Implant space

The different bone cuts (at the required level and the desired orientation), and the necessary soft tissue releases will have created a space that will be filled by the prosthesis. This is the implant space (fig. 9).

The implant space may be divided into a number of subunits or subspaces – a tibial subspace, a femoral subspace, and a patellar subspace.

These subspaces are separated from each other by the line between the implant components, which constitutes the new joint line. The distance between this line and the bone cuts allows the tibial, femoral (distal, anterior, posterior), and patellar implant spaces to be defined.

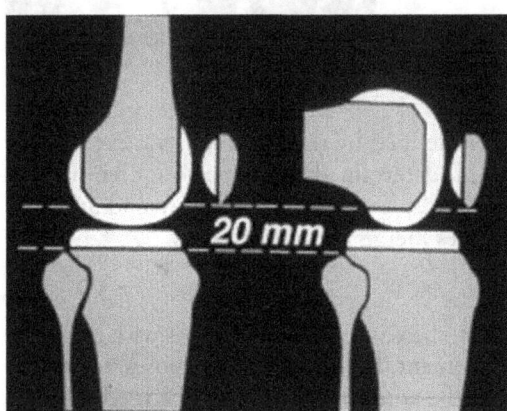

Fig. 9 – Implant space.

Insertion stages

Bone cuts

The bone cuts may be made with a conventional set of instruments, or using a navigation system. Conventional instrumentation will provide an extramedullary alignment system that works off the mechanical axis, or an intramedullary alignment system that references from the anatomical axes.

Navigation systems allow the centres of rotation to be calculated, and to determine the mechanical axes. These axes may also be determined with reference to anatomical landmarks.

Each bone cut will have a level and an orientation.

Orientation of bone cuts

This aspect needs to be dealt with separately for the tibial and for the femoral cuts.

Tibial cut

The orientation of the tibial cut will affect the varus or valgus positioning of the implant in extension as well as throughout flexion. A cut other than at right angles to the mechanical limb axis in the coronal plane will affect the knee replacement both in flexion and in extension. The tibial slope will affect the extension space as well as the flexion space.

Extramedullary, intramedullary, or extra- and intramedullary alignment guides may be used to determine the tibial bone cut. In the majority of cases, the surgeon will aim at a cut at right angles to the mechanical axis in the coronal plane (fig. 10 **a.**), and at right angles to the tibia in the sagittal plane.

In the HLS system, extra- and intramedullary alignment guides may be used together, to allow a 90° sagittal-plane cut to be made.

Other authors have proposed additional target values, e.g. a tibial 3° varus cut, as advocated by Hungerford and Krackow (fig. 10 **b.**), or the 5-10° sagittal-plane cut of the tibia recommended by Galante.

a.

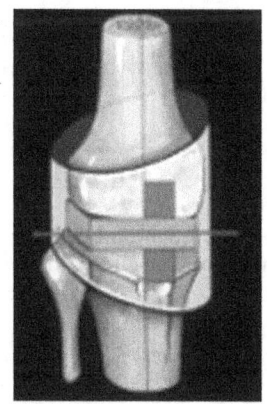

b.

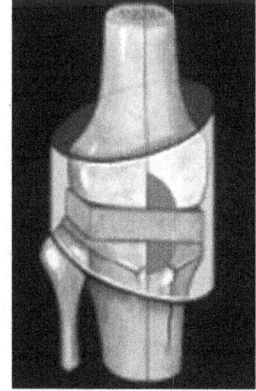

Fig. 10 – a. Coronal-plane cuts at right angles to the mechanical axis.
b. Tibial 3° varus cut, as advocated by Krackow and Hungerford.

Femoral cut

• Distal femoral cut

The orientation of the distal femoral cut will affect the varus / valgus position of the implant.

The cut may be referenced from various axes:

– *The femoral anatomical axis II* described by Moreland *et al.* (9). This axis is constituted by a line linking two points (called shaft centres I and II) situated halfway up the femoral shaft and 10cm above the surface of the knee joint, respectively, and midway between the medial and lateral surfaces of the shaft. This line normally passes through the medial condyle. If this axis, which extends the line of the shaft, is used for intramedullary alignment, the surgeon should be aware of the need for offsetting the implant during the subsequent stages of implantation, so as to obtain correct positioning on the distal end of the femur. The offset will affect the final femoral mechanical angle of the implant.

– *The femoral mechanical axis* is defined as a straight line from the centre of the femoral head to the centre of the knee. This axis is difficult to establish using conventional extramedullary guides. Even with fluoroscopy, the centre of the femoral head may not be established with absolute accuracy. With navigation systems, accurate determination of the axis becomes possible. The femoral mechanical axis is becoming increasingly important as computer-assisted surgery is being more widely used.

– *The femoral anatomical axis I* described by Moreland *et al.* (9) is currently the most frequently used. It is defined as a line drawn between the femoral shaft centre I and the knee centre. This femoral anatomical axis I allows the use of an intramedullary guide that does not take a high femoral deformity into account if a fixed angle of the instrumentation jig (e.g., 5° of valgus in a preoperative valgus deformity, or 7° of valgus in a preoperative varus deformity) is used. If the amount of valgus to be used in the insertion system is calculated beforehand from the HKS angle (between the femoral mechanical axis and the femoral anatomical axis II) or the angle α (between the femoral mechanical axis and the femoral anatomical axis I), proximal femoral deformity is taken into account. It should be remembered that HKS and α are affected by femoral rotation, and are, therefore, difficult to calculate (8) (fig. 11).

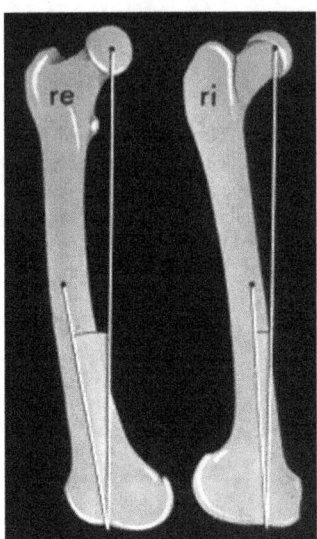

Fig. 11 – The HKS angle (enclosed by the femoral mechanical axis and the femoral anatomical axis II) is affected by femoral rotation.
re = external rotation ; ri = internal rotation

• Posterior femoral cut

The posterior femoral cut will affect the rotation of the femoral component (3), and, hence, the varus / valgus positioning of the femoral component in flexion. In a given implant, the tilt of the patella will depend upon the orientation of the posterior femoral cut (fig. 12).

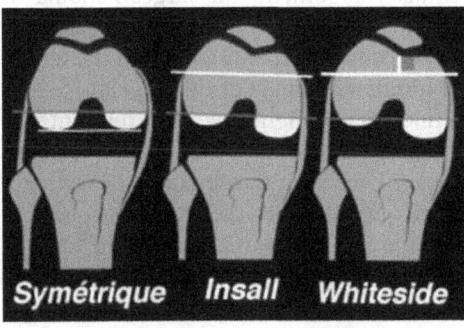

Fig. 12 – The patellar tilt of a given implant will be influenced by the orientation of the posterior femoral cut, which may be symmetrical, parallel to the biepicondylar axis, or at right angles to the anteroposterior axis.
Symétrique = symmetrical

Patellar cut

The orientation of this cut will also affect patellar tilt. Various parameters may be used to measure this orientation, the most important being the angles α and β (6).

In the light of more recent research, however, it would appear that the orientation of the trochlear groove is the most critical parameter affecting patellar tilt.

The cutting jigs provided are calipers or slotted guides that take a sawblade or a rotary milling blade. However, some surgeons prefer to "eyeball" the cut, working off the posterior attachments of the patellar tendon and the quadriceps tendon. These landmarks allow the orientation as well as the level of the patellar cut to be determined. Other surgeons go by the measured thickness of the patella before and after resection.

Level of the cuts

The level of the cut is guided by a reference, which may be a point or a side. Bone that is removed on the reference side will be replaced by the implant. This reference is usually situated on the convex side. The most commonly used principle involves a soft tissue release in the concavity, in order to restore sufficient height on the concave side. This release allows a rectangular space to be created. Regardless of whether soft tissue release is required because of asymmetrical bone cuts or because of contraction of the ligaments, the end result will always be a lengthening, which may be described as unilateral, since only the concave side will have been changed (fig. 13).

There are, however, cases in which the amount of bone resected will not be accurately replaced by the thickness of the implant. The specific problems posed by such cases must be carefully considered. The pattern is encountered, for instance, in lateral tibiofemoral compartment OA, in RA, and in patients who have previously undergone high tibial valgus osteotomy. In these cases, there will be cartilage wear or a lowering of the tibial plateau, as a result of which less bone will need resecting on the reference side. Under these circumstances, we follow the rule of resecting 6mm of bone on the tibial reference side, to allow a tibial plateau thickness of 9mm to be used.

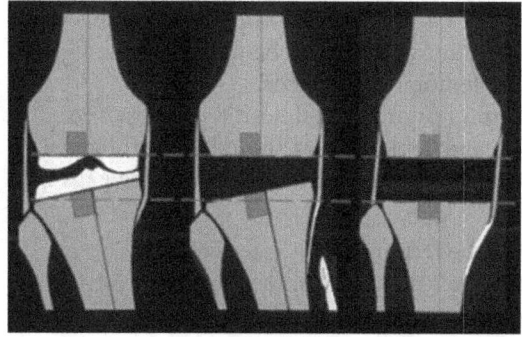

Fig. 13 – "Unilateral lengthening": only the concave side has been "lengthened".

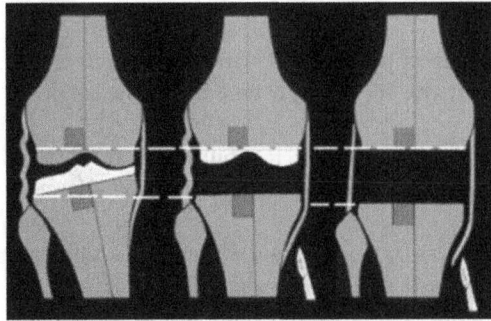

Fig. 14 – "Bilateral lengthening", with release in the concavity and taking up of slack on the convexity.

The problem is different, and more complex, if the convex side is stretched. In this case, both sides of the joint will need to be addressed: on the concave side, soft tissue release will need to be performed, while the slack on the convex side will need to be taken up. This will result in bilateral lengthening, with an increase in limb length by a few millimetres (fig. 14).

The different patterns encountered, and their implications, may be summed up as follows:

– If the reference side is not stretched (i.e., if only unilateral lengthening is required), the thickness of the bone cut on the convex side will be equal to the implant space. If the reference side is stretched, there will be bilateral lengthening, and the space created by the bone cuts plus the amount of soft tissue slack will be equal to the implant space.

– These facts should be taken into account in selecting the level of the bone cuts, remembering that the minimum implant space is the sum of the thicknesses of the two components – usually 9mm on the tibial side, and 10mm on the femoral side. However, the height of these components may be increased: the thickness of the tibial component may be 11, 13, or 15mm; on the femoral side, distal (2-, 4-, or 6-mm) augments, or posterior (2-, 4-, or 6-mm) augments may be used. In other words, the tibial and femoral implant spaces will need to be considered.

Gaps

Gap geometry is determined by the orientation of the bone cuts on the one hand, and by soft tissue releases on the other hand.

The height of the space that will be filled by the implant depends on the amount of bone resected. This amount will need to be judged in the light of the thickness of the tibial and the femoral component.

In the creation of the gaps, certain priorities will need to be observed.

As discussed above, the tibial and femoral cuts should be orthogonal in extension. Our order of priorities concerning the fashioning of the gaps is as follows:

– Priority No. 1: The gap must be rectangular in extension;
– Priority No. 2: The gap must be rectangular in flexion;
– Priority No. 3: The height of the gap must be the same in flexion and in

extension; in other words, the flexion gap must equal the extension gap. The extension gap must always match the implant space;

– Priority No. 4: The implant joint line must be at the level of the native joint line, both in flexion and in extension. (This point will need to be considered in the selection of the tibial and femoral component thicknesses.)

Priority No. 1: Rectangular extension gap

Our aim is to have two orthogonal cuts, at 90° in the femur and at 90° in the tibia (fig. 10A), with a rectangular space (i.e., without any laxity in extension). This is the ideal pattern, which would produce a straight (180°) mechanical axis. The most important factor within this objective is the absence of laxity in the coronal plane, especially with weight bearing. Once this priority has been established, the bone cuts may be made in such a way as to attain the overall goal of arthroplasty.

Priority No. 2: Rectangular flexion gap

Dennis (5) has stressed the deleterious effects of lift-off in flexion. There are several ways in which the soft tissues may be tightened.

In the CORES™ (CORrespondance des ESpaces) system, the lateral and the medial collaterals are tightened asymmetrically and independently of each other, using a tensor that will tension the medial and lateral soft tissues separately. In this system, the flexion gap is made to match the extension gap, and the orientation of the posterior femoral cuts is determined by the tensioning of the ligaments (fig. 15).

In the HLS system, the posterior femoral cuts are symmetrical, and ligament balancing is used to produce a rectangular flexion gap.

Other systems produce asymmetrical bone cuts, involving such features as routine external rotation; a cut at right angles to Whiteside's AP axis (2); or a cut parallel to the Insall's biepicondylar axis (7) (fig. 12).

Whenever asymmetrical resection is being used, it is important to decide whether more bone is being removed from the medial condyle (medial over-resection) or less bone is being removed from the lateral condyle (lateral under-resection).

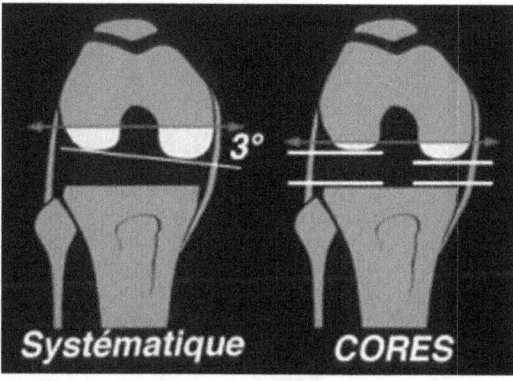

Fig. 15 – Unlike systems that apply 3° of external rotation to all femurs, the CORES™ system tensions the ligaments symmetrically, addressing the medial and lateral structures independently.
Systématique = all femurs

Medial over-resection may be linked with lateral under-resection if the tensor has a central axis of rotation. Medial over-resection and lateral under-resection may be independent of each other if the tensor does not have an axis of symmetry. In this case, the level of the bone cut in one compartment will need to be established without reference to the other compartment. This is an important, though rarely mentioned, concept, which is mainly a function of the tensor used. Navigation systems have the necessary accuracy and precision to cope with these details.

Priority No. 3: Flexion gap equals extension gap

Where the flexion gap is too small, there will be a flexion deficit; where the extension gap is too small, extension will be restricted.

If the flexion gap is larger than the extension gap, the knee will be lax in flexion. This is acceptable, providing that the amount of laxity is small, and that there is posterior stabilization to provide protection against dislocation.

If the extension gap is larger than the flexion gap, the knee will be lax in extension. This form of laxity is unacceptable. In order to prevent it, a thicker implant would need to be used, which would, however, restrict flexion.

It follows from the above that the flexion gap and the extension gap must be equal. The flexion gap may be adjusted to the gap produced in extension; alternatively, the extension gap may be made to match the flexion gap. The choice made will affect the sequence of bone cuts.

1. The flexion gap is adjusted to the extension gap. This is the case, for instance, with the CORES™ system, which relies upon ligament tensioning. The femoral component will be rotated.

2. The extension gap is adjusted to the flexion gap. This is the case with the HLS system. The use of the spreader in extension allows the height of the flexion gap measured with a spacer to be applied to the extension gap. Balancing is done in extension, and the femoral component is not rotated. This may result in insufficient balancing in flexion.

The Zimmer system (NexGen®) also adjusts the extension gap to the flexion gap. A variable soft tissue alignment tensor is provided, which allows asymmetrical bone cuts to be made, especially in flexion. However, the transfer of these bone cuts parallel to the biepicondylar axis from flexion to extension may result in suboptimal femoral component positioning with regard to the femoral mechanical axis (figs. 16-18).

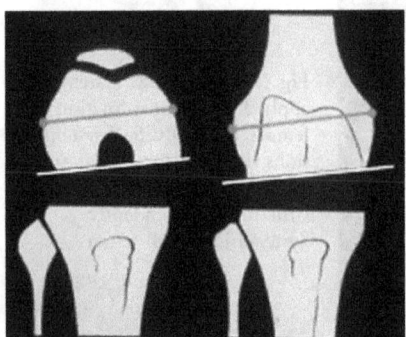

Fig. 16 – Posterior femoral cut parallel to biepicondylar axis.

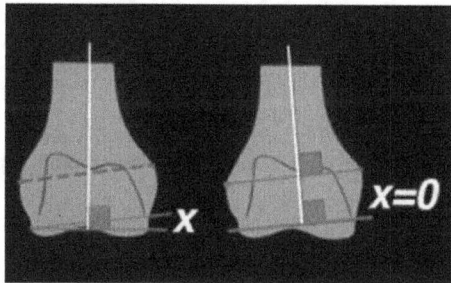

Fig. 17 – The angle x between the distal femoral cut and the biepicondylar axis is not always perpendicular.

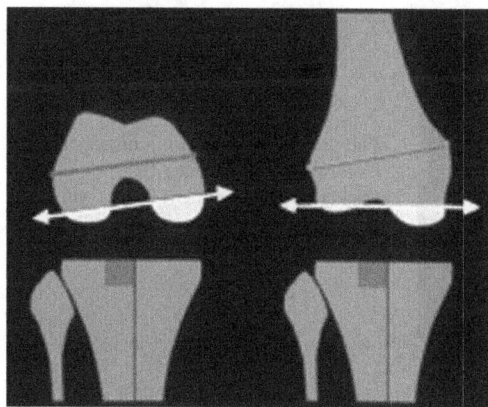

Fig. 18 – Starting with a cut in flexion, parallel to the biepicondylar axis, makes sense only if the femoral mechanical axis is at right angles to the biepicondylar axis, which is not always the case.

Priority No. 4: Level of implant joint line

For the sake of clarity, the joint line in extension will be considered separately from the joint line in flexion.

• Level of joint line in extension

Where the implant thickness exactly matches the volume of bone resected, keeping the implant joint line at the level of the native joint line is straightforward.

Where unilateral lengthening has to be performed, the level of the implant joint line may be established from the reference side (fig. 13).

Where the lengthening is bilateral, thicker implants will need to be used, or bone resection will have to be more sparing.

If less bone is removed from the tibial side, or if a thicker polyethylene component is used, the tibial subspace will be increased, i.e., there will be a greater distance between the implant joint line and all the soft tissue insertions on the tibia (MCL, patellar tendon, capsule) and on the fibula (LCL) (fig. 19).

If less bone is removed from the femoral side, or if the bearing surface of the femoral component is moved more distally by the use of augments, the femoral subspace will be increased, i.e., there will be a greater distance between the implant joint line and the ligament insertions on the distal end of the femur (MCL, LCL, capsule), and, to a lesser extent, between the implant joint line and the elastic, muscular portion of the extensor apparatus (fig. 20).

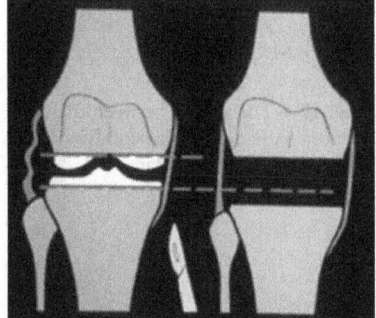

Fig. 19 – With bilateral lengthening, a thicker implant or more sparing bone cuts should be used.

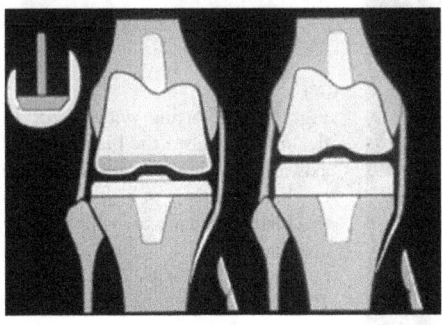

Fig. 20 – In extension: distalizing the femoral bearing surface (left) or using a thicker tibial component (right) will affect the implant joint line.

• Level of joint line in flexion

This level is a function of the implant space in flexion. Once again, there are two subspaces – a tibial subspace, and a femoral subspace.

As regards the anterior and posterior femoral cuts, most implant systems come in six sizes, with ca. 3mm between sizes in the anteroposterior plane. The different implant systems use different references: some key off the anterior cortex, thereby allowing to define the anterior space more accurately; others reference from the posterior condyles or the tibial plateaus, which gives better control of the flexion gap and stability in flexion, albeit sometimes at the expense of the anterior space.

Sequence of cuts, and strategy

Sequence of cuts

Option No. 1: Tibia-first preparation

The object of joint replacement is to substitute an implant for the bone that has been resected. This is feasible, provided there is no extra-articular bony deformity (straight tibia). If there is a tibial bony deformity (e.g., tibia vara), only the convex side will be accurately replaced by the implant, and even that is contingent upon the absence of laxity on the convex side.

Making the tibial cut first allows balancing to be started either in extension or in flexion. This gives rise to two different sequences – balancing first in flexion, and balancing first in extension, respectively.

Option No. 2: Distal femur-first preparation

This option has the advantage of establishing the level of the cut and the orientation in the femur. However, this advantage is turned into a disadvantage if there is laxity on the convex side. Such cases of bilateral lengthening will need managing in special ways:

1. a thicker plateau may be used (which would, however, place the patella more distally);
2. distal augments may be used on the femoral condyles;
3. a more sparing distal femoral cut may be made, although it is difficult to assess accurately how much (e.g., 2mm) more distally the cut should be made.

Depending on the sequence adopted, the flexion gap will need to be adjusted to the extension gap, or vice versa.

Our current principles of knee assessment

Traditionally, the knee has been assessed in the light of its anatomical pattern and the stages of OA. Currently, our analysis is based upon a consideration of the following factors:
1. the soft tissue (capsular and ligamentous) envelope;
2. the absence or presence of deformity, as well as the site of any deformity, which may be intra- or extra-articular, and in the tibia or in the femur.

Contraction, laxity, or lengthening of the soft tissue envelope

When it comes to soft tissue release, two things must be borne in mind.

If the soft tissues are contracted, release is performed in order to restore the tissues to their "normal" length.

If there is laxity on the convex side, release is performed in order to lengthen the soft tissues in the concavity. This lengthening is also required (in cases of extra-articular deformity) in order to balance laxity that has been created by resection (fig. 21).

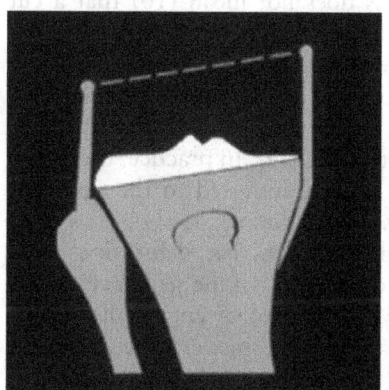

Fig. 21 – An asymmetrical bone cut will produce "resection-related laxity", which is balanced by ligament lengthening in the concavity.

Where the required lengthening of the soft tissue envelope exceeds a certain limit, the medial collateral ligament will need to be released in knees with a varus deformity, while the lateral collateral ligament will need to be released in knees with a valgus deformity.

Lengthening of the soft tissue envelope may be performed in several ways.

Lengthening will be unilateral in cases of resection-related laxity, or where hypoplasia of the lateral femoral condyle is to be addressed. In this case, the soft tissue envelope would be "lengthened" on the lateral side.

Lengthening will be bilateral in cases of laxity on the convex side (what actually happens is lengthening in the concavity, and tightening on the convex side) (fig. 22).

The pattern encountered in the individual knee will dictate the soft tissue releases. Thus, release of the MCL should, obviously, be considered in knees with a constitutional deformity, even where there is no major wear. Conversely, major deformity that is purely wear-related will very rarely require release of the MCL, providing that there is no extra-articular deformity.

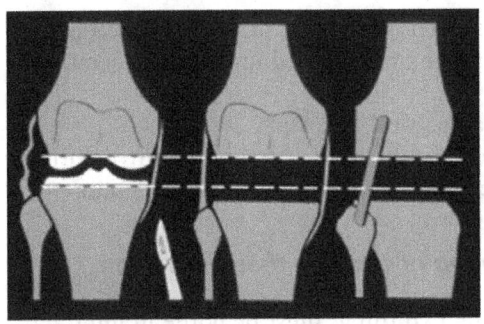

Fig. 22 – Lengthening is bilateral when the convex side is slack. (What actually happens is lengthening in the concavity, and tightening on the convex side.)

Extra-articular deformity

Absence of extra-articular deformity

The orthogonal tibial cut will usually remove 3° more bone laterally than medially.

The distal femoral cut will also be asymmetrical. This asymmetry of the femoral cut is transferred into flexion. This does not mean (10) that a cut should be made in 3° external rotation in order to obtain matching flexion and extension gaps (fig. 23). The principle to be applied consists in cutting each condyle, at the same distance ratio from the epicondyles (collateral ligament insertions) medially and laterally, in flexion and in extension. If this is done, the collateral ligaments will be isometric (fig. 24). In practice, the asymmetry of the distal femoral cut will have to be transferred to the posterior femoral cut (taking wear and osteophytes into account). It should also be remembered that, in simple cases without extra-articular deformity, equal flexion and extension gaps may be produced regardless of the sequence of cuts and the actual technique (e.g., CORES™, HLS) used. A cut parallel to the posterior condyles will have virtually the same effect, since it will exploit the elasticity of the collateral ligaments.

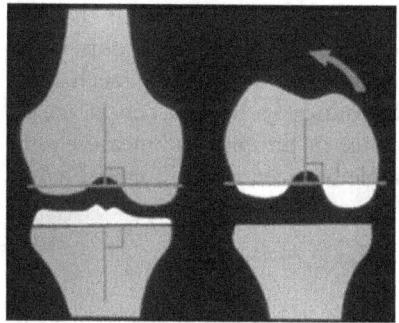

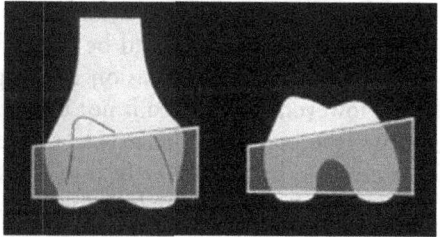

Fig. 24 – Collateral ligament isometry will be obtained if the distal and the posterior femoral cut have the same ratio of distance from the epidocndyles on the medial and on the lateral side.

Fig. 23 – External rotation of the femoral cut is not applied because of the asymmetrical tibial cut. The only valid reason for femoral component rotation is an asymmetrical cut of the distal femur.

Presence of extra-articular deformity

Where there is extra-articular deformity, a distinction must be made between tibial deformity and femoral deformity.

Extra-articular deformity in the tibia

The tibial bone cut will affect the extension gap and the flexion gap. Releases that produce a rectangular extension gap will also result in a rectangular flexion gap, and vice versa. Thus, in the case of a varus deformity of tibial origin, balancing of the "resection-related laxity" (the functional laxity resulting from resection) is brought about by a release of the structure that controls the valgus positioning of the tibial segment, i.e., the MCL. If the resection-related laxity is slight, one may rely largely on the elasticity of the soft tissues, and perform a minimal or partial release. Contrary to the view advanced by some surgeons, femoral component rotation has nothing to do with this balancing. The only justification for a "femoral component rotation" is an asymmetrical cut of the distal femur (fig. 23). This is the only situation in which a posterior femoral cut to keep the flexion gap rectangular and preserve ligament isometry would be justified.

Extra-articular deformity in the femur

Where the deformity is in the femur, matters are far less straightforward. An asymmetrical cut of the distal femur will necessitate a rotation of the femoral component if the flexion gap is to match the extension gap.

It has been suggested that the cut in flexion should be referenced from the biepicondylar axis (fig. 16).

The situation can be readily assessed: the distal femoral cut will need to be at right angles to the femoral mechanical axis.

This cut encloses an angle x (which may be zero) with the biepicondylar axis (fig. 17). This angle must, in all cases, be applied to the posterior femoral cut.

To say that the biepicondylar axis is the reference (which means that the posterior femoral cut should be parallel to this axis) makes sense only if the biepicondylar axis in extension is at right angles to the femoral mechanical axis. However, this pattern is not universally found (1). For this reason, we do not use the biepicondylar axis as the reference in flexion. The measurement that needs to be applied in flexion is the angle between the orthogonal femoral cut and the biepicondylar axis.

Objectives of the sequence of cuts

Our *objective No. 1* is to create a rectangular extension gap at right angles to the mechanical axis (where an implant with symmetrical condyles is to be used). For this objective to be attained, three conditions have to be met.

Firstly, the tibial mechanical axis must be at 90°. Any asymmetry of the bone cut may be compensated for in flexion and extension, by soft tissue releases. (Release may be facilitated by a preliminary posterior femoral cut, especially where there is a fixed flexion deformity.)

Secondly, the extension gap must be rectangular. The necessary balancing is obtained by soft tissue release.

Thirdly, the femoral mechanical axis must be at 90°. To our way of thinking, this condition is less essential than the first two conditions described above; a very slight amount of residual femoral varus would not constitute a violation of the objective.

Our *objective No. 2* is to create a rectangular flexion gap. If it is decided to have a rectangular flexion gap, the posterior femoral cut will have to have the same orientation or angulation with regard to the biepicondylar axis as the cut in extension, rather than the other way round. Any departure from this sequence may lead to problems with rotation and imbalance in flexion.

Referencing may also be done using bony landmarks.

The angle measured (during preoperative planning and at surgery) between the biepicondylar axis and the perpendicular to the mechanical femoral angle is applied.

Posterior femoral cuts referenced from the posterior condyles or the biepicondylar axis using a predetermined amount of 3° external rotation (or a cut parallel to one of the two references) will not allow the objective to be attained consistently. If it is decided to use these bony landmarks (posterior condyles or biepicondylar axis), the angulation of the cut with regard to these landmarks will need to be determined individually, in the light of the pattern encountered in the particular patient.

The CORES™ system is based upon a different concept. It allows the cut to be defined using equal medial and lateral soft tissue tension as the reference (fig. 15).

Our *objective No. 3* is the correct establishment of the implant joint line. This requires an understanding of the concepts of the tibial and femoral implant subspaces discussed above. The tensor is used (in the light of the priorities and objectives established by the surgeon) as a means to equalizing the spaces in flexion and extension.

Every attempt should be made to attain the three objectives set out above without any compromise: any decision to go for less than the ideal will have repercussions on the result of arthroplasty.

Examples

1. Medial compartment OA in a knee with a constitutional varus deformity of tibial origin

The mechanical tibiofemoral angle is 10°. The constitutional portion is 8° in the tibial metaphysis. The bony femoral valgus is 3°. Medial compartment wear is slight. The tibia is cut at an angle of 90°. This cut will remove more bone laterally than medially. The orthogonal distal femoral cut will remove 3° more bone medially than laterally. The laxity in extension thus created will be taken care of by subsequent soft tissue balancing. However, in order to obtain rectangular flexion and extension gaps, equal posterior femoral cuts will need to be made on the distal and on the posterior femur.

Since femoral condylar wear may be asymmetrical, it may be preferable to define this equal of bone to be removed using a reference other than the posterior condyles – e.g., the bicondylar axis.

Another, more straightforward option is to reference from the posterior condyles, which provide a simple and handy landmark for the surgeon to use. However, in doing so, consideration must be given to cartilage wear, which may be between 0 and 3mm. We routinely use this reference.

In this case (and only in this case), the flexion and extension gaps will be equal. Several points need to be remembered:

– The position in rotation is determined by the angle between the biepicondylar axis and the femoral mechanical axis;

– The rotation or asymmetry of the femoral cuts is not dictated by the tibial deformity or the asymmetrical bone removal from the tibia as a result of the extra-articular deformity;

– Major extra-articular tibial deformity will not affect the rotation of femoral component;

– The asymmetry of the tibial cut can be converted into balanced flexion and extension gaps only by soft tissue release. This rule applies regardless of the actual amount of asymmetry.

If there is no extra-articular deformity in the femur, an orthogonal cut of the femur at 90° will produce a 3° asymmetry of the femoral cut, which may be transferred to the posterior femoral condyles.

2. Medial compartment OA in a knee with a varus deformity of femoral origin

This pattern confronts the surgeon with a near insoluble problem (4, 10). The orthogonal femoral cut will remove more bone laterally. If this asymmetry of the cut is transferred to the flexion gap, it will be possible to make the flexion and extension gaps equal (creating rectangular and symmetrical gaps by means of a medial release); however, the price to pay will be internal rotation of the femoral component, which is known to affect the patellofemoral joint adversely.

There are two things that the surgeon can do:

– Abandon the essential requirement of a femoral mechanical angle of 90°, and accept a femoral cut in very slight varus, with less bone removed from the lateral compartment, and a symmetrical posterior femoral bone cut;

– Perform an orthogonal (and hence asymmetrical) distal femoral cut, and accept a symmetrical posterior femoral cut, which will result in slight medial laxity in flexion.

It follows that in a varus knee resulting from malunion of a femoral fracture, the surgeon should be prepared to perform an osteotomy as part of the procedure.

Consequences of the choices made

The different techniques available to the surgeon must be carefully weighed and meticulously performed, even though any adverse results may not show up for a long time. Minor defects may add up and lead to implant failure. The surgeon must therefore, at all times, consider the eventual outcome and understand what he or she is proposing to do.

Femoral component rotation

Rotating the femoral component will obviously affect the tibiofemoral and the patellofemoral stress patterns. Several studies have shown that external rotation of the femoral component is beneficial in that it decreases patellofemoral stresses. However, there is nothing in the literature to date regarding the repercussions on the medial compartment stress pattern of an external rotation of the femoral component. It is, however, well known that malunion in external rotation of the femoral shaft or metaphysis will raise the medial compartment stress levels, and thus lead to medial compartment OA, albeit over an extended period of time. It will take more than ten years for degenerative joint lesions to develop in a femur with 10° torsion. It is not known how much femoral component rotation will be harmful, or how long the adverse effects will take to manifest themselves. All that can be said with certainty is that external rotation of the femoral component causes a rise in medial compart-

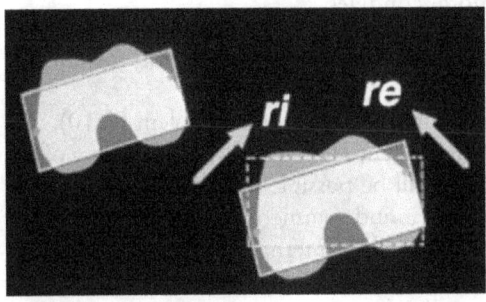

Fig. 25 – Positioning the femoral component in external rotation will affect the anterior space as well as the tibiofemoral stress pattern in flexion. ri = internal rotation ; re = external rotation

ment stress, while internal rotation of the femoral component causes a rise in lateral compartment stress. It follows that implanting the femoral component in external rotation in a patient with medial compartment OA does not make sense. Conversely, implanting the femoral component in external rotation in a patient with lateral compartment OA would be perfectly acceptable (fig. 25).

Implant design

Implant design and insertion technique are interrelated: the implant must be designed in such a way as to allow the technique to be performed; while the choice of technique will need to be made in the light of the implant pattern. The design of the implant will have a direct bearing on the bone cuts, the soft tissue releases, ligament balancing, and the rotation / non-rotation of the femoral component (fig. 26). Where an asymmetrical implant pattern is to be used, the bone cuts must be made in such a way as to match this pattern. However, the mere fact that the implant design is asymmetrical does not mean that all the problems discussed above will be resolved without any further action having to be taken. With an asymmetrical implant, too, the way in which the bone cuts are made must take into account the other factors mentioned above. Merely using an implant with 3° asymmetry is not a cure-all. 3° of asymmetry in the implant would presuppose that the distal femoral cut will always be 3° asymmetrical, which is not the case. It should also be noted that this asymmetry will elevate the lateral condyle, which is undesirable except in cases of valgus knees with a hypoplastic lateral condyle.

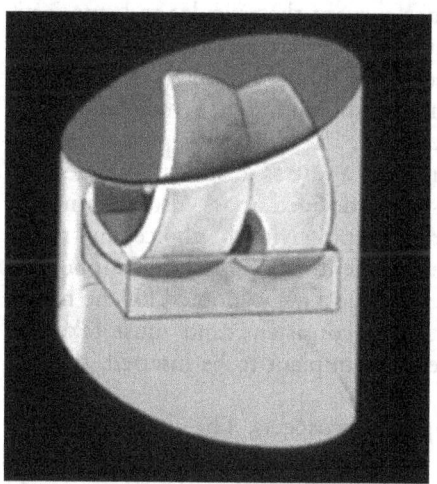

Fig. 26 – The implant is seated within its soft tissue envelope.

Conclusion

This chapter has been concerned with some of the problems that confront the surgeon performing a total knee replacement. From the above discussion, it will be clear that, while the design of an implant is an important factor, the instruments used and the order of the bone cuts will also affect the result of arthro-plasty. The long-term results of the choices made by the implanting surgeon are not currently known. However, we feel that it is crucial for the surgeon to be able to use a spreader or a tensor, even if the overwhelming majority of total knee replacements may be performed without recourse to a tensor. Whenever there is evidence of major deformity, such as advanced OA or, especially, an extra-articular malalignment, the availability of a tensor is an added bonus.

From the points discussed in this chapter, we may also distil a number of questions that should be further researched over the next few years:

How does femoral component rotation affect the tibiofemoral stress pat-tern?

Is there, in the light of our analysis, still a rationale for using implants with asymmetrical posterior condyles?

What are the effects of the different soft tissue releases? They have been found to work in two very different situations: when the ligaments are contracted, and when the bone cuts have resulted in resection-related laxity. How – in these apparently very different patterns – can one create a perfectly rectangular flexion and extension space?

In some cases of medial compartment OA in knees with excessive constitu-tional varus (preoperative tibiofemoral mechanical angles of between 15° and 20°), we have opted for a medial opening-wedge osteotomy in the tibia, as a one-stage procedure with total knee replacement, in order to correct the constitutional bony deformity. This procedure allows a symmetrical cut of the tibia to be made, once the bony deformity has been corrected. As a result, there is no need for a major medial release; in particular, the MCL does not need to be detached. This is why, prior to surgery, the articular and extra-arti-cular contributions to a given deformity must be very carefully analyzed.

The priorities and objectives will need to be thought through carefully, and a considered choice will need to be made. It should also be remembered that, in some cases, a compromise will be required.

The instruments must be designed in such a way as to allow the surgeon to perform the technical steps that he or she has decided upon. Also, the implant design features must be compatible and in keeping with the choices and trade-offs made by the surgeon. Total knee replacement may be performed following a number of different strategies. However, the strategy adopted for the mana-gement of the individual patient must be consistent, and must take full account of the objectives to be attained, the implant to be inserted, the ins-truments available, etc. (fig. 27).

Surgical navigation systems open up new prospects. The challenge at this point in time is how to integrate this new tool into the surgeon's analysis of the case and the decision-making process. Ideally, the new systems should work from the kinematic centres and / or the bony landmarks of a normal knee, regardless of the fact that the joint to be replaced is affected by defor-mity and degenerative disease. They should allow the surgeon not only to make better bone cuts, but also to assess the soft tissue releases.

The points raised in this chapter need to be addressed in the specification of any contemporary instrumentation system (be it mechanical or computer-

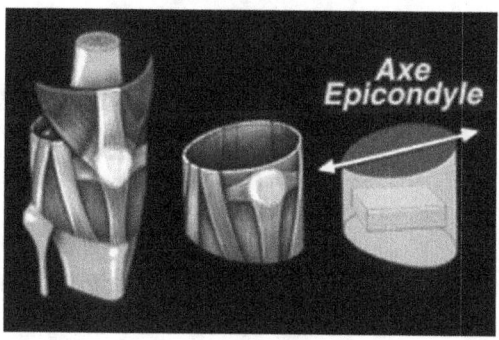

Fig. 27 – Any insertion technique will need to be consistent, and take account of the goals of arthroplasty, the implant, and the instruments. Axe épicondyle = epicondylar axis.

based), in order to ensure that the implant will be optimally inserted within its soft tissue envelope.

Acknowledgements

The authors wish to thank Éditions Sauramps Médical, for permission to use line drawings originally published in Chirurgie prothétique du genou, and Nicole Walch, for providing the drawings.

References

1. Akagi M, Yamashita E, Nakagawa T *et al.* (20001) Relationship between frontal knee alignment and reference axes in the distal femur. Clin Orthop, 388: 147-56
2. Arima J, Whiteside LA, McCarthy DS *et al.* (1995) Femoral rotational alignment, based on the anteroposterior axis, in total knee arthroplasty in a valgus knee. A technical note. J Bone Joint Surg Am 77 (9): 1331-4
3. Berger RA, Rubash HE, Seel MJ *et al.* (1993) Determining the rotational alignment of the femoral component in total knee arthroplasty using biepicondylar axis. Chir Orthop 286: 40-7
4. Dejour H, Neyret P (1991) Les gonarthroses. Journées Lyonnaises du Genou (personal communications)
5. Dennis D (2001) *In vivo* fluoroscopic evaluation of kinematics after TKA: anteroposterior translation. ISAKOS Knee Committee, Florence 11-13 January 2001, Book of Abstracts: 241-60
6. Deroche P (1992) La prothèse totale à glissement du genou HLS1. Thesis, University of Lyon
7. Griffin FM, Math K, Scuderi GR (2000) Anatomy of the epicondyles of the distal femur: MRI analysis of normal knees. J Arthroplasty, 15: 354-9
8. Jiang CL, Insall JN (1989) Effect of rotation on the axial alignment of the femur. Chir Orthop, 248: 50-6
9. Moreland JR, Bassett LW, Hanker GJ (1987) Radiographic analysis of the axial alignment of the lower extremity. J Bone Joint Surg, 69-A: 745-9
10. Rivat P, Neyret P, Aït Si Selmi T (1999) Influence de l'ordre des coupes – Coupes dépendantes et indépendantes – Rôle du tenseur. Chirurgie prothétique du genou, Éd. Sauramps Médical: 41-76

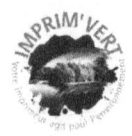 Composition, mise en pages et impression : Imprimerie BARNÉOUD
BP 44 - 53960 BONCHAMP-LÈS-LAVAL
Dépôt légal : avril 2008 - N° d'imprimeur : 707004
Imprimé en France